Where There Is No Doctor
a village health care handbook

~revised edition~

by

David Werner

with

Carol Thuman and Jane Maxwell

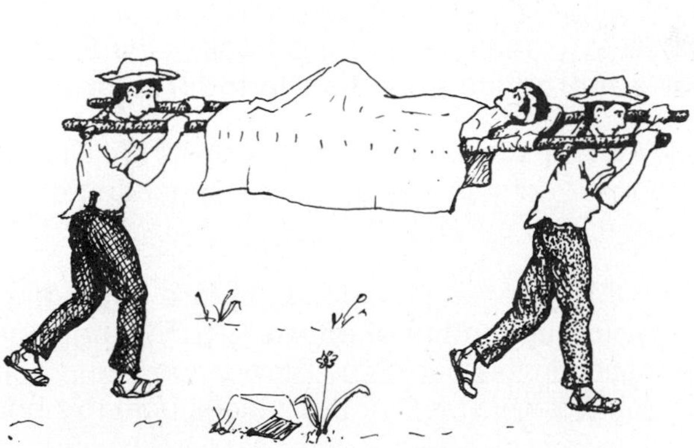

with drawings by David Werner

Library of Congress Cataloging-in-Publication Data

Werner, David, 1934–

Where there is no doctor: a village health care handbook / by David Werner; with Carol Thuman and Jane Maxwell. — Rev. ed.

Includes Index.

ISBN 0-942364-15-5

1. Medicine, Popular. 2. Rural health. I. Thuman, Carol, 1959– . II. Maxwell, Jane, 1941– . III. Title.

[DNLM: 1. Community Health Aides—handbooks.
2. Medicine—popular works. 3. Rural Health—handbooks.
WA 39 W492w]
RC81.W4813 1992 610—dc20
DNLM/DLC 92-1539
for Library of Congress CIP

Published by:

The Hesperian Foundation
PO Box 11577
Berkeley, California 94712-2577
United States of America

First English edition: October 1977

Revised English edition: May 1992

Sixth printing, January 2002

The original English version of this book was produced in 1977 as a revised translation of the Spanish edition, *Donde no hay doctor.*

Please contact the Hesperian Foundation **before beginning any translation or adaptation to avoid duplication of efforts,** and for suggestions about adapting the information in this book. The Foundation would appreciate receiving a copy of any materials in which text or illustrations from this book have been used.

THIS REVISED EDITION CAN BE IMPROVED WITH YOUR HELP. If you are a village health worker, doctor, mother, or anyone with ideas or suggestions for ways this book could be changed to better meet the needs of your people, please write to the Hesperian Foundation at the above address. Thank you for your help.

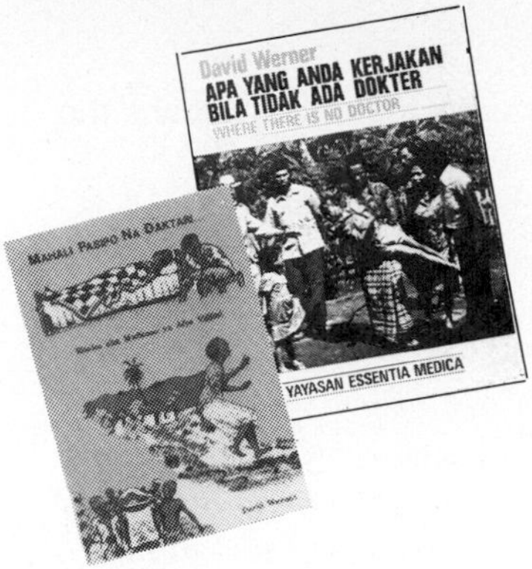

Thanks to the work and dedication of many groups and individuals around the world, *Where There Is No Doctor* has been translated into more than 80 languages. The following are some of the translations and the addresses where you can obtain them.

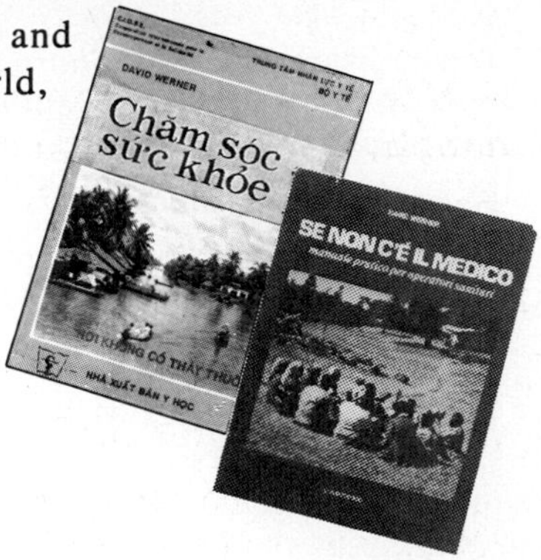

SPANISH AND ENGLISH:

The Hesperian Foundation
PO Box 11577
Berkeley, California 94712-2577
United States of America

FRENCH:

ENDA
Publications Dept.
B.P. 3370
Dakar, SENEGAL

ARABIC:

Arab Resource Collective
P.O. Box 7380
Nicosia, CYPRUS

HINDI:

VHAI
40, Institutional Area
(Near Qutab Hotel, S. of I.T.T.)
New Delhi, 110016
INDIA

INDONESIAN:

Yayasan Essentia Medica
P.O. Box 1058
Yogyakarta, INDONESIA 55010

SPANISH:

Editorial Pax-México
Ave. Cuauhtémoc 1434
México, D.F. 03310
MEXICO

NEPALI:

Health Learning Materials Ctr.
Institute of Medicine
P.O. Box 2533
Kathmandu, NEPAL

RUSSIAN:

Mercy Corps International
3030 SW 1st Avenue
Portland, Oregon 97201
United States of America

UZBEK:

Andijon Development Center
Sh. Rashidov Ko'chasi 1 A
Andijon City, 710000
UZBEKISTAN

ITALIAN:

Aldo Benevelli
Universitá Della Pace "Giorgio La Pira"
C.so IV Novembre, 28
12100 Cuneo, ITALY

Please write to the Hesperian Foundation for information on other editions, including Aymara, Bengali, Chinese, Creole, Dari, German, Kannada, Korean, Lao, Marathi, Nepali, Pushtu, Quechua, Shuar, Sindhi, Sinhala, Tamil, Thai, Tigre, Tigrina, Tswana, and Urdu, as well as English editions adapted for specific countries.

We are looking for ways to get this book to those it can serve best—namely persons in isolated villages and fringe communities of poor countries. If you are able to help or have suggestions, please contact the Hesperian Foundation. We offer this book at a lower price to persons of low income living in poor countries.

THANKS

This revision of ***Where There Is No Doctor*** has been a cooperative effort. We thank the many users of the book around the world who have written us over the years with comments and suggestions—these have guided us in updating this information.

David Werner is the author of the original Spanish and English versions of the book. His vision, caring, and commitment are present on every page. Carol Thuman and Jane Maxwell share credit for most of the research, writing, and preparation of this revised version. We are deeply grateful for their excellent and very careful work.

Thanks also to others who researched portions of this revised edition: Suellen Miller, Susan Klein, Ronnie Lovich, Mary Ellen Guroy, Shelley Kahane, Paula Elster, and George Kent. For information taken from the African edition, our thanks to Andrew Pearson and the other authors at Macmillan Publishers.

Many doctors and health care specialists from around the world generously reviewed portions of the book. We cannot list them all here, but the help of the following was exceptional: David Sanders, Richard Laing, Bill Bower, Greg Troll, Deborah Bickel, Tom Frieden, Jane Zucker, David Morley, Frank Catchpool, Lonny Shavelson, Rudolph Bock, Joseph Cook, Sadja Greenwood, Victoria Sheffield, Sherry Hilaski, Pam Zinkin, Fernando Viteri, Jordan Tapero, Robert Gelber, Ted Greiner, Stephen Gloyd, Barbara Mintzes, Rainer Arnhold, Michael Tan, Brian Linde, Davida Coady, and Alejandro de Avila. Their expert advice and help have been of great value.

We warmly thank the dedicated members of the Hesperian Foundation for their help in preparing the manuscript: Kyle Craven for computer graphic arts and layout, Stephen Babb and Cynthia Roat for computer graphics, and Lisa de Avila for editorial assistance. We are also grateful to many others who helped in this book's preparation: Kathy Alberts, Mary Klein, Evan Winslow-Smith, Jane Bavelas, Kim Gannon, Heidi Park, Laura Gibney, Nancy Ogaz, Martín Bustos, Karen Woodbury, and Trude Bock. Our special thanks to Keith and Luella McFarland for being there when we needed them most.

For helping in updating this book, we thank Manisha Aryal, Marcos Burgos, Todd Jailer, Erika Leemann, Malcolm Lowe, Elena Metcalf, Lora Santiago, Peter Small, and Fred Strauss.

Artwork for the new edition was created by David Werner, Kyle Craven, Susan Klein, Regina Faul-Jansen, and Sandy Frank. We also thank the following persons and groups for permission to use their artwork: Dale Crosby, Carl Werner, Macmillan Publishers (for some of Felicity Shepherd's drawings in the African edition of this book), the "New Internationalist" (for the picture of the VIP latrine), James Ogwang (for the drawings on page 417) and McGraw-Hill Book Company (for drawings appearing on pages 85 and 104 taken from ***Emergency Medical Guide*** by John Henderson, illustrated by Niel Hardy).

The fine work of those who helped in the creation of the original version is still reflected on nearly every page. Our thanks to Val Price, Al Hotti, Rodney Kendall, Max Capestany, Rudolf Bock, Kent Benedict, Alfonzo Darricades, Carlos Felipe Soto Miller, Paul Quintana, David Morley, Bill Bower, Allison Orozco, Susan Klein, Greg Troll, Carol Westburg, Lynn Gordon, Myra Polinger, Trude Bock, Roger Bunch, Lynne Coen, George Kent, Jack May, Oliver Bock, Bill Gonda, Ray Bleicher, and Jesús Manjarrez.

For this new edition, we are grateful for financial support from the Carnegie Corporation, Gladys and Merrill Muttart Foundation, Myra Polinger, the Public Welfare Foundation, Misereor, the W.K. Kellogg Foundation, the Sunflower Foundation, and the Edna McConnell Clark Foundation.

Finally, our warm thanks to the village health workers of Project Piaxtla in rural Mexico—especially Martín Reyes, Miguel Angel Manjarrez, Miguel Angel Alvarez, and Roberto Fajardo—whose experience and commitment have provided the foundation for this book.

CONTENTS

A list of what is discussed in each chapter

INTRODUCTION

NOTE ABOUT THIS NEW EDITION

WORDS TO THE VILLAGE HEALTH WORKER (Brown Pages) w1

Health Needs and Human Needs w2
Many Things Relate to Health Care w7
Take a Good Look at Your Community w8
Using Local Resources to Meet Needs w12
Deciding What to Do and Where to Begin w13
Trying a New Idea w15
A Balance Between People and Land w16
A Balance Between Prevention and Treatment w17
Sensible and Limited Use of Medicines w18
Finding Out What Progress Has Been Made w20
Teaching and Learning Together w21
Tools for Teaching w22
Making the Best Use of This Book w28

Chapter 1

HOME CURES AND POPULAR BELIEFS 1

Home Cures That Help 1
Beliefs That Can Make People Well 2
Beliefs That Can Make People Sick 4
Witchcraft—Black Magic—and the Evil Eye 5
Questions and Answers 6
Sunken Fontanel or Soft Spot 9
Ways to Tell Whether a Home Remedy Works or Not 10
Medicinal Plants 12
Homemade Casts—for Broken Bones 14
Enemas, Laxatives, and Purges 15

Chapter 2

SICKNESSES THAT ARE OFTEN CONFUSED 17

What Causes Sickness? 17
Different Kinds of Sicknesses and Their Causes 18
Non-infectious Diseases 18
Infectious Diseases 19
Sicknesses That Are Hard to Tell Apart 20
Examples of Local Names for Sicknesses 22
Misunderstandings Due to Confusion of Names 25
Confusion between Different Illnesses That Cause Fever 26

Chapter 3

HOW TO EXAMINE A SICK PERSON 29

Questions 29
General Condition of Health 30
Temperature 30
How to Use a Thermometer 31
Breathing (Respiration) 32
Pulse (Heartbeat) 32
Eyes 33
Ears 34
Skin 34
The Belly (Abdomen) 35
Muscles and Nerves 37

Chapter 4

HOW TO TAKE CARE OF A SICK PERSON 39

The Comfort of the Sick Person 39
Special Care for a Person Who Is Very Ill 40
Liquids 40
Food 41
Cleanliness and Changing Position in Bed 41
Watching for Changes 41
Signs of Dangerous Illness 42
When and How to Look for Medical Help 43
What to Tell the Health Worker 43
Patient Report 44

Chapter 5

HEALING WITHOUT MEDICINES 45

Healing with Water 46
When Water Is Better than Medicines 47

Chapter 6

RIGHT AND WRONG USE OF MODERN MEDICINES 49

Guidelines for the Use of Medicine 49
The Most Dangerous Misuse of Medicine 50
When Should Medicine Not Be Taken? 54

Chapter 7

ANTIBIOTICS: WHAT THEY ARE AND HOW TO USE THEM 55

Guidelines for the Use of Antibiotics 56
What to Do if an Antibiotic Does Not Seem to Help 57
Importance of Limited Use of Antibiotics 58

Chapter 8

HOW TO MEASURE AND GIVE MEDICINE 59

Medicine in Liquid Form 61
How to Give Medicines to Small Children 62
How to Take Medicines 63
Dosage Instructions for Persons Who Cannot Read 63

Chapter 9

INSTRUCTIONS AND PRECAUTIONS FOR INJECTIONS 65

When to Inject and When Not To 65
Emergencies When It Is Important to Give Injections 66
Medicines Not to Inject 67
Risks and Precautions 68
Dangerous Reactions From Injecting Certain Medicines 70
Avoiding Serious Reactions to Penicillin 71
How to Prepare a Syringe for Injection 72
How to Inject 73
How Injections Can Disable Children 74
How to Sterilize Equipment 74

Chapter 10

FIRST AID 75

Fever 75
Shock 77
Loss of Consciousness 78
When Something Gets Stuck in the Throat 79
Drowning 79
When Breathing Stops: Mouth-to-Mouth Breathing 80
Emergencies Caused by Heat 81
How to Control Bleeding from a Wound 82
How to Stop Nosebleeds 83
Cuts, Scrapes, and Small Wounds 84
Large Cuts: How to Close Them 85
Bandages 87
Infected Wounds 88
Bullet, Knife, and Other Serious Wounds 90
Emergency Problems of the Gut (Acute Abdomen) 93
Appendicitis, Peritonitis 94
Burns 96
Broken Bones (Fractures) 98
How to Move a Badly Injured Person 100
Dislocations (Bones out of Place at a Joint) 101
Strains and Sprains 102
Poisoning 103
Snakebite 104
Other Poisonous Bites and Stings 106

Chapter 11

NUTRITION: WHAT TO EAT TO BE HEALTHY 107

Sicknesses Caused by Not Eating Well 107
Why It Is Important to Eat Right 109
Preventing Malnutrition 109
Main Foods and Helper Foods 110
Eating Right to Stay Healthy 111
How to Recognize Malnutrition 112
Eating Better When You Do Not Have Much Money or Land 115
Where to Get Vitamins: In Pills or in Foods? 118
Things to Avoid in Our Diet 119
The Best Diet for Small Children 120
Harmful Ideas about Diet 123
Special Diets for Specific Health Problems 124
Anemia 124
Rickets 125
High Blood Pressure 125
Fat People 126
Constipation 126
Diabetes 127
Acid Indigestion, Heartburn, and Stomach Ulcers 128
Goiter (A Swelling or Lump on the Throat) 130

Chapter 12

PREVENTION: HOW TO AVOID MANY SICKNESSES 131

Cleanliness—and Problems from Lack of Cleanliness 131
Basic Guidelines of Cleanliness 133
Sanitation and Latrines 137
Worms and Other Intestinal Parasites 140
Roundworm (Ascaris) 140
Pinworm (Threadworm, Enterobius) 141
Whipworm (Trichuris) 142
Hookworm 142
Tapeworm 143
Trichinosis 144
Amebas 144
Giardia 145
Blood Flukes (Schistosomiasis, Bilharzia) 146
Vaccinations (Immunizations)—Simple, Sure Protection 147
Other Ways to Prevent Sickness and Injury 148
Habits That Affect Health 148

Chapter 13

SOME VERY COMMON SICKNESSES 151

Dehydration 151
Diarrhea and Dysentery 153
The Care of a Person with Acute Diarrhea 160
Vomiting 161
Headaches and Migraines 162
Colds and the Flu 163
Stuffy and Runny Noses 164
Sinus Trouble (Sinusitis) 165
Hay Fever (Allergic Rhinitis) 165
Allergic Reactions 166
Asthma 167
Cough 168
Bronchitis 170
Pneumonia 171
Hepatitis 172
Arthritis (Painful, Inflamed Joints) 173
Back Pain 173
Varicose Veins 175
Piles (Hemorrhoids) 175
Swelling of the Feet and Other Parts of the Body 176
Hernia (Rupture) 177
Fits (Convulsions) 178

Chapter 14

SERIOUS ILLNESSES THAT NEED SPECIAL MEDICAL ATTENTION . . . 179

Tuberculosis (TB, Consumption) 179
Rabies 181
Tetanus (Lockjaw) 182
Meningitis 185
Malaria 186
Dengue (Breakbone Fever, Dandy Fever) 187
Brucellosis (Undulant Fever, Malta Fever) 188
Typhoid Fever 188
Typhus 190
Leprosy (Hansen's Disease) 191

Chapter 15

SKIN PROBLEMS 193

General Rules for Treating Skin Problems 193
Instructions for Using Hot Compresses 195
Identifying Skin Problems 196
Scabies 199
Lice 200
Bedbugs 200
Ticks and Chiggers 201
Small Sores with Pus 201
Impetigo 202
Boils and Abscesses 202
Itching Rash, Welts, or Hives 203
Things That Cause Itching or Burning of the Skin 204
Shingles (Herpes Zoster) 204
Ringworm, Tinea (Fungus Infections) 205
White Spots on the Face and Body 206
Mask of Pregnancy 207
Pellagra and Other Skin Problems Due to Malnutrition 208
Warts (Verrucae) 210
Corns 210
Pimples and Blackheads (Acne) 211
Cancer of the Skin 211
Tuberculosis of the Skin or Lymph Nodes 212
Erysipelas and Cellulitis 212
Gangrene (Gas Gangrene) 213
Ulcers of the Skin Caused by Poor Circulation 213
Bed Sores 214
Skin Problems of Babies 215
Eczema (Red Patches with Little Blisters) 216
Psoriasis 216

Chapter 16

THE EYES 217

Danger Signs 217
Injuries to the Eye 218
How to Remove a Speck of Dirt from the Eye 218
Chemical Burns of the Eye 219
Red, Painful Eyes—Different Causes 219
'Pink Eye' (Conjunctivitis) 219
Trachoma 220
Infected Eyes in Newborn Babies (Neonatal Conjunctivitis) 221
Iritis (Inflammation of the Iris) 221
Glaucoma 222
Infection of the Tear Sac (Dacryocystitis) 223
Trouble Seeing Clearly 223
Cross-Eyes and Wandering Eyes 223
Sty (Hordeolum) 224
Pterygium 224
A Scrape, Ulcer, or Scar on the Cornea 224
Bleeding in the White of the Eye 225
Bleeding behind the Cornea (Hyphema) 225
Pus behind the Cornea (Hypopyon) 225
Cataract 225
Night Blindness and Xerophthalmia 226
Spots or 'Flies' before the Eyes 227
Double Vision 227
River Blindness (Onchocerciasis) 227

Chapter 17

THE TEETH, GUMS, AND MOUTH 229

Care of Teeth and Gums 229
If You Do Not Have A Toothbrush 230
Toothaches and Abscesses 231
Pyorrhea, a Disease of the Gums 231
Sores or Cracks at the Corners of the Mouth 232
White Patches or Spots in the Mouth 232
Cold Sores and Fever Blisters 232

Chapter 18

THE URINARY SYSTEM AND THE GENITALS 233

Urinary Tract Infections 234
Kidney or Bladder Stones 235
Enlarged Prostate Gland 235
Diseases Spread by Sexual Contact (Sexually Transmitted Diseases) 236
Gonorrhea (Clap, VD, the Drip) and Chlamydia 236
Syphilis 237
Bubos: Bursting Lymph Nodes in the Groin 238
Use of a Catheter to Drain Urine 239
Problems of Women 241
Vaginal Discharge 241
How a Woman Can Avoid Many Infections 242
Pain or Discomfort in a Woman's Belly 243
Men and Women Who Cannot Have Children (Infertility) 244

Chapter 19

INFORMATION FOR MOTHERS AND MIDWIVES 245

The Menstrual Period (Monthly Bleeding in Women) 245
The Menopause (When Women Stop Having Periods) 246
Pregnancy 247
How to Stay Healthy during Pregnancy 247
Minor Problems during Pregnancy 248
Danger Signs in Pregnancy 249
Check-ups during Pregnancy (Prenatal Care) 250

Record of Prenatal Care 253
Things to Have Ready before the Birth 254
Preparing for Birth 256
Signs That Show Labor Is Near 258
The Stages of Labor 259
Care of the Baby at Birth 262
Care of the Cut Cord (Navel) 263
The Delivery of the Placenta (Afterbirth) 264
Hemorrhaging (Heavy Bleeding) 264
The Correct Use of Oxytocics: Ergonovine, Oxytocin, Pitocin, etc. 266
Difficult Births 267
Tearing of the Birth Opening 269
Care of the Newborn Baby 270
Illnesses of the Newborn 272
The Mother's Health after Childbirth 276
Childbirth Fever (Infection after Giving Birth) 276
Care of the Breasts 277
Lumps or Growths in the Lower Part of the Belly 280
Miscarriage (Spontaneous Abortion) 281
High Risk Mothers and Babies 282

Chapter 20

FAMILY PLANNING— HAVING THE NUMBER OF CHILDREN YOU WANT 283

Is Birth Control Good—and Is It Safe? 284
Choosing a Method of Birth Control 285
Birth Control Pills (Oral Contraceptives) 286
Other Methods of Birth Control 290
Combined Methods 292
Methods for Those Who Never Want to Have More Children 293
Home Methods for Preventing Pregnancy 294

Chapter 21

HEALTH AND SICKNESSES OF CHILDREN 295

What to Do to Protect Children's Health 295
Children's Growth— and the 'Road to Health' 297
Child Health Chart 298
Review of Children's Health Problems Discussed in Other Chapters 305
Health Problems of Children Not Discussed in Other Chapters 309
Earache and Ear Infections 309
Sore Throat and Inflamed Tonsils 309
Rheumatic Fever 310
Infectious Diseases of Childhood 311
Chickenpox 311
Measles (Rubeola) 311
German Measles (Rubella) 312
Mumps 312
Whooping Cough 313
Diphtheria 313
Infantile Paralysis (Polio) 314
How to Make Simple Crutches 315
Problems Children Are Born With 316
Dislocated Hip 316
Umbilical Hernia (Belly Button That Sticks Out) 317
A 'Swollen Testicle' (Hydrocele or Hernia) 317
Mentally Slow, Deaf, or Deformed Children 318
The Spastic Child (Cerebral Palsy) 320
Retardation in the First Months of Life 321
Sickle Cell Disease 321
Helping Children Learn 322

Chapter 22

HEALTH AND SICKNESSES OF OLDER PEOPLE 323

Summary of Health Problems Discussed in Other Chapters 323
Other Important Illnesses of Old Age 325
Heart Trouble 325
Words to Younger Persons Who Want to Stay Healthy When Older 326
Stroke (Apoplexy, Cerebro-Vascular Accident, CVA) 327
Deafness 327
Loss of Sleep (Insomnia) 328
Diseases Found More Often in People over Forty 328
Cirrhosis of the Liver 328
Gallbladder Problems 329
Accepting Death 330

Chapter 23

THE MEDICINE KIT 331

How to Care for Your Medicine Kit 332
Buying Supplies for the Medicine Kit 333
The Home Medicine Kit 334
The Village Medicine Kit 336
Words to the Village Storekeeper (or Pharmacist) 338

THE GREEN PAGES—The Uses, Dosage, and Precautions for Medicines . 339

List of Medicines in the Green Pages 341
Index of Medicines in the Green Pages 345
Information on Medicines 351

THE BLUE PAGES—New Information 399

AIDS 399
Sores on the Genitals 402
Circumcision and Excision 404
Special Care for Small, Early, and Underweight Babies 405
Ear Wax 405
Leishmaniasis 406
Guinea Worm 406
Emergencies Caused by Cold 408
How to Measure Blood Pressure 410
Poisoning from Pesticides 412
Complications from Abortion 414
Drug Abuse and Addiction 416

VOCABULARY—Explaining Difficult Words 419

ADDRESSES FOR TEACHING MATERIALS 429

INDEX (Yellow Pages) 433

Dosage Instructions for Persons Who Cannot Read
Making Medical Reports
Information About Vital Signs

INTRODUCTION

This handbook has been written primarily for those who live far from medical centers, in places where there is no doctor. But even where there are doctors, people can and should take the lead in their own health care. So this book is for everyone who cares. It has been written in the belief that:

1. **Health care is not only everyone's right, but everyone's responsibility.**
2. **Informed self-care should be the main goal of any health program or activity.**
3. **Ordinary people provided with clear, simple information can prevent and treat most common health problems in their own homes—earlier, cheaper, and often better than can doctors.**
4. **Medical knowledge should not be the guarded secret of a select few, but should be freely shared by everyone.**
5. **People with little formal education can be trusted as much as those with a lot. And they are just as smart.**
6. **Basic health care should not be delivered, but encouraged.**

Clearly, a part of informed self-care is knowing one's own limits. Therefore guidelines are included not only for **what to do,** but for **when to seek help.** The book points out those cases when it is important to see or get advice from a health worker or doctor. But because doctors or health workers are not always nearby, the book also suggests **what to do in the meantime**—even for very serious problems.

This book has been written in fairly basic English, so that persons without much formal education (or whose first language is not English) can understand it. The language used is simple but, I hope, not childish. A few more difficult words have been used where they are *appropriate* or fit well. Usually they are used in ways that their meanings can be easily guessed. This way, those who read this book have a chance to increase their language skills as well as their medical skills.

Important words the reader may not understand are explained in a word list or *vocabulary* at the end of the book. The first time a word listed in the vocabulary is mentioned in a chapter it is usually written in *italics.*

Where There Is No Doctor was first written in Spanish for farm people in the mountains of Mexico where, 27 years ago, the author helped form a health care network now run by the villagers themselves. *Where There Is No Doctor* has been translated into more than 50 languages and is used by village health workers in over 100 countries.

The first English edition was the result of many requests to adapt it for use in Africa and Asia. I received help and suggestions from persons with experience in many parts of the world. But the English edition seems to have lost much of the flavor and usefulness of the original Spanish edition, which was written for a specific area, and for people who have for years been my neighbors and friends. In rewriting the book to serve people in many parts of the world, it has in some ways become too general.

To be fully useful, this book should be adapted by persons familiar with the health needs, customs, special ways of healing, and local language of specific areas.

Persons or programs who wish to use this book, or portions of it, in preparing their own manuals for villagers or health workers are encouraged to do so. Permission from the author or publisher is not needed—**provided the parts reproduced are distributed free or at cost—not for profit.** It would be appreciated if you would (1) include a note of credit and (2) send a copy of your production to The Hesperian Foundation, Box 1692, Palo Alto, California 94302, U.S A.

For local or regional health programs that do not have the resources for revising this book or preparing their own manuals, it is strongly suggested that if the present edition is used, leaflets or inserts be supplied with the book to provide additional information as needed.

In the **Green Pages** (the Uses, Dosage, and Precautions for Medicines) blank spaces have been left to write in common brand names and prices of medicines. Once again, local programs or organizations distributing the book would do well to make up a list of generic or low-cost brand names and prices, to be included with each copy of the book.

This book was written for anyone who wants to do something about his or her own and other people's health. However, it has been widely used as a training and work manual for community health workers. For this reason, an introductory section has been added for the health worker, making clear that **the health worker's first job is to share her knowledge and help educate people.**

Today in over-developed as well as under-developed countries, existing health care systems are in a state of crisis. Often, human needs are not being well met. There is too little fairness. Too much is in the hands of too few.

Let us hope that through a more generous sharing of knowledge, and through learning to use what is best in both traditional and modern ways of healing, people everywhere will develop a kinder, more sensible approach to caring—for their own health, and for each other.

—D.W.

NOTE ABOUT THIS NEW EDITION

In this revised edition of *Where There Is No Doctor,* we have added new information and updated old information, based on the latest scientific knowledge. Health care specialists from many parts of the world have generously given advice and suggestions.

When it would fit without having to change page numbers, we have added new information to the main part of the book. (This way, the numbering stays the same, so that page references in our other books, such as *Helping Health Workers Learn,* will still be correct.)

The **Blue Pages**—a completely new section at the end of the book (p. 399)—has information about health problems of growing or special concern: AIDS, sores on the genitals, leishmaniasis, complications from abortion, guinea worm, and others. Here also are new topics such as measuring blood pressure, misuse of pesticides, drug addiction, and a method of caring for early and underweight babies.

New ideas and information can be found throughout the book—medical knowledge is always changing! For example:

- **Nutrition** advice has changed. Experts used to tell mothers to give children more foods rich in proteins. But it is now known that what most poorly nourished children need is more energy-rich foods. Many low-cost energy foods, especially grains, provide enough protein *if the child eats enough of them.* Finding ways to give enough energy foods is now emphasized, instead of the 'four food groups'. (See Chapter 11.)

- Advice for treatment of **stomach ulcer** is different nowadays. For years doctors recommended drinking lots of milk. But according to recent studies, it is better to drink lots of water, not milk. (See p. 129.)

- Knowledge about **special drinks for diarrhea** (oral rehydration therapy) has also changed. Not long ago experts thought that drinks made with sugar were best. But we now know that drinks made with cereals do more to prevent water loss, slow down diarrhea, and combat malnutrition than do sugar-based drinks or "ORS" packets. (See p. 152.)

- A section has been added on **sterilizing equipment.** This is important to prevent the spread of certain diseases, such as AIDS. (See p. 74.)

- We have also added sections on **dengue** (p. 187), **sickle cell disease** (p. 321), and **contraceptive implants** (p. 293). Page 105 contains revised information about **treatment of snakebite.**

- See page 139 for details on building the fly-killing **VIP latrine.**

If you have suggestions for improving this book, please let us know. Your ideas are very important to us!

The **Green Pages** now include some additional medicines. This is because some diseases have become resistant to the medicines that were used in the past. So it is now harder to give simple medical advice for certain diseases—especially malaria, tuberculosis, typhoid, and sexually spread diseases. Often we give several possibilities for treatment. But **for many infectious diseases you will need local advice** about which medicines are available and effective in your area.

In updating the information on medicines, we mostly include only those on the World Health Organization's *List of Essential Drugs.* (However, we also discuss some widely used but dangerous medicines to give warnings and to discourage their use—see also pages 50 to 52.) In trying to cover health needs and variations in many parts of the world, we have listed more medicines than will be needed for any one area. To persons preparing adaptations of this book, we strongly suggest that the Green Pages be shortened and modified to meet the specific needs and treatment patterns in your country.

In this new edition of *Where There Is No Doctor* we continue to stress the value of traditional forms of healing, and have added some more "home remedies." However, since many folk remedies depend on local plants and customs, we have added only a few which use commonly found items such as garlic. We hope those adapting this book will add home remedies useful to their area.

Community action is emphasized throughout this book. For example, today it is often not enough to explain to mothers that 'breast is best'. Communities must organize to make sure that mothers are able to breast feed their babies at work. Likewise, problems such as misuse of pesticides (p. 412), drug abuse (p. 416), and unsafe abortions (p. 414) are best solved by people working together to make their communities safer, healthier, and more fair.

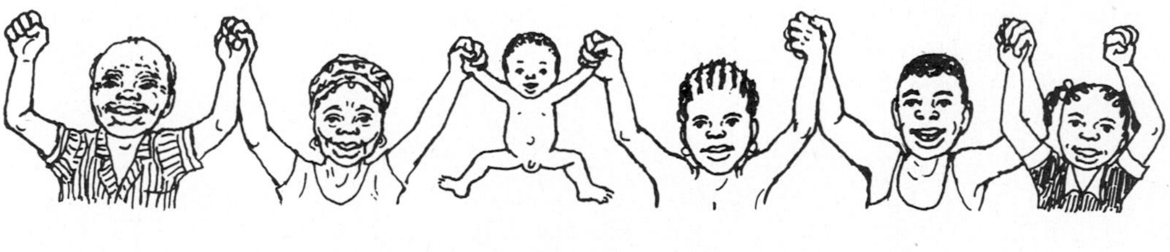

"Health for all" can be achieved only through the organized demand by people for greater equality in terms of land, wages, services, and basic rights. More power to the people!

WORDS TO THE VILLAGE HEALTH WORKER

Who is the village health worker?

A village health worker is a person who helps lead family and neighbors toward better health. Often he or she has been selected by the other villagers as someone who is especially able and kind.

Some village health workers receive training and help from an organized program, perhaps the Ministry of Health. Others have no official position, but are simply members of the community whom people respect as healers or leaders in matters of health. Often they learn by watching, helping, and studying on their own.

In the larger sense, **a village health worker is anyone who takes part in making his or her village a healthier place to live.**

This means almost everyone can and should be a health worker:

- Mothers and fathers can show their children how to keep clean;
- Farm people can work together to help their land produce more food;
- Teachers can teach schoolchildren how to prevent and treat many common sicknesses and injuries;
- Schoolchildren can share what they learn with their parents;
- Shopkeepers can find out about the correct use of medicines they sell and give sensible advice and warning to buyers (see p. 338);
- Midwives can counsel parents about the importance of eating well during pregnancy, breast feeding, and family planning.

This book was written for the health worker in the larger sense. It is for anyone who wants to know and do more for his own, his family's or his people's well-being.

If you are a community health worker, an auxiliary nurse, or even a doctor, remember: this book is not just for you. It is for **all the people.** Share it!

Use this book to help explain what you know to others. Perhaps you can get small groups together to read a chapter at a time and discuss it.

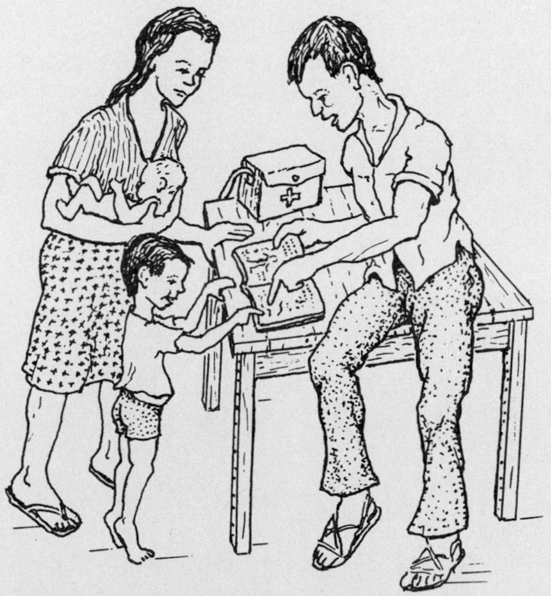

THE VILLAGE HEALTH WORKER LIVES AND WORKS AT THE LEVEL OF HIS PEOPLE. HIS FIRST JOB IS TO SHARE HIS KNOWLEDGE.

Dear Village Health Worker,

This book is mostly about people's **health needs**. But to help your village be a healthy place to live, you must also be in touch with their **human needs**. Your understanding and concern for people are just as important as your knowledge of medicine and sanitation.

Here are some suggestions that may help you serve your people's human needs as well as health needs:

1. BE KIND. A friendly word, a smile, a hand on the shoulder, or some other sign of caring often means more than anything else you can do. **Treat others as your equals.** Even when you are hurried or worried, try to remember the feelings and needs of others. Often it helps to ask yourself, "What would I do if this were a member of my own family?"

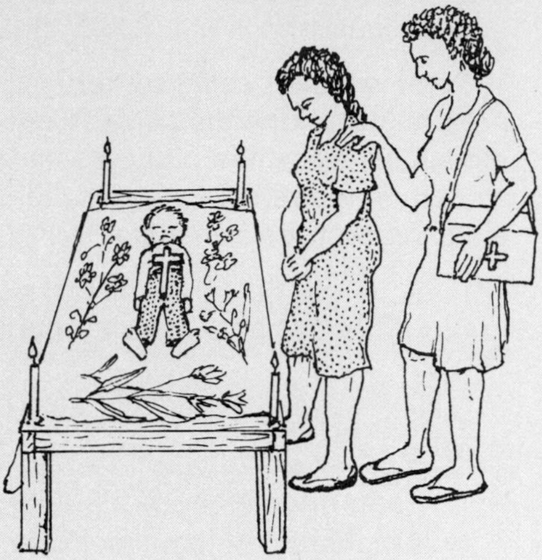

HAVE COMPASSION.

Kindness often helps more than medicine. Never be afraid to show you care.

Treat the sick as people. Be especially kind to those who are very sick or dying. And be kind to their families. Let them see that you care.

2. SHARE YOUR KNOWLEDGE. As a health worker, your first job is to teach. This means helping people learn more about how to keep from getting sick. It also means helping people learn how to recognize and manage their illnesses—including the sensible use of home remedies and common medicines.

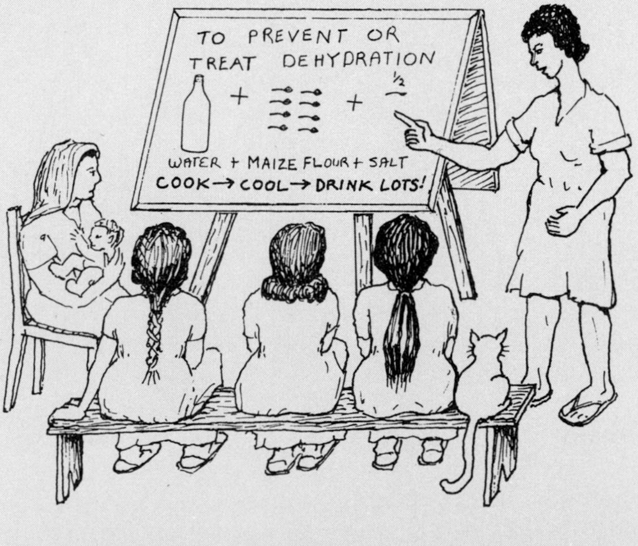

LOOK FOR WAYS TO SHARE YOUR KNOWLEDGE.

There is nothing you have learned that, if carefully explained, should be of danger to anyone. Some doctors talk about **self-care** as if it were dangerous, perhaps because they like people to depend on their costly services. But in truth, **most common health problems could be handled earlier and better by people in their own homes.**

3. RESPECT YOUR PEOPLE'S TRADITIONS AND IDEAS.

Because you learn something about modern medicine does not mean you should no longer appreciate the customs and ways of healing of your people. Too often the human touch in the art of healing is lost when medical science moves in. This is too bad, because . . .

If you can use what is best in modern medicine, together with what is best in traditional healing, the combination may be better than either one alone.

In this way, you will be adding to your people's culture, not taking away.

Of course, if you see that some of the home cures or customs are harmful (for example, putting excrement on the freshly cut cord of a newborn baby), you will want to do something to change this. But do so carefully, with respect for those who believe in such things. Never just tell people they are wrong. Try to help them understand WHY they should do something differently.

People are slow to change their attitudes and traditions, and with good reason. They are true to what they feel is right. And this we must respect.

Modern medicine does not have all the answers either. It has helped solve some problems, yet has led to other, sometimes even bigger ones. People quickly come to depend too much on modern medicine and its experts, to overuse medicines, and to forget how to care for themselves and each other.

So go slow—and always keep a deep respect for your people, their traditions, and their human dignity. Help them build on the knowledge and skills they already have.

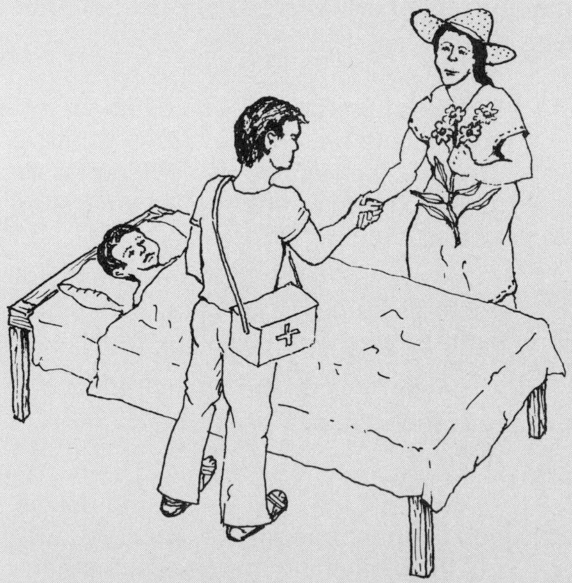

WORK WITH TRADITIONAL HEALERS AND MIDWIVES—NOT AGAINST THEM.

Learn from them and encourage them to learn from you.

4. KNOW YOUR OWN LIMITS.

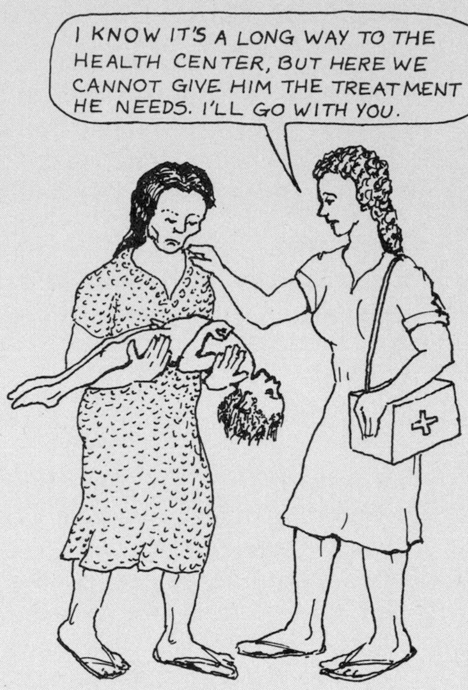
I KNOW IT'S A LONG WAY TO THE HEALTH CENTER, BUT HERE WE CANNOT GIVE HIM THE TREATMENT HE NEEDS. I'LL GO WITH YOU.

KNOW YOUR LIMITS.

No matter how great or small your knowledge and skills, you can do a good job as long as you know and work within your limits. This means: **Do what you know how to do.** Do not try things you have not learned about or have not had enough experience doing, if they might harm or endanger someone.

But use your judgment.

Often, what you decide to do or not do will depend on how far you have to go to get more expert help.

For example, a mother has just given birth and is bleeding more than you think is normal. If you are only half an hour away from a medical center, it may be wise to take her there right away. But if the mother is bleeding very heavily and you are a long way from the health center, you may decide to massage her womb (see p. 265) or inject an oxytocic (see p. 266) even if you were not taught this.

Do not take unnecessary chances. But when the danger is clearly greater if you do nothing, do not be afraid to try something you feel reasonably sure will help.

Know your limits—but also use your head. Always do your best to protect the sick person rather than yourself.

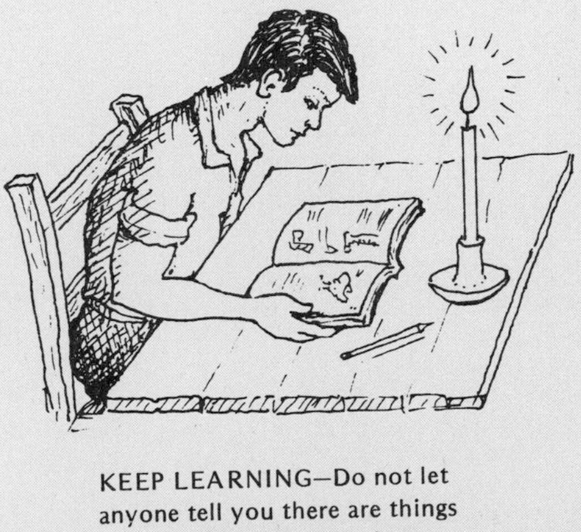

KEEP LEARNING—Do not let anyone tell you there are things you should not learn or know.

5. KEEP LEARNING. Use every chance you have to learn more. Study whatever books or information you can lay your hands on that will help you be a better worker, teacher, or person.

Always be ready to ask questions of doctors, sanitation officers, agriculture experts, or anyone else you can learn from.

Never pass up the chance to take refresher courses or get additional training.

Your first job is to teach, and unless you keep learning more, soon you will not have anything new to teach others.

6. PRACTICE WHAT YOU TEACH.

People are more likely to pay attention to what you do than what you say. As a health worker, you want to take special care in your personal life and habits, so as to set a good example for your neighbors.

Before you ask people to make latrines, be sure your own family has one.

Also, if you help organize a work group—for example, to dig a common garbage hole—be sure you work and sweat as hard as everyone else.

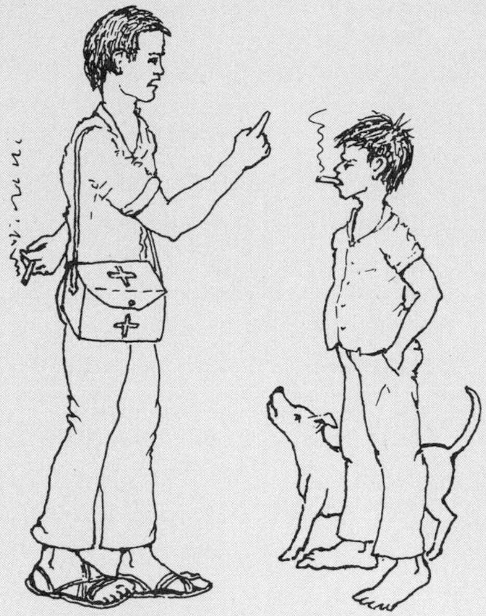

PRACTICE WHAT YOU TEACH
(or who will listen to you?)

Good leaders do not tell people what to do. They set the example.

7. WORK FOR THE JOY OF IT.

If you want other people to take part in improving their village and caring for their health, you must enjoy such activity yourself. If not, who will want to follow your example?

Try to make community work projects fun. For example, fencing off the public water hole to keep animals away from where people take water can be hard work. But if the whole village helps do it as a 'work festival'—perhaps with refreshments and music—the job will be done quickly and can be fun. Children will work hard and enjoy it, if they can turn work into play.

You may or may not be paid for your work. But never refuse to care, or care less, for someone who is poor or cannot pay.

This way you will win your people's love and respect. These are worth far more than money.

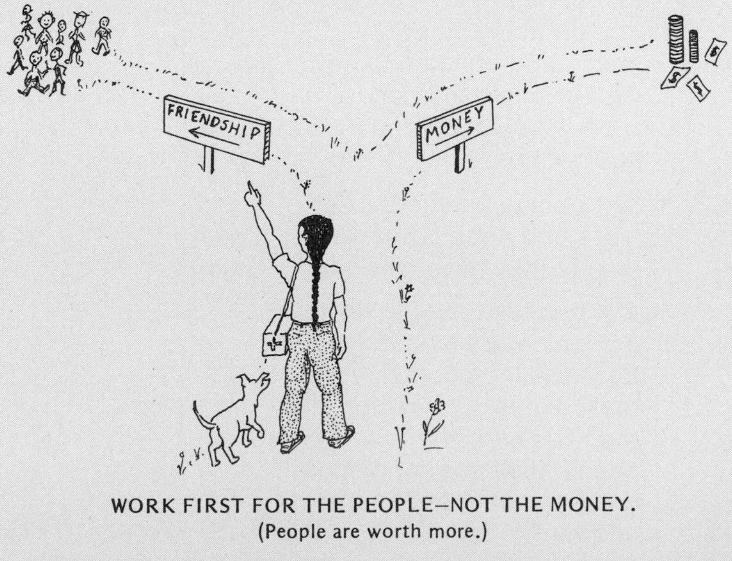

WORK FIRST FOR THE PEOPLE—NOT THE MONEY.
(People are worth more.)

8. LOOK AHEAD—AND HELP OTHERS TO LOOK AHEAD.

A responsible health worker does not wait for people to get sick. She tries to stop sickness before it starts. She encourages people to take action **now** to protect their health and well-being in the future.

Many sicknesses can be prevented. Your job, then, is to help your people understand the causes of their health problems and do something about them.

Most health problems have many causes, one leading to another. To correct the problem in a lasting way, you must look for and deal with the **underlying causes.** You must get to the root of the problem.

For example, in many villages diarrhea is the most common cause of death in small children. The spread of diarrhea is caused in part by lack of cleanliness (poor *sanitation* and *hygiene*). You can do something to correct this by digging latrines and teaching basic guidelines of cleanliness (p. 133).

But the children who suffer and die most often from diarrhea are those who are poorly nourished. Their bodies do not have strength to fight the infections. So to prevent death from diarrhea we must also prevent poor nutrition.

And why do so many children suffer from poor nutrition?

- Is it because mothers do not realize what foods are most important (for example, breast milk)?
- Is it because the family does not have enough money or land to produce the food it needs?
- Is it because a few rich persons control most of the land and the wealth?
- Is it because the poor do not make the best use of land they have?
- Is it because parents have more children than they or their land can provide for, and keep having more?
- Is it because fathers lose hope and spend the little money they have on drink?
- Is it because people do not look or plan ahead? Because they do not realize that by working together and sharing they can change the conditions under which they live and die?

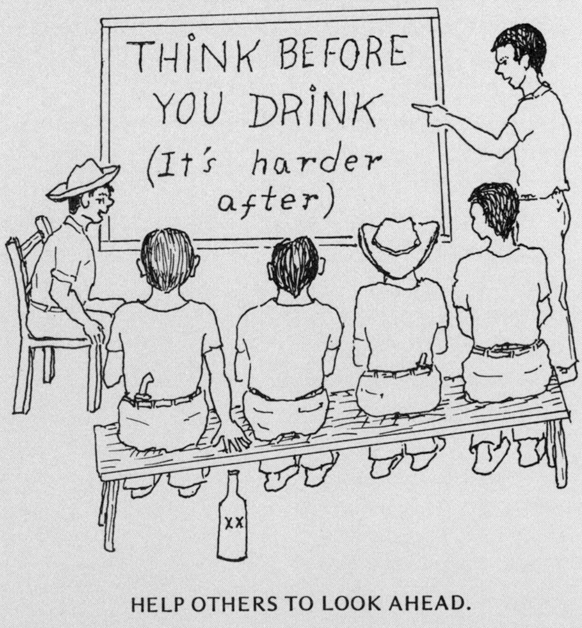

HELP OTHERS TO LOOK AHEAD.

You may find that many, if not all, of these things lie behind infant deaths in your area. You will, no doubt, find other causes as well. As a health worker it is your job to help people understand and do something about as many of these causes as you can.

But remember: to prevent frequent deaths from diarrhea will take far more than latrines, pure water, and 'special drink' (oral rehydration). You may find that child spacing, better land use, and fairer distribution of wealth, land, and power are more important in the long run.

The causes that lie behind much sickness and human suffering are short-sightedness and greed. If your interest is your people's well-being, you must help them learn to share, to work together, and to look ahead.

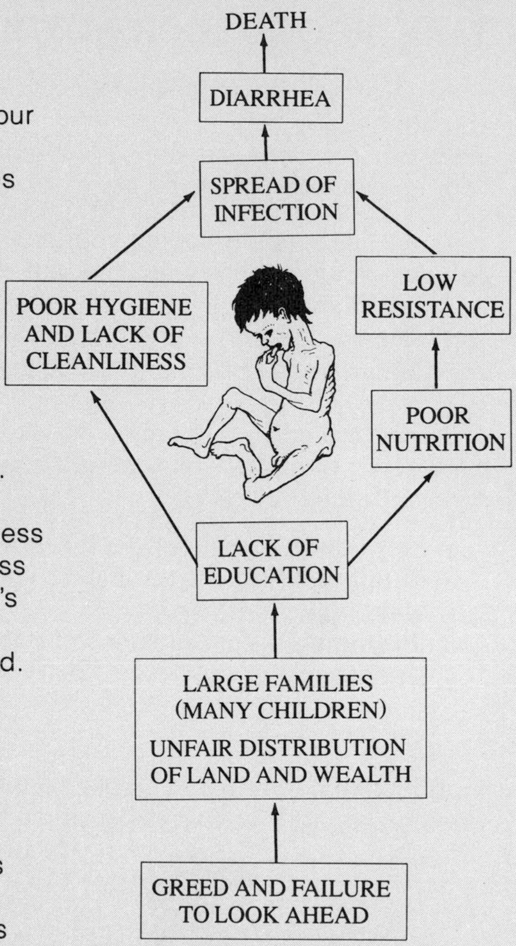

The chain of causes leading to death from diarrhea.

MANY THINGS RELATE TO HEALTH CARE

We have looked at some of the causes that underlie diarrhea and poor nutrition. Likewise, you will find that such things as **food production, land distribution, education,** and **the way people treat or mistreat each other** lie behind many different health problems.

If you are interested in the long-term welfare of your whole community, you must help your people look for answers to these larger questions.

Health is more than not being sick. It is well-being: in body, mind, and community. People live best in healthy surroundings, in a place where they can trust each other, work together to meet daily needs, share in times of difficulty and plenty, and help each other learn and grow and live, each as fully as he or she can.

Do your best to solve day-to-day problems. But remember that your greatest job is to help your community become a more healthy and more human place to live.

You as a health worker have a big responsibility.

Where should you begin?

TAKE A GOOD LOOK AT YOUR COMMUNITY

Because you have grown up in your community and know your people well, you are already familiar with many of their health problems. You have an inside view. But in order to see the whole picture, you will need to look carefully at your community from many points of view.

As a village health worker, your concern is for the well-being of **all the people**—not just those you know well or who come to you. Go to your people. Visit their homes, fields, gathering places, and schools. Understand their joys and concerns. Examine with them their habits, the things in their daily lives that bring about good health, and those that may lead to sickness or injury.

Before you and your community attempt any project or activity, carefully think about what it will require and how likely it is to work. To do this, you must consider **all** the following:

1. **Felt needs**—what people feel are their biggest problems.
2. **Real needs**—steps people can take to correct these problems in a lasting way.
3. **Willingness**—or readiness of people to plan and take the needed steps.
4. **Resources**—the persons, skills, materials, and/or money needed to carry out the activities decided upon.

As a simple example of how each of these things can be important, let us suppose that a man who smokes a lot comes to you complaining of a cough that has steadily been getting worse.

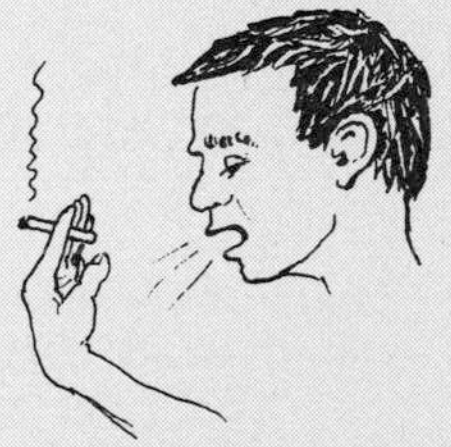

1. His **felt need** is to get rid of his cough.

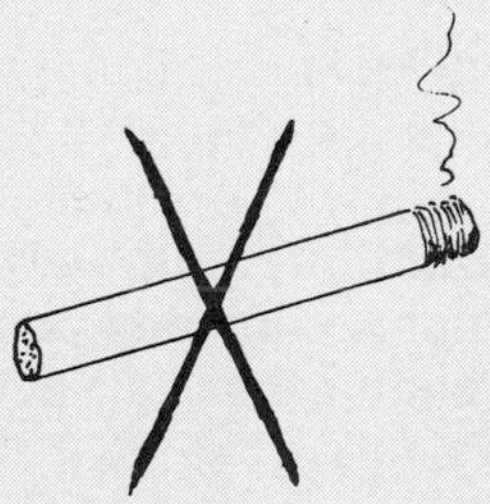

2. His **real need** (to correct the problem) is to give up smoking.

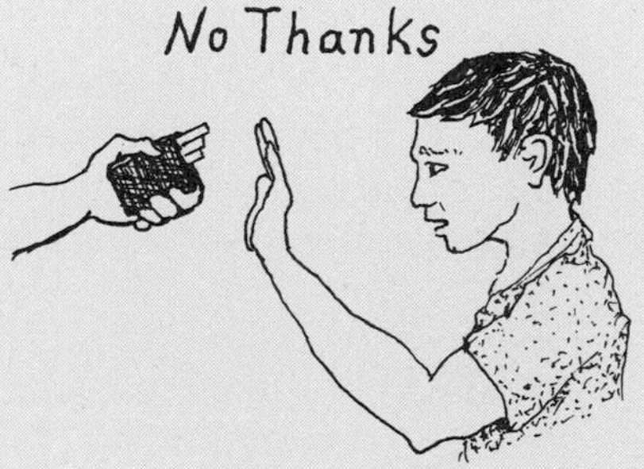

3. To get rid of his cough will require his **willingness** to give up smoking. For this he must understand how much it really matters.

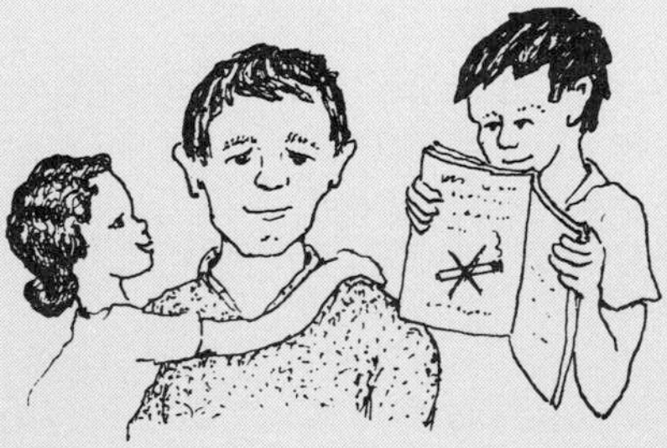

4. One **resource** that may help him give up smoking is information about the harm it can do him and his family (see p. 149). Another is the support and encouragement of his family, his friends, and you.

Finding Out the Needs

As a health worker, you will first want to find out your people's most important health problems and their biggest concerns. To gather the information necessary to decide what the greatest needs and concerns really are, it may help to make up a list of questions.

On the next 2 pages are samples of the kinds of things you may want to ask. But think of questions that are important **in your area.** Ask questions that not only help you get information, but that get others asking important questions themselves.

Do not make your list of questions too long or complicated—especially a list you take from house to house. Remember, **people are not numbers** and do not like to be looked at as numbers. As you gather information, be sure your first interest is always in what individuals want and feel. It may be better not even to carry a list of questions. But in considering the needs of your community, you should keep certain basic questions in mind.

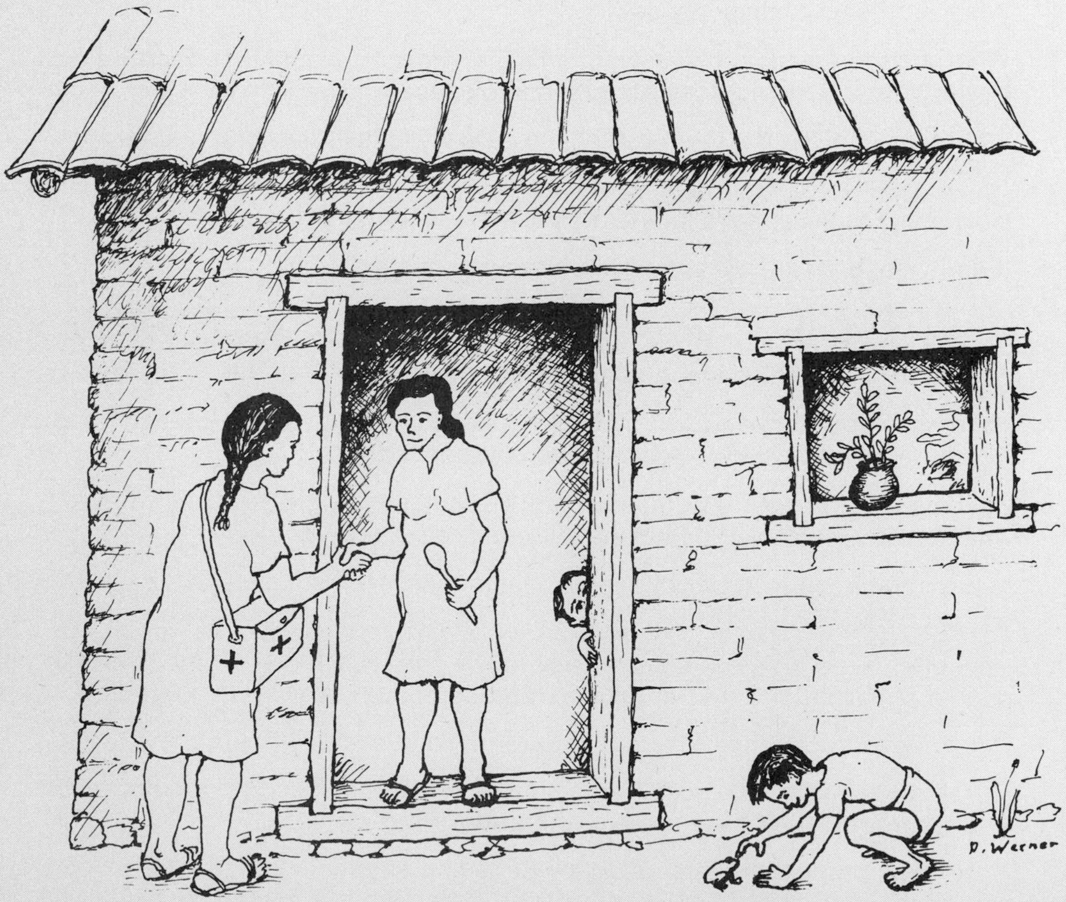

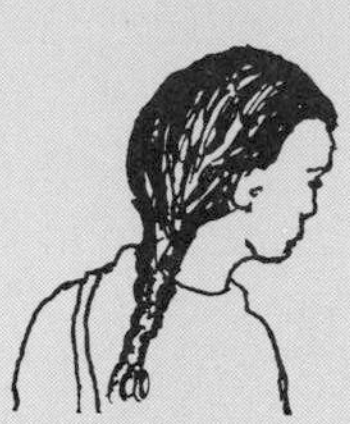

Sample Lists of Questions

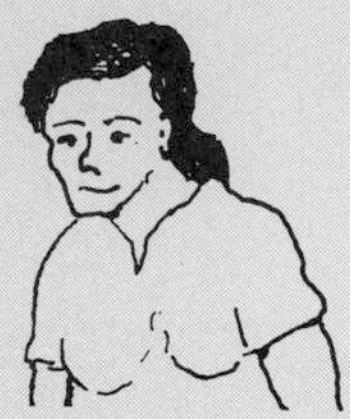

To Help Determine Community Health Needs And at the Same Time Get People Thinking

FELT NEEDS

What things in your people's daily lives (living conditions, ways of doing things, beliefs, etc.) do they feel help them to be healthy?

What do people feel to be their major problems, concerns, and needs—not only those related to health, but in general?

HOUSING AND SANITATION

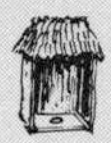

What are different houses made of? Walls? Floors? Are the houses kept clean? Is cooking done on the floor or where? How does smoke get out? On what do people sleep?

Are flies, fleas, bedbugs, rats, or other pests a problem? In what way? What do people do to control them? What else could be done?

Is food protected? How could it be better protected?

What animals (dogs, chickens, pigs, etc.), if any, are allowed in the house? What problems do they cause?

What are the common diseases of animals? How do they affect people's health? What is being done about these diseases?

Where do families get their water? Is it safe to drink? What precautions are taken?

How many families have latrines? How many use them properly?

Is the village clean? Where do people put garbage? Why?

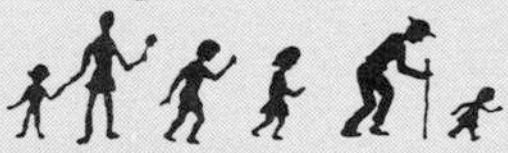

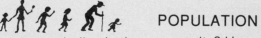

POPULATION

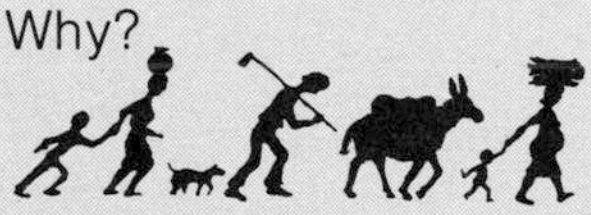

How many people live in the community? How many are under 15 years old?

How many can read and write? What good is schooling? Does it teach children what they need to know? How else do children learn?

How many babies were born this year? How many people died? Of what? At what ages? Could their deaths have been prevented? How?

Is the population (number of people) getting larger or smaller? Does this cause any problems?

How often were different persons sick in the past year? How many days was each sick? What sickness or injuries did each have? Why?

How many people have chronic (long-term) illnesses? What are they?

How many children do most parents have? How many children died? Of what? At what ages? What were some of the **underlying** causes?

How many parents are interested in not having any more children or in not having them so often? For what reasons? (See Family Planning, p. 283.)

NUTRITION

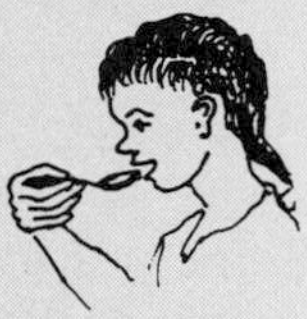

How many mothers breast feed their babies? For how long? Are these babies healthier than those who are not breast fed? Why?

What are the main foods people eat? Where do they come from?

Do people make good use of all foods available?

How many children are underweight (p. 109) or show signs of poor nutrition? How much do parents and schoolchildren know about nutritional needs?

How many people smoke a lot? How many drink alcoholic or soft drinks very often? What effect does this have on their own and their families' health? (See p. 148 to 150.)

LAND AND FOOD

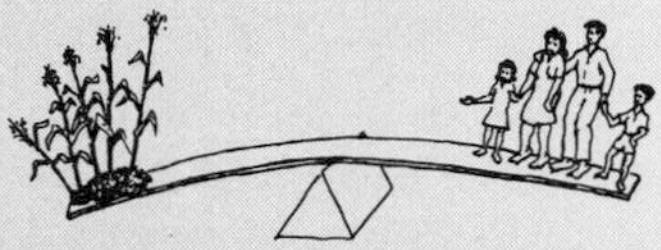

Does the land provide enough food for each family? How long will it continue to produce enough food if families keep growing?

How is farm land distributed? How many people own their land?

What efforts are being made to help the land produce more?

How are crops and food stored? Is there much damage or loss? Why?

HEALING, HEALTH

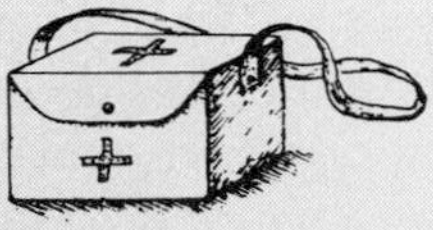

What role do local midwives and healers play in health care?

What traditional ways of healing and medicines are used? Which are of greatest value? Are any harmful or dangerous?

What health services are nearby? How good are they? What do they cost? How much are they used?

How many children have been vaccinated? Against what sicknesses?

What other preventive measures are being taken? What others might be taken? How important are they?

SELF-HELP

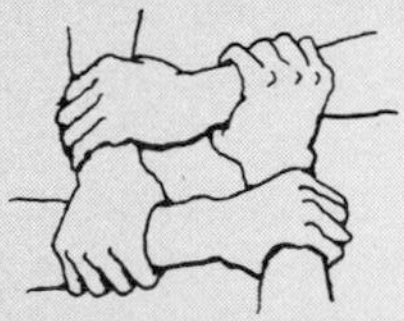

What are the most important things that affect your people's health and well-being—now and in the future?

How many of their common health problems can people care for themselves? How much must they rely on outside help and medication?

Are people interested in finding ways of making self-care safer, more effective, and more complete? Why? How can they learn more? What stands in the way?

What are the rights of rich people? Of poor people? Of men? Of women? Of children? How is each of these groups treated? Why? Is this fair? What needs to be changed? By whom? How?

Do people work together to meet common needs? Do they share or help each other when needs are great?

What can be done to make your village a better, healthier place to live? Where might you and your people begin?

USING LOCAL RESOURCES TO MEET NEEDS

How you deal with a problem will depend upon what resources are available.

Some activities require outside resources (materials, money, or people from somewhere else). For example, a vaccination program is possible only if vaccines are brought in—often from another country.

Other activities can be carried out completely with local resources. A family or a group of neighbors can fence off a water hole or build simple latrines using materials close at hand.

Some outside resources, such as vaccines and a few important medicines, can make a big difference in people's health. You should do your best to get them. But as a general rule, it is in the best interest of your people to

Use local resources whenever possible.

The more you and your people can do for yourselves, and the less you have to depend on outside assistance and supplies, the healthier and stronger your community will become.

Not only can you count on local resources to be on hand when you need them, but often they do the best job at the lowest cost. For example, if you can encourage mothers to breast feed rather than bottle feed their babies, this will build self-reliance through a top quality local resource—breast milk! It will also prevent needless sickness and death of many babies.

In your health work always remember:

Encourage people to make the most of local resources.

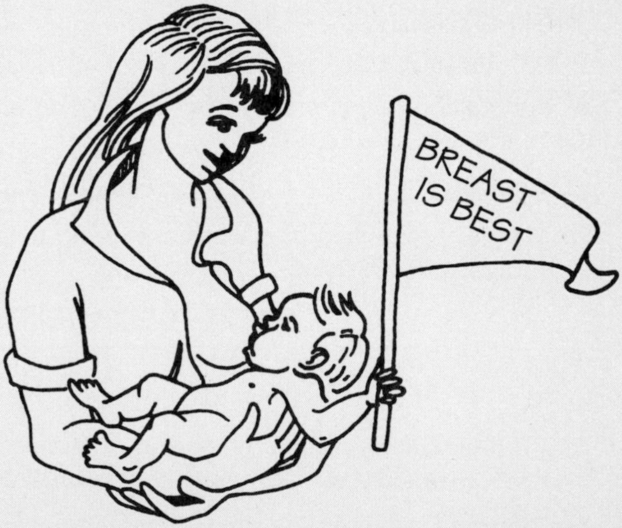

BREAST MILK—A TOP QUALITY LOCAL RESOURCE—BETTER THAN ANYTHING MONEY CAN BUY!

The most valuable resource for the health of the people is the people themselves.

DECIDING WHAT TO DO AND WHERE TO BEGIN

After taking a careful look at needs and resources, you and your people must decide which things are more important and which to do first. You can do many different things to help people be healthy. Some are important immediately. Others will help determine the future well-being of individuals or the whole community.

In a lot of villages, poor nutrition plays a part in other health problems. **People cannot be healthy unless there is enough to eat.** Whatever other problems you decide to work with, if people are hungry or children are poorly nourished, better nutrition must be your first concern.

There are many different ways to approach the problem of poor nutrition, for many different things join to cause it. You and your community must consider the possible actions you might take and decide which are most likely to work.

Here are a few examples of ways some people have helped meet their needs for better nutrition. Some actions bring quick results. Others work over a longer time. You and your people must decide what is most likely to work in your area.

POSSIBLE WAYS TO WORK TOWARD BETTER NUTRITION

FAMILY GARDENS

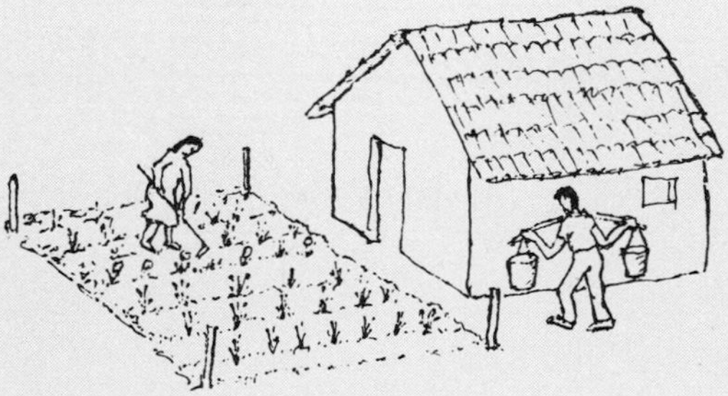

CONTOUR DITCHES
to prevent soil from washing away

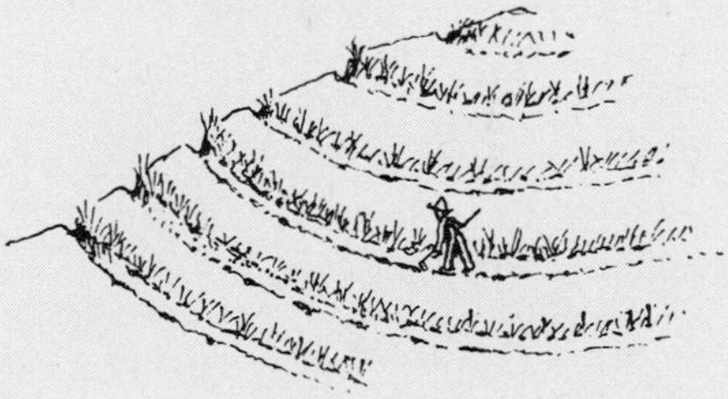

ROTATION OF CROPS
Every other planting season plant a crop that returns strength to the soil—like beans, peas, lentils, alfalfa, peanuts or some other plant with seed in pods (legumes).

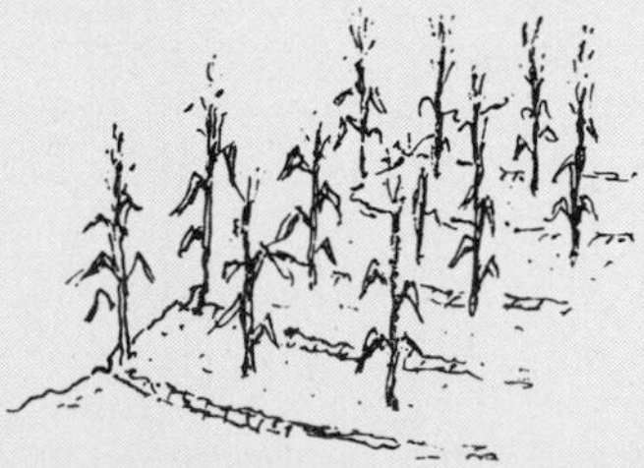

This year **maize**

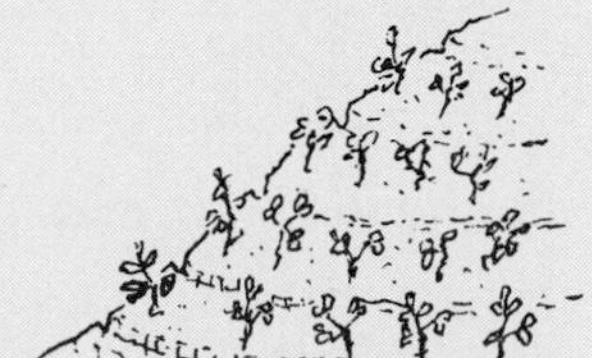

Next year **beans**

MORE WAYS TO WORK TOWARD BETTER NUTRITION

IRRIGATION OF LAND

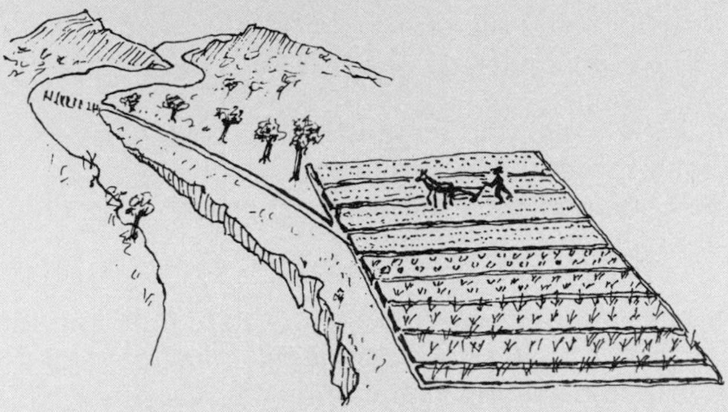

FISH BREEDING

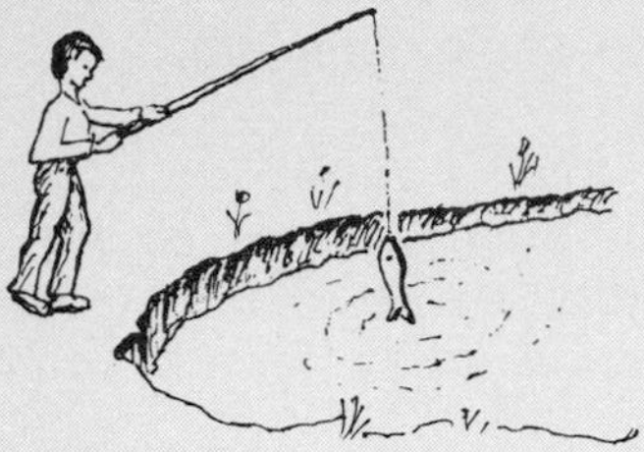

BEEKEEPING

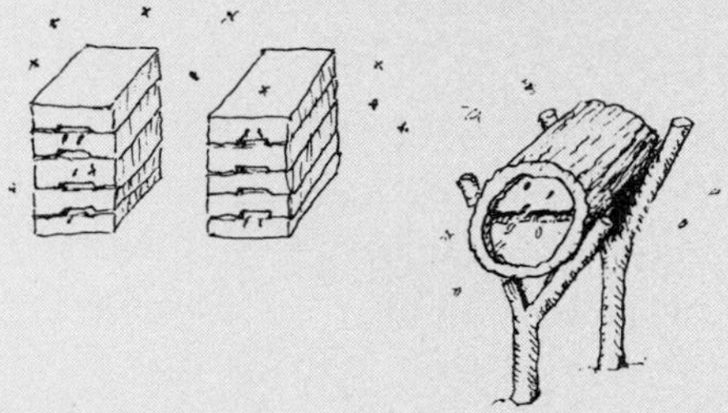

NATURAL FERTILIZERS

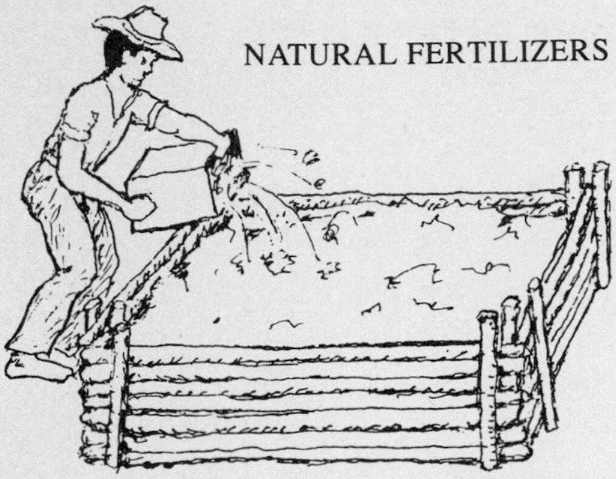

Compost pile

BETTER FOOD STORAGE

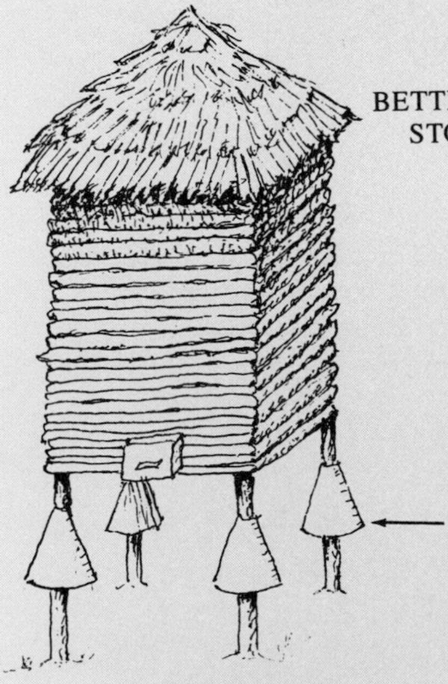

Metal sleeves to keep out rats

SMALLER FAMILIES

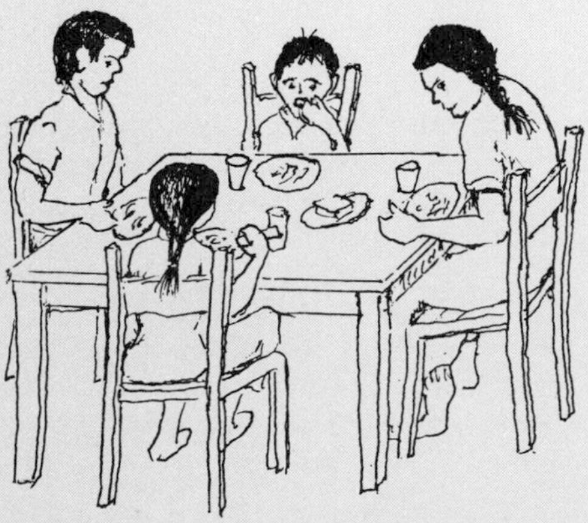

THROUGH FAMILY PLANNING
(p. 283)

TRYING A NEW IDEA

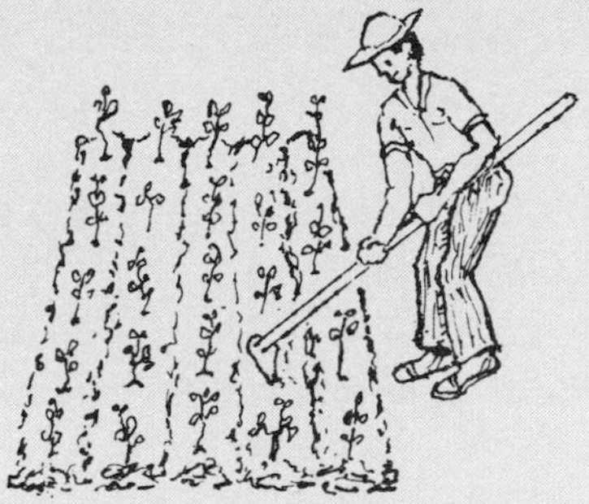
START SMALL

Not all the suggestions on the last pages are likely to work in your area. Perhaps some will work if changed for your particular situation and resources at hand. Often you can only know whether something will work or not by trying it. That is, by experiment.

When you try out a new idea, **always start small.** If you start small and the experiment fails, or something has to be done differently, you will not lose much. If it works, people will see that it works and can begin to apply it in a bigger way.

Do not be discouraged if an experiment does not work. Perhaps you can try again with certain changes. You can learn as much from your failures as your successes. But start small.

Here is an example of experimenting with a new idea.

You learn that a certain kind of bean, such as soya, is an excellent body-building food. But will it grow in your area? And if it grows, will people eat it?

Start by planting a small patch—or 2 or 3 small patches in different conditions of soil or water. If the beans do well, try preparing them in different ways, and see if people will eat them. If so, try planting more beans in the conditions where you found they grew best. But try out still other conditions in more small patches to see if you can get an even better crop.

There may be several conditions you want to try changing. For example, type of soil, addition of fertilizer, amount of water, or different varieties of seed. To best understand what helps and what does not, be sure to change only **one** condition at a time and keep all the rest the same.

For example, to find out if animal fertilizer (manure) helps the beans grow, and how much to use, plant several small bean patches side by side, under the same conditions of water and sunlight, and using the same seed. But before you plant, mix each patch with a different amount of manure, something like this:

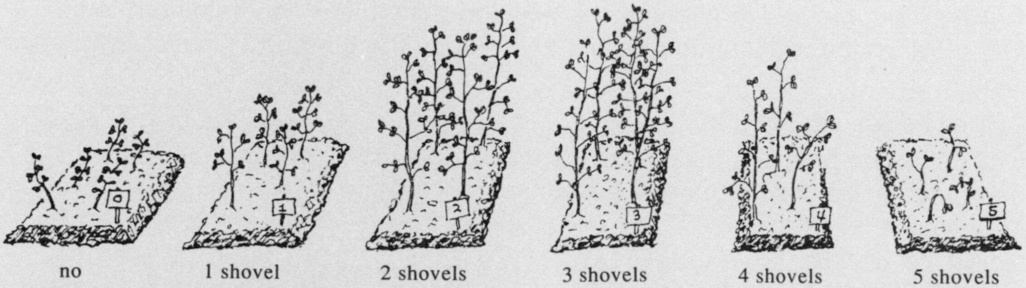

This experiment shows that a certain amount of manure helps, but that too much can harm the plants. This is only an example. Your experiments may give different results. Try for yourself!

WORKING TOWARD A BALANCE BETWEEN PEOPLE AND LAND

Health depends on many things, but above all it depends on whether people have enough to eat.

Most food comes from the land. Land that is used well can produce more food. A health worker needs to know ways to help the land better feed the people—now and in the future. But even the best used piece of land can only feed a certain number of people. And today, **many of the people who farm do not have enough land to meet their needs or to stay healthy.**

In many parts of the world, the situation is getting worse, not better. Parents often have many children, so year by year there are more mouths to feed on the limited land that the poor are permitted to use.

Many health programs try to work toward a balance between people and land through 'family planning', or helping people have only the number of children they want. Smaller families, they reason, will mean more land and food to go around. But family planning by itself has little effect. As long as people are very poor, they often want many children. Children help with work without having to be paid, and as they get bigger may even bring home a little money. When the parents grow old, some of their children—or grandchildren—will perhaps be able to help care for them.

For a poor country to have many children may be an economic disaster. But for a poor family to have many children is often an economic necessity—especially when many die young. In the world today, **for most people, having many children is the surest form of social security they can hope for.**

Some groups and programs take a different approach. They recognize that hunger exists not because there is too little land to feed everyone, but because most of the land is in the hands of a few selfish persons. The balance they seek is a fairer distribution of land and wealth. They work to help people gain greater control over their health, land, and lives.

It has been shown that, where land and wealth are shared more fairly and people gain greater economic security, they usually choose to have smaller families. Family planning helps when it is truly the people's choice. A balance between people and land can more likely be gained through helping people work toward fairer distribution and social justice than through family planning alone.

It has been said that the social meaning of *love* is *justice.* The health worker who loves her people should help them work toward a balance based on a more just distribution of land and wealth.

A LIMITED AMOUNT OF LAND CAN ONLY SUPPORT A LIMITED NUMBER OF PEOPLE.

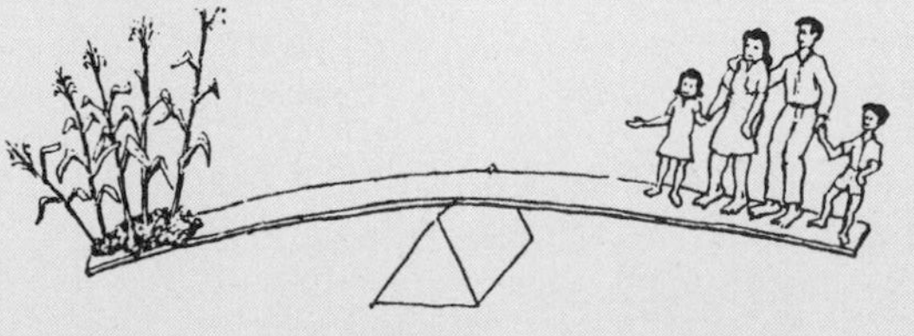

A LASTING BALANCE BETWEEN PEOPLE AND LAND MUST BE BASED ON FAIR DISTRIBUTION.

WORKING TOWARD A BALANCE BETWEEN Prevention and Treatment

A balance between treatment and prevention often comes down to a balance between immediate needs and long-term needs.

As a health worker you must go to your people, work with them on their terms, and help them find answers to the needs they feel most. People's first concern is often to find relief for the sick and suffering. Therefore, **one of your first concerns must be to help with healing.**

But also look ahead. While caring for people's immediate felt needs, also help them look to the future. Help them realize that much sickness and suffering can be prevented and that they themselves can take preventive actions.

But be careful! Sometimes health planners and workers go too far. In their eagerness to prevent future ills, they may show too little concern for the sickness and suffering that already exist. By failing to respond to people's present needs, they may fail to gain their cooperation. And so they fail in much of their preventive work as well.

Treatment and prevention go hand in hand. Early treatment often prevents mild illness from becoming serious. If you help people to recognize many of their common health problems and to treat them early, in their own homes, much needless suffering can be prevented.

Early treatment is a form of preventive medicine.

If you want their cooperation, **start where your people are.** Work toward a balance between prevention and treatment that is acceptable to them. Such a balance will be largely determined by people's present attitudes toward sickness, healing, and health. As you help them look farther ahead, as their attitudes change, and as more diseases are controlled, you may find that the balance shifts naturally in favor of prevention.

You cannot tell the mother whose child is ill that prevention is more important than cure. Not if you want her to listen. But you can tell her, while you help her care for her child, that prevention is equally important.

Work toward prevention—do not force it.

Use treatment as a doorway to prevention. One of the best times to talk to people about prevention is when they come for treatment. For example, if a mother brings a child with worms, carefully explain to her how to treat him. But also take time to explain to both the mother and child how the worms are spread and the different things they can do to prevent this from happening (see Chapter 12). Visit their home from time to time, not to find fault, but to help the family toward more effective self-care.

Use treatment as a chance to teach prevention.

SENSIBLE AND LIMITED USE OF MEDICINES

One of the most difficult and important parts of preventive care is to educate your people in the sensible and limited use of medicines. A few modern medicines are very important and can save lives. But **for most sicknesses no medicine is needed.** The body itself can usually fight off sickness with rest, good food, drinking lots of liquid, and perhaps some simple home remedies.

People may come to you asking for medicine when they do not need any. You may be tempted to give them some medicine just to please. But if you do, when they get well, they will think that you and the medicine cured them. Really their bodies cured themselves.

Instead of teaching people to depend on medicines they do not need, take time to explain **why** they should not be used. Also tell people **what they can do themselves** to get well.

This way you are helping people to rely on local resources (themselves), rather than on an outside resource (medicine). Also, you are protecting their health, for **there is no medicine that does not have some risk in its use.**

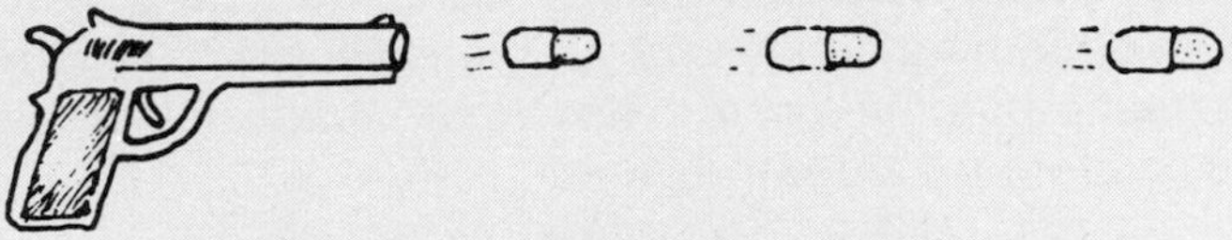

REMEMBER: *MEDICINES CAN KILL*

Three common health problems for which people too often request medicines they do not need are (1) the common cold, (2) minor cough, and (3) diarrhea.

The **common cold** is best treated by resting, drinking lots of liquids, and at the most taking aspirin. Penicillin, tetracycline, and other antibiotics do not help at all (see p. 163).

For **minor coughs,** or even more severe coughs with thick mucus or *phlegm,* drinking a lot of water will loosen mucus and ease the cough faster and better than cough syrup. Breathing warm water vapor brings even greater relief (see p. 168). Do not make people dependent on cough syrup or other medicines they do not need.

For most **diarrhea** of children, medicines do not make them get well. Many commonly used medicines (neomycin, streptomycin, kaolin-pectin, *Lomotil,* chloramphenicol) may even be harmful. **What is most important is that the child get *lots of liquids* and *enough food*** (see p. 155 to 156). **The key to the child's recovery is the mother, not the medicine.** If you can help mothers understand this and learn what to do, many children's lives can be saved.

Medicines are often used too much, both by doctors and by ordinary people. This is unfortunate for many reasons:

- It is wasteful. Most money spent on medicine would be better spent on food.
- It makes people depend on something they do not need (and often cannot afford).
- Every medicine has some risk in its use. There is always a chance that an unneeded medicine may actually do the person harm.
- What is more, when some medicines are used too often for minor problems, they lose their power to fight dangerous sicknesses.

An example of a medicine losing its power is chloramphenicol. The extreme overuse of this important but risky antibiotic for minor infections has meant that in some parts of the world chloramphenicol no longer works against typhoid fever, a very dangerous infection. Frequent overuse of chloramphenicol has allowed typhoid to become *resistant* to it (see p. 58).

For all the above reasons the use of medicines should be limited.

But how? Neither rigid rules and restrictions nor permitting only highly trained persons to decide about the use of medicines has prevented overuse. Only when the people themselves are better informed will the limited and careful use of medicines be common.

To educate people about sensible and limited use of medicines is one of the important jobs of the health worker.

This is especially true in areas where modern medicines are already in great use.

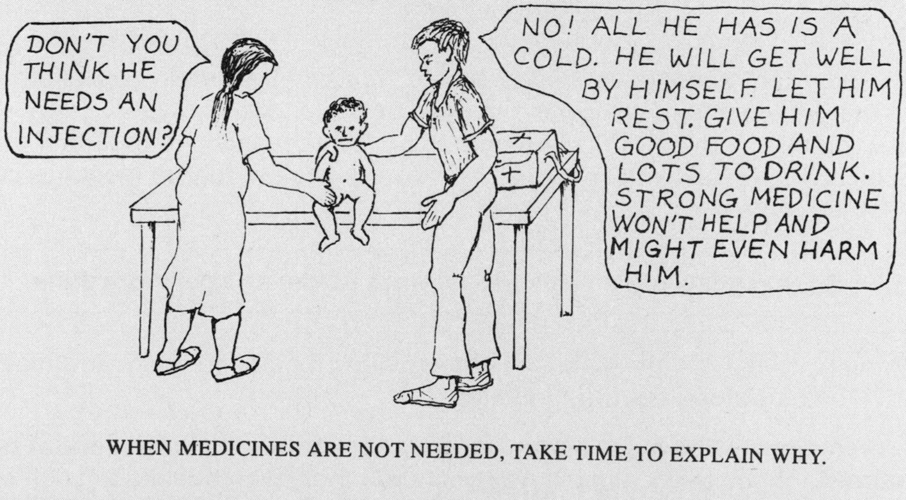
DON'T YOU THINK HE NEEDS AN INJECTION?
NO! ALL HE HAS IS A COLD. HE WILL GET WELL BY HIMSELF. LET HIM REST. GIVE HIM GOOD FOOD AND LOTS TO DRINK. STRONG MEDICINE WON'T HELP AND MIGHT EVEN HARM HIM.

WHEN MEDICINES ARE NOT NEEDED, TAKE TIME TO EXPLAIN WHY.

For more information about the use and misuse of medicines, see Chapter 6, page 49. For the use and misuse of injections, see Chapter 9, page 65. For sensible use of home remedies, see Chapter 1.

FINDING OUT WHAT PROGRESS HAS BEEN MADE (EVALUATION)

From time to time in your health work, it helps to take a careful look at **what** and **how much** you and your people have succeeded in doing. What changes, if any, have been made to improve health and well-being in your community?

You may want to record each month or year the health activities that can be measured. For example:

- How many families have put in latrines?
- How many farmers take part in activities to improve their land and crops?
- How many mothers and children take part in an *Under-Fives Program* (regular check-ups and learning)?

This kind of question will help you measure **action taken.** But to find out the result or **impact** of these activities on health, you will need to answer other questions such as:

- How many children had diarrhea or signs of worms in the past month or year—as compared to before there were latrines?
- How much was harvested this season (corn, beans, or other crops)—as compared to before improved methods were used?
- How many children show normal weight and weight-gain on their Child Health Charts (see p. 297)—as compared to when the Under-Fives Program was started?
- Do fewer children die now than before?

To be able to judge the success of any activity you need to collect certain information both before and after. For example, if you want to teach mothers how important it is to breast feed their babies, first take a count of how many mothers are doing so. Then begin the teaching program and each year take another count. This way you can get a good idea as to how much effect your teaching has had.

You may want to set goals. For example, you and the health committee may hope that 80% of the families have latrines by the end of one year. Every month you take a count. If, by the end of six months, only one-third of the families have latrines, you know you will have to work harder to meet the goal you set for yourselves.

Setting goals often helps people work harder and get more done.

To evaluate the results of your health activities it helps to count and measure certain things **before, during,** and **after.**

But remember: **The most important part of your health work cannot be measured.** It has to do with the way you and other people relate to each other; with people learning and working together; with the growth of kindness, responsibility, sharing, and hope. It depends on the growing strength and unity of the people to stand up for their basic rights. You cannot measure these things. But weigh them well when you consider what changes have been made.

TEACHING AND LEARNING TOGETHER— THE HEALTH WORKER AS AN EDUCATOR

As you come to realize how many things affect health, you may think the health worker has an impossibly large job. And true, you will never get much done if you try to deliver health care by yourself.

Only when the people themselves become actively responsible for their own and their community's health, can important changes take place.

Your community's well-being depends on the involvement not of one person, but of nearly everyone. For this to happen, responsibility and knowledge must be shared.

This is why **your first job as a health worker is to teach**—to teach children, parents, farmers, schoolteachers, other health workers—everyone you can.

The art of teaching is the most important skill a person can learn. To teach is to help others grow, and to grow with them. **A good teacher is not someone who puts ideas into other people's heads; he or she is someone who helps others build on their own ideas, to make new discoveries for themselves.**

Teaching and learning should not be limited to the schoolhouse or health post. They should take place in the home and in the fields and on the road. As a health worker one of your best chances to teach will probably be when you treat the sick. But you should look for every opportunity to exchange ideas, to share, to show, and to help your people think and work together.

On the next few pages are some ideas that may help you do this. They are only suggestions. You will have many other ideas yourself.

TWO APPROACHES TO HEALTH CARE

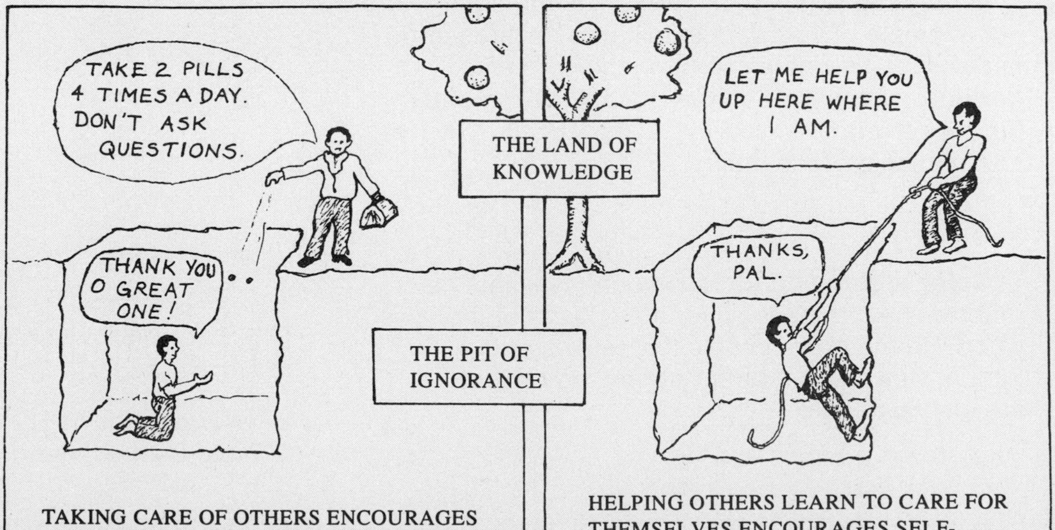

TAKING CARE OF OTHERS ENCOURAGES DEPENDENCY AND LOSS OF FREEDOM.

HELPING OTHERS LEARN TO CARE FOR THEMSELVES ENCOURAGES SELF-RELIANCE AND EQUALITY.

Tools for Teaching

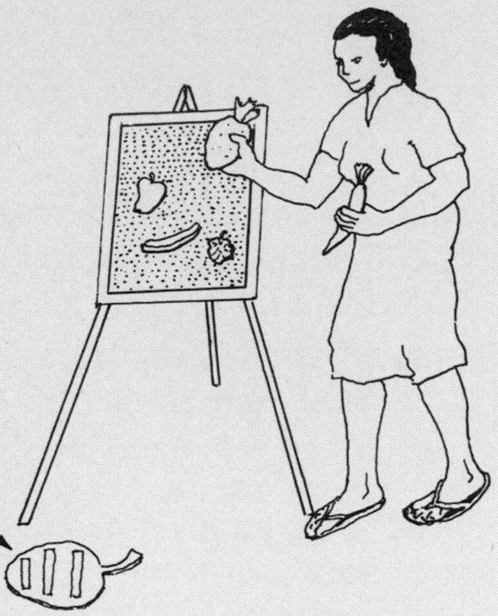

Flannel-graphs are good for talking with groups because you can keep making new pictures. Cover a square board or piece of cardboard with a flannel cloth. You can place different cutout drawings or photos on it. Strips of sandpaper or flannel glued to the backs of cutouts help them stick to the flannelboard.

Posters and displays. "A picture is worth a thousand words." Simple drawings, with or without a few words of information, can be hung in the health post or anywhere that people will look at them. You can copy some of the pictures from this book.

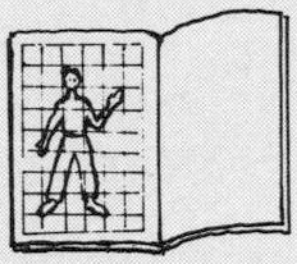

If you have trouble getting sizes and shapes right, draw light, even squares in pencil over the picture you want to copy.

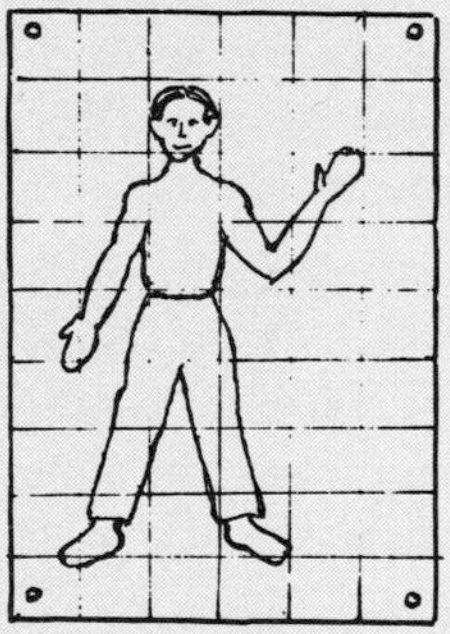

Now draw the same number of squares lightly, but larger, on the poster paper or cardboard. Then copy the drawing, square for square.

If possible, ask village artists to draw or paint posters. Or have children make posters on different subjects.

Models and demonstrations help get ideas across. For example, if you want to talk with mothers and midwives about care in cutting the cord of a newborn child, you can make a doll for the baby. Pin a cloth cord to its belly. Experienced midwives can demonstrate to others.

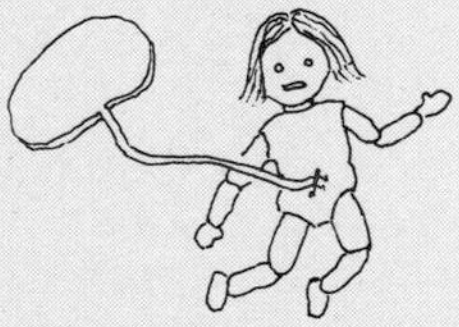

Color slides and filmstrips are available on different health subjects for many parts of the world. Some come in sets that tell a story. Simple viewers and battery-operated projectors are also available.

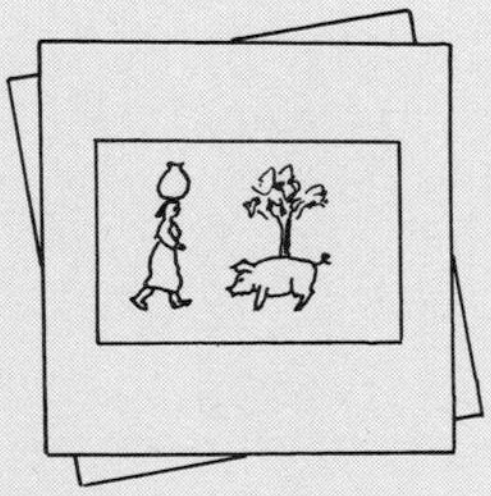

A list of addresses where you can send for teaching materials to use for health education in your village can be found on pages 429 to 432.

Other Ways to Get Ideas Across

Story telling. When you have a hard time explaining something, a story, especially a true one, will help make your point.

For example, if I tell you that sometimes a village worker can make a better diagnosis than a doctor, you may not believe me. But if I tell you about a village health worker called Irene, who runs a small nutrition center in Central America, you may understand.

> One day a small sickly child arrived at the nutrition center. He had been sent by the doctor at a nearby health center because he was badly malnourished. The child also had a cough, and the doctor had prescribed a cough medicine. Irene was worried about the child. She knew he came from a very poor family and that an older brother had died a few weeks before. She went to visit the family and learned that the older brother had been very sick for a long time and had coughed blood. Irene went to the health center and told the doctor she was afraid the child had tuberculosis. Tests were made, and it turned out that Irene was right. . . . So you see, the health worker spotted the real problem before the doctor—because she knew her people and visited their homes.

Stories also make learning more interesting. It helps if health workers are good story tellers.

Play acting. Stories that make important points can reach people with even more force if they are acted out. Perhaps you, the schoolteacher, or someone on the health committee can plan short plays or 'skits' with the schoolchildren.

For example, to make the point that food should be protected from flies to prevent the spread of disease, several small children could dress up as flies and buzz around food. The flies dirty the food that has not been covered. Then children eat this food and get sick. But the flies cannot get at food in a box with a wire screen front. So the children who eat this food stay well.

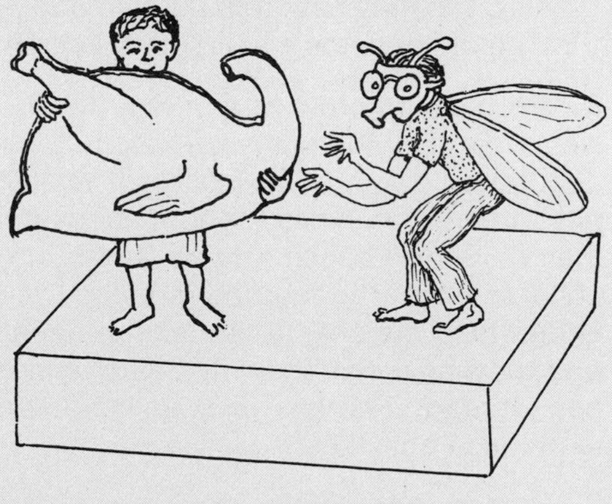

The more ways you can find to share ideas, the more people will understand and remember.

Working and Learning Together for the Common Good

There are many ways to interest and involve people in working together to meet their common needs. Here are a few ideas:

1. **A village health committee.** A group of able, interested persons can be chosen by the village to help plan and lead activities relating to the well-being of the community—for example, digging garbage pits or latrines. The health worker can and should share much of his responsibility with other persons.

2. **Group discussions.** Mothers, fathers, schoolchildren, young people, folk healers, or other groups can discuss needs and problems that affect health. Their chief purpose can be to help people share ideas and build on what they already know.

3. **Work festivals.** Community projects such as putting in a water system or cleaning up the village go quickly and can be fun if everybody helps. Games, races, refreshments, and simple prizes help turn work into play. Use imagination.

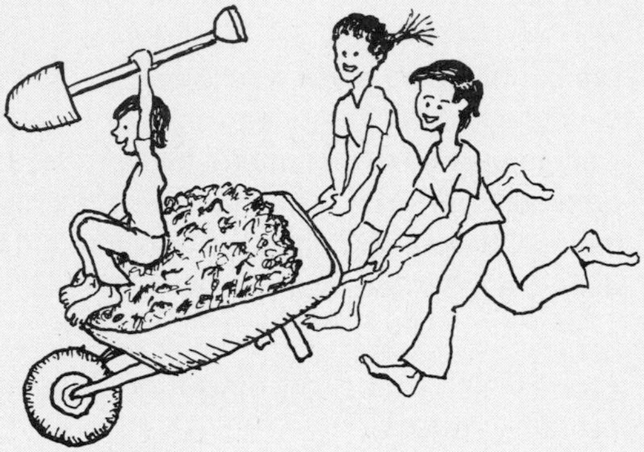

CHILDREN CAN DO AN AMAZING AMOUNT OF WORK WHEN IT IS TURNED INTO A GAME!

4. **Cooperatives.** People can help keep prices down by sharing tools, storage, and perhaps land. Group cooperation can have a big influence on people's well-being.

5. **Classroom visits.** Work with the village schoolteacher to encourage health-related activities, through demonstrations and play acting. Also invite small groups of students to come to the health center. Children not only learn quickly, but they can help out in many ways. If you give children a chance, they gladly become a valuable resource.

6. **Mother and child health meetings.** It is especially important that pregnant women and mothers of small children (under five years old) be well informed about their own and their babies' health needs. Regular visits to the health post are opportunities for both check-ups and learning. Have mothers keep their children's health records and bring them each month to have their children's growth recorded (see the Child Health Chart, p. 297). Mothers who understand the chart often take pride in making sure their children are eating and growing well. They can learn to understand these charts even if they cannot read. Perhaps you can help train interested mothers to organize and lead these activities.

7. **Home visits.** Make friendly visits to people's homes, especially homes of families who have special problems, who do not come often to the health post, or who do not take part in group activities. But respect people's privacy. If your visit cannot be friendly, do not make it—unless children or defenseless persons are in danger.

Ways to Share and Exchange Ideas in a Group

As a health worker you will find that the success you have in improving your people's health will depend far more on your skills as a teacher than on your medical or technical knowledge. For only when the whole community is involved and works together can big problems be overcome.

People do not learn much from what they are told. They learn from what they think, feel, discuss, see, and do together.

So the good teacher does not sit behind a desk and talk **at** people. He talks and works **with** them. He helps his people to think clearly about their needs and to find suitable ways to meet them. He looks for every opportunity to share ideas in an open and friendly way.

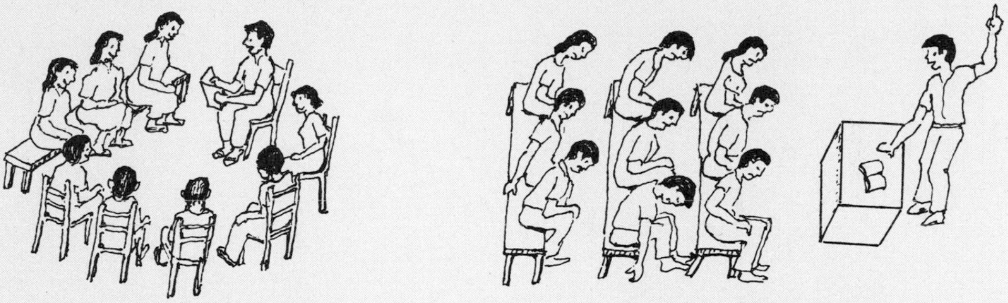

TALK WITH PEOPLE .... NOT AT THEM

Perhaps the most important thing you can do as a health worker is to awaken your people to their own possibilities . . . to help them gain confidence in themselves. Sometimes villagers do not change things they do not like because they do not try. Too often they may think of themselves as ignorant and powerless. But they are not. Most villagers, including those who cannot read or write, have remarkable knowledge and skills. They already make great changes in their surroundings with the tools they use, the land they farm, and the things they build. They can do many important things that people with a lot of schooling cannot.

If you can help people realize how much they already know and have done to change their surroundings, they may also realize that they can learn and do even more. By working together it is within their power to bring about even bigger changes for their health and well-being.

Then how do you tell people these things?

Often you cannot! But you can help them find out some of these things for themselves—by bringing them together for discussions. Say little yourself, but start the discussion by asking certain questions. Simple pictures like the drawing on the next page of a farm family in Central America may help. You will want to draw your own picture, with buildings, people, animals, and crops that look as much as possible like those in your area.

USE PICTURES TO GET PEOPLE TALKING AND THINKING TOGETHER

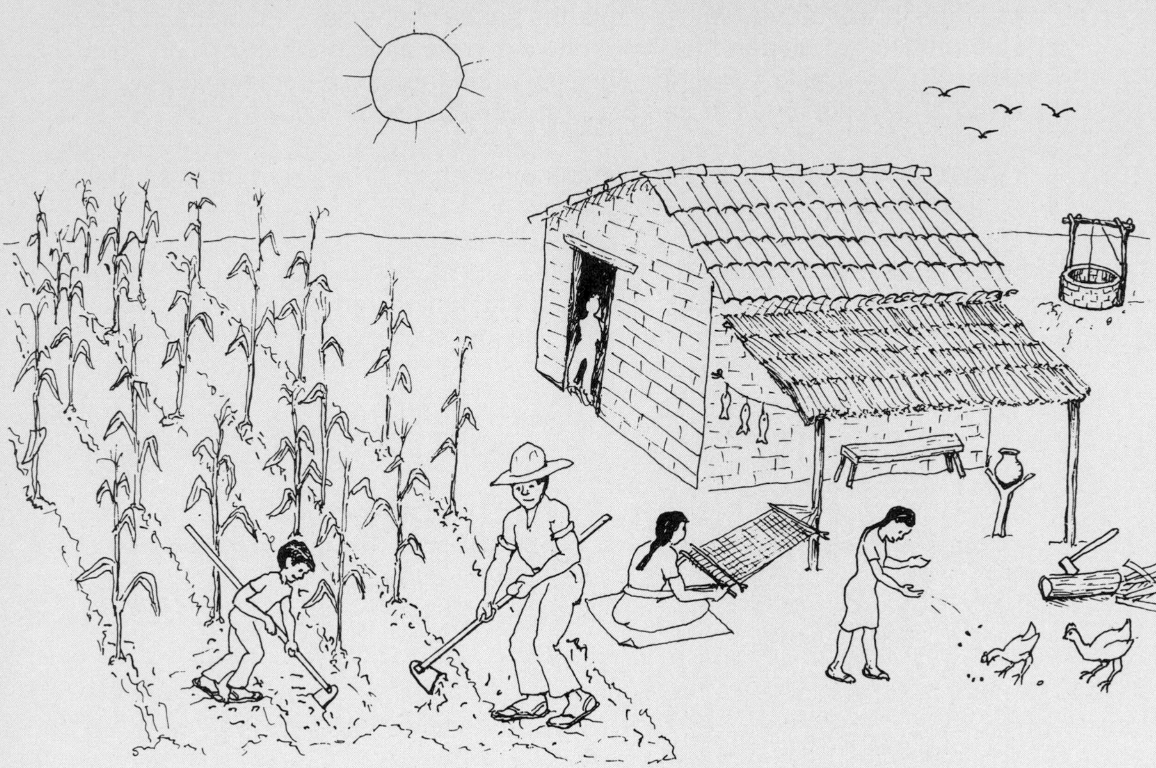

Show a group of people a picture similar to this and ask them to discuss it. Ask questions that get people talking about what they know and can do. Here are some sample questions:

- Who are the people in the picture and how do they live?
- What was this land like before the people came?
- In what ways have they changed their surroundings?
- How do these changes affect their health and well-being?
- What other changes could these people make? What else could they learn to do? What is stopping them? How could they learn more?
- How did they learn to farm? Who taught them?
- If a doctor or a lawyer moved onto this land with no more money or tools than these people, could he farm it as well? Why or why not?
- In what ways are these people like ourselves?

This kind of group discussion helps build people's confidence in themselves and in their ability to change things. It can also make them feel more involved in their community.

At first you may find that people are slow to speak out and say what they think. But after a while they will usually begin to talk more freely and ask important questions themselves. Encourage everyone to say what he or she feels and to speak up without fear. Ask those who talk most to give a chance to those who are slower to speak up.

You can think of many other drawings and questions to start discussions that can help people look more clearly at problems, their causes, and possible solutions.

What questions can you ask to get people thinking about the different things that lead to the condition of the child in the following picture?

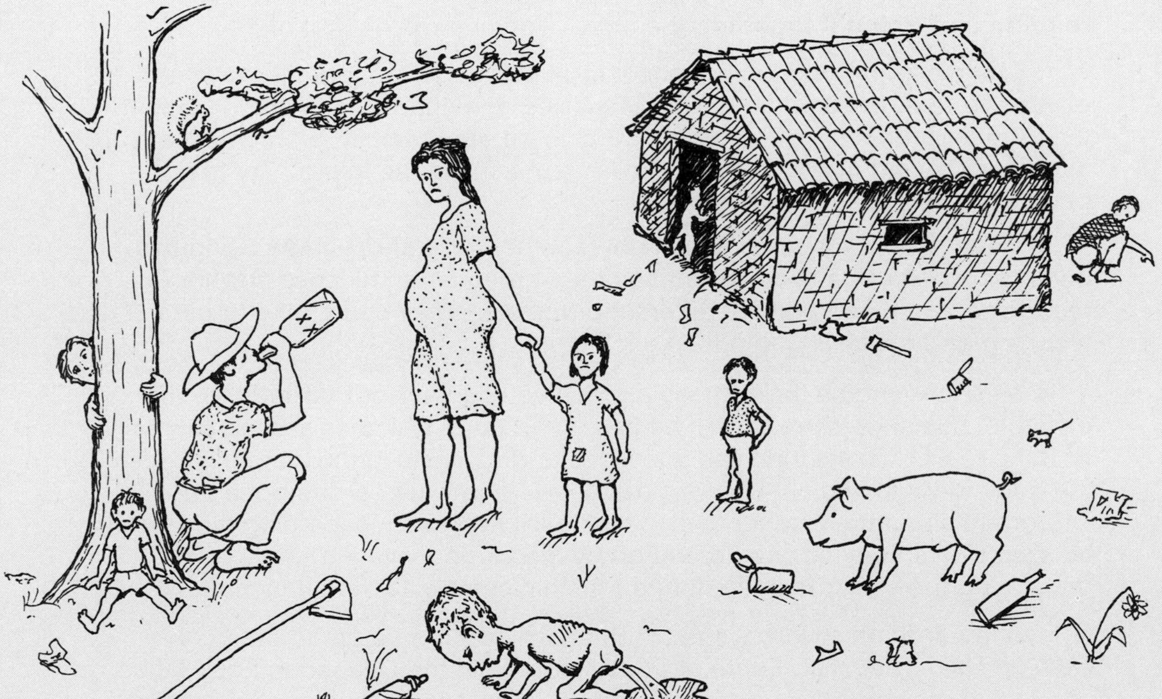

Try to think of questions that lead to others and get people asking for themselves. How many of the causes underlying death from diarrhea (see p. w7) will your people think of when they discuss a picture like this?

MAKING THE BEST USE OF THIS BOOK

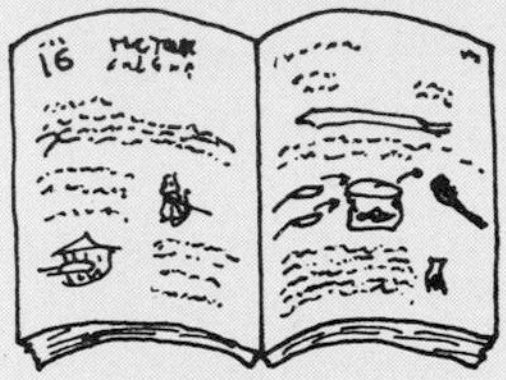

Anyone who knows how to read can use this book in her own home. Even those who do not read can learn from the pictures. But to make the fullest and best use of the book, people often need some instruction. This can be done in several ways.

A health worker or anyone who gives out the book should make sure that people understand how to use the list of Contents, the Index, the Green Pages and the Vocabulary. Take special care to give examples of **how to look things up.** Urge each person to carefully read the sections of the book that will help her understand **what may be helpful to do, what could be harmful or dangerous,** and **when it is important to get help** (see especially Chapters 1, 2, 6, and 8, and also the SIGNS OF DANGEROUS ILLNESS, p. 42). Point out how important it is to **prevent sickness** before it starts. Encourage people to pay special attention to Chapters 11 and 12, which deal with **eating right** (nutrition) and **keeping clean** (hygiene and sanitation).

Also **show and mark the pages that tell about the most common problems in your area.** For example, you can mark the pages on **diarrhea** and be sure mothers with small children understand about **'special drink'** (oral rehydration, p. 152). Many problems and needs can be explained briefly. But the more time you spend with people **discussing** how to use the book or **reading and using it together,** the more everyone will get out of it.

You as a health worker might encourage people to get together in **small groups** to read through the book, discussing one chapter at a time. Look at the biggest problems in your area—what to do about health problems that already exist and how to prevent similar problems in the future. Try to get people looking ahead.

Perhaps interested persons can get together for a **short class** using this book (or others) as a text. Members of the group could discuss how to recognize, treat, and prevent different problems. They could take turns teaching and explaining things to each other.

To help learning be fun in these classes you can **act out situations.** For example, someone can act as if he has a particular sickness and can explain what he feels. Others then ask questions and examine him (Chapter 3). Use the book to try to find out what his problem is and what can be done about it. The group should remember to involve the 'sick' person in learning more about his own sickness—and should end up by discussing with him ways of preventing the sickness in the future. All this can be acted out in class.

Exciting and effective ways to teach about health care are in the book *Helping Health Workers Learn,* also available from the Hesperian Foundation.

As a health worker, one of the best ways you can help people use this book correctly is this: When persons come to you for treatment, have them look up their own or their child's problem in the book and find out how to treat it. This takes more time, but helps much more than doing it for them. Only when someone makes a mistake or misses something important do you need to step in and help him learn how to do it better. In this way, **even sickness gives a chance to help people learn.**

Dear village health worker—whoever and wherever you are, whether you have a title or official position, or are simply someone, like myself, with an interest in the well-being of others—make good use of this book. It is for you and for everyone.

But remember, the most important part of health care you will not find in this book or any other. The key to good health lies within you and your people, in the care, the concern, and appreciation you have for each other. If you want to see your community be healthy, build on these.

Caring and sharing are the key to health.

Yours truly,

David

David Werner

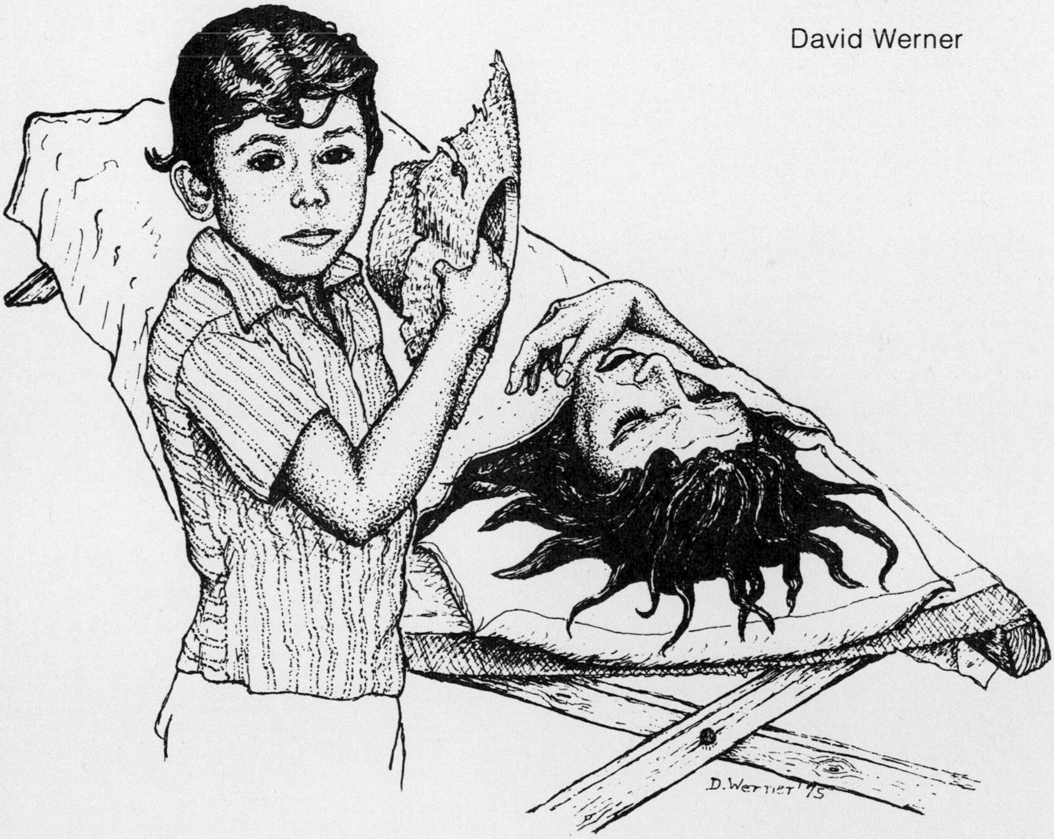

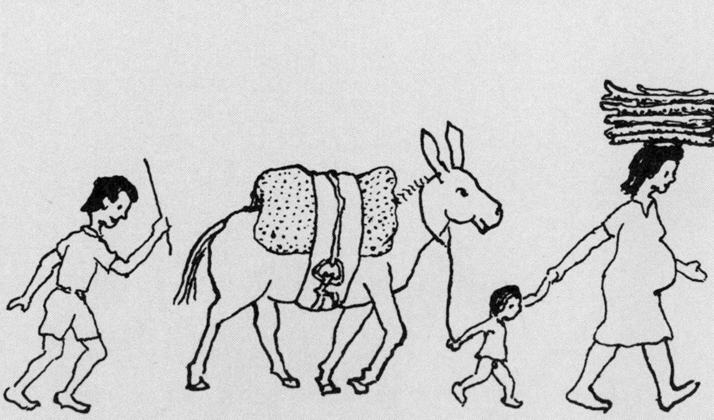

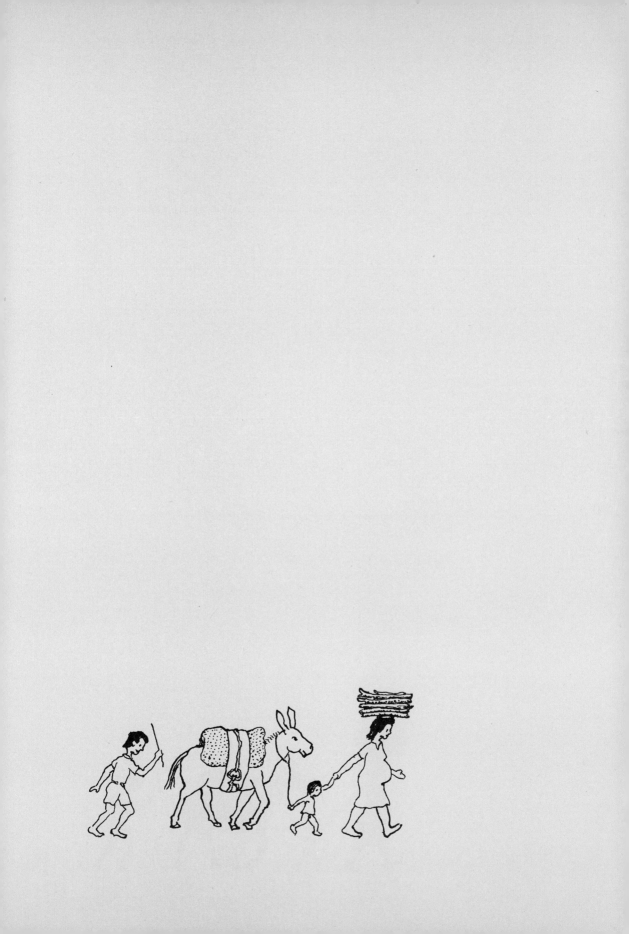

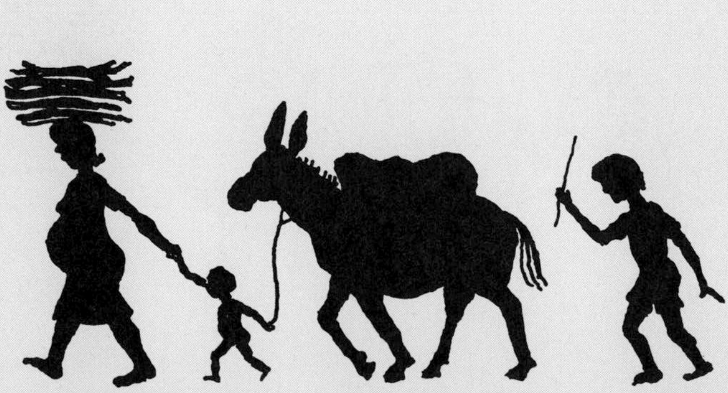

NOTICE

This book is to help people meet most of their common health needs for and by themselves. But it does not have all the answers. In case of serious illness or if you are uncertain about how to handle a health problem, get advice from a health worker or doctor whenever possible.

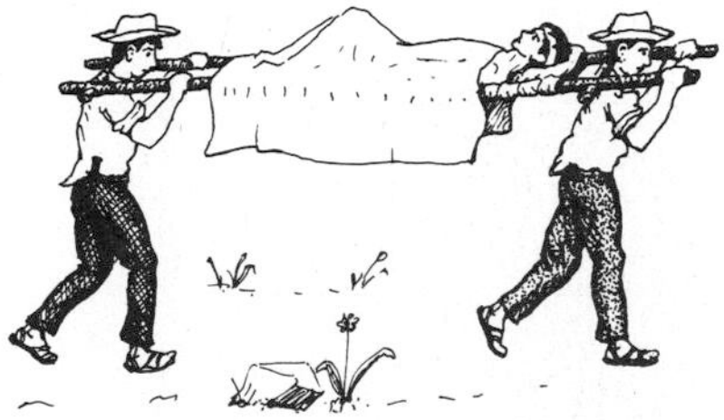

CHAPTER

HOME CURES AND POPULAR BELIEFS

1

Everywhere on earth people use home remedies. In some places, the older or *traditional* ways of healing have been passed down from parents to children for hundreds of years.

Many home remedies have great value. Others have less. And some may be risky or harmful. Home remedies, like modern medicines, must be used with caution.

Try to ***do no harm.***
Only use home remedies if you are sure they are safe and know exactly how to use them.

HOME CURES THAT HELP

For many sicknesses, time-tested home remedies work as well as modern medicines —or even **better.** They are often **cheaper.** And in some cases they are **safer.**

For example, many of the herbal teas people use for home treatment of coughs and colds do more good and cause fewer problems than cough syrups and strong medicines some doctors prescribe.

Also, the 'rice water', teas, or sweetened drinks that many mothers give to babies with diarrhea are often safer and do more good than any modern medicine. What matters most is that a baby with diarrhea get plenty of liquids (see p. 151).

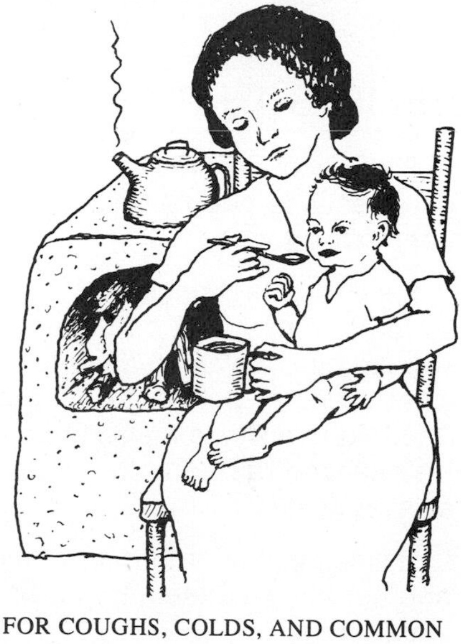

FOR COUGHS, COLDS, AND COMMON DIARRHEA, HERBAL TEAS ARE OFTEN *BETTER, CHEAPER,* AND *SAFER* THAN MODERN MEDICINES.

The Limitations of Home Remedies

Some diseases are helped by home remedies. Others can be treated better with modern medicine. This is true for most serious infections. Sicknesses like pneumonia, tetanus, typhoid, tuberculosis, appendicitis, diseases caused by sexual contact, and fever after childbirth should be treated with modern medicines as soon as possible. For these diseases, do not lose time trying to treat them first with home remedies only.

It is sometimes hard to be sure which home remedies work well and which do not. More careful studies are needed. For this reason:

It is often safer to treat very serious illnesses with modern medicines—following the advice of a health worker if possible.

Old Ways and New

Some modern ways of meeting health needs work better than old ones. But at times the older, traditional ways are best. For example, traditional ways of caring for children or old people are often kinder and work better than some newer, less personal ways.

Not many years ago everyone thought that mother's milk was the best food for a young baby. They were right! Then the big companies that make canned and artificial milk began to tell mothers that bottle feeding was better. This is not true, but many mothers believed them and started to bottle feed their babies. As a result, thousands of babies have suffered and died needlessly from infection or hunger. For the reasons **breast is best,** see p. 271.

Respect your people's traditions and build on them.

For more ideas for building on local traditions, see *Helping Health Workers Learn,* Chapter 7.

BELIEFS THAT CAN MAKE PEOPLE WELL

Some home remedies have a direct effect on the body. Others seem to work only because people believe in them. **The healing power of belief can be very strong.**

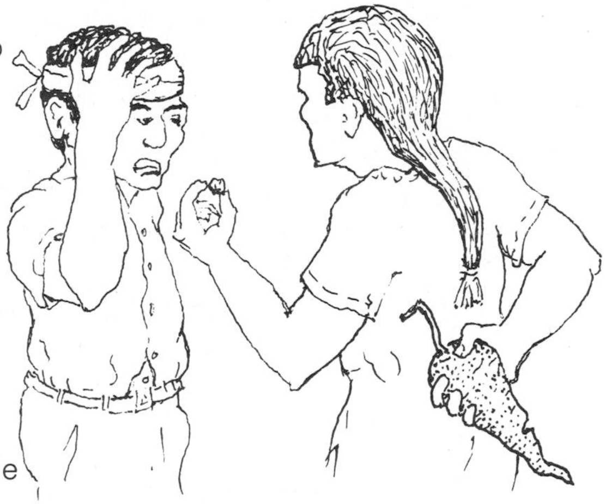

For example, I once saw a man who suffered from a very bad headache. To cure him, a woman gave him a small piece of yam, or sweet potato. She told him it was a strong painkiller. He believed her—and the pain went away quickly.

It was his faith in her treatment, and not the yam itself, that made him feel better.

Many home remedies work in this way. They help largely because people have faith in them. For this reason, they are **especially useful to cure illnesses that are partly in people's minds, or those caused in part by a person's beliefs, worry, or fears.**

Included in this group of sicknesses are: bewitchment or hexing, unreasonable or hysterical fear, uncertain 'aches and pains' (especially in persons going through stressful times, such as teenage girls or older women), and anxiety or nervous worry. Also included are some cases of asthma, hiccups, indigestion, stomach ulcers, migraine headaches, and even warts.

For all of these problems, **the manner or 'touch' of the healer can be very important.** What it often comes down to is showing you care, helping the sick person believe he will get well, or simply helping him relax.

Sometimes a person's belief in a remedy can help with problems that have completely physical causes.

For example, Mexican villagers have the following home cures for poisonous snakebite:

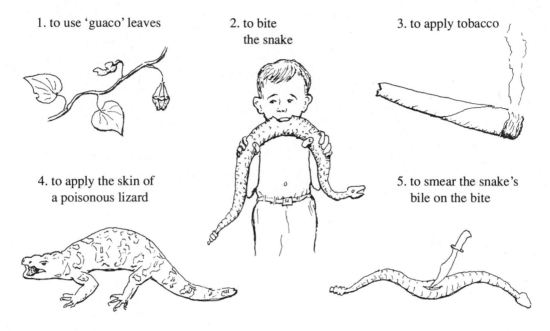

1. to use 'guaco' leaves

2. to bite the snake

3. to apply tobacco

4. to apply the skin of a poisonous lizard

5. to smear the snake's bile on the bite

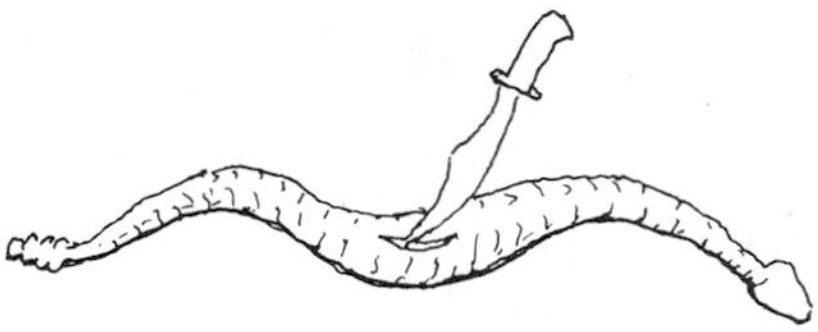

In other lands people have their own snakebite remedies—often many different ones. As far as we know, **none of these home remedies has any direct effect against snake poison.** The person who says that a home remedy kept a snake's poison from harming him at all was probably bitten by a non-poisonous snake!

Yet any of these home remedies may do some good if a person believes in it. If it makes him less afraid, his pulse will slow down, he will move and tremble less, and as a result, the poison will spread through his body more slowly. So there is less danger!

But the benefit of these home remedies for snakebite is limited. In spite of their common use, may people still become very ill or die. As far as we know:

No home cure for poisonous bites
(whether from snakes, scorpions, spiders, or other poisonous animals)
has much effect beyond that of the healing power of belief.

For snakebite it is usually better to use modern treatment. Be prepared: obtain *'antivenoms'* or 'serums' for poisonous bites **before** you need them (see p. 105). Do not wait until it is too late.

BELIEFS THAT CAN MAKE PEOPLE SICK

The power of belief can help heal people. But it can also harm them. If a person believes strongly enough that something will hurt him, his own fear can make him sick. For example:

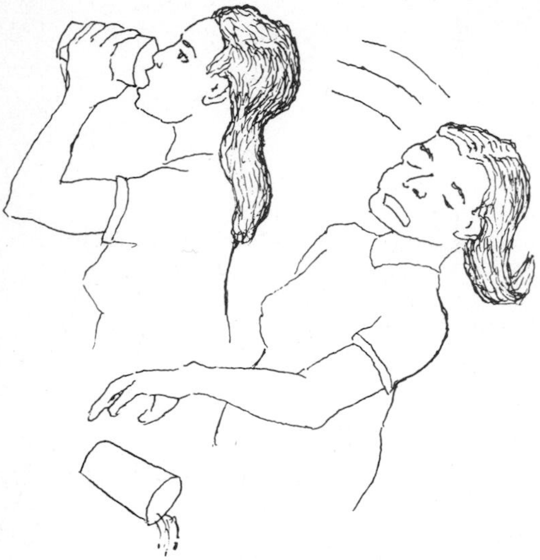

Once I was called to see a woman who had just had a *miscarriage* and was still bleeding a little. There was an orange tree near her house. So I suggested she drink a glass of orange juice. (Oranges have vitamin C which helps strengthen blood vessels.) She drank it—even though she was afraid it would harm her.

Her fear was so great that soon she became very ill. I examined her, but could find nothing physically wrong. I tried to comfort her, telling her she was not in danger. But she said she was going to die. At last I gave her an injection of distilled (completely pure) water. Distilled water has no medical effect. But since she had great faith in injections, she quickly got better.

Actually, the juice did not harm her. What harmed her was her **belief that it would make her sick.** And what made her well was her faith in injections!

In this same way, many persons go on believing false ideas about witchcraft, injections, diet, and many other things. Much needless suffering is the result.

Perhaps, in a way, I had helped this woman. But the more I thought about it, the more I realized I had also wronged her; I had led her to believe things that were not true.

I wanted to set this right. So a few days later, when she was completely well, I went to her home and apologized for what I had done. I tried to help her understand that not the orange juice, but her **fear** had made her so sick. And that not the injection of water, but her **freedom from fear** had helped her get well.

By understanding the truth about the orange, the injection, and the tricks of her own mind, perhaps this woman and her family will become freer from fear and better able to care for their health in the future. For **health** is closely related to **understanding** and **freedom from fear.**

Many things do harm only because people believe they are harmful.

WITCHCRAFT—BLACK MAGIC—AND THE EVIL EYE

If a person believes strongly enough that someone has the power to harm him, he may actually become ill. Anyone who believes he is bewitched or has been given the ***evil eye*** is really the victim of his own fears (see Susto, p. 24).

A 'witch' has no power over other people, except for her ability to make them believe that she has. For this reason:

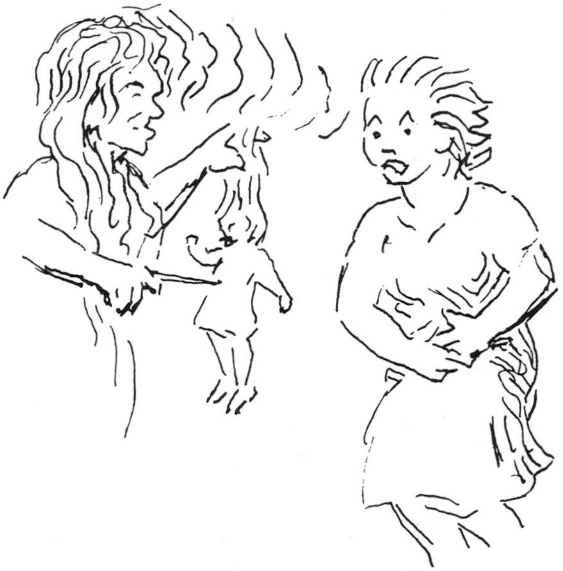

It is impossible to bewitch a person who does not believe in witchcraft.

Some people think that they are 'bewitched' when they have strange or frightening illnesses (such as ***tumors*** of the ***genitals*** or ***cirrhosis*** of the liver, see p. 328). Such sicknesses have nothing to do with witchcraft or black magic. Their causes are natural.

Do not waste your money at 'magic centers' that claim to cure witchcraft. And do not seek revenge against a witch, because it will not solve anything. If you are seriously ill, go for medical help.

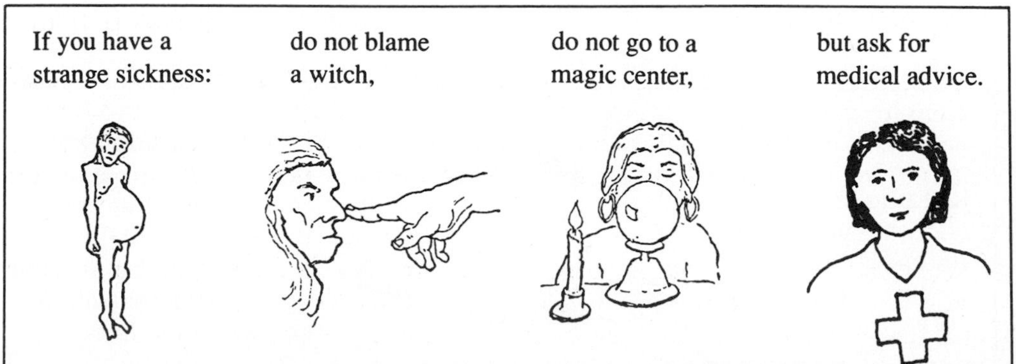

If you have a strange sickness:
do not blame a witch,
do not go to a magic center,
but ask for medical advice.

QUESTIONS AND ANSWERS ON SOME FOLK BELIEFS AND HOME REMEDIES

These examples are from the mountains of Mexico, the area that I know best. Perhaps some of the beliefs of your people are similar. Think about ways to learn which beliefs in your area lead to better health and which do not.

When people think someone is bewitched, is it true that he will get well if his relatives harm or kill the witch?

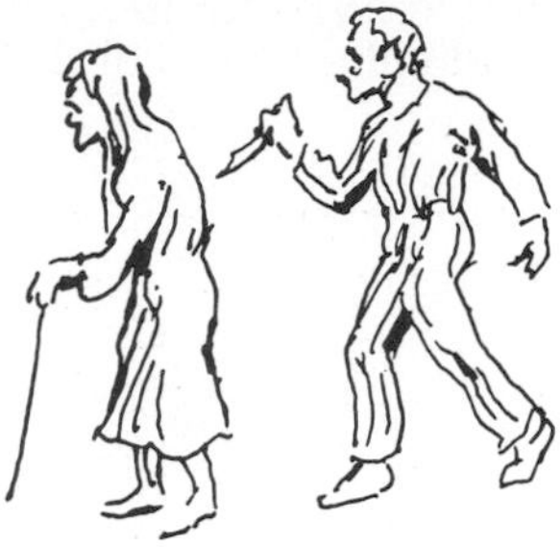

FALSE! No one is ever helped by harming someone else.

Is it true that when the 'soft spot' on top of a baby's head sinks inward this means the baby will die of diarrhea unless he gets special treatment?

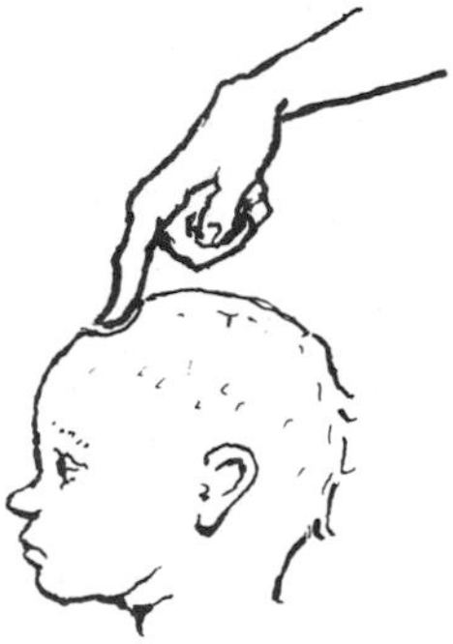

This is often true. The 'soft spot' sinks because the baby has lost too much liquid (see p. 151). Unless he gets more liquid soon, he may die (see p. 152).

Is it true that if the light of the eclipsing moon falls on a pregnant mother, her child will be born deformed or retarded?

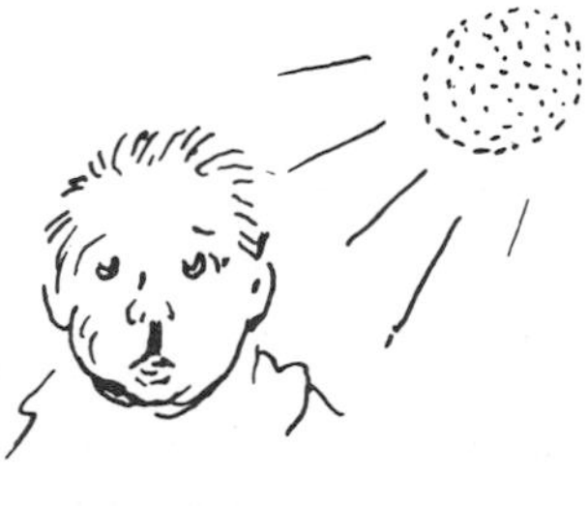

This is not true! But children may be born retarded, deaf, or deformed if the mother does not use iodized salt, if she takes certain medicines, or for other reasons (see p. 318).

Is it true that mothers should give birth in a darkened room?

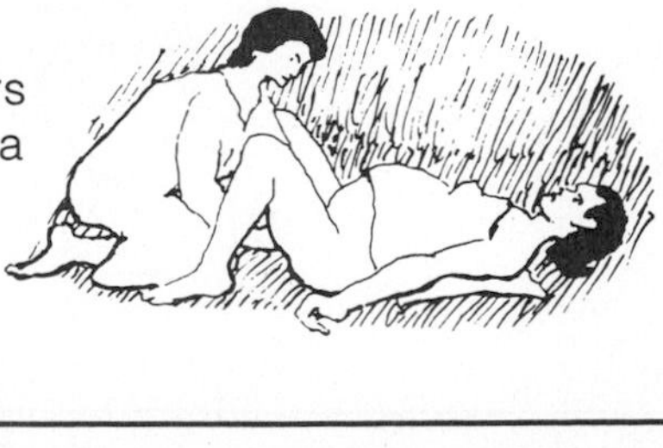

It is true that soft light is easier on the eyes of both the mother and the newborn child. But there should be enough light for the midwife to see what she is doing.

Is it true that a newborn baby should not be bathed until the cord falls off?

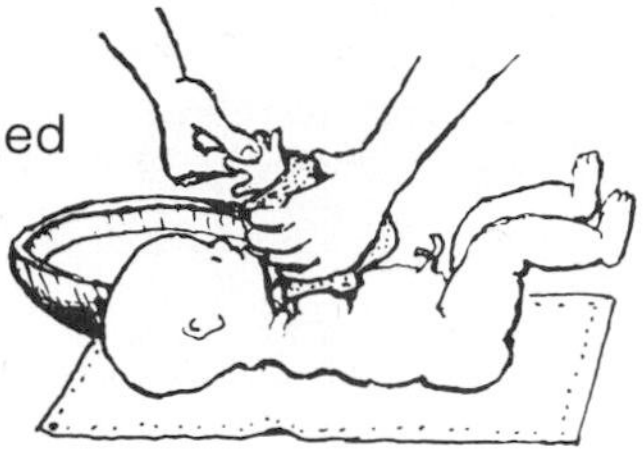

True! The stump of the cord should be kept dry until it falls off. But the baby can be gently cleaned with a clean, soft, damp cloth.

How many days after giving birth should a mother wait before she bathes?

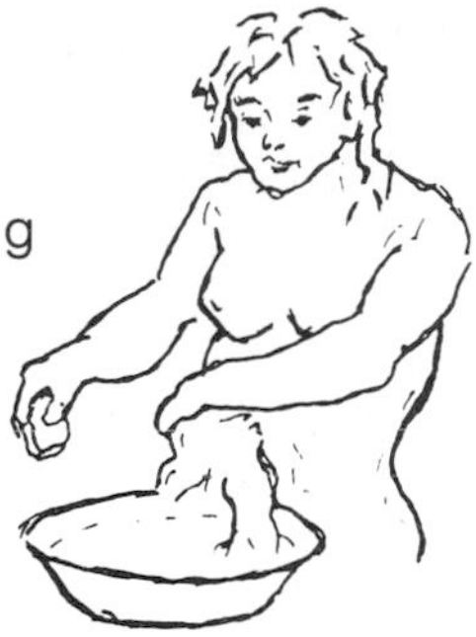

A mother should wash with warm water the **day after giving birth.** The custom of not bathing for weeks following childbirth can lead to infections.

Is it true that traditional breast feeding is better than 'modern' bottle feeding?

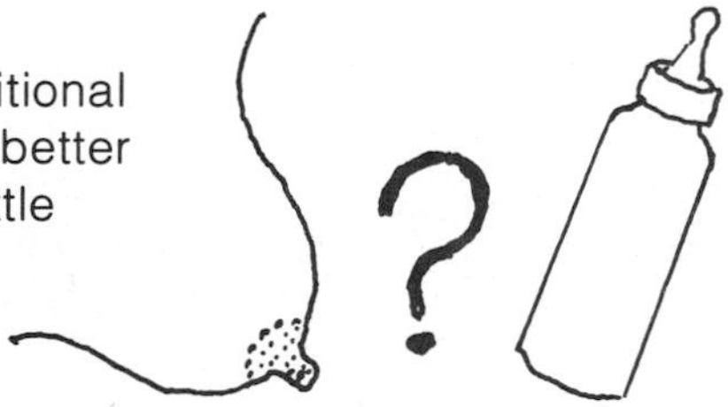

TRUE! Breast milk is better food and also helps protect the baby against infection.

What foods should women avoid in the first few weeks after childbirth?

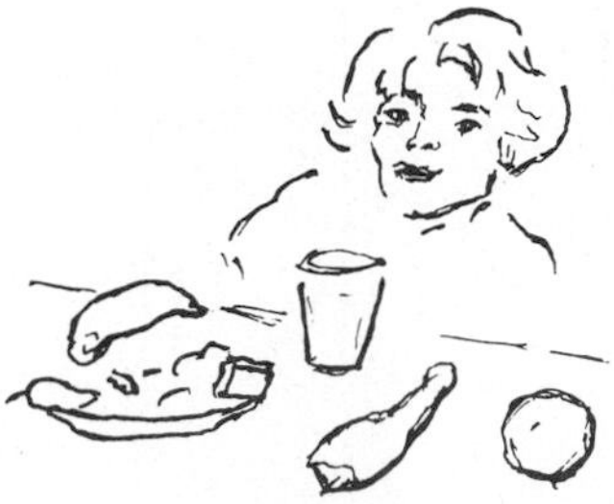

In the weeks following childbirth, women should not avoid any nutritious foods. Instead, they should eat plenty of fruit, vegetables, meat, milk, eggs, whole grains, and beans (see p. 276).

Is it a good idea to bathe a sick person, or will it do him harm?

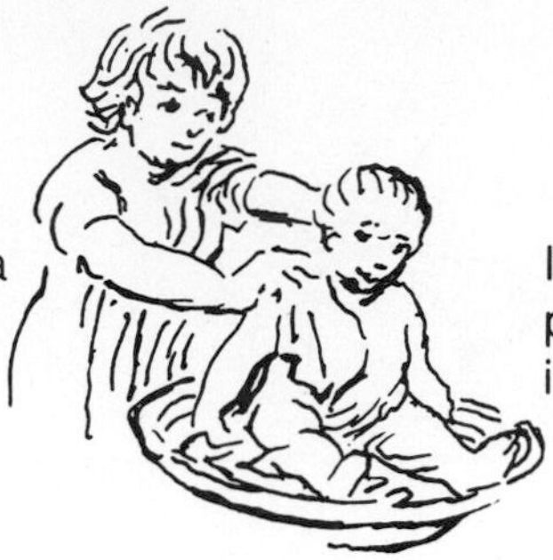

It is a good idea. Sick people should be bathed in warm water every day.

Is it true that oranges, guavas, and other fruits are harmful when one has a cold or a fever?

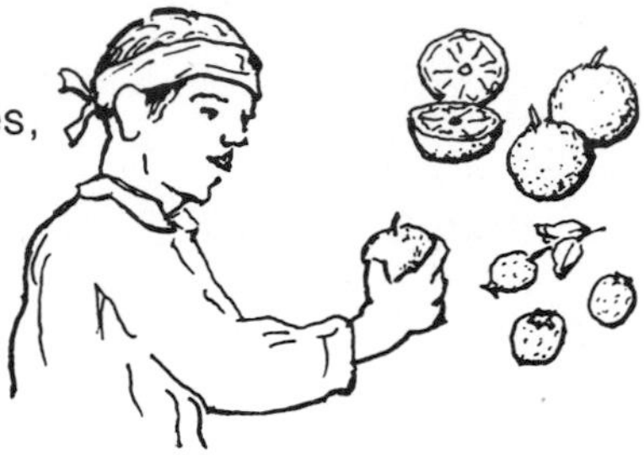

NO! All fruits and juices are helpful when one has a cold or fever. They do not cause congestion or harm of any kind.

Is it true that when a person has a high fever, he should be wrapped up so that the air will not harm him?

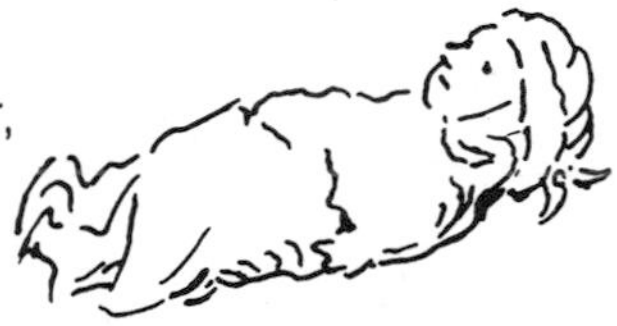

NO! When a person has a high fever, take off all covers and clothing. Let the air reach his body. This will help the fever go down (see p. 76).

Is it true that tea made from willow bark will help bring fever down and stop pain?

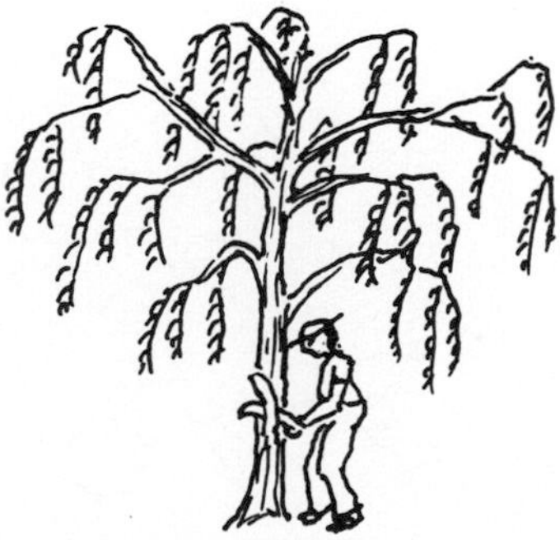

True. It helps. Willow bark has a natural medicine in it very much like aspirin.

SUNKEN FONTANEL OR SOFT SPOT

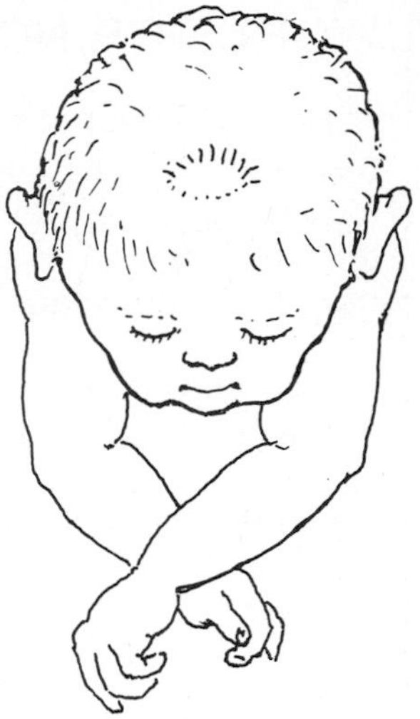

The *fontanel* is the soft spot on the top of a newborn baby's head. It is where the bones of his skull have not formed completely. Normally it takes a year to a year and a half for the soft spot to close completely.

Mothers in different lands realize that when the soft spot sinks inward their babies are in danger. They have many beliefs to explain this. In Latin America mothers think the baby's brains have slipped downward. They try to correct this by sucking on the soft spot, by pushing up on the roof of the mouth, or by holding the baby upside down and slapping his feet. This does not help because . . . **A sunken soft spot is really caused by dehydration** (see p. 151).

This means **the child is losing more liquid than he is drinking.** He is too dry—usually because he has diarrhea, or diarrhea with vomiting.

Treatment:

1. Give the child plenty of liquid: Rehydration Drink (see p. 152), breast milk, or boiled water.
2. If necessary, treat the causes of the diarrhea and vomiting (see p. 152 to 161). For most diarrheas, medicine is not needed, and may do more harm than good.

TO CURE A SUNKEN SOFT SPOT . . .

DO NOT DO THIS

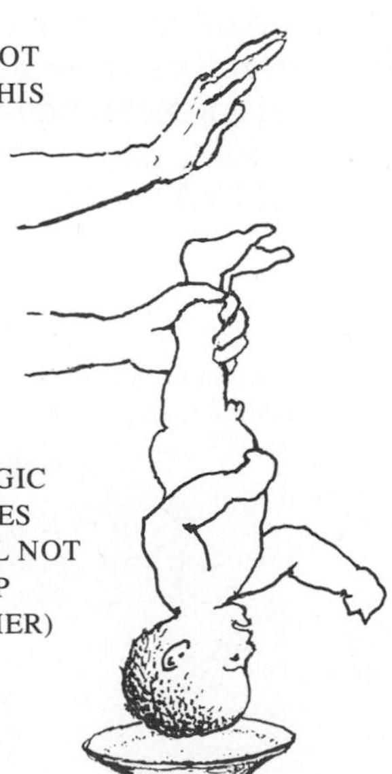

(MAGIC CURES WILL NOT HELP EITHER)

DO THIS

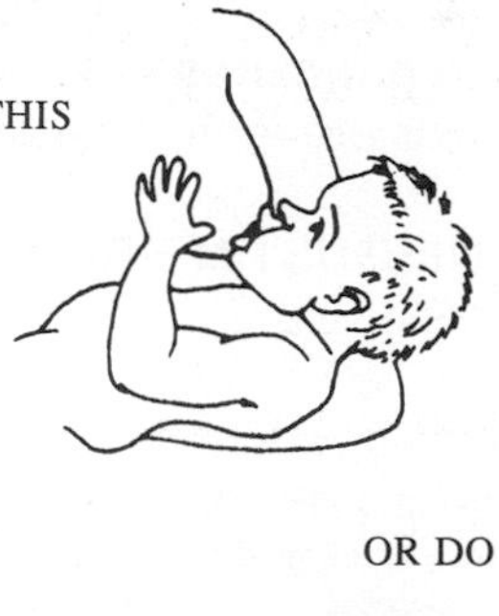

OR DO THIS

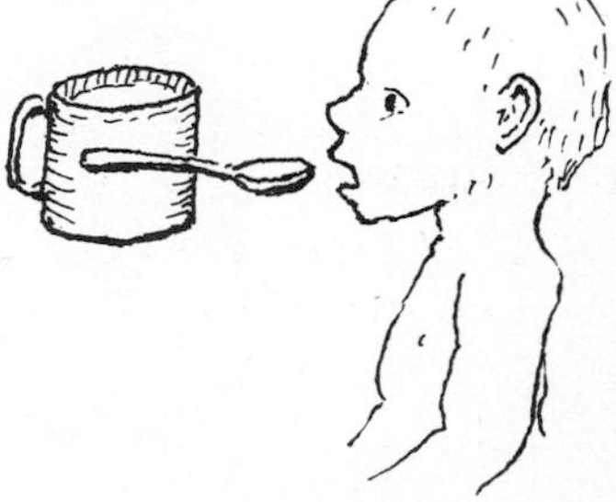

Note: If the soft spot is swollen or bulges **upward,** this may be a sign of meningitis. Begin treatment at once (see p. 185), and get medical help.

WAYS TO TELL WHETHER A HOME REMEDY WORKS OR NOT

Because a lot of people use a home cure does not necessarily mean it works well or is safe. It is often hard to know which remedies are helpful and which may be harmful. Careful study is needed to be sure. Here are four rules to help tell which remedies are least likely to work, or are dangerous. (Examples are from Mexican villages.)

1. THE MORE REMEDIES THERE ARE FOR ANY ONE ILLNESS, THE LESS LIKELY IT IS THAT ANY OF THEM WORKS.

For example: In rural Mexico there are **many** home remedies for goiter, **none** of which does any real good. Here are some of them:

1. to tie a crab on the goiter

DON'T

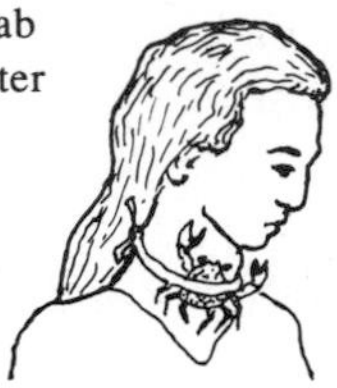

2. to rub the goiter with the hand of a dead child

DON'T

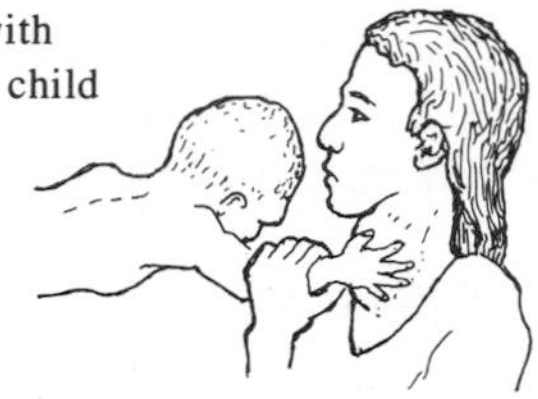

3. to smear the brains of a vulture on the goiter

DON'T

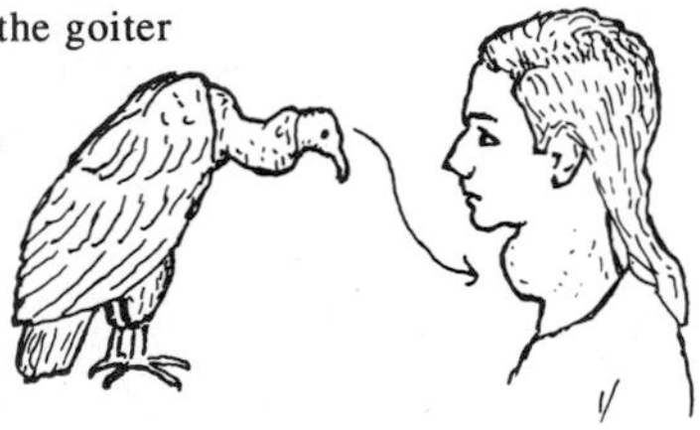

4. to smear human feces on the goiter

DON'T

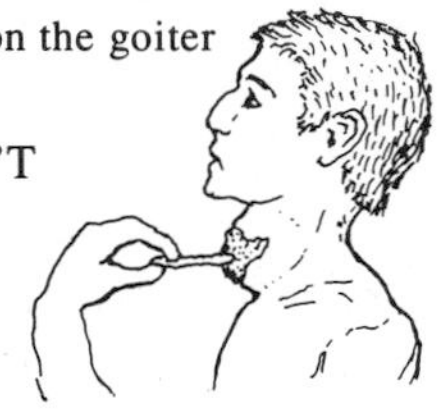

Not one of these many remedies works. If it did, the others would not be needed. **When a sickness has just one popular cure, it is more likely to be a good one.** For prevention and treatment of goiter use iodized salt (p. 130).

2. FOUL OR DISGUSTING REMEDIES ARE NOT LIKELY TO HELP—AND ARE OFTEN HARMFUL.

For example:

1. the idea that leprosy can be cured by a drink made of rotting snakes

DON'T

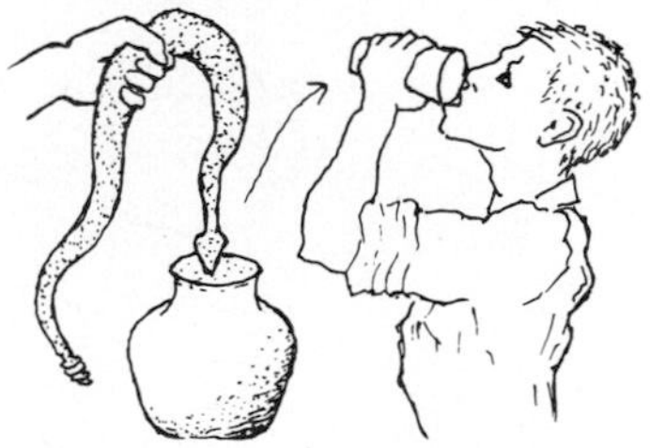

2. the idea that syphilis can be cured by eating a vulture

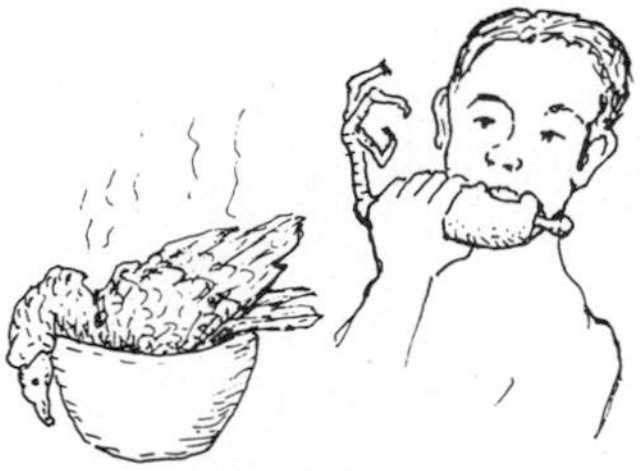

DON'T

These two remedies do not help at all. The first one can cause dangerous infections. Belief in remedies like these sometimes causes delay in getting proper medical care.

3. REMEDIES THAT USE ANIMAL OR HUMAN WASTE DO NO GOOD AND CAN CAUSE DANGEROUS INFECTIONS. NEVER USE THEM.

Examples:

1. Putting human feces around the eye does not cure blurred vision and can cause infections.

2. Smearing cow dung on the head to fight ringworm can cause tetanus and other dangerous infections.

DON'T

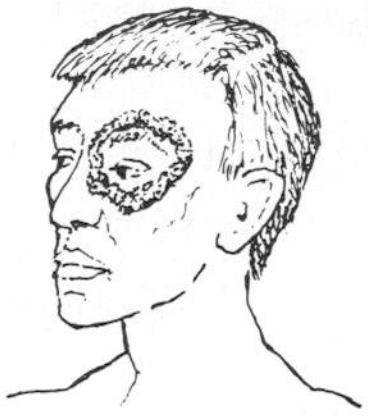

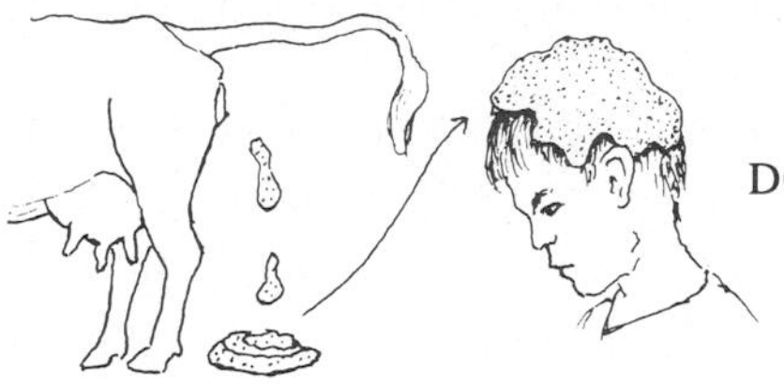

DON'T!

Also, the droppings of rabbits or other animals do not help heal burns. To use them is very dangerous. Cow dung, held in the hand, cannot help control fits. Teas made from human, pig, or any other animal feces do not cure anything. They can make people sicker. **Never** put feces on the navel of a newborn baby. This can cause tetanus.

4. THE MORE A REMEDY RESEMBLES THE SICKNESS IT IS SAID TO CURE, THE MORE LIKELY ITS BENEFITS COME ONLY FROM THE POWER OF BELIEF.

The association between each of the following illnesses and its remedy is clear in these examples from Mexico:

1. for a nosebleed, using *yesca* (a bright red mushroom)

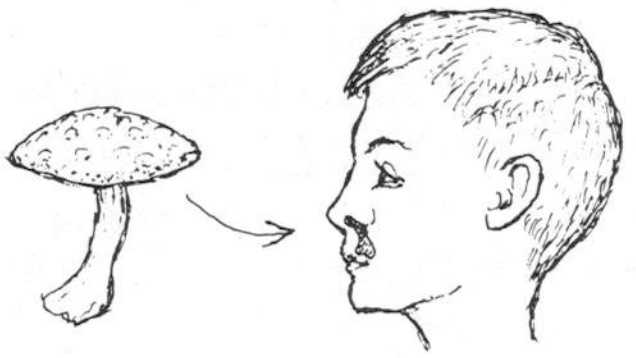

2. for deafness, putting powdered rattlesnake's rattle in the ear

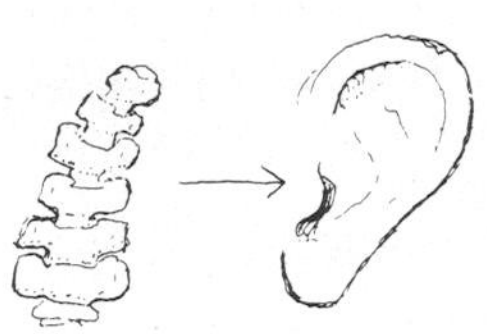

3. for dog bite, drink tea made from the dog's tail

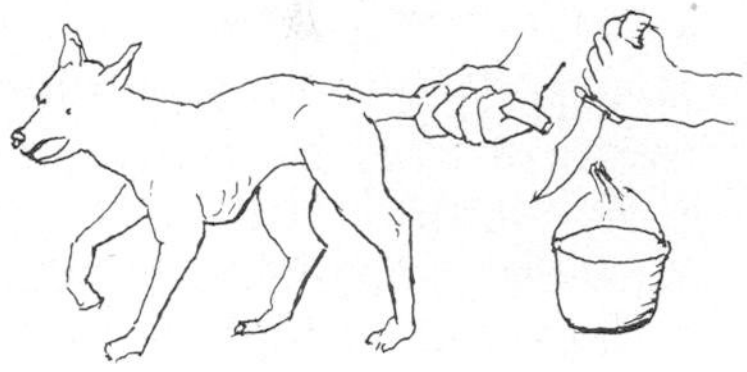

4. for scorpion sting, tying a scorpion against the stung finger

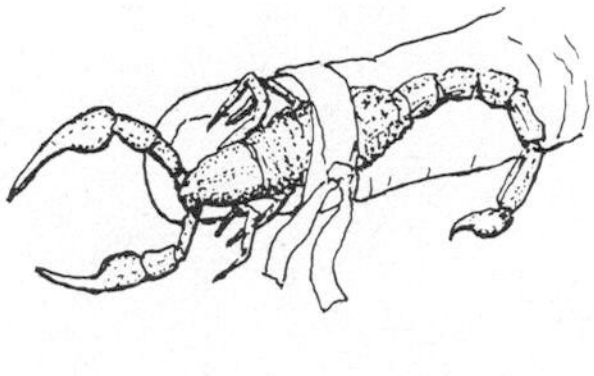

5. to prevent diarrhea when a child is teething, putting a necklace of snake's fangs around the baby's neck

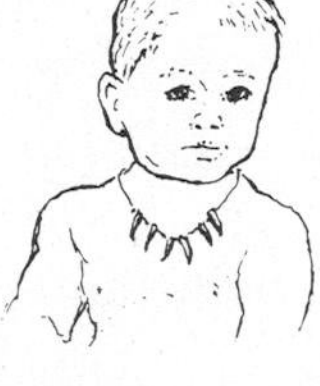

6. to 'bring out' the rash of measles, making tea from kapok bark

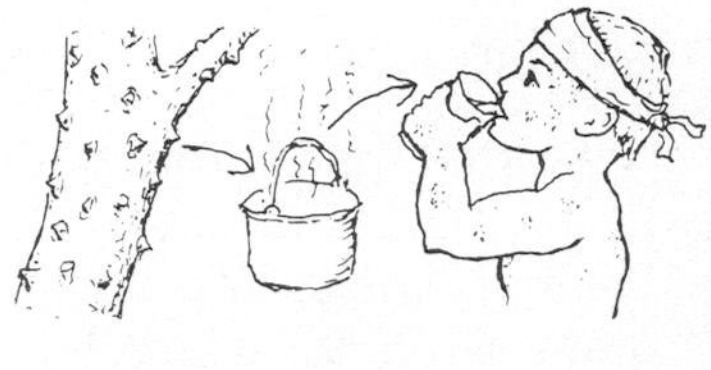

These remedies, and many other similar ones, have no curative value in themselves. They may be of some benefit if people believe in them. But for serious problems, be sure their use does not delay more effective treatment.

MEDICINAL PLANTS

Many plants have curative powers. Some of the best modern medicines are made from wild herbs.

Nevertheless, not all 'curative herbs' people use have medical value . . . and those that have are sometimes used the wrong way. Try to learn about the herbs in your area and find out which ones are worthwhile.

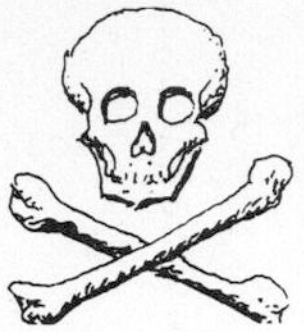

CAUTION! Some medicinal herbs are very poisonous if taken in more than the recommended dose. For this reason it is often safer to use modern medicine, since the dosage is easier to control.

Here are a few examples of plants that can be useful if used correctly:

ANGEL'S TRUMPET *(Datura arborea)*

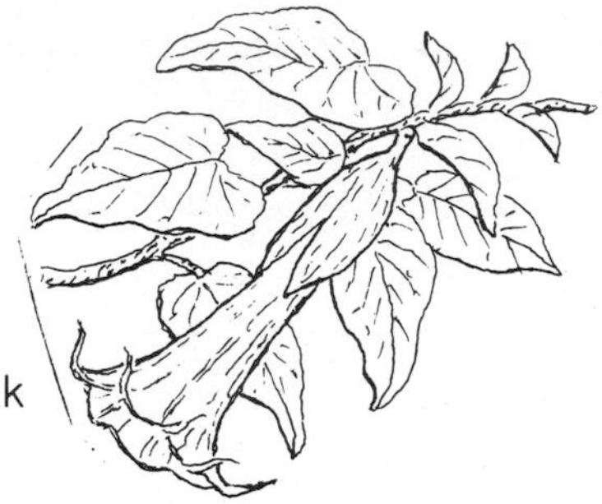

The leaves of this and certain other members of the nightshade family contain a drug that helps to calm intestinal cramps, stomach-aches, and even gallbladder pain.

Grind up 1 or 2 leaves of Angel's Trumpet and soak them for a day in 7 tablespoons (100 ml.) of water.

Dosage: Between 10 and 15 drops every 4 hours (adults only).

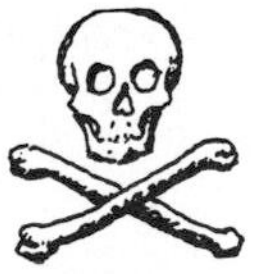

WARNING: Angel's Trumpet is very poisonous if you take more than the recommended dose.

CORN SILK (the tassels or 'silk' from an ear of maize)

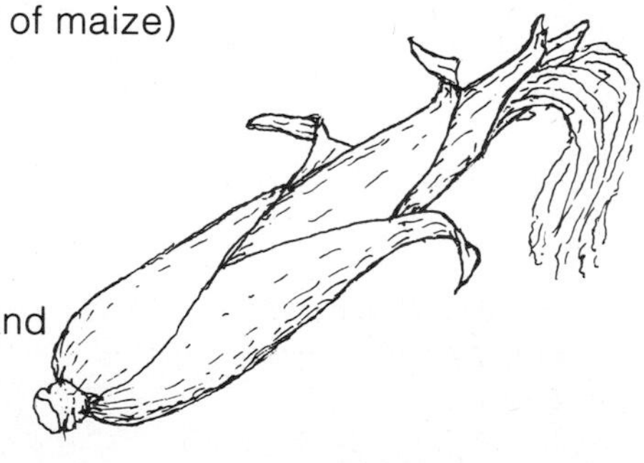

A tea made from corn silk makes a person pass more urine. This can help reduce swelling of the feet—especially in pregnant women (see p. 176 and 248).

Boil a large handful of corn silk in water and drink 1 or 2 glasses. It is not dangerous.

GARLIC

A drink made from garlic can often get rid of pinworms.

Chop finely, or crush, 4 cloves of garlic and mix with 1 glass of liquid (water, juice, or milk).

Dosage: Drink 1 glass daily for 3 weeks.

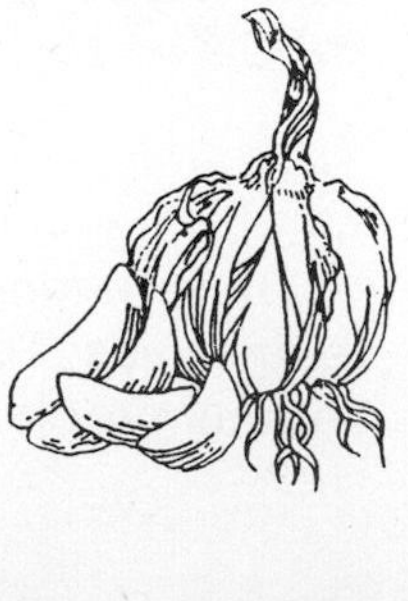

To treat vaginal infections with garlic, see p. 241 and 242.

CARDON CACTUS *(Pachycerius pectin-aboriginum)*

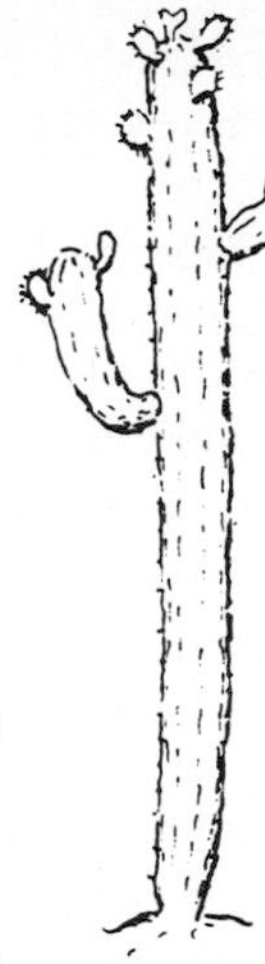

Cactus juice can be used to clean wounds when there is no boiled water and no way to get any. Cardon cactus also helps stop a wound from bleeding, because the juice makes the cut blood vessels squeeze shut.

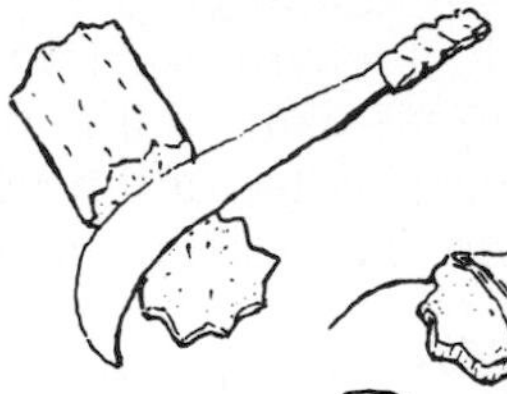

Cut a piece of the cactus with a clean knife and press it firmly against the wound.

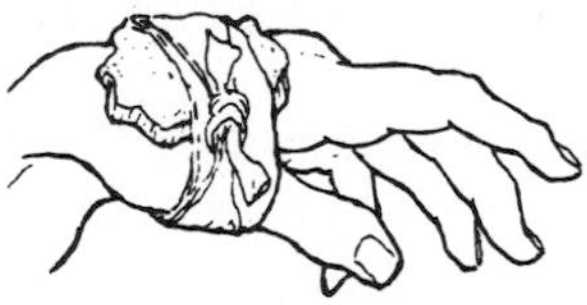

When the bleeding is under control, tie a piece of the cactus to the wound with a strip of cloth.

After 2 or 3 hours, take off the cactus and clean the wound with boiled water and soap. There are more instructions on how to care for wounds and control bleeding on pages 82 to 87.

ALOE VERA *(Sabila)*

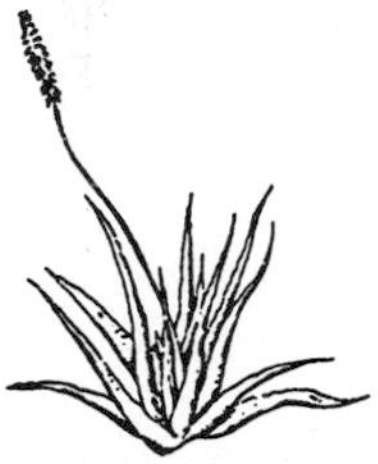

Aloe vera can be used to treat minor burns and wounds. The thick, slimy juice inside the plant calms pain and itching, aids healing, and helps prevent infection. Cut off a piece of the plant, peel back the outer layer, and apply the fleshy leaf or juice directly to the burn or wound.

Aloe can also help treat stomach ulcers and gastritis. Chop the spongy leaves into small pieces, soak them in water overnight, and then drink one glass of the slimy, bitter liquid every 2 hours.

PAPAYA

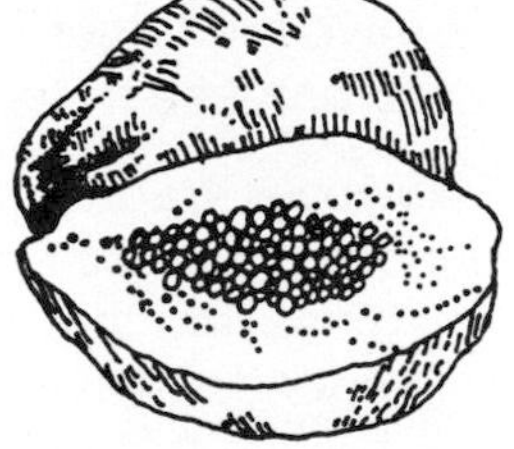

Ripe papayas are rich in vitamins and also aid digestion. Eating them is especially helpful for weak or old people who complain of upset stomach when they eat meat, chicken, or eggs. Papaya makes these foods easier to digest.

Papaya can also help get rid of intestinal worms, although modern medicines often work better. Collect 3 or 4 teaspoons (15-20 ml.) of the 'milk' that comes out when the green fruit or trunk of the tree is cut. Mix this with an equal amount of sugar or honey and stir it into a cup of hot water. If possible, drink along with a laxative.

Or, dry and crush to a powder the papaya seeds. Take 3 teaspoons mixed with 1 glass water or some honey 3 times a day for 7 days.

Papayas can also be used for treating pressure sores. The fruit contains chemicals that help soften and make dead flesh easier to remove. First clean and wash out a pressure sore that has dead flesh in it. Then soak a sterile cloth or gauze with 'milk' from the trunk or green fruit of a papaya plant and pack this into the sore. Repeat cleaning and repacking 3 times a day.

HOMEMADE CASTS—
FOR KEEPING BROKEN BONES IN PLACE

In Mexico several different plants such as ***tepeguaje*** (a tree of the bean family) and ***solda con solda*** (a huge, tree-climbing arum lily) are used to make casts. However, any plant will do if a syrup can be made from it that will dry hard and firm and will not irritate the skin. In India, traditional bone-setters make casts using a mixture of egg whites and herbs instead of a syrup made from plant juices. But the method is similar. Try out different plants in your area.

For a cast using tepeguaje: Put 1 kilogram of the bark into 5 liters of water and boil until only 2 liters are left. Strain and boil until a thick syrup is formed. Dip strips of flannel or clean sheet in the syrup and carefully use as follows.

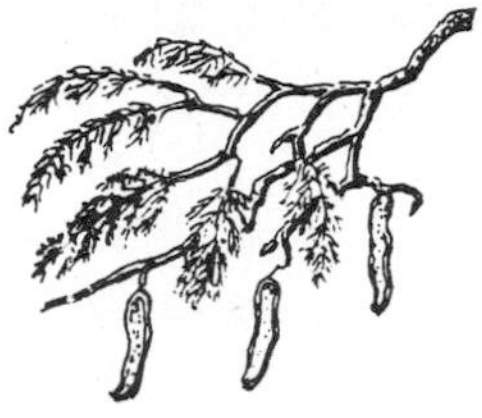

Make sure the bones are in a good position (p. 98).

Do **not** put the cast directly against the skin.

Wrap the arm or leg in a soft cloth.

Then follow with a layer of cotton or wild kapok.

Finally, put on the wet cloth strips so that they form a cast that is firm but not too tight.

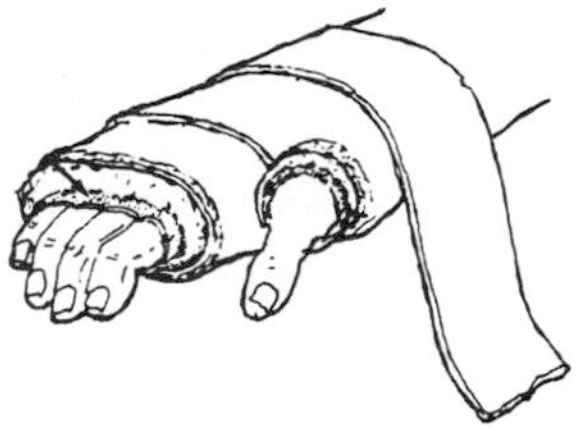

Most doctors recommend that the cast cover the joint above and the joint below the break, to keep the broken bones from moving.

This would mean that, for a broken wrist, the cast should cover almost the whole arm, like this:

Leave the finger tips uncovered so that you can see if they keep a good color.

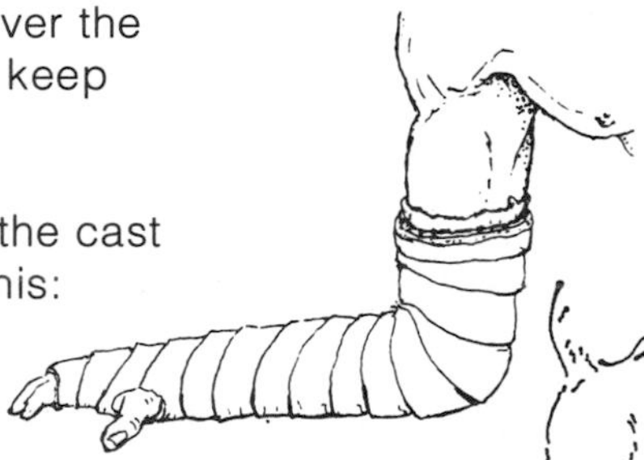

However, traditional bone-setters in China and Latin America use a short cast on a *simple* break of the arm saying that a little movement of the bone-ends speeds healing. Recent scientific studies have proven this to be true.

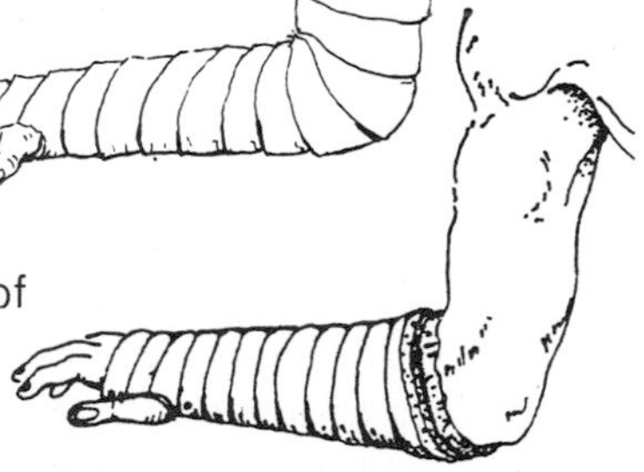

A temporary leg or arm splint can be made of cardboard, folded paper, or the thick curved stem of dried banana leaf, or palm leaf.

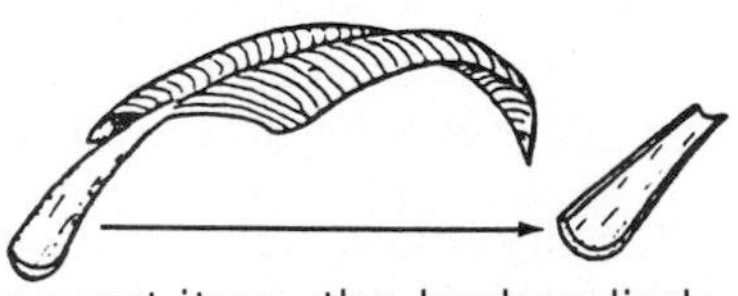

CAUTION: Even if the cast is not very tight when you put it on, the broken limb may swell up later. If the person complains that the cast is too tight, or if his fingers or toes become cold, white, or blue, take the cast off and put on a new, looser one.

Never put on a cast over a cut or a wound.

ENEMAS, LAXATIVES, AND PURGES: WHEN TO USE THEM AND WHEN NOT TO

Many people give enemas and take laxatives far too often. The 'urge to purge' is world wide.

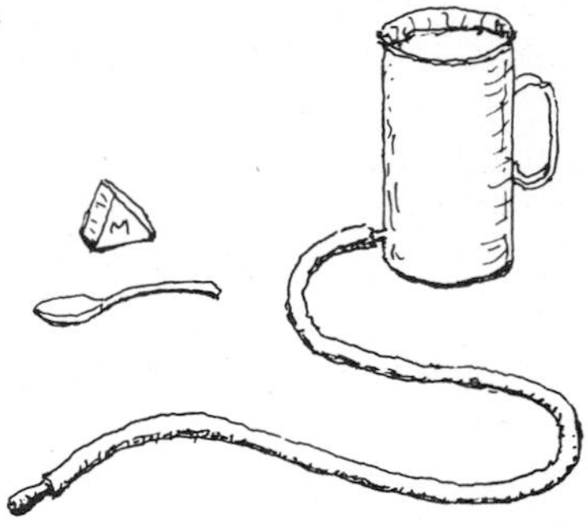

Enemas and purges are very popular home cures. And they are often very harmful. Many people believe fever and diarrhea can be 'washed out' by giving an **enema** (running water into the gut through the anus) or by using a ***purge,*** or strong laxative. Unfortunately, such efforts to clean or purge the sick body often cause more injury to the already damaged gut.

Rarely do enemas or laxatives do any good at all.
Often they are dangerous—especially strong laxatives.

CASES IN WHICH IT IS DANGEROUS TO USE ENEMAS OR LAXATIVES

Never use an enema or laxative if a person has a severe stomach-ache or any other sign of appendicitis or 'acute abdomen' (see p. 93), even if he passes days without a bowel movement.

Never give an enema or laxative to a person with a bullet wound or other injury to the gut.

Never give a strong laxative to a weak or sick person. It will weaken him more.

Never give an enema or purge to a baby less than 2 years old.

Never give a laxative or purge to a child with high fever, vomiting, diarrhea or signs of dehydration (see p. 151). It can increase dehydration and kill the child.

Do not make a habit of using laxatives often (see Constipation, p. 126).

THE CORRECT USES OF ENEMAS

1. Simple enemas can help relieve constipation (dry, hard, difficult stools). Use warm water only, or water with a little soap in it.

2. When a person with severe vomiting is dehydrated, you can try replacing water by giving an enema of Rehydration Drink **very slowly** (see p. 152).

PURGES AND LAXATIVES THAT ARE OFTEN USED

CASTOR OIL SENNA LEAF CASCARA (cascara sagrada)	These are irritating purges that often do more harm than good. It is better not to use them.
MAGNESIUM HYDROXIDE MILK OF MAGNESIA EPSOM SALTS (magnesium sulfate) (see p. 383)	These are salt purges. Use them only in low doses, as laxatives for constipation. Do not use them often and **never when there is pain in the belly.**
MINERAL OIL (see p. 383)	This is sometimes used for constipation in persons with piles... but it is like passing greased rocks. Not recommended.

CORRECT USES OF LAXATIVES AND PURGES

Laxatives are like purges but weaker. All the products listed above are laxatives when taken in small doses and purges when taken in large doses. Laxatives soften and hurry the bowel movement; purges cause diarrhea.

Purges: The only time a person should use a strong dose of a purge is when he has taken a poison and must clean it out quickly (see p. 103). At any other time a purge is harmful.

Laxatives: One can use milk of magnesia or other magnesium salts in small doses, as laxatives, in some cases of constipation. People with ***hemorrhoids*** (piles, p. 175) who have constipation can take mineral oil but this only makes their stools slippery, not soft. The dose for mineral oil is 3 to 6 teaspoons at bedtime (never with a meal because the oil will rob the body of important vitamins in the food). This is not the best way.

Suppositories, or bullet-shaped pills that can be pushed up the rectum, can also be used to relieve constipation or piles (see pages 175, 383, and 392).

A BETTER WAY

Foods with fiber. The healthiest and most gentle way to have softer, more frequent stools is to *drink a lot of water* and to *eat more foods with lots of natural fiber,* or 'roughage' like *cassava, yam,* or *bran* (wheat husks) and other whole grain cereals (see p. 126). Eating plenty of fruits and vegetables also helps.

People who traditionally eat lots of food with natural fiber suffer much less from piles, constipation, and cancer of the gut than do people who eat a lot of refined 'modern' foods. For better bowel habits, avoid refined foods and eat foods prepared from unpolished or unrefined grains.

CHAPTER 2

Sicknesses That Are Often Confused

WHAT CAUSES SICKNESS?

Persons from different countries or backgrounds have different ways to explain what causes sickness.

A baby gets diarrhea. But why?

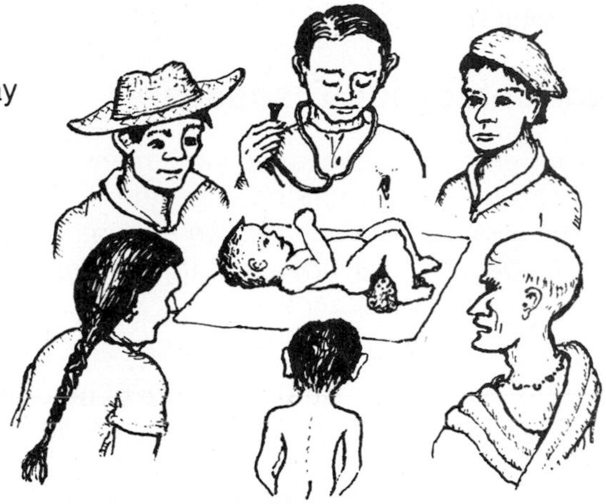

People in small villages may say it is because the parents did something wrong, or perhaps because they made a god or spirit angry.

A doctor may say it is because the child has an infection.

A public health officer may say it is because the villagers do not have a good water system or use latrines.

A social reformer may say the unhealthy conditions that lead to frequent childhood diarrhea are caused by an unfair distribution of land and wealth.

A teacher may place the blame on lack of education.

People see the cause of sickness in terms of their own experience and point of view. Who then is right about the cause? Possibly everyone is right, or partly right. This is because . . .

Sickness usually results from a combination of causes.

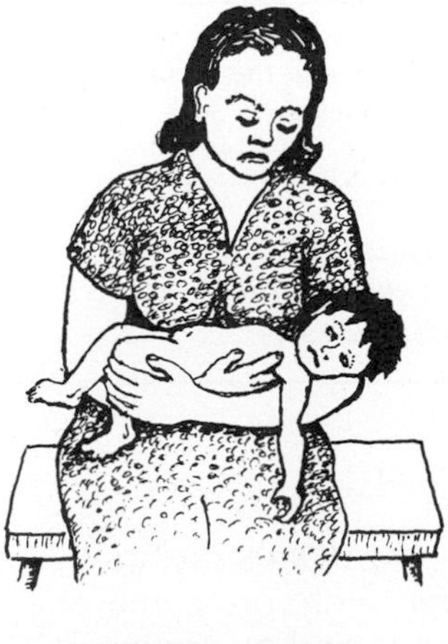

"Why my child?"

Each of the causes suggested above may be a part of the reason why a baby gets diarrhea.

To prevent and treat sickness successfully, it helps to have as full an understanding as possible about the common sicknesses in your area and the combination of things that causes them.

In this book, different sicknesses are discussed mostly according to the systems and terms of modern or scientific medicine.

To make good use of this book, and safe use of the medicines it recommends, you will need some understanding of sicknesses and their causes according to medical science. Reading this chapter may help.

DIFFERENT KINDS OF SICKNESSES AND THEIR CAUSES

When considering how to prevent or treat different sicknesses, it helps to think of them in two groups: infectious and non-infectious.

Infectious diseases are those that spread from one person to another. Healthy persons must be protected from people with these sicknesses.

Non-infectious diseases do not spread from person to person. They have other causes. Therefore, it is important to know which sicknesses are infectious and which are not.

Non-infectious Diseases

Non-infectious diseases have many different causes. But they are never caused by germs, bacteria, or other living organisms that attack the body. They never spread from one person to another. It is important to realize that *antibiotics,* or medicines that fight germs (see p. 55), do not help cure non-infectious diseases.

> *Remember:* **Antibiotics are of no use for non-infectious diseases.**

EXAMPLES OF NON-INFECTIOUS DISEASES

Problems caused by something that wears out or goes wrong within the body:	**Problems caused by something from outside that harms or troubles the body:**	**Problems caused by a lack of something the body needs:**
rheumatism heart attack epileptic fits stroke migraine headaches cataract cancer	allergies asthma poisons snakebite cough from smoking stomach ulcer alcoholism	malnutrition anemia pellagra night blindness and xerophthalmia goiter and cretinism cirrhosis of the liver (part of the cause)

Problems people are born with:		**Problems that begin in the mind (mental 'illnesses'):**
harelip crossed or wall-eyes (squint) other deformities	epilepsy (some kinds) retarded (backward) children birthmarks	fear that something is harmful when it is not (paranoia) nervous worry (anxiety) belief in hexes (witchcraft) uncontrolled fear (hysteria)

Infectious Diseases

Infectious diseases are caused by bacteria and other *organisms* (living things) that harm the body. They are spread in many ways. Here are some of the most important kinds of organisms that cause infections and examples of sicknesses they cause:

EXAMPLES OF INFECTIOUS DISEASES

Organism that causes the sickness	Name of the sickness	How it is spread or enters the body	Principal medicine
bacteria (microbes or germs)	tuberculosis	through the air (coughing)	different antibiotics for different bacterial infections
	tetanus	dirty wounds	
	some diarrhea	dirty fingers, water, flies	
	pneumonia (some kinds)	through the air (coughing)	
	gonorrhea, chlamydia, and syphillis	sexual contact	
	earache	with a cold	
	infected wounds	contact with dirty things	
	sores with pus	direct contact (by touch)	
virus (germs smaller than bacteria)	colds, flu, measles, mumps, chickenpox, infantile paralysis, virus diarrhea	from someone who is sick, through the air, by coughing, flies, etc.	aspirin and other painkillers (There are no medicines that fight viruses effectively. Antibiotics do not help.) Vaccinations help prevent some virus infections.
	rabies	animal bites	
	warts	touch	
fungus	ringworm athlete's foot jock itch	by touch or from clothing	sulfur and vinegar ointments: undecylenic, benzoic, salicylic acid griseofulvin
internal parasites (harmful animals living in the body)	In the gut: worms amebas (dysentery)	feces-to-mouth lack of cleanliness	different specific medicines
	In the blood: malaria	mosquito bite	chloroquine (or other malaria medicine)
external parasites (harmful animals living on the body)	lice fleas bedbugs scabies	by contact with infected persons or their clothes	insecticides, lindane

Bacteria, like many of the organisms that cause infections, are so small you cannot see them without a microscope—an instrument that→ makes tiny things look bigger. Viruses are even smaller than bacteria.

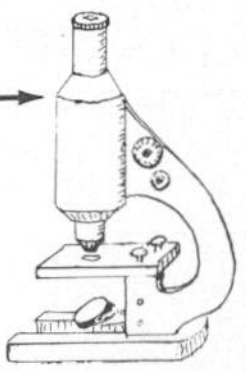

Antibiotics (penicillin, tetracycline, etc.) are medicines that help cure certain illnesses caused by bacteria. **Antibiotics have no effect on illnesses caused by most viruses,** such as colds, flu, mumps, chickenpox, etc. **Do not treat virus infections with antibiotics.** They will not help and may be harmful (see **Antibiotics,** p. 55).

SICKNESSES THAT ARE HARD TO TELL APART

Sometimes diseases that have different causes and require different treatment result in problems that look very much alike. For example:

1. **A child who slowly becomes thin and wasted, while his belly gets more and more swollen, could have any (or several) of the following problems:**

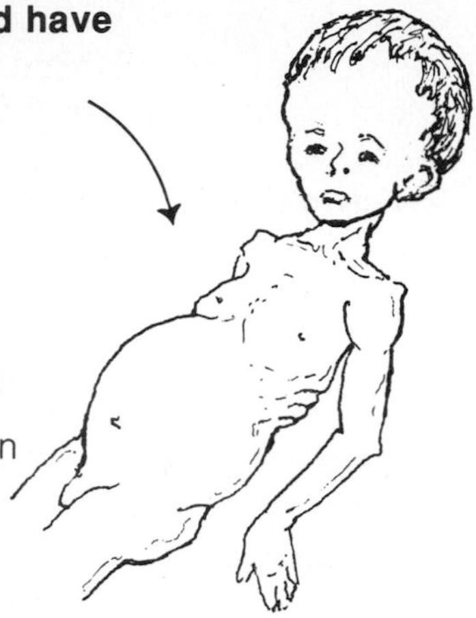

- malnutrition (see p. 112)
- a lot of roundworms, p. 140, (usually together with malnutrition)
- advanced tuberculosis (p. 179)
- a long-term severe urinary infection (p. 234)
- any of several problems of the liver or spleen
- leukemia (cancer of the blood)

2. **An older person with a big, open, slowly growing sore on the ankle could have:**

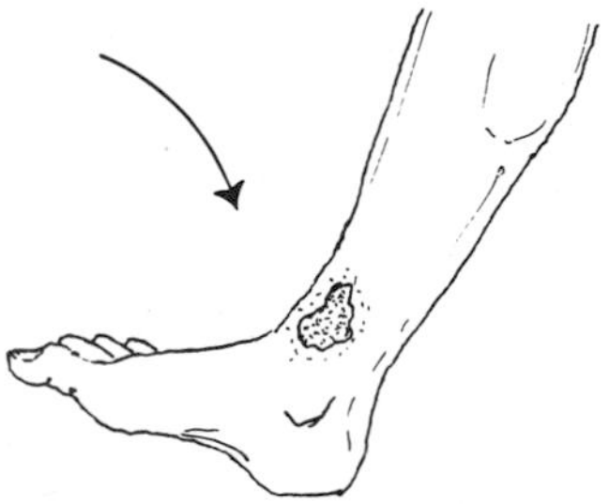

- bad circulation that results from varicose veins or other causes (p. 213)
- diabetes (p. 127)
- infection of the bone (osteomyelitis)
- leprosy (p. 191)
- tuberculosis of the skin (p. 212)
- advanced syphilis (p. 237)

The medical treatment for each of these diseases is different, so to treat them correctly it is important to tell them apart.

Many illnesses at first seem very similar. But if you ask the right questions and know what to look for, you can often learn information and see certain signs that will help tell you what illness a person has.

This book describes the typical history and signs for many illnesses. But be careful! Diseases do not always show the signs described for them—or the signs may be confusing. **For difficult cases, the help of a skilled health worker or doctor is often needed.** Sometimes special tests or analyses are necessary.

Work within your limits!
In using this book, remember it is easy to make mistakes.
Never pretend you know something you do not.
If you are not fairly sure what an illness is and how to treat it, or if the illness is very serious—get medical help.

SICKNESSES THAT ARE OFTEN CONFUSED OR GIVEN THE SAME NAME

Many of the common names people use for their sicknesses were first used long before anyone knew about germs or bacteria or the medicines that fight them. Different diseases that caused more or less similar problems—such as 'high fever' or 'pain in the side'—were often given a single name. In many parts of the world, these common names are still used. City-trained doctors often neither know nor use these names. For this reason, people sometimes think they apply to 'sicknesses doctors do not treat'. So they treat these **home sicknesses** with herbs or home remedies.

Actually, most of these home sicknesses or 'folk diseases' are the same ones known to medical science. Only the names are different.

For many sicknesses, home remedies work well. But for some sicknesses, treatment with modern medicine works much better and may be life-saving. This is especially true for dangerous infections like pneumonia, typhoid, tuberculosis, or infections after giving birth.

To know which sicknesses definitely require modern medicines and to decide what medicine to use, it is important that you try to **find out what the disease is in the terms used by trained health workers and in this book.**

If you cannot find the sickness you are looking for in this book, look for it under a different name or in the chapter that covers the same sort of problem. Use the list of CONTENTS and the INDEX.

If you are unsure what the sickness is—expecially if it seems serious—try to get medical help.

The rest of this chapter gives examples of common or *traditional* names people use for various sicknesses. Often a single name is given to diseases that are different according to medical science.

Examples cannot be given for each country or area where this book may be used. Therefore, I have kept those from the Spanish edition, with names used by villagers in western Mexico. They will not be the same names you use. However, people in many parts of the world see and speak of their illnesses in a similar way. So the examples may help you think about how people name diseases in your area.

Can you think of a name your people use for the following 'folk diseases'? If you can, write it in after the Spanish name, where it says,

Name in Your Area: ______________________________

EXAMPLES OF LOCAL NAMES FOR SICKNESSES

Spanish Name: ***EMPACHO*** **(STOPPED-UP GUT)** Name in Your Area:_______________

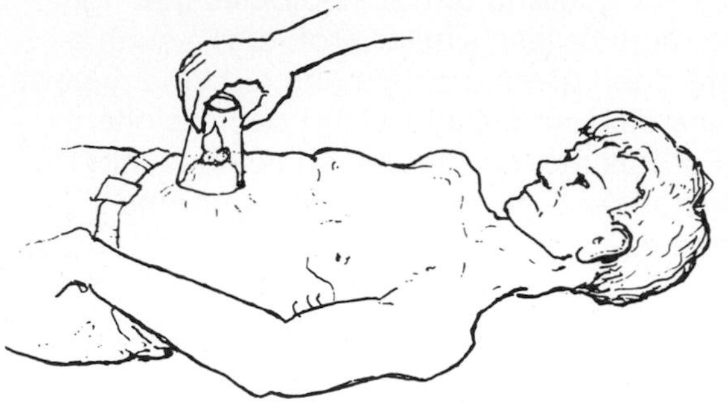

In medical terms ***empacho*** (impaction) means that the gut is stopped up or ***obstructed*** (see p. 94). But in Mexican villages any illness causing stomach-ache or diarrhea may be called ***empacho.*** It is said that a ball of hair or something else blocks a part of the gut. People put the blame on witches or evil spirits, and treat with magic cures and ***cupping*** (see picture). Sometimes folk healers pretend to take a ball of hair and thorns out of the gut by sucking on the belly.

Different illnesses that cause stomach pain or discomfort and are sometimes called ***empacho*** are:

- diarrhea or dysentery with cramps (p. 153)
- worms (p. 140)
- swollen stomach due to malnutrition (p. 112)
- indigestion or stomach ulcer (p. 128)
- and rarely, true gut obstruction or appendicitis (p. 94)

Most of these problems are not helped much by magic cures or cupping. To treat ***empacho,*** try to identify and treat the sickness that causes it.

Spanish Name: ***DOLOR DE IJAR*** **(SIDE PAINS)** Name in Your Area:_______________

This name is used for any pain women get in one side of their belly. Often the pain goes around to the mid or lower back. Possible causes of this kind of pain include:

- an infection of the urinary system (the kidneys, the bladder, or the tubes that join them, see p. 234)
- cramps or gas pains (see diarrhea, p. 153)
- menstrual pains (see p. 245)
- appendicitis (see p. 94)
- an infection, cyst, or tumor in the womb or ovaries (p. 243) or an out-of-place pregnancy (see p. 280)

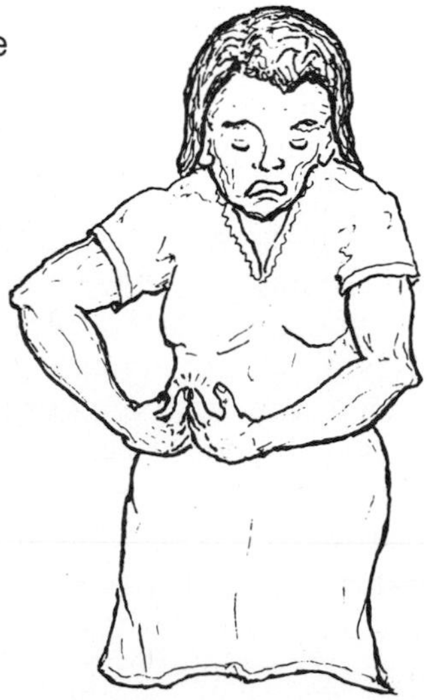

Spanish Name: *LA CONGESTION* (CONGESTION) Name in Your Area:______________

Any sudden upset or illness that causes great distress is called *la congestión* by Mexican villagers. People speak of *congestión* of:

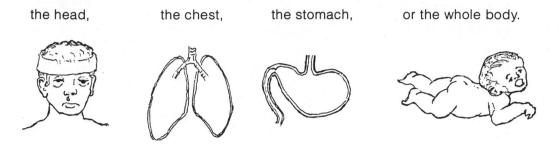

the head, the chest, the stomach, or the whole body.

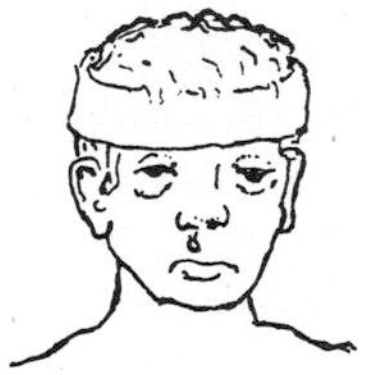

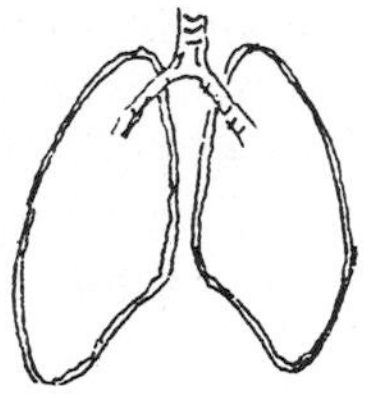

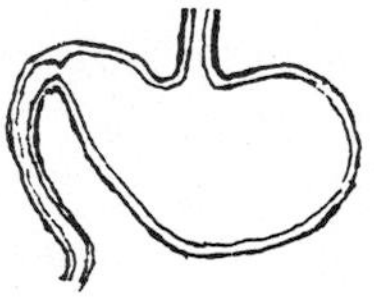

It is said that *la congestión* strikes persons who break 'the diet' (see p. 123), by eating foods that are forbidden or *taboo* after childbirth, while taking a medicine, or when they have a cold or cough. Although **these foods usually cause no harm** and are sometimes just what their bodies need, many people will not touch them because they are so afraid of getting *la congestión.*

Different illnesses that are sometimes called *la congestión* are:

- Food poisoning, from eating spoiled food: causes sudden vomiting followed by diarrhea, cramps, and weakness (see p. 135).
- A severe allergic reaction, in allergic persons after they eat certain foods (shellfish, chocolate, etc.), take certain medicines, or are injected with penicillin. May cause vomiting, diarrhea, cold sweat, breathing trouble, itchy rash, and severe distress (see p. 166).
- Any sudden upset of the stomach or gut: see diarrhea (p. 153), vomiting (p. 161), and acute abdomen (p. 93).
- Sudden or severe difficulty breathing: caused by asthma (p. 167), pneumonia (p. 171), or something stuck in the throat (p. 79).
- Illnesses that cause fits or paralysis: see fits (p. 178), tetanus (p. 182), meningitis (p. 185), polio (p. 314), and stroke (p. 327).
- Heart attacks: mostly in older persons (p. 325).

Spanish Name: *LATIDO* (PULSING) Name in Your Area:______________

Latido is a name used in Latin America for a pulsing or 'jumping' in the pit of the stomach. It is really the pulse *of the aorta* or big blood vessel coming from the heart. This pulse can be seen and felt on a person who is very thin and hungry. *Latido* is often a sign of malnutrition (p. 112)—or hunger! Eating enough good food is the only real treatment (see p. 110 and 111).

Spanish Name: *SUSTO* (HYSTERIA, FRIGHT) Name in Your Area:________________

According to Mexican villagers, ***susto*** is caused by a sudden fright a person has had, or by witchcraft, black magic, or evil spirits. A person with ***susto*** is very nervous and afraid. He may shake, behave strangely, not be able to sleep, lose weight, or even die.

Possible medical explanations for *susto:*

1. In many people, ***susto*** is a state of fear or ***hysteria,*** perhaps caused by the 'power of belief' (see p. 4). For example, a woman who is afraid someone will hex her becomes nervous and does not eat or sleep well. She begins to grow weak and lose weight. She takes this as a sign she has been hexed, so she becomes still more nervous and frightened. Her ***susto*** gets worse and worse.

2. In babies or small children, ***susto*** is usually very different. Bad dreams may cause a child to cry out in his sleep or wake up frightened. High fevers from any illness can cause very strange speech and behavior ***(delirium).*** A child that often looks and acts worried may be malnourished (p. 112). Sometimes early signs of tetanus (p. 182) or meningitis (p. 185) are also called ***susto.***

Treatment:

When the ***susto*** is caused by a specific illness, treat the illness. Help the person understand its cause. Ask for medical advice, if needed.

When the ***susto*** is caused by fright, try to comfort the person and help him understand that his fear itself is the cause of his problem. Magic cures and home remedies sometimes help.

If the frightened person is breathing very hard and fast, his body may be getting too much air—which may be part of the problem:

EXTREME FRIGHT OR HYSTERIA WITH FAST HEAVY BREATHING (HYPERVENTILATION)

Signs:

- person very frightened
- breathing fast and deep
- fast, pounding heartbeat
- numbness or tingling of face, hands, or feet
- muscle cramps

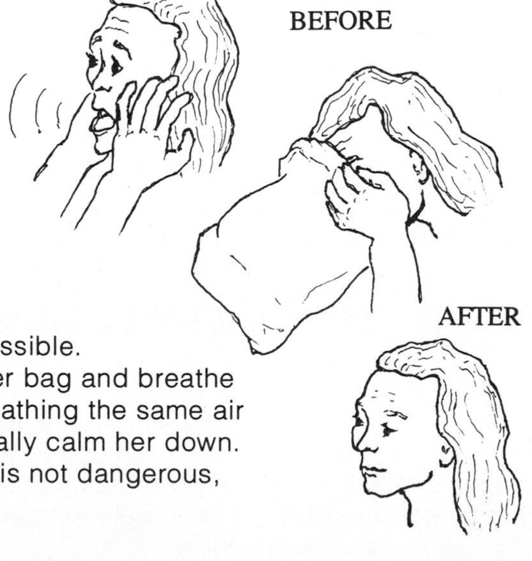

Treatment:

- Keep the person as quiet as possible.
- Have her put her face in a paper bag and breathe slowly. She should continue breathing the same air for 2 or 3 minutes. This will usually calm her down.
- Explain to her that the problem is not dangerous, and she will soon be all right.

MISUNDERSTANDINGS DUE TO CONFUSION OF NAMES

This page shows 2 examples of misunderstandings that can result when certain names like 'cancer' and 'leprosy' mean one thing to medical workers and something else to villagers. In talking with health workers—and in using this book:

Avoid misunderstanding—go by the signs and history of a person's sickness, not the name people give it!

Spanish Name: *CANCER* (CANCER) Name in Your Area:____________________

Mexican villagers use the word ***cancer*** for any severe infection of the skin, especially badly infected wounds (p. 88) or gangrene (p. 213).

In modern medical language, cancer is not an infection, but an abnormal growth or lump in any part of the body. Common types of cancer that you should watch out for are:

cancer of the skin (p. 211)

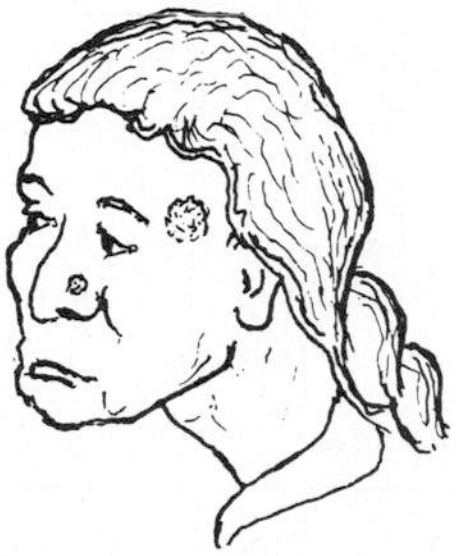

breast cancer (p. 279)

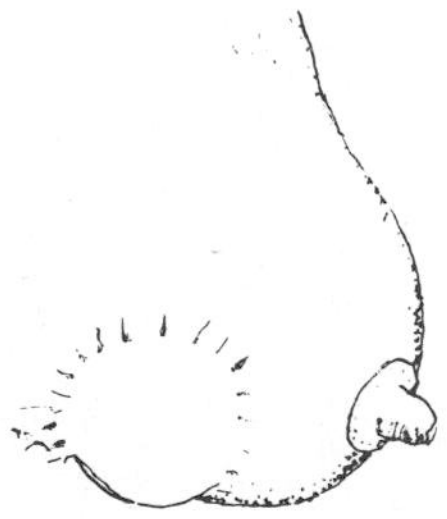

cancer of the womb or ovaries (p. 280)

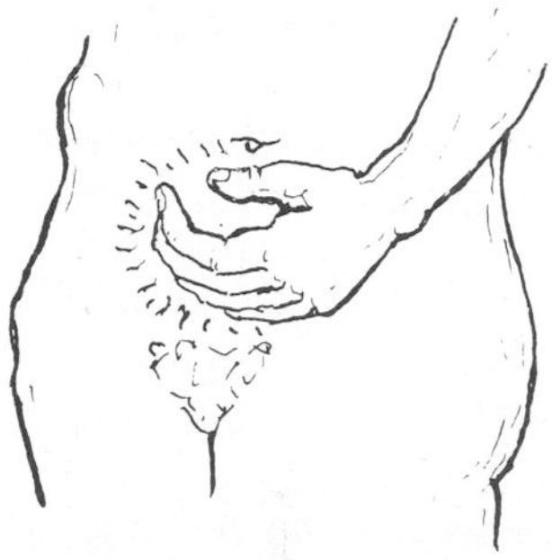

Any hard, painless, slowly growing lump in any part of your body may be cancer. Cancer is often dangerous and may need surgery.

At the first suspicion of cancer seek medical help.

Spanish Name: *LEPRA* (LEPROSY) Name in Your Area:____________________

Mexican villagers call any open spreading sore ***lepra.*** This leads to confusion, because medical workers use this term only for true leprosy (Hansen's disease, p. 191). Sores commonly called *lepra* are:

- impetigo and other skin infections (p. 202)
- sores that come from insect bites or scabies (p. 199)
- chronic sores or skin ulcers such as those caused by poor circulation (p. 213)
- skin cancer (p. 211)
- less commonly, leprosy (p. 191) or tuberculosis of the skin (p. 212)

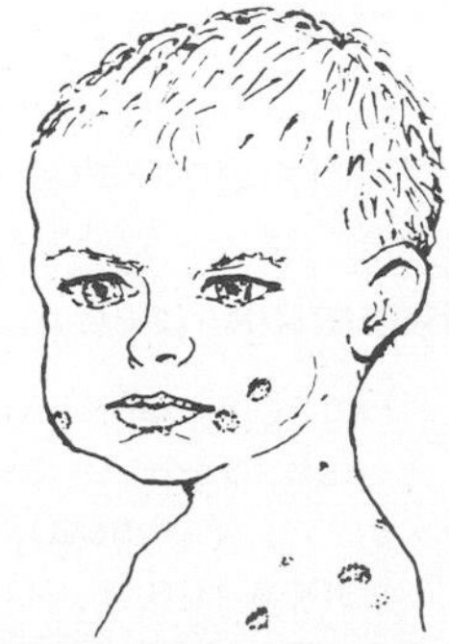

This child has impetigo, not leprosy.

CONFUSION BETWEEN DIFFERENT ILLNESSES THAT CAUSE FEVER

Spanish Name: *LA FIEBRE* (THE FEVER) Name in Your Area:____________________

Correctly speaking, a *fever* is a **body temperature higher than normal.** But in Latin America, a number of serious illnesses that cause high temperatures are all called *la fiebre*—or 'the fever'.

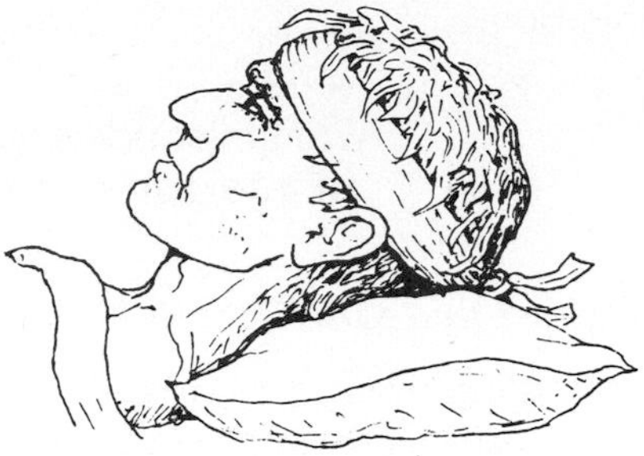

To prevent or treat these diseases successfully, it is important to know how to tell one from another.

Here are some of the important acute illnesses in which fever is an outstanding sign. The drawings show the **fever pattern** (rise and fall of temperature) that is typical for each disease.

Malaria: (see p. 186)

Begins with weakness, chills and fever. Fever may come and go for a few days, with shivering (chills) as the temperature rises, and sweating as it falls. Then, fever may come for a few hours every second or third day. On other days, the person may feel more or less well.

MALARIA—TYPICAL FEVER PATTERN

The solid line shows the rise and fall of temperature.

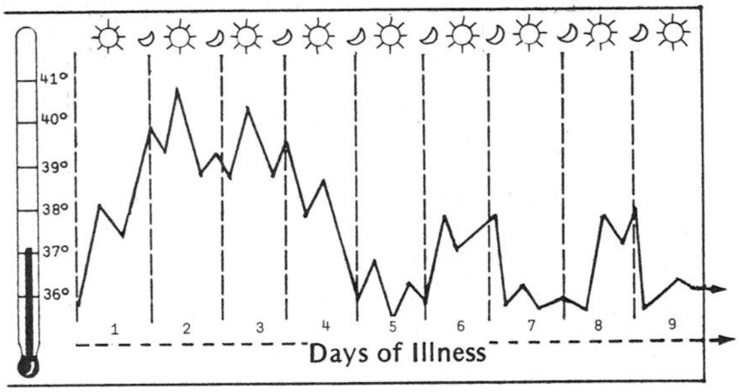

Typhoid: (see p. 188)

Begins like a cold. Temperature goes up a little more each day. Pulse relatively slow. Sometimes diarrhea and dehydration. Trembling or delirium (mind wanders). Person very ill.

TYPHOID—TYPICAL FEVER PATTERN

The fever goes up a little each day.

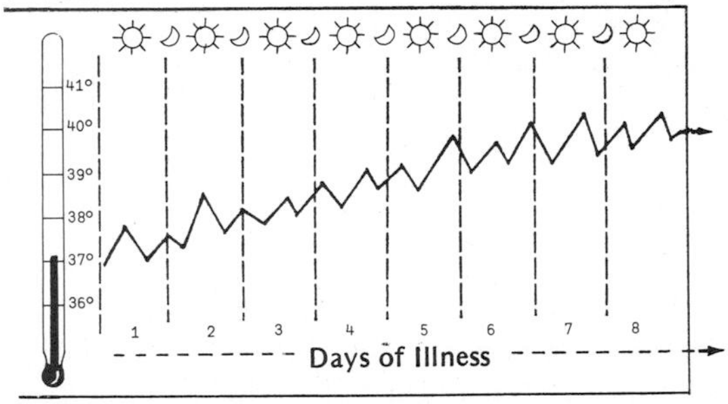

Typhus: (see p. 190)

Similar to typhoid. Rash similar to that of measles, with tiny bruises.

Hepatitis: (see p. 172)

Person loses appetite. Does not wish to eat or smoke. Wants to vomit (nausea). Eyes and skin turn yellow; urine orange or brown; stools whitish. Sometimes liver becomes large, tender. Mild fever. Person very weak.

HEPATITIS—TYPICAL FEVER PATTERN

Usually the fever is mild.

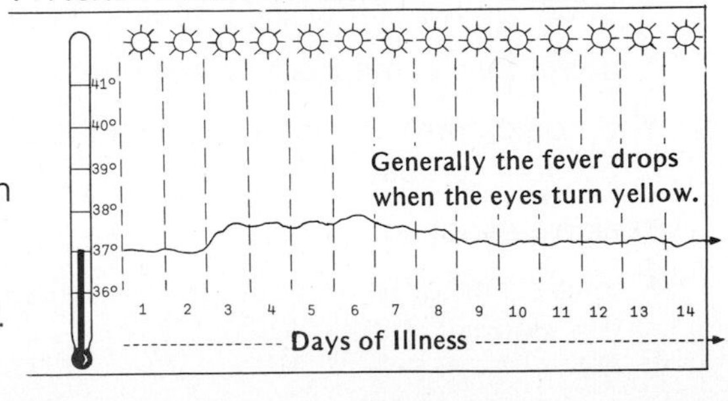

Pneumonia: **(see p. 171)**

Fast, shallow breathing. Temperature rises quickly. Cough with green, yellow, or bloody mucus. May be pain in chest. Person very ill.

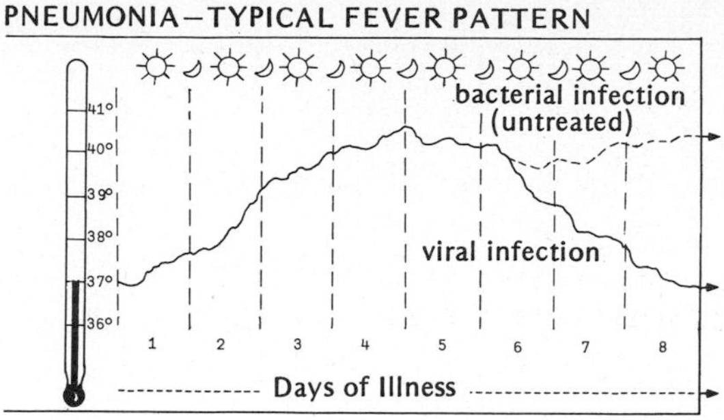

Rheumatic fever: **(see p. 310)**

Most common in children and teenagers. Pain in joints. High fever. Often comes after a sore throat. May be pain in the chest with shortness of breath. Or uncontrolled movements of arms and legs.

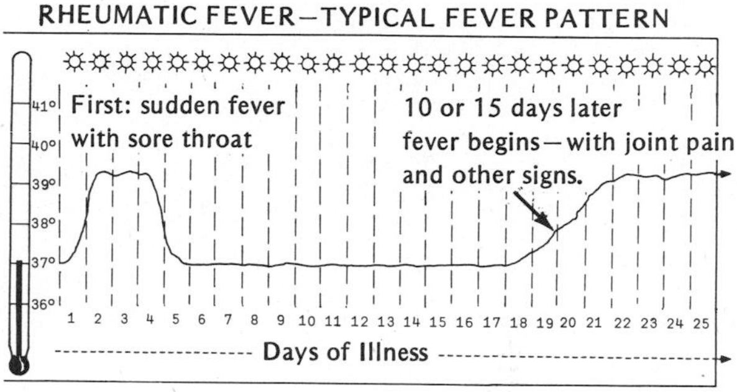

Brucellosis (undulant fever, Malta fever): **(see p. 188)**

Begins slowly with tiredness, headache, and pains in the bones. Fever and sweating most common at night. Fever disappears for a few days only to come back again. This may go on for months or years.

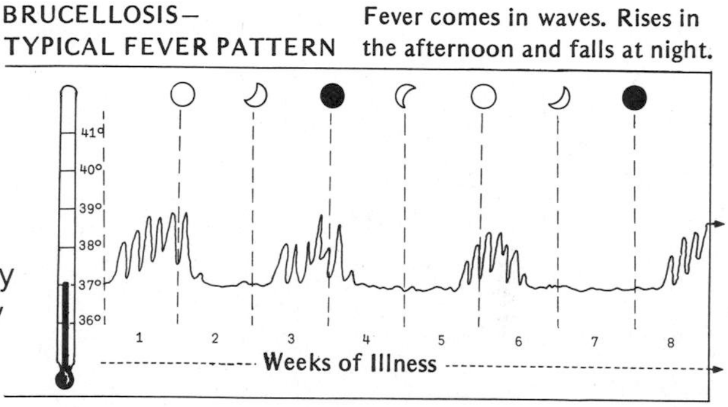

Childbirth fever: **(see p. 276)**

Begins a day or more after giving birth. Starts with a slight fever, which often rises later. Foul-smelling vaginal *discharge.* Pain and sometimes bleeding.

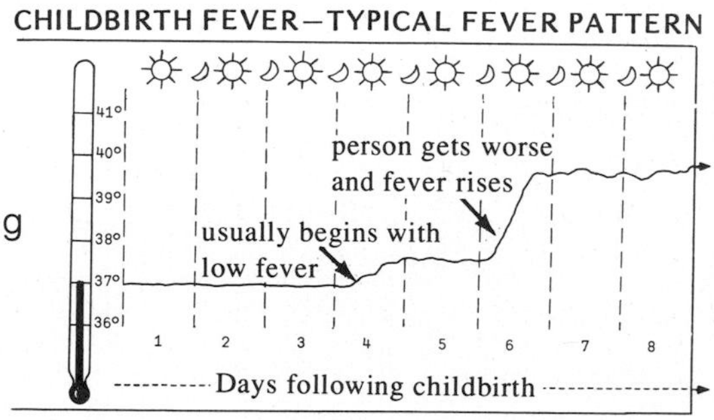

All of these illnesses can be dangerous. In addition to those shown here, there are many other diseases that may cause similar signs and fever. For example, fevers that last for more than 1 month, or night sweats, may be caused by the HIV/AIDS virus (see p. 399). When possible, seek medical help.

CHAPTER

HOW TO EXAMINE A SICK PERSON

3

To find out the needs of a sick person, first you must ask important questions and then examine him carefully. You should look for ***signs*** and ***symptoms*** that help you tell how ill the person is and what kind of sickness he may have.

Always examine the person where there is good light, preferably in the sunlight—**never** in a dark room.

There are certain basic things to ask and to look for in anyone who is sick. These include things the sick person feels or reports (symptoms), as well as things **you** notice on examining him (signs). These signs can be especially important in babies and persons unable to talk. In this book the word 'signs' is used for both symptoms and signs.

When you examine a sick person, write down your findings and keep them for the health worker in case he is needed (see p. 44).

QUESTIONS

Start by asking the person about her sickness. Be sure to ask the following:

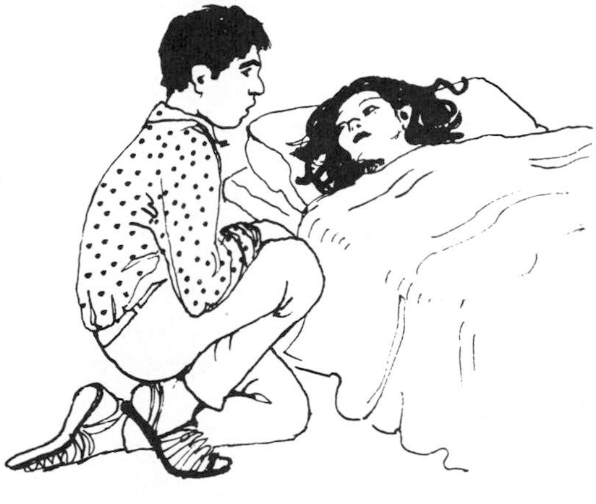

What bothers you most right now?

What makes you feel better or worse?

How and when did your sickness begin?

Have you had this same trouble before, or has anyone else in your family or neighborhood had it?

Continue with other questions in order to learn the details of the illness.

For example, if the sick person has a pain, ask her:

Where does it hurt? (Ask her to point to the exact place with one finger.)

Does it hurt all the time, or off and on?

What is the pain like? (sharp? dull? burning?)

Can you sleep with the pain?

If the sick person is a baby who still does not talk, look for signs of pain. Notice his movements and how he cries. (For example, a child with an earache sometimes rubs the side of his head or pulls at his ear.)

GENERAL CONDITION OF HEALTH

Before touching the sick person, look at him carefully. Observe how ill or weak he looks, the way he moves, how he breathes, and how clear his mind seems. Look for signs of dehydration (see p. 151) and of shock (p. 77).

Notice whether the person looks well nourished or poorly nourished. Has he been losing weight? When a person has lost weight slowly over a long period of time, he may have a ***chronic illness*** (one that lasts a long time).

Also note the color of the skin and eyes. These sometimes change when a person is sick. (Dark skin can hide color changes. So look at parts of the body where the skin is pale, such as palms of the hands or soles of the feet, the fingernails, or the insides of the lips and eyelids.)

- Paleness, especially of the lips and inside the eyelids, is a sign of anemia (p. 124). Skin may also go lighter as a result of tuberculosis (p.179), or kwashiorkor (p. 113).
- Darkening of the skin may be a sign of starvation (see p. 112).
- Bluish skin, especially blueness or darkness of the lips and fingernails, may mean serious problems with breathing (p. 79, 167, and 313) or with the heart (p. 325). Blue-gray color in an unconscious child may be a sign of cerebral malaria (p. 186).
- A gray-white coloring, with cool moist skin, often means a person is in shock (p. 77).
- Yellow color (jaundice) of the skin and eyes may result from disease in the liver (hepatitis, p. 172, cirrhosis, p. 328, or amebic abscess, p. 145) or gallbladder (p. 329). It may also occur in newborn babies (p. 274), and in children born with sickle cell disease (p. 321).

Look also at the skin when a light is shining across it from one side. This can show the earliest sign of measles rash on the face of a feverish child (p. 311).

TEMPERATURE

It is often wise to take a sick person's temperature, even if he does not seem to have a fever. If the person is very sick, take the temperature at least 4 times each day and write it down.

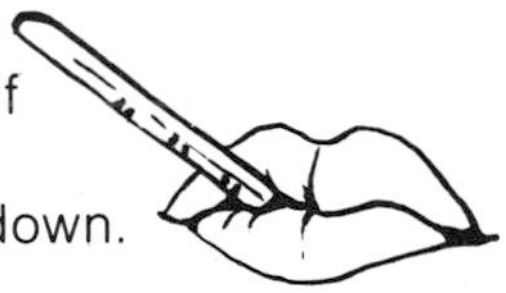

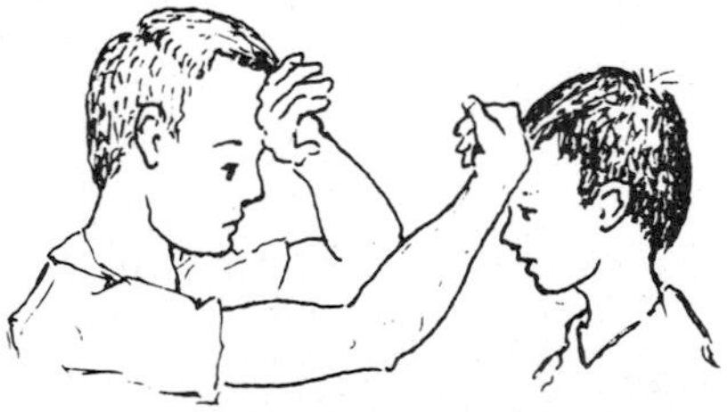

If there is no thermometer, you can get an idea of the temperature by putting the back of one hand on the sick person's forehead and the other on your own or that of another healthy person. If the sick person has a fever, you should feel the difference.

It is important to find out when and how the fever comes, how long it lasts, and how it goes away. This may help you identify the disease. Not every fever is malaria, though in some countries it is often treated as such. Remember other possible causes. For example:

- Common cold, and other virus infections (p. 163). The fever is usually mild.
- Typhoid causes a fever that goes on rising for 5 days. Malaria medicine does not help.
- Tuberculosis sometimes causes a mild fever in the afternoon. At night the person often sweats, and the fever goes down.

How to Use a Thermometer

Every family should have a thermometer. Take the temperature of a sick person 4 times a day and always write it down.

How to read the thermometer (using one marked in degrees *centigrade*—°C):

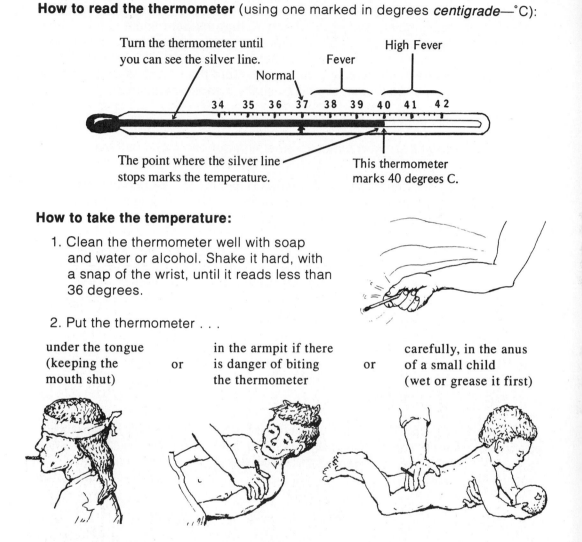

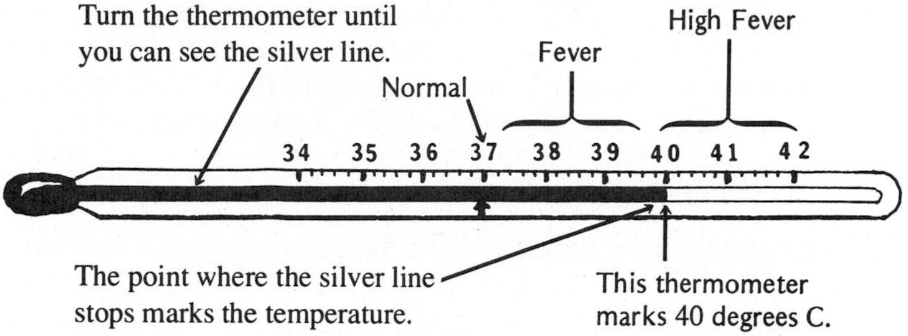
Turn the thermometer until you can see the silver line.
High Fever
Fever
Normal
34 35 36 37 38 39 40 41 42
The point where the silver line stops marks the temperature.
This thermometer marks 40 degrees C.

How to take the temperature:

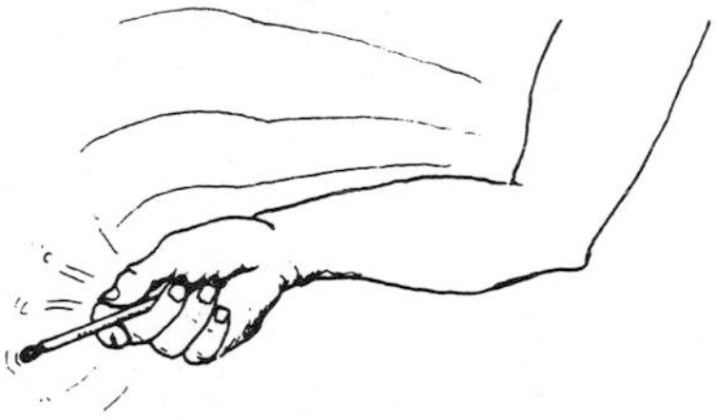

1. Clean the thermometer well with soap and water or alcohol. Shake it hard, with a snap of the wrist, until it reads less than 36 degrees.

2. Put the thermometer . . .

under the tongue (keeping the mouth shut) or in the armpit if there is danger of biting the thermometer or carefully, in the anus of a small child (wet or grease it first)

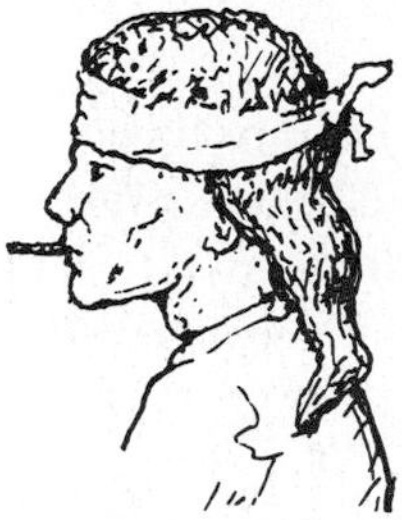

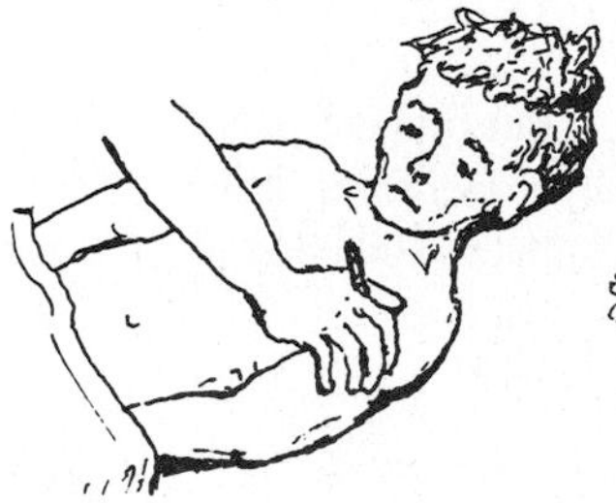

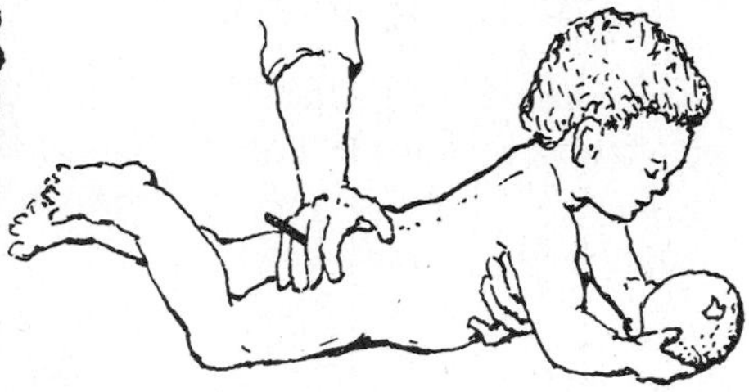

3. Leave it there for 3 or 4 minutes.

4. Read it. (An armpit temperature will read a little lower than a mouth reading; in the anus it will read a little higher.)

5. Wash the thermometer well with soap and water.

Note: In newborn babies a temperature that is unusually high **or unusually low** (below 36°) may mean a serious infection (see p. 275).

- To learn about other fever patterns, see p. 26 to 27.
- To learn what to do for a fever, see p. 75.

BREATHING (RESPIRATION)

Pay special attention to the way the sick person breathes—the depth (deep or shallow), rate (how often breaths are taken), and difficulty. Notice if both sides of the chest move equally when she breathes.

If you have a watch or simple timer, count the number of breaths per minute (when the person is quiet). Between 12 and 20 breaths per minute is normal for adults and older children. Up to 30 breaths a minute is normal for children, and 40 for babies. People with a high fever or serious respiratory illnesses (like pneumonia) breathe more quickly than normal. More than 40 **shallow** breaths a minute in an adult, or 60 in a small child, usually means pneumonia.

Listen carefully to the sound of the breaths. For example:

- A whistle or wheeze and difficulty breathing out can mean asthma (see p. 167).
- A gurgling or snoring noise and difficult breathing in an unconscious person may mean the tongue, mucus (slime or pus), or something else is stuck in the throat and does not let enough air get through.

Look for 'sucking in' of the skin between ribs and at the angle of the neck (behind the collar bone) when the person breathes in. This means air has trouble getting through. Consider the possibility of something stuck in the throat (p. 79), pneumonia (p. 171), asthma (p. 167), or bronchitis (mild sucking in, see p. 170).

If the person has a cough, ask if it keeps her from sleeping. Find out if she coughs up mucus, how much, its color, and if there is blood in it.

PULSE (HEARTBEAT)

To take the person's pulse, put your fingers on the wrist as shown. (Do not use your thumb to feel for the pulse.)

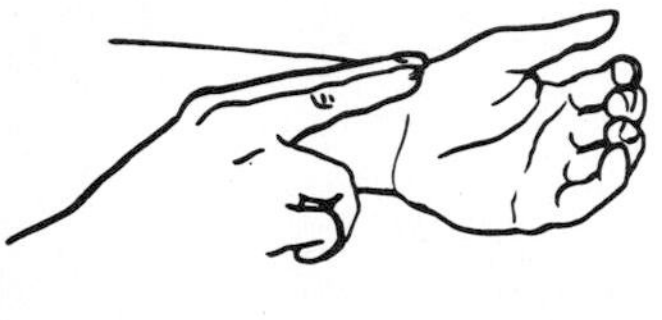

If you cannot find the pulse in the wrist, feel for it in the neck beside the voicebox,

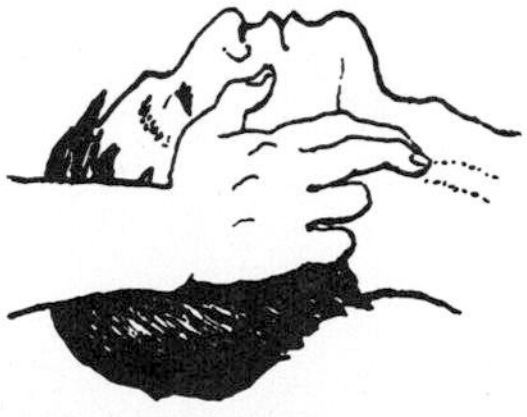

or put your ear directly on the chest and listen for the heartbeat (or use a stethoscope if you have one).

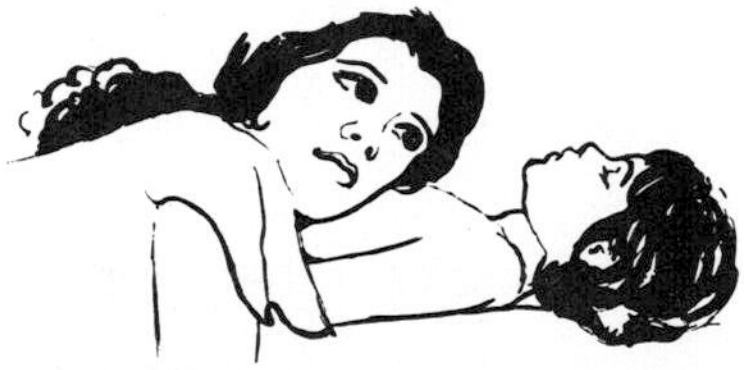

Pay attention to the strength, the rate, and the regularity of the pulse. If you have a watch or timer, count the pulses per minute.

NORMAL PULSE FOR PEOPLE AT REST

adults	from 60 to 80 per minute
children	80 to 100
babies	100 to 140

The pulse gets much faster with exercise and when a person is nervous, frightened, or has a fever. As a general rule, the pulse increases 20 beats per minute for each degree (°C) rise in fever.

When a person is very ill, take the pulse often and write it down along with the temperature and rate of breathing.

It is important to notice changes in the pulse rate. For example:

- A weak, rapid pulse can mean a state of shock (see p. 77).
- A very rapid, very slow, or irregular pulse could mean heart trouble (see p. 325).
- A relatively slow pulse in a person with a high fever may be a sign of typhoid (see p. 188).

EYES

Look at the color of the white part of the eyes. Is it normal, red (p. 219), or yellow? Also note any changes in the sick person's vision.

Have the person slowly move her eyes up and down and from side to side. Jerking or uneven movement may be a sign of brain damage.

Pay attention to the size of the ***pupils*** (the black 'window' in the center of the eye). If they are very large, it can mean a state of shock (see p. 77). If they are very large, or very small, it can mean poison or the effect of certain drugs.

Look at both eyes and note any difference between the two, especially in the size of the pupils:

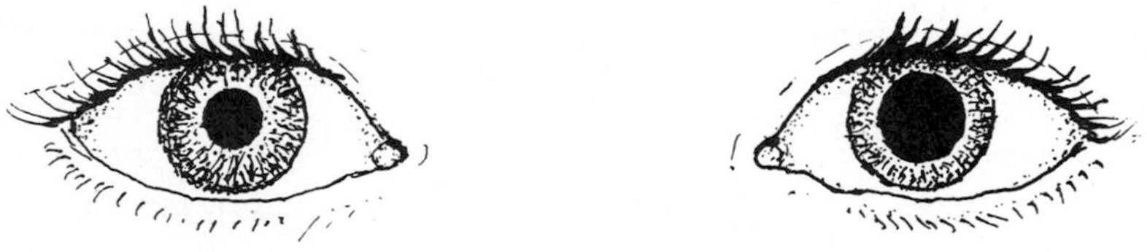

A big difference in the size of the pupils is almost always a medical emergency.

- If the eye with the larger pupil hurts so badly it causes vomiting, the person probably has GLAUCOMA (see p. 222).
- If the eye with the smaller pupil hurts a great deal, the person may have IRITIS, a very serious problem (see p. 221).
- Difference in the size of the pupils of an unconscious person or a person who has had a recent head injury may mean brain damage. It may also mean STROKE (see p. 327).

Always compare the pupils of a person who is unconscious or has had a head injury.

EARS, THROAT, AND NOSE

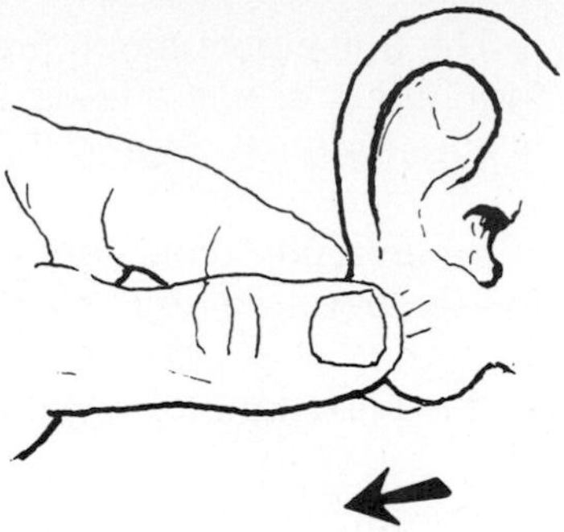

Ears: Always check for signs of pain and infection in the ears—especially in a child with fever or a cold. A baby who cries a lot or pulls at his ear often has an ear infection (p. 309).

Pull the ear gently. If this increases pain, the infection is probably in the tube of the ear (ear canal). Also look for redness or pus inside the ear. A small flashlight or penlight will help. But never put a stick, wire, or other hard object inside the ear.

Find out if the person hears well, or if one side is more deaf than the other. Rub your thumb and fingers together near the person's ear to see if he can hear it. For deafness and ringing of the ears see page 327.

Throat and Mouth: With a torch (flashlight) or sunlight examine the mouth and throat. To do this hold down tongue with a spoon handle or have the person say 'ahhhhh...' Notice if the throat is red and if the tonsils (2 lumps at the back of the throat) are swollen or have spots with pus (see p. 309). Also examine the mouth for sores, inflamed gums, sore tongue, rotten or abscessed teeth and other problems. (Read Chapter 17.)

Nose: Is the nose runny or plugged? (Notice if and how a baby breathes through his nose.) Shine a light inside and look for mucus, pus, blood; also look for redness, swelling, or bad smell. Check for signs of sinus trouble or hayfever (p. 165).

SKIN

It is important to examine the sick person's whole body, no matter how mild the sickness may seem. Babies and children should be undressed completely. Look carefully for anything that is not normal, including:

- sores, wounds, or splinters
- rashes or welts
- spots, patches, or any unusual markings
- *inflammation* (sign of infection with redness, heat, pain and swelling)
- swelling or puffiness
- swollen *lymph nodes* (little lumps in the neck, the armpits, or the groin, see p. 88)
- abnormal lumps or masses
- unusual thinning or loss of hair, or loss of its color or shine (p. 112)
- loss of eyebrows (leprosy? p. 191)

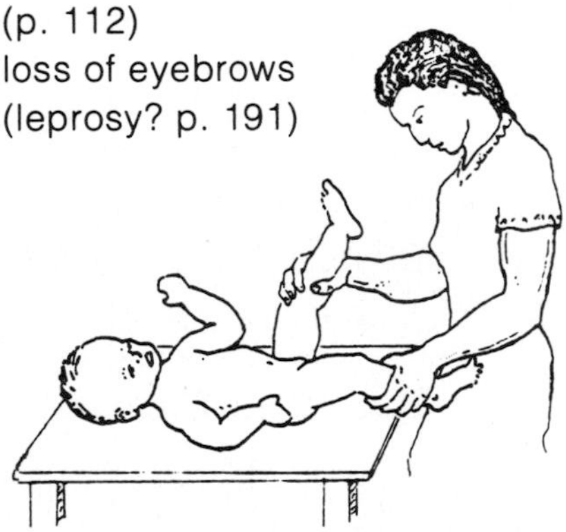

Always examine little children between the buttocks, in the genital area, between the fingers and toes, behind the ears, and in the hair (for lice, scabies, ringworm, rashes, and sores).

For identification of different skin problems, see pages 196–198.

THE BELLY (ABDOMEN)

If a person has pain in the belly, try to find out exactly where it hurts.

Learn whether the pain is steady or whether it suddenly comes and goes, like cramps or *colic.*

When you examine the belly, first look at it for any unusual swelling or lumps.

The location of the pain often gives a clue to the cause (see the following page).

First, ask the person to point with one finger where it hurts.

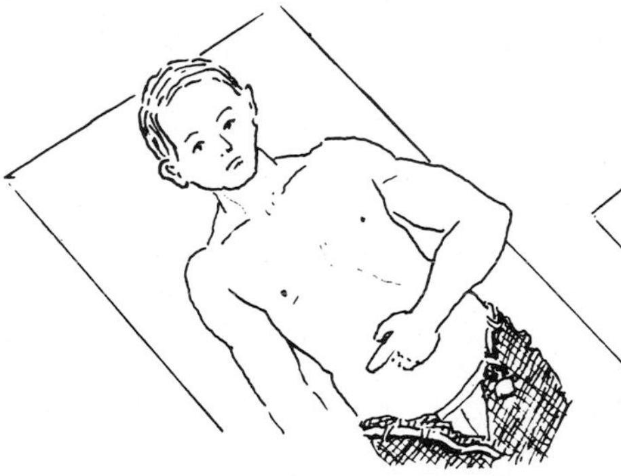

Then, beginning on the opposite side from the spot where he has pointed, press gently on different parts of the belly to see where it hurts most.

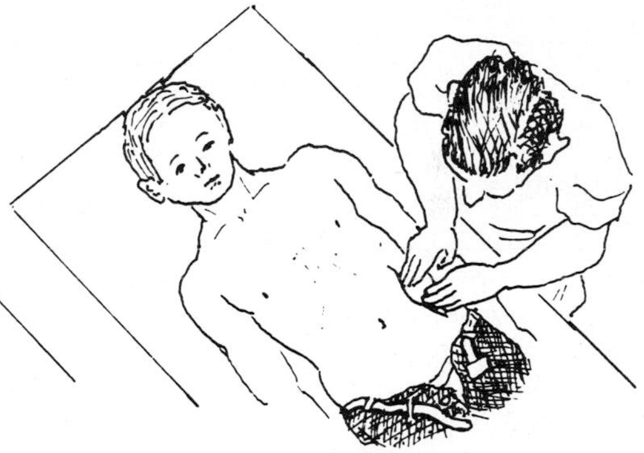

See if the belly is soft or hard and whether the person can relax his stomach muscles. A very hard belly could mean an acute abdomen—perhaps appendicitis or peritonitis (see p. 94).

If you suspect peritonitis or appendicitis, do the test for ***rebound pain*** described on page 95.

Feel for any abnormal lumps and hardened areas in the belly.

If the person has a constant pain in the stomach, with nausea, and has not been able to move her bowels, put an ear (or stethoscope) on the belly, like this:

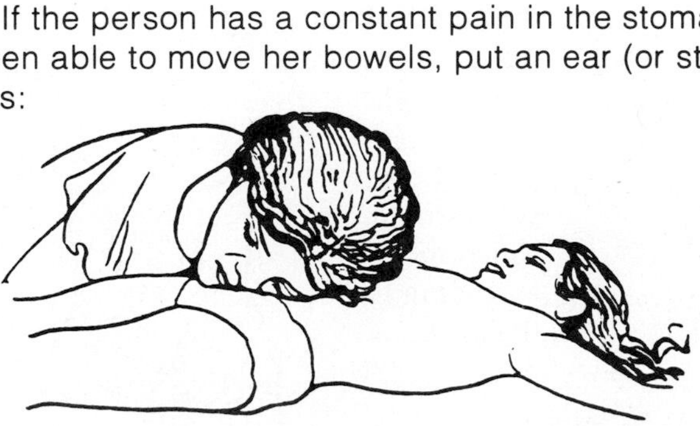

Listen for gurgles in the intestines. If you hear nothing after about 2 minutes, this is a danger sign. (See Emergency Problems of the Gut, p. 93.)

A silent belly is like a silent dog. Beware!

These pictures show the areas of the belly that usually hurt when a person has the following problems:

Ulcer
(see p. 128)

pain in the 'pit of the stomach'

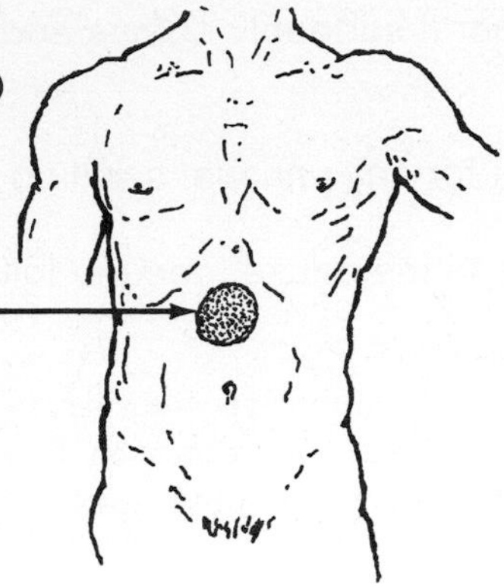

Appendicitis
(see p. 94)

first it hurts here

later it hurts here

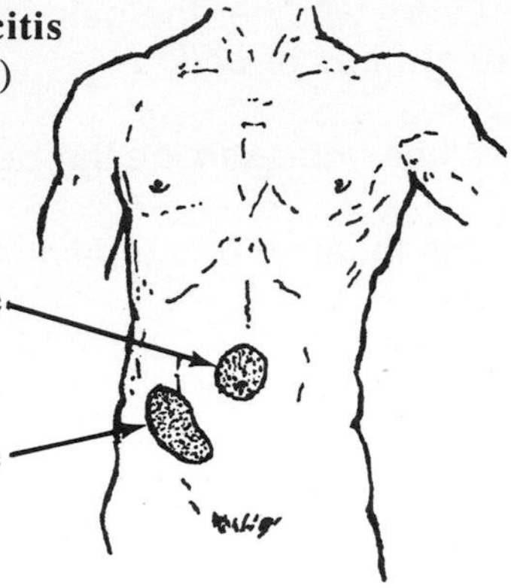

Gallbladder
(see p. 329)

the pain often reaches to the back

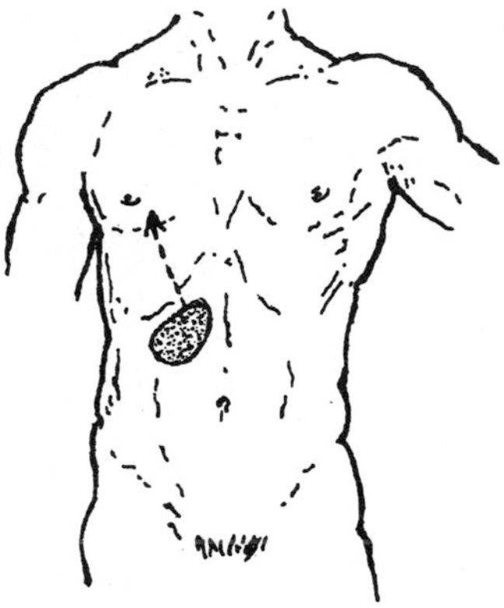

Liver
(see p. 172, 144, and 328)

pain here, at times it spreads to the chest

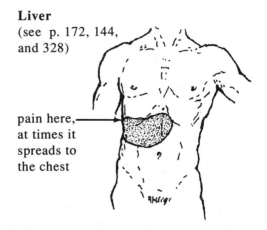

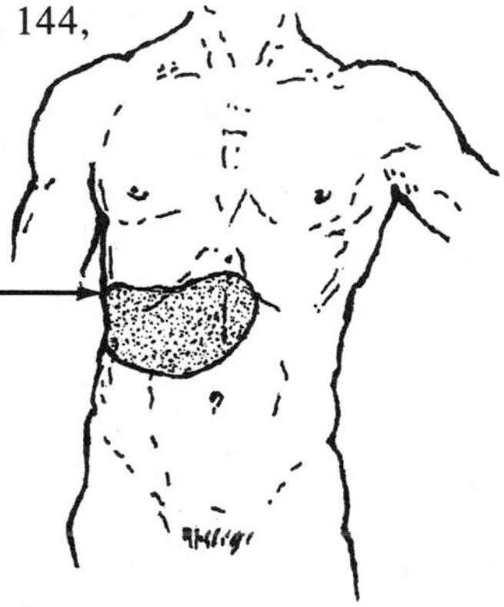

Urinary system
(see p. 234)

mid or low back pain; often goes around the waist to the lower part of the belly

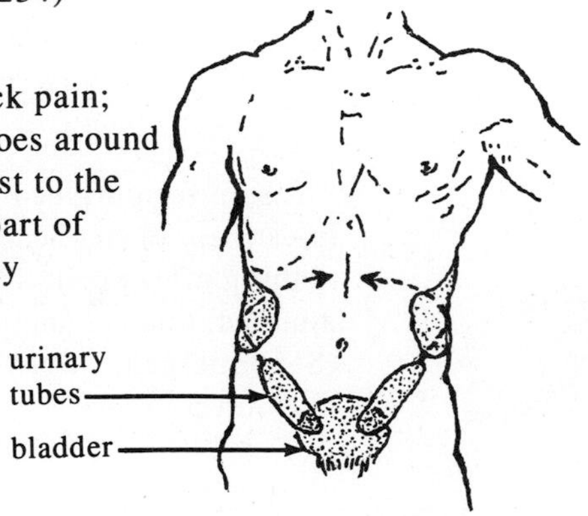

Inflammation or tumor of the ovaries, or out-of-place pregnancy , etc.
(see p. 280)

pain on one side or both, sometimes spreading to the back

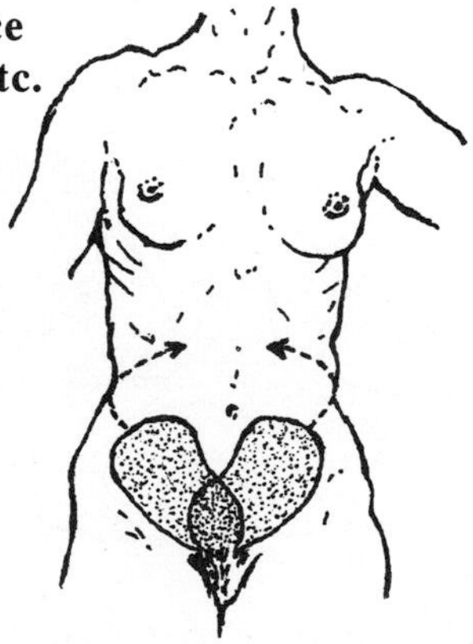

Note: For different causes of back pain see p. 173.

MUSCLES AND NERVES

If a person complains of numbness, weakness, or loss of control in part of his body, or you want to test it: notice the way he walks and moves. Have him stand, sit, or lie completely straight, and carefully compare both sides of his body.

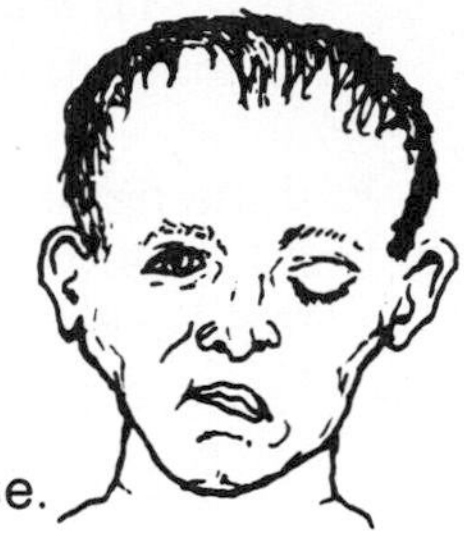

Face: Have him smile, frown, open his eyes wide, and squeeze them shut. Notice any drooping or weakness on one side.

If the problem began more or less suddenly, think of a head injury (p. 91), stroke (p. 327), or Bell's palsy (p. 327).

If it came slowly, it may be a brain tumor. Get medical advice.

Also check for normal eye movement, size of pupils (p. 217), and how well he can see.

Arms and legs: Look for loss of muscle. Notice—or measure—difference in thickness of arms or legs.

Have him squeeze your fingers to compare strength in his hands

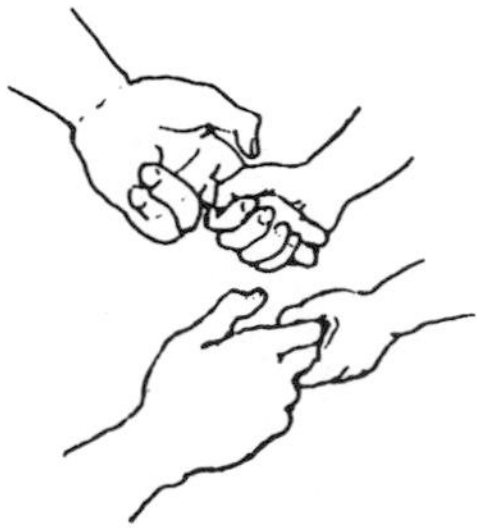

and push and pull with his feet against your hand.

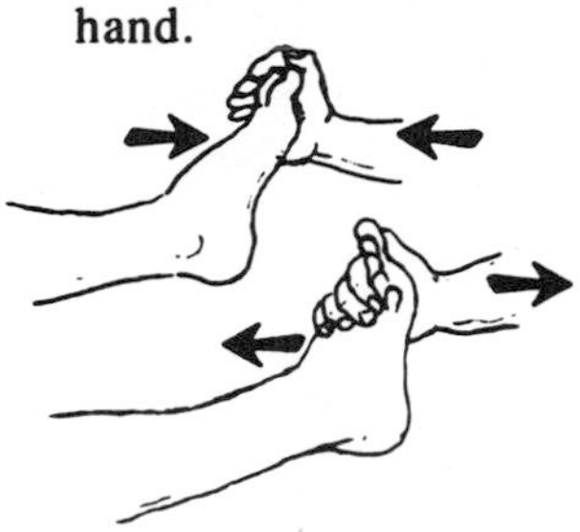

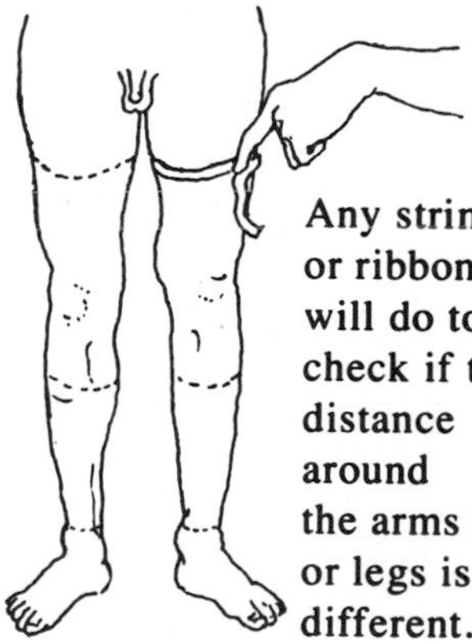

Any string or ribbon will do to check if the distance around the arms or legs is different.

Also have him hold his arms straight out and turn his hands up and down.

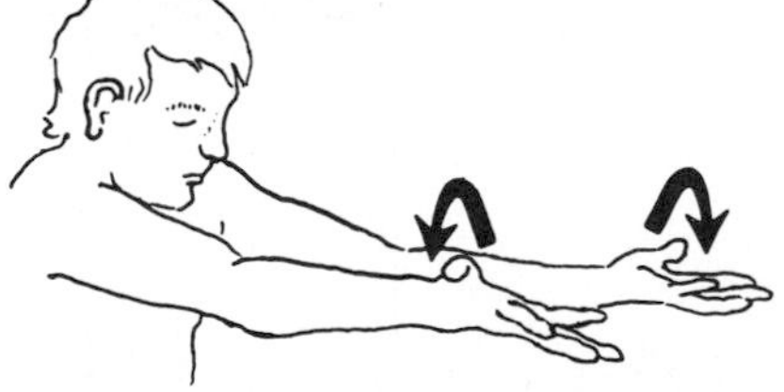

Note any weakness or trembling.

Have him lie down and lift one leg and then the other.

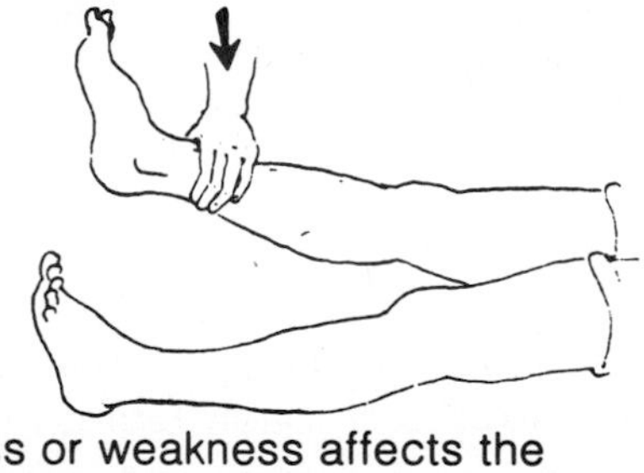

Watch how he moves and walks. If muscle loss or weakness affects the whole body, suspect malnutrition (p. 112) or a chronic (long-term) illness like tuberculosis.

If muscle loss and weakness is uneven or worse on one side, in children, think first of polio (p. 314); in adults, think of a back problem, a back or head injury, or stroke.

For more information on muscle testing and physical examination of disabled persons, see ***Disabled Village Children***, Chapter 4.

Check for stiffness or tightness of different muscles:

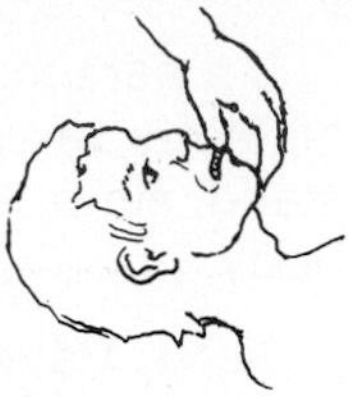

- If the jaw is stiff or will not open, suspect tetanus (p. 182) or a severe infection of the throat (p. 309) or of a tooth (p. 231). If the problem began after he yawned or was hit in the jaw, he may have a dislocated jaw.

- If the neck or back is stiff and bent backwards, in a very sick child, suspect meningitis. If the head will not bend forward or cannot be put between the knees, meningitis is likely (p. 185).

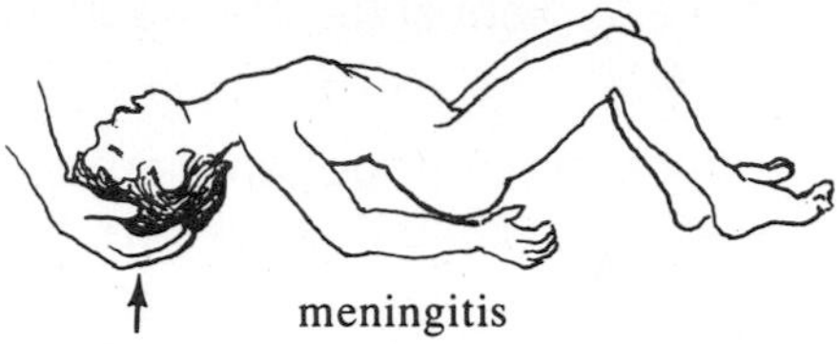

meningitis

- If a child **always** has some stiff muscles and makes strange or jerky movements, he may be ***spastic*** (p. 320).

- If strange or jerky movements come suddenly, with loss of consciousness, he may have fits (p. 178). If fits happen often, think of epilepsy. If they happen when he is ill, the cause may be high fever (p. 76) or dehydration (p. 151) or tetanus (p. 182) or meningitis (p. 185).

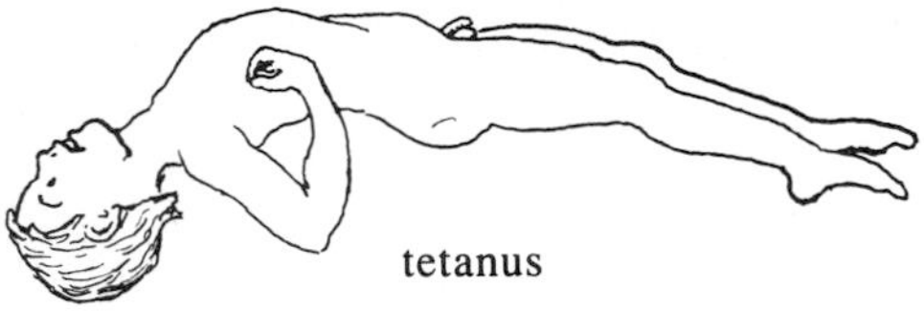

tetanus

To test a person's reflexes when you suspect tetanus, see p. 183.

To check for loss of feeling in the hands, feet, or other parts of the body:

Have the person cover his eyes. Lightly touch or prick the skin in different places. Ask him to say 'yes' when he feels it.

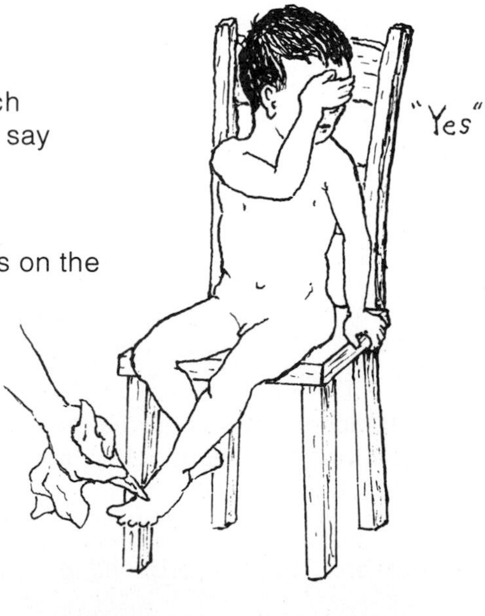

- Loss of feeling in or near spots or patches on the body is probably leprosy (p. 191).

- Loss of feeling in both hands or feet may be due to diabetes (p. 127) or leprosy.

- Loss of feeling on one side only could come from a back problem (p. 174) or injury.

CHAPTER 4

HOW TO TAKE CARE OF A SICK PERSON

Sickness weakens the body. To gain strength and get well quickly, special care is needed.

The care a sick person receives is frequently the most important part of his treatment.

Medicines are often not necessary. But good care is always important. The following are the basis of good care:

1. The Comfort of the Sick Person

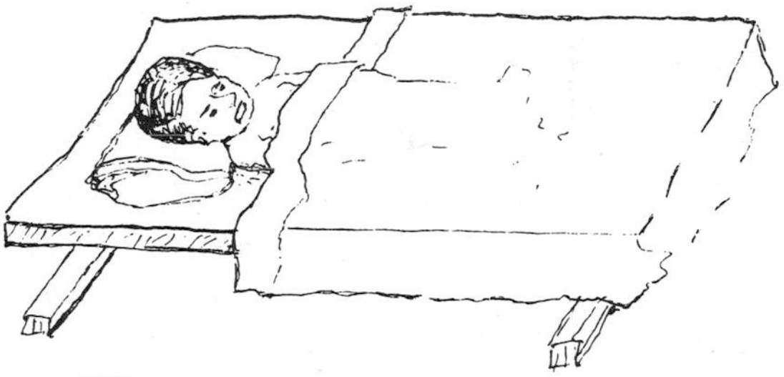

A person who is sick should rest in a quiet, comfortable place with plenty of fresh air and light. He should keep from getting too hot or cold. If the air is cold or the person is chilled, cover him with a sheet or blanket. But if the weather is hot or the person has a fever, do not cover him at all (see p. 75).

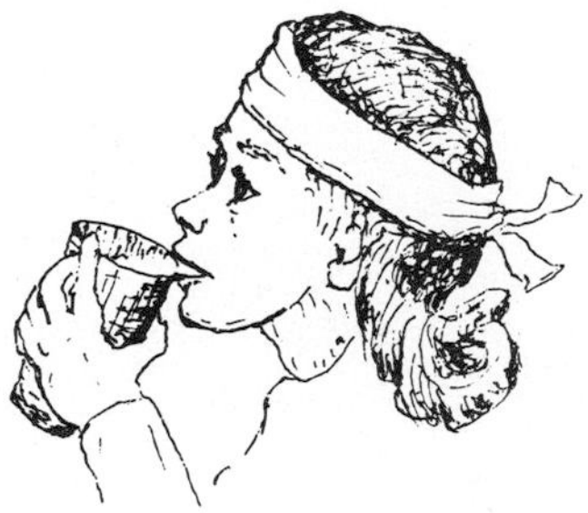

2. Liquids

In nearly every sickness, especially when there is fever or diarrhea, the sick person should drink plenty of liquids: water, tea, juices, broths, etc.

3. Personal Cleanliness

It is important to keep the sick person clean. He should be bathed every day. If he is too sick to get out of bed, wash him with a sponge or cloth and lukewarm water. His clothes, sheets, and covers must also be kept clean. Take care to keep crumbs and bits of food out of the bed.

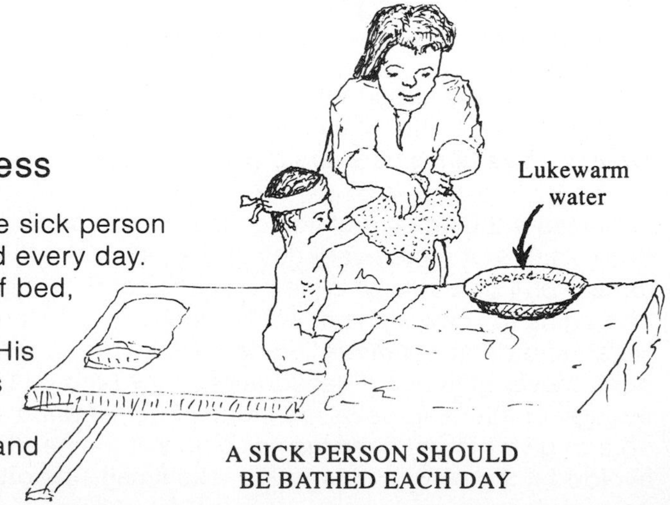

A SICK PERSON SHOULD BE BATHED EACH DAY

4. Good Food

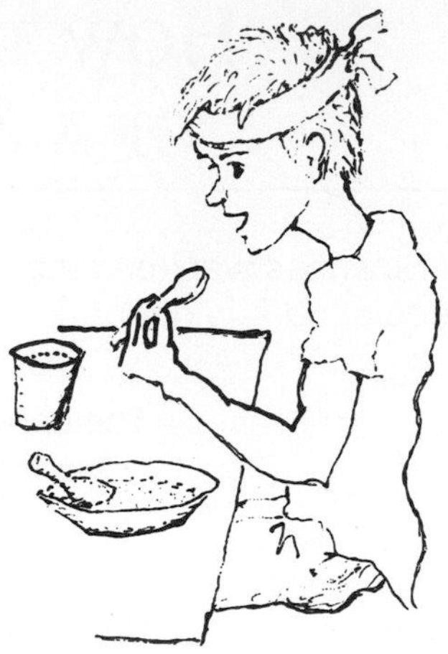

If the sick person feels like eating, let him. Most sicknesses do not require special diets.

A sick person should drink plenty of liquids and eat a lot of nourishing food (see Chapter 11).

If the person is very weak, give him as much nourishing food as he can eat, many times a day. If necessary, mash the foods, or make them into soups or juices.

Energy foods are especially important—for example, porridges of rice, wheat, oatmeal, potato, or cassava. Adding a little sugar and vegetable oil will increase the energy. Also encourage the sick person to drink plenty of sweetened drinks, especially if he will not eat much.

A few problems do require special diets. These are explained on the following pages:

stomach ulcers and heartburn . . . . .p. 128
appendicitis, gut obstruction, acute abdomen
(in these cases take no food at all) p. 93
diabetes . . . . .p. 127
heart problems .p. 325
gallbladder problems . . . . .p. 329

SPECIAL CARE FOR A PERSON WHO IS VERY ILL

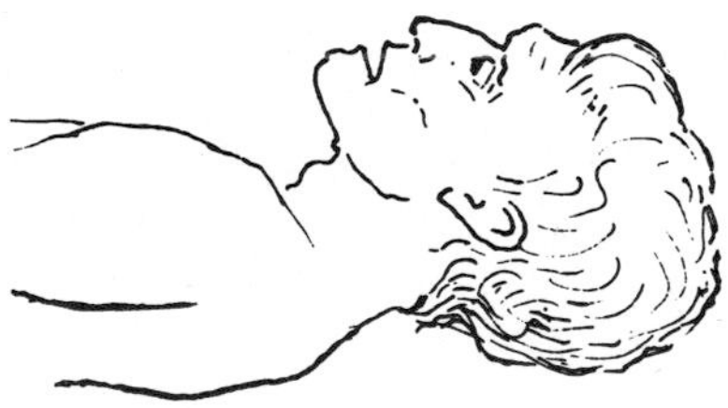

1. Liquids

It is extremely important that a very sick person drink enough liquid. If he only can drink a little at a time, give him small amounts often. If he can barely swallow, give him sips every 5 or 10 minutes.

Measure the amount of liquids the person drinks each day. An adult needs to drink 2 liters or more every day and should urinate at least a cup (60 cc.) of urine 3 or 4 times daily. If the person is not drinking or urinating enough, or if he begins to show signs of dehydration (p. 151), encourage him to drink more. He should drink ***nutritious*** liquids, usually with a little salt added. If he will not drink these, give him a Rehydration Drink (see p. 152). If he cannot drink enough of this, and develops signs of ***dehydration,*** a health worker may be able to give him ***intravenous solution.*** But the need for this can usually be avoided if the person is urged to take small sips often.

2. Food

If the person is too sick to eat solid foods, give her soups, milk, juices, broths, and other nutritious liquids (see Chapter 11). A porridge of cornmeal, oatmeal, or rice is also good, but should be given together with body-building foods. Soups can be made with egg, beans, or well-chopped meat, fish, or chicken. If the person can eat only a little at a time, she should eat several small meals each day.

3. Cleanliness

Personal cleanliness is very important for a seriously ill person. She should be bathed every day with warm water.

Change the bed clothes daily and each time they become dirty. Soiled or bloodstained clothes, bedding, and towels of a person with an infectious disease should be handled with care. To kill any viruses or germs, wash these in hot soapy water, or add some chlorine bleach.

4. Changing Position in Bed

A person who is very weak and cannot turn over alone should be helped to change position in bed many times each day. This helps prevent bed sores (see p. 214).

A child who is sick for a long time should be held often on her mother's lap.

Frequent changing of the person's position also helps to prevent pneumonia, a constant danger for anyone who is very weak or ill and must stay in bed for a long time. If the person has a fever, begins to cough, and breathes with fast, shallow breaths, she probably has pneumonia (see p. 171).

5. Watching for Changes

You should watch for any change in the sick person's condition that may tell you whether he is getting better or worse. Keep a record of his 'vital signs'. Write down the following facts 4 times a day:

temperature
(how many degrees)

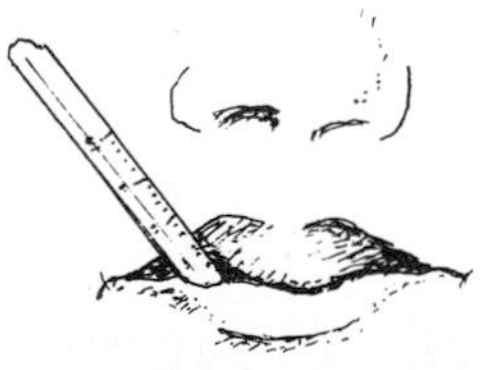

pulse
(beats per minute)

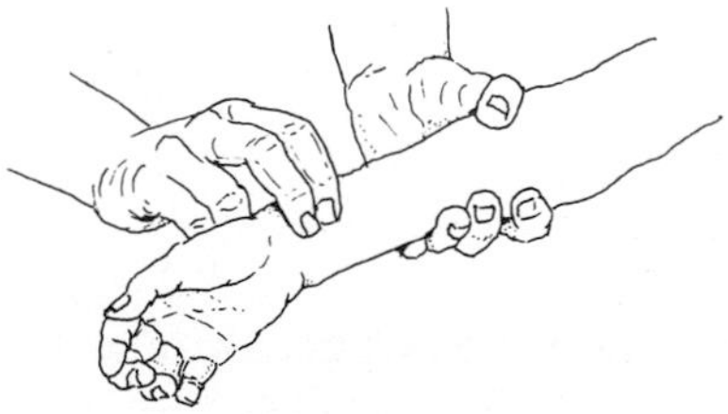

breathing
(breaths per minute)

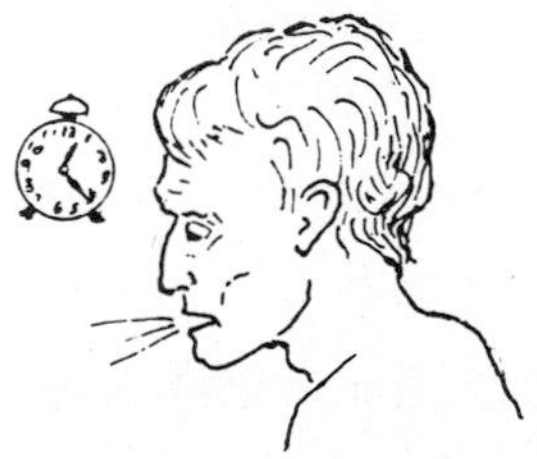

Also write down the amount of liquids the person drinks and how many times a day he urinates and has a bowel movement. Save this information for the health worker or doctor.

It is very important to look for signs that warn you that the person's sickness is serious or dangerous. A list of **Signs of Dangerous Illness** is on the next page. If the person shows any of these signs, **seek medical help immediately**.

SIGNS OF DANGEROUS ILLNESS

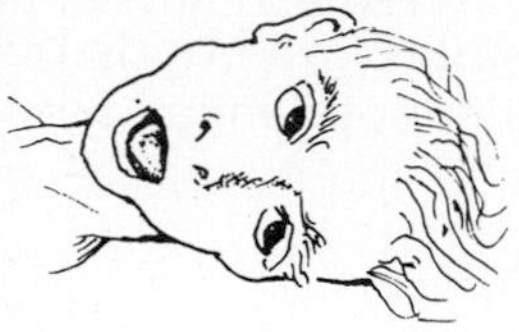

A person who has one or more of the following signs is probably too sick to be treated at home without skilled medical help. His life may be in danger. **Seek medical help as soon as possible.** Until help comes, follow the instructions on the pages indicated.

	page
1. Loss of large amounts of blood from anywhere in the body	82, 264, 281
2. Coughing up blood	179
3. Marked blueness of lips and nails (if it is new)	30
4. Great difficulty in breathing; does not improve with rest	167, 325
5. The person cannot be wakened (coma)	78
6. The person is so weak he faints when he stands up	325
7. A day or more without being able to urinate	234
8. A day or more without being able to drink any liquids	151
9. Heavy vomiting or severe diarrhea that lasts for more than one day or more than a few hours in babies	151
10. Black stools like tar, or vomit with blood or feces	128
11. Strong, continuous stomach pains with vomiting in a person who does not have diarrhea or cannot have a bowel movement	93
12. Any strong continuous pain that lasts for more than 3 days	29 to 38
13. Stiff neck with arched back, with or without a stiff jaw	182, 185
14. More than one fit (convulsions) in someone with fever or serious illness	76, 185
15. High fever (above 39°C) that cannot be brought down or that lasts more than 4 or 5 days	75
16. Weight loss over an extended time	20, 400
17. Blood in the urine	146, 234
18. Sores that keep growing and do not go away with treatment	191, 196, 211, 212
19. A lump in any part of the body that keeps getting bigger	196, 280
20. Problems with pregnancy and childbirth:	
any bleeding during pregnancy	249, 281
swollen face and trouble seeing in the last months	249
long delay once the waters have broken and labor has begun	267
severe bleeding	264

WHEN AND HOW TO LOOK FOR MEDICAL HELP

Seek medical help at the first sign of a dangerous illness. Do not wait until the person is so sick that it becomes difficult or impossible to take him to a health center or hospital.

If a sick or injured person's condition could be made worse by the difficulties in moving him to a health center, try to bring a health worker to the person. But in an emergency when very special attention or an operation may be needed (for example, appendicitis), do not wait for the health worker. Take the person to the health center or the hospital at once.

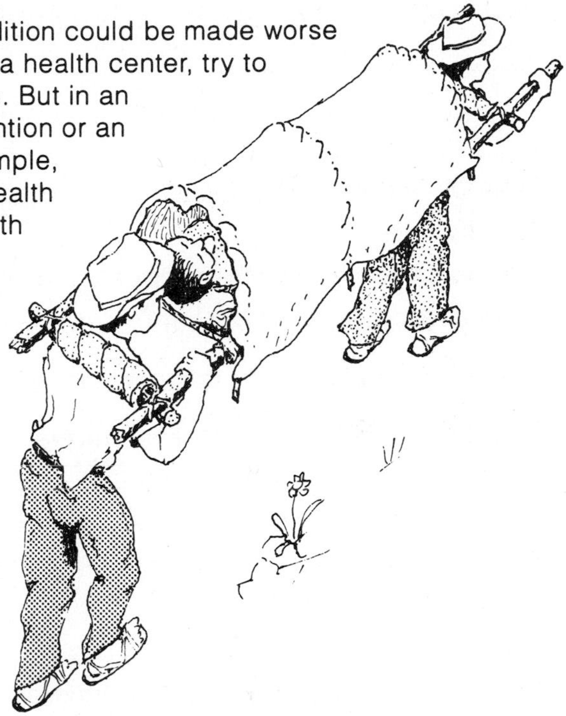

When you need to carry a person on a stretcher, make sure he is as comfortable as possible and cannot fall out. If he has any broken bones, splint them before moving him (see p. 99). If the sun is very strong, rig a sheet over the stretcher to give shade yet allow fresh air to pass underneath

WHAT TO TELL THE HEALTH WORKER

For a health worker or doctor to recommend treatment or prescribe medicine wisely, she should see the sick person. If the sick person cannot be moved, have the health worker come to him. If this is not possible, send a responsible person who knows the details of the illness. **Never send a small child or a fool.**

Before sending for medical help, examine the sick person carefully and completely. Then write down the details of his disease and general condition (see Chapter 3).

On the next page is a form on which you can make a PATIENT REPORT. Several copies of this form are at the end of this book. Tear out one of these forms and carefully complete the report, giving all the details you can.

When you send someone for medical help, always send a completed information form with him.

PATIENT REPORT

TO USE WHEN SENDING FOR MEDICAL HELP

Name of the sick person:______________________________Age:______

Male _____Female_____ Where is he (she)? ________________________

What is the main sickness or problem right now? __________________

____

____

____

When did it begin?____

How did it begin? ____

Has the person had the same problem before? _______ When? __________

Is there fever? _______How high? ______° When and for how long? __________

Pain?_________Where?____________________ What kind? ____________

What is wrong or different from normal in any of the following?

Skin: ________________________ **Ears:** ________________________

Eyes:________________________ **Mouth and throat:**________________

Genitals:____

Urine: Much or little?___________ Color?___________ Trouble urinating?_____

Describe: ____________________ Times in 24 hours:______ Times at night: ____

Stools: Color?____________ Blood or mucus?____________ Diarrhea?_______

Number of times a day:_______ Cramps?________ Dehydration?________ Mild or severe?_____________ Worms?_________ What kind? ______________

Breathing: Breaths per minute:________Deep, shallow, or normal? __________

Difficulty breathing (describe):__________________ Cough (describe): _______

_________________Wheezing?_________ Mucus?__________ With blood?_____

Does the person have any of the SIGNS OF DANGEROUS ILLNESS listed on page 42?________ Which? (give details)____________________________

____

Other signs: ____

Is the person taking medicine?________ What? _______________________

Has the person ever used medicine that has caused a rash, hives (or bumps) with itching, or other allergic reactions?________ What? _______________

The state of the sick person is: Not very serious:___________ Serious: _______

Very serious:________________

CHAPTER

5

HEALING WITHOUT MEDICINES

For most sicknesses no medicines are needed. Our bodies have their own defenses, or ways to resist and fight disease. In most cases, these natural defenses are far more important to our health than are medicines.

People will get well from most sicknesses —including the common cold and 'flu' — by themselves, without need for medicines.

To help the body fight off or overcome a sickness, often all that is needed is to:

keep clean

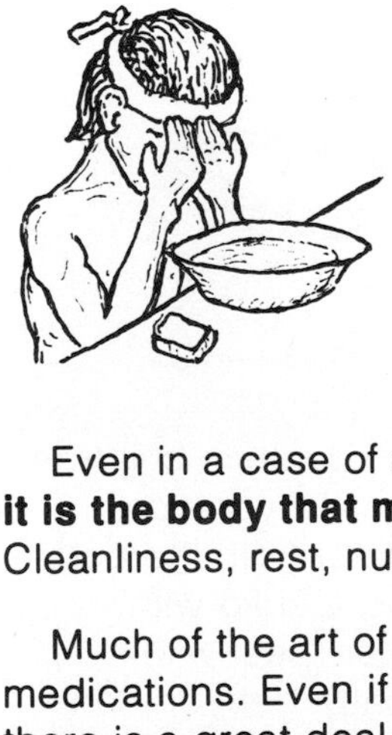

get plenty of rest

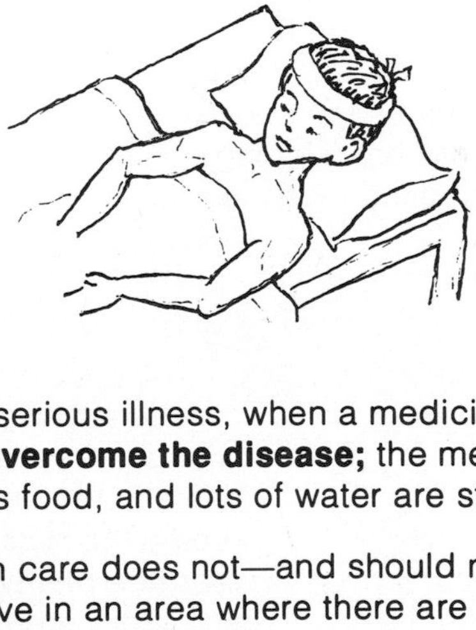

eat well and drink a lot of liquid

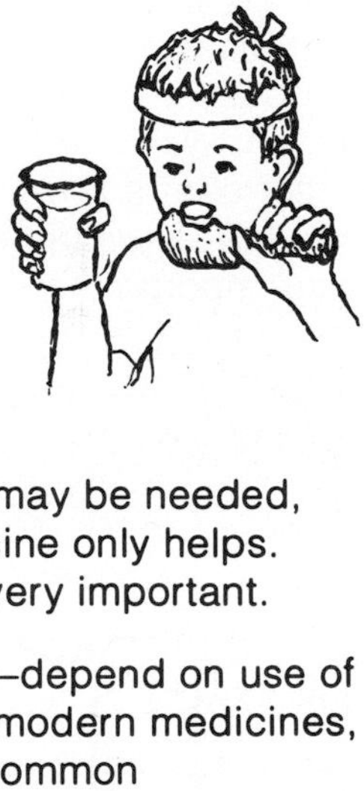

Even in a case of more serious illness, when a medicine may be needed, **it is the body that must overcome the disease;** the medicine only helps. Cleanliness, rest, nutritious food, and lots of water are still very important.

Much of the art of health care does not—and should not—depend on use of medications. Even if you live in an area where there are no modern medicines, there is a great deal you can do to prevent and treat most common sicknesses—if you learn how.

Many sicknesses can be prevented or treated without medicines.

If people simply learned how to use **water** correctly, this alone might do more to prevent and cure illnesses than all the medicines they now use . . . and misuse.

HEALING WITH WATER

Most of us could live without medicines. But no one can live without water. In fact, over half (57%) of the human body is water. If everyone living in farms and villages made the best use of water, the amount of sickness and death —especially of children—could be reduced.

For example, correct use of water is basic both in the prevention and treatment of diarrhea. In many areas diarrhea is the most common cause of sickness and death in small children. ***Contaminated*** (unclean) water is often part of the cause.

An important part of the prevention of diarrhea and many other illnesses is to make sure that drinking water is safe. Protect wells and springs from dirt and animals by putting fences or walls around them. Use cement or rock to provide good drainage around the well or spring, so that rain or spilled water runs away from it.

Where water may be contaminated, an important part of the prevention of diarrhea is to boil or filter the water used for drinking or for preparing foods. This is especially important for babies. Babies' bottles and eating utensils should also be boiled. If regular boiling of bottles is not possible, it is safer to use a cup and spoon. Washing hands with soap and water after a bowel movement (shitting) and before eating or handling foods is also important.

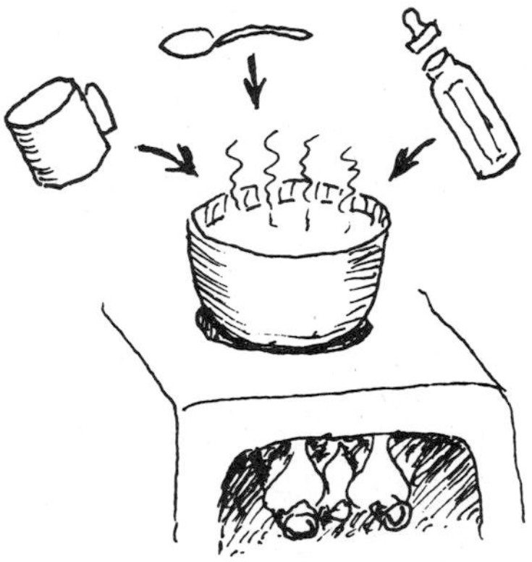

PREVENTION

TREATMENT

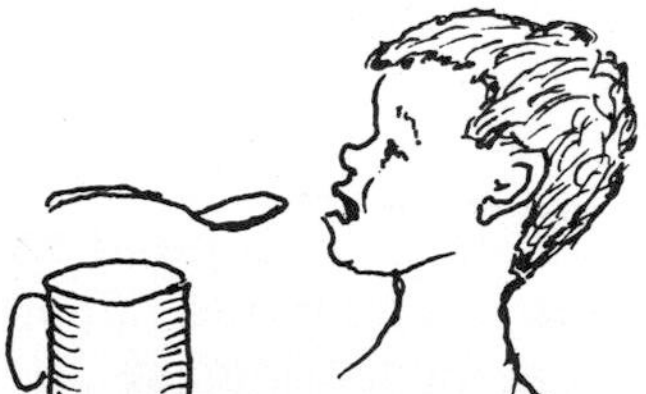

A common cause of death in children with diarrhea is severe ***dehydration,*** or loss of too much water from the body (see p. 151). By giving a child with diarrhea plenty of water (best with sugar or cereal and salt), dehydration can often be prevented or corrected (see Rehydration Drink, p. 152).

Giving lots of liquids to a child with diarrhea is more important than any medicine. In fact, if enough liquid is given, no medicine is usually needed in the treatment of diarrhea.

On the next 2 pages are a number of other situations in which **it is often more important to use water correctly than to use medicines.**

Times When the Right Use of Water May Do More Good than Medicines

PREVENTION

to help prevent	use water	see page
1. diarrhea, worms, gut infections	boil or filter drinking water, wash hands, etc.	135
2. skin infections	bathe often	133
3. wounds becoming infected; tetanus	wash wounds well with soap and clean water	84, 89

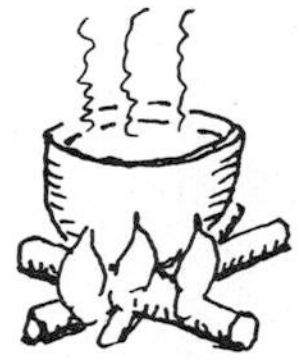

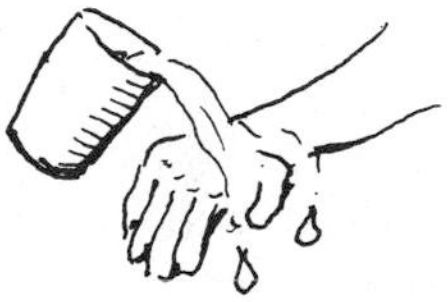

TREATMENT

to treat	use water	see page
1. diarrhea, dehydration	drink plenty of liquids	152
2. illnesses with fever	drink plenty of liquids	75
3. high fever	remove clothing and soak body with cool water	76
4. minor urinary infections (common in women)	drink plenty of water	235
5. cough, asthma, bronchitis, pneumonia, whooping cough	drink a lot of water and breathe hot water vapors (to loosen mucus)	168

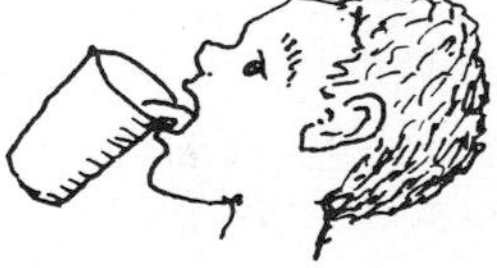

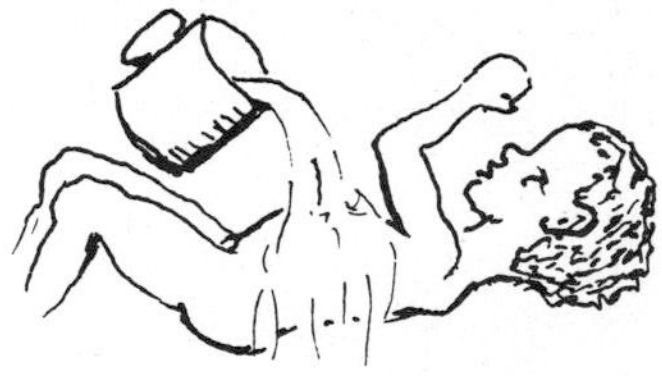

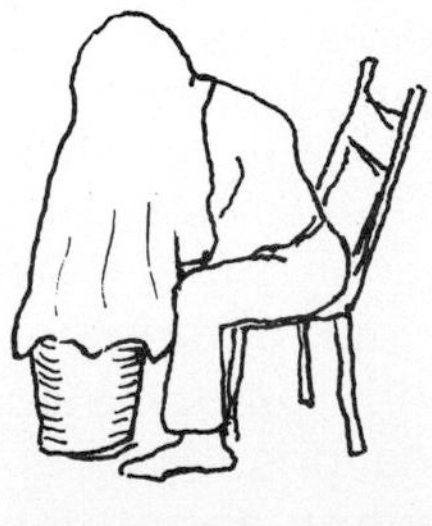

to treat	use water	see page	
6. sores, impetigo, ringworm of skin or scalp, cradle cap, pimples	scrub with soap and clean water	201, 202, 205, 211, 215	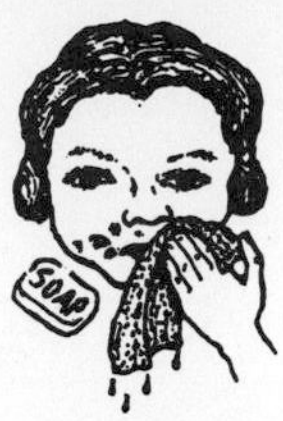
7. infected wounds, abscesses, boils	hot soaks or compresses	88, 202	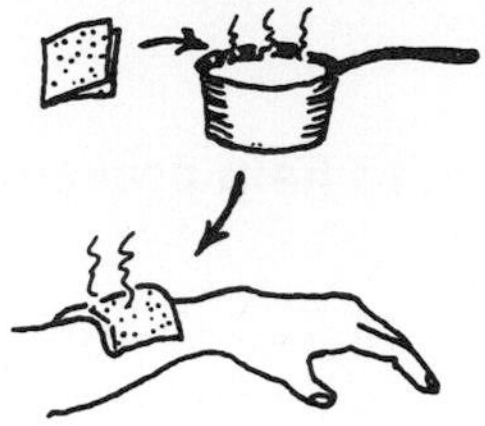
8. stiff, sore muscles and joints	hot compresses	102, 173, 174	
9. strains and sprains	the first day: soak joint in cold water; then use hot soaks	102	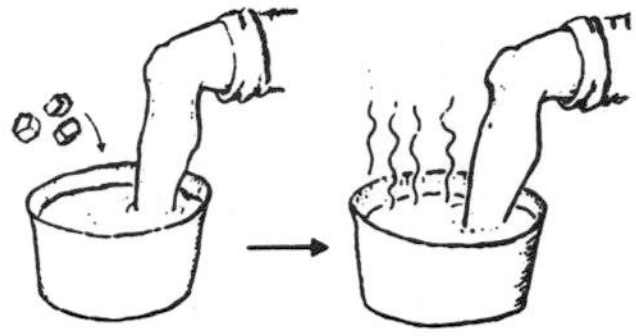
10. itching, burning, or weeping irritations of the skin	cold compresses	193, 194	
11. minor burns	hold in cold water at once	96	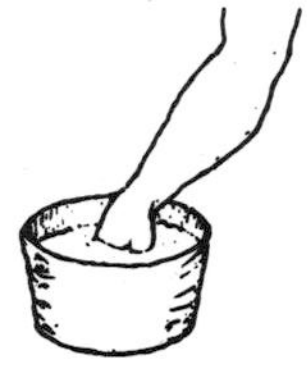
12. sore throat or tonsillitis	gargle with warm salt water	309	
13. acid, lye, dirt, or irritating substance in eye	flood eye with cool water at once, and continue for 30 minutes	219	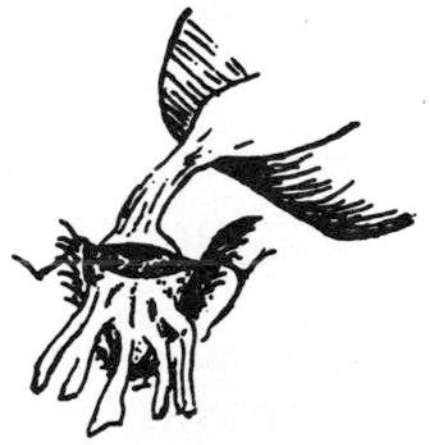
14. stuffed up nose	sniff salt water	164	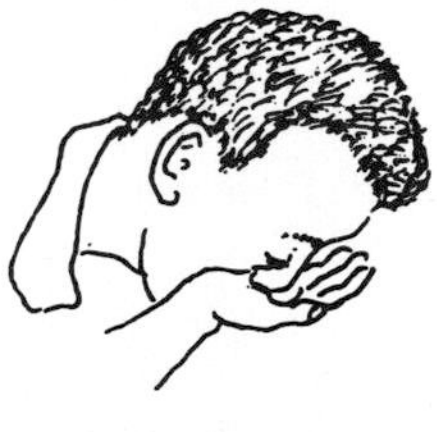
15. constipation, hard stools	drink lots of water (also, enemas are safer than laxatives, but do not overuse)	15, 126	
16. cold sores or fever blisters	hold ice on blister for 1 hr. at first sign	232	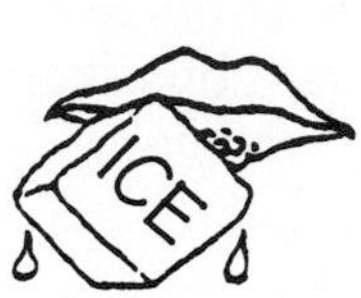

In each of the above cases (except pneumonia) when water is used correctly, often medicines are not needed. In this book you will find many suggestions for ways of healing without need for medicine. **Use medicines only when absolutely necessary.**

CHAPTER 6

RIGHT AND WRONG USES OF MODERN MEDICINES

Some medicines sold in pharmacies or village stores can be very useful. But many are of no value. Of the 60,000 medicines sold in most countries, the World Health Organization says that only about 200 are necessary.

Also, people sometimes use the best medicines in the wrong way, so that they do more harm than good. **To be helpful, medicine must be used correctly.**

Many people, including most doctors and health workers, prescribe far more medicines than are needed—and by so doing cause much needless sickness and death.

There is some danger in the use of any medicine.

Some medicines are much more dangerous than others. Unfortunately, people sometimes use very dangerous medicines for mild sicknesses. (I have seen a baby die because his mother gave him a dangerous medicine, chloramphenicol, for a cold.) **Never use a dangerous medicine for a mild illness.**

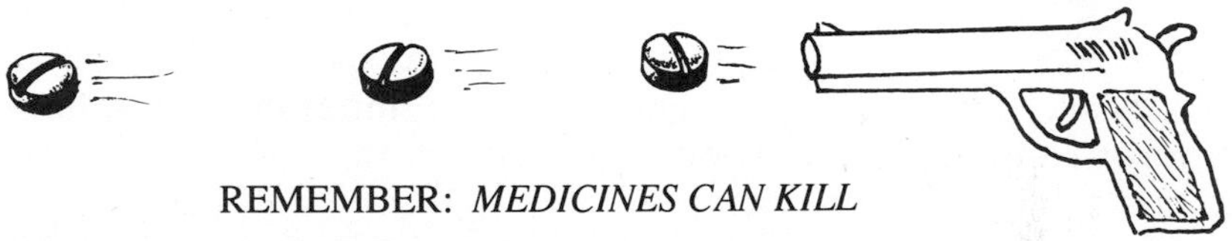

REMEMBER: *MEDICINES CAN KILL*

Guidelines for the use of medicine:

1. Use medicines only when necessary.
2. Know the correct use and precautions for any medicine you use (see the GREEN PAGES).
3. Be sure to use the right dose.
4. If the medicine does not help, or causes problems, stop using it.
5. When in doubt, seek the advice of a health worker.

Note: Some health workers and many doctors give medicines when none is needed, often because they think patients expect medicine and will not be satisfied until they get some. Tell your doctor or health worker you only want medicine if it is definitely needed. This will save you money and be safer for your health.

Only use a medicine when you are sure it is needed and when you are sure how to use it.

THE MOST DANGEROUS MISUSE OF MEDICINE

Here is a list of the most common and dangerous errors people make in using modern medicines. The improper use of the following medicines causes many deaths each year. BE CAREFUL!

1. Chloramphenicol *(Chloromycetin)* (p. 357)

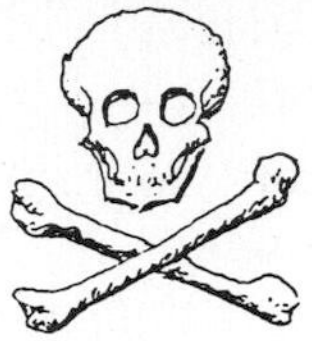

The popular use of this medicine for simple diarrhea and other mild sicknesses is extremely unfortunate, because it is so risky. Use chloramphenicol only for very severe illnesses, like typhoid (see p. 188). Never give it to newborn babies.

2. Oxytocin *(Pitocin)*, **Pituitrin, and Ergonovine** *(Ergotrate)* (p. 391)

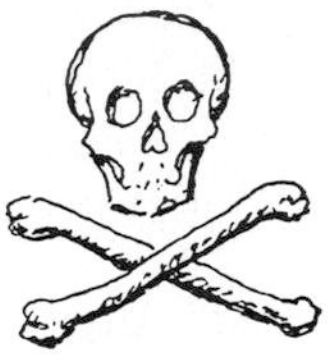

Unfortunately, some midwives use these medicines to speed up childbirth or 'give strength' to the mother in labor. This practice is very dangerous. It can kill the mother or the child. Use these medicines **only** to control bleeding **after** the child is born (see p. 266).

3. Injections of any medicine

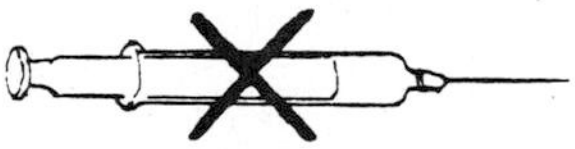

The common belief that injections are usually better than medicine taken by mouth is **not** true. Many times medicines taken by mouth work as well as or better than injections. Also, **most medicine is more dangerous injected than when taken by mouth.** Injections given to a child who has a mild polio infection (with only signs of a cold) can lead to paralysis (see p. 74). Use of injections should be **very limited** (read Chapter 9 carefully).

4. Penicillin (p. 351)

Penicillin works only against certain types of *infections.* Use of penicillin for sprains, bruises, or any pain or fever is a great mistake. As a general rule, injuries that do not break the skin, even if they make large bruises, have no danger of infection; they do not need to be treated with penicillin or any other antibiotic. Neither penicillin nor other antibiotics helps colds (see p. 163).

Penicillin is dangerous for some people. Before using it, know its risks and the precautions you must take—see pages 70 and 351.

5. Kanamycin and Gentamicin *(Garamycin)* (p. 359)

Too much use of these antibiotics for babies has caused permanent hearing loss (deafness) in millions of babies. Give to babies only for life-threatening infections. For many infections of the newborn, ampicillin works as well and is much less dangerous.

6. Anti-diarrhea medicines with hydroxyquinolines (Clioquinol, di-iodohydroxyquinoline, halquinol, broxyquinoline: *Diodoquin, Enteroquinol, Amicline, Quogyl,* and many other brand names) (p. 370)

In the past **clioquinols** were widely used to treat diarrhea. These dangerous medicines are now prohibited in many countries—but in others are still sold. They can cause permanent paralysis, blindness, and even death. For treatment of diarrhea, see Chapter 13.

7. Cortisone and cortico-steroids (Prednisolone, dexamethasone, and others)

These are powerful anti-inflammatory drugs that are occasionally needed for severe attacks of asthma, arthritis, or severe allergic reactions. But in many countries, steroids are prescribed for minor aches and pains because they often give quick results. This is a big mistake. Steroids cause serious or dangerous side effects—especially if used in high doses or for more than a few days. They lower a person's defenses against infection. They can make tuberculosis much worse, cause bleeding of stomach ulcers, and make bones so weak that they break easily.

8. Anabolic steroids (Nandrolone decanoate, *Durabolin, Deca-Durabolin, Orabolin;* **stanozolol,** *Cetabon;* **oxymetholone,** *Anapolon;* **ethylestrenol,** *Organaboral.* There are many other brand names.)

Anabolic steroids are made from male hormones and are mistakenly used in tonics to help children gain weight and grow. At first the child may grow faster, but he will stop growing sooner and end up shorter than he would have if he had not taken the medicine. Anabolic steroids cause very dangerous side effects. Girls grow hair on their faces like boys, which does not go away, even when the child stops taking the medicine. **Do not give growth tonics to children.** Instead, to help your child grow, use the money to buy food.

9. Arthritis medicines (Butazones: oxyphenbutazone, *Amidozone;* **and phenylbutazone,** *Butazolidin)*

These medicines for joint pain (arthritis) can cause a dangerous, sometimes deadly, blood disease (agranulocytosis). They can also damage the stomach, liver, and kidneys. **Do not use these dangerous medicines.** For arthritis, aspirin (p. 379) or ibuprofen (p. 380) is much safer and cheaper. For pain and fever only, acetaminophen (p. 380) can be used.

10. Vitamin B_{12}, liver extract, and iron injections (p. 393)

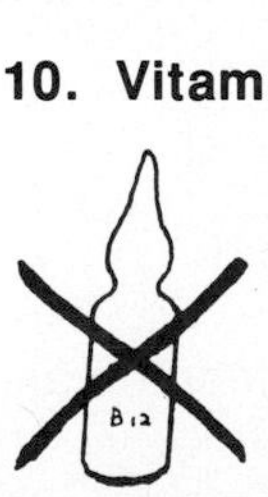

Vitamin B_{12} and liver extract do not help anemia or 'weakness' except in rare cases. Also, they have certain risks when injected. They should only be used when a specialist has prescribed them **after testing the blood.** Also, avoid injectable iron, such as *Inferon.* To combat anemia, iron pills are safer and work as well (see p. 124).

11. Other vitamins (p. 392)

As a general rule, DO NOT INJECT VITAMINS. Injections are more dangerous, more expensive, and usually no more effective than pills.

Unfortunately, many people waste their money on syrups, tonics, and 'elixirs' that contain vitamins. Many lack the most important vitamins (see p. 118). But even when they contain them, it is wiser to buy more and better food. Body-building and protective foods like beans, eggs, meat, fruit, vegetables, and whole grains are rich in vitamins and other nutrients (see p. 111). Giving a thin, weak person good food more often will usually help him far more than giving him vitamin and mineral supplements.

A person who eats well does not need extra vitamins.

THE BEST WAY TO GET VITAMINS:

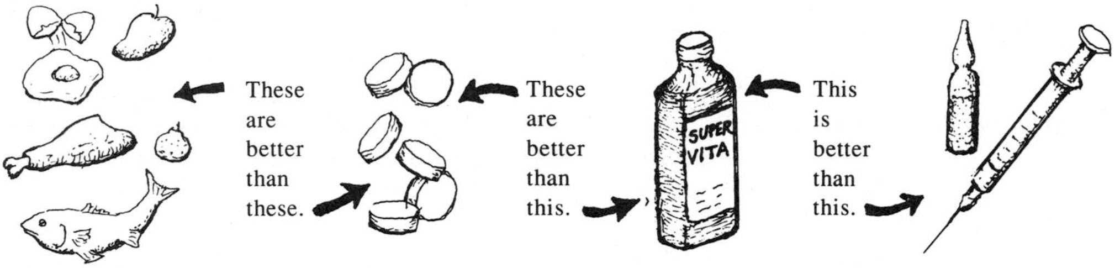
These are better than these.
These are better than this.
SUPER VITA
This is better than this.

For more information about vitamins, when they are necessary, and the foods that have them, read Chapter 11, especially pages 111 and 118.

12. Combination medicines

Sometimes, 2 or more medicines are combined in the same pill or tonic. Usually they are less effective, and more expensive, when prepared this way. Sometimes **they do more harm than good.** If someone wants to prescribe combination medicines, ask him or her to prescribe only the medicine that is really necessary. Do not waste your money on these medicines.

Some common combination medicines that should be **avoided** are:

- **cough medicines** which contain medicines both to suppress a cough and also to get rid of mucus. (Cough medicines are almost always useless and a waste of money, whether or not they combine medicines.)
- **antibiotics** combined with **anti–diarrhea medicine**
- **antacids** to treat stomach ulcers together with medicine to prevent stomach cramps
- 2 or more **pain medicines** (aspirin with acetaminophen—sometimes also with caffeine)

13. Calcium

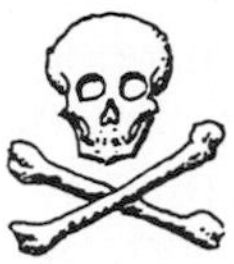

Injecting calcium into a vein can be extremely dangerous. It can quickly kill someone if not injected **very slowly.** Injecting calcium into the buttocks sometimes causes very serious abscesses or infections.

Never inject calcium without first seeking medical advice!

Note: In Mexico and other countries where people eat a lot of corn tortillas or other foods prepared with lime, it is foolish to use calcium injections or tonics (as is often done to 'give strength' or 'help children grow'). The body gets all the calcium it needs from the lime.

14. 'Feeding' through the veins (Intravenous or 'I.V.' solutions)

In some areas, persons who are anemic or very weak spend their last penny to have a liter of I.V. solution put into their veins. They believe that this will make them stronger or their blood richer. But they are wrong! Intravenous solution is nothing more than pure water with some salt or sugar in it. It gives less energy than a large candy bar and makes the blood thinner, not richer. It does not help anemia or make the weak person stronger.

Also when a person who is not well trained puts the I.V. solution into a vein, there is danger of an infection entering the blood. This can kill the sick person.

Intravenous solution should be used only when a person can take nothing by mouth, or when she is badly dehydrated (see p. 151).

If the sick person can swallow, give her a liter of water with sugar (or cereal) and salt (see Rehydration Drink, p. 152). It will do as much for her as injecting a liter of I.V. solution. For people who are able to eat, nutritious foods do more to strengthen them than any type of I.V. fluid.

If a sick person is able to swallow and keep down liquids . . .

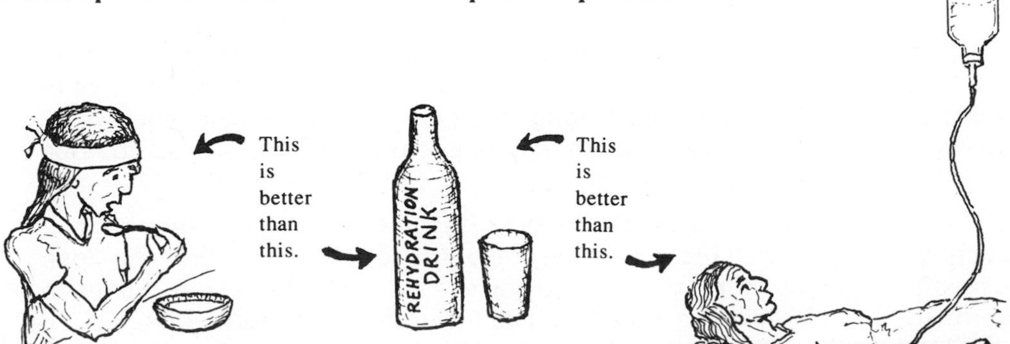

This is better than this.
REHYDRATION DRINK
This is better than this.

WHEN SHOULD MEDICINE NOT BE TAKEN?

Many people have beliefs about things they should not do or eat when taking medicines. For this reason they may stop taking a medicine they need. In truth, no medicine causes harm just because it is taken with certain foods—whether pork, chili pepper, guava, oranges, or any other food. But foods with lots of grease or spices can make problems of the stomach or gut worse—whether or not any medicine is being taken (see p. 128). Certain medicines will cause bad reactions if a person drinks alcohol (see metronidazole, p. 369).

There are situations when, without a doubt, it is best **not** to use certain medicines:

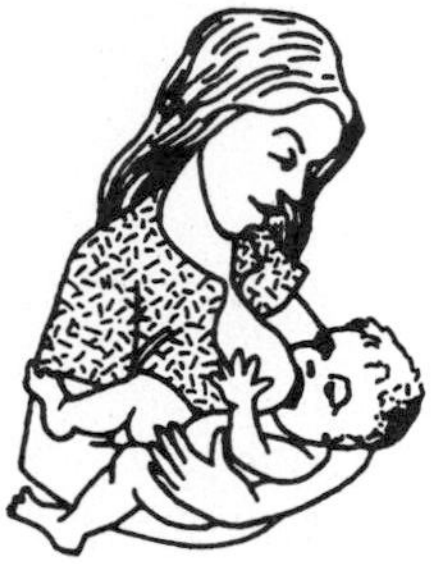

1. Pregnant women or women who are breast feeding should avoid all medicines that are not absolutely necessary. (However, they can take limited amounts of vitamins or iron pills without danger.)

2. With newborn children, be very careful when using medicines. Whenever possible look for medical help before giving them any type of medicine. Be sure not to give too much.

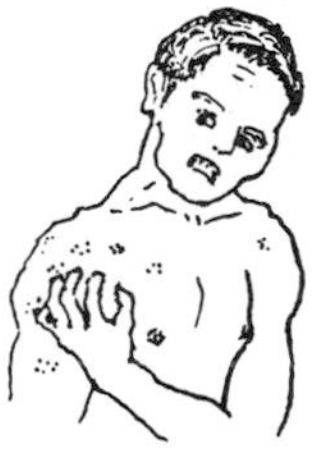

3. A person who has ever had any sort of allergic reaction—***hives,*** itching, etc.—after taking penicillin, ampicillin, a sulfonamide, or other medicines, **should never use that medicine again for the rest of his life** because it would be dangerous (see Dangerous reactions from injections of certain medicines, p. 70).

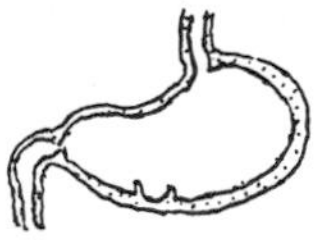

4. Persons who have stomach ulcers or heartburn should avoid medicines that contain aspirin. Most painkillers, and all steroids (see p. 51) make ulcers and acid indigestion worse. One painkiller that does not irritate the stomach is acetaminophen (paracetamol, see p. 380).

5. There are specific medicines that are harmful or dangerous to take when you have certain illnesses. For example, persons with hepatitis should not be treated with antibiotics or other strong medicines, because their liver is damaged, and the medicines are more likely to poison the body (see p. 172).

6. Persons who are dehydrated or have disease of the kidneys should be especially careful with medicines they take. Do not give more than one dose of a medicine that could poison the body unless (or until) the person is urinating normally. For example, if a child has high fever and is dehydrated (see p. 76), do not give him more than one dose of acetaminophen or aspirin until he begins to urinate. **Never give sulfa to a person who is dehydrated.**

CHAPTER

7

ANTIBIOTICS: WHAT THEY ARE AND HOW TO USE THEM

When used correctly, antibiotics are extremely useful and important medicines. They fight certain infections and diseases caused by *bacteria.* Well-known antibiotics are penicillin, tetracycline, streptomycin, chloramphenicol, and the sulfa drugs, or sulfonamides.

The different antibiotics work in different ways against specific infections. All antibiotics have dangers in their use, but some are far more dangerous than others. Take great care in choosing and using antibiotics.

There are many kinds of antibiotics, and each kind is sold under several 'brand names'. This can be confusing. However, the most important antibiotics fall into a few major groups:

antibiotic group (generic name)	examples of brand names	brand names in your area (write in)	see page
PENICILLINS	*Pen-V-K*	________________	351
AMPICILLINS*	*Penbritin*	________________	353
TETRACYCLINES	*Terramycin*	________________	356
SULFAS (SULFONAMIDES)	*Gantrisin*	________________	358
CO-TRIMOXAZOLE	*Bactrim*	________________	358
STREPTOMYCIN, etc.	*Ambistryn*	________________	363, 359
CHLORAMPHENICOL	*Chloromycetin*	________________	357
ERYTHROMYCIN	*Erythrocin*	________________	355
CEPHALOSPORINS	*Keflex*	________________	359

***Note:** Ampicillin is a type of penicillin that kills more kinds of bacteria than do ordinary penicillins.

If you have a brand-name antibiotic and do not know to which group it belongs, read the fine print on the bottle or box. For example, if you have some *Paraxin 'S'* but do not know what is in it, read the fine print. It says 'chloramphenicol'.

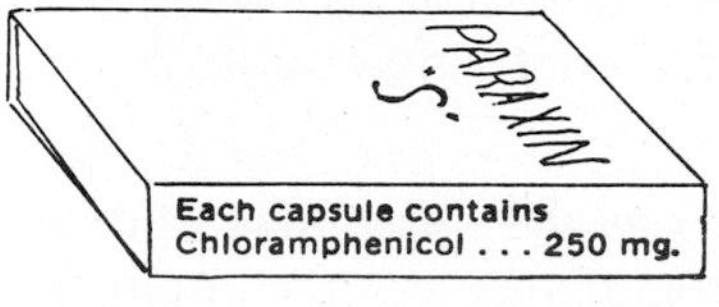

Look up chloramphenicol in the GREEN PAGES (p. 357). You will find it must be used only for a few very serious illnesses, like typhoid, and is especially dangerous when given to the newborn.

Never use an antibiotic unless you know to what group it belongs, what diseases it fights, and the precautions you must take to use it safely.

Information on the uses, dosage, risks, and precautions for the antibiotics recommended in this book can be found in the GREEN PAGES. Look for the name of the medicine in the alphabetical list at the beginning of those pages.

GUIDELINES FOR THE USE OF *ALL* ANTIBIOTICS

1. If you do not know exactly how to use the antibiotic and what infections it can be used for, do not use it.

2. Use only an antibiotic that is recommended for the infection you wish to treat. (Look for the illness in this book.)

3 . Know the risks in using the antibiotic and take all the recommended precautions (see the GREEN PAGES).

4. Use the antibiotic only in the recommended dose—no more, no less. The dose depends on the illness and the age or weight of the sick person.

5. Never use injections of antibiotics if taking them by mouth is likely to work as well. Inject only when absolutely necessary.

6. Keep using the antibiotics until the illness is completely cured, or for at least 2 days after the fever and other signs of infection have gone. (Some illnesses, like tuberculosis and leprosy, need to be treated for many months or years after the person feels better. Follow the instructions for each illness.)

7. If the antibiotic causes a skin rash, itching, difficult breathing, or any serious reactions, the person must stop using it and **never use it again** (see p. 70).

8. **Only use antibiotics when the need is great.** When antibiotics are used too much they begin not to work as well.

GUIDELINES FOR THE USE OF *CERTAIN* ANTIBIOTICS

1. Before you inject penicillin or ampicillin, always have ready ampules of *Adrenalin* (epinephrine) to control an allergic reaction if one occurs (p. 70).

2. For persons who are allergic to penicillin, use another antibiotic such as erythromycin or a sulfa (see p. 355 and 358).

3. Do not use tetracycline, ampicillin, or another ***broad-spectrum*** antibiotic for an illness that can probably be controlled with penicillin or another *narrow-spectrum* antibiotic (see p. 58). Broad-spectrum antibiotics attack many more kinds of bacteria than narrow-spectrum antibiotics.

4. As a rule, use chloramphenicol only for certain severe or life-threatening illnesses like typhoid. It is a dangerous drug. **Never** use it for mild illness. And never give it to newborn children (except perhaps for whooping cough, p. 313).

5. Never inject tetracycline or chloramphenicol. They are safer, less painful, and do as much or more good when taken by mouth.

6. Do not give tetracycline to pregnant women or to children under 8 years old. It can damage new teeth and bones (see p. 356).

7. As a general rule, use streptomycin, and products that contain it, only for tuberculosis—and always together with other anti-tuberculosis medicines (see p. 363). Streptomycin in combination with penicillin can be used for deep wounds to the gut, appendicitis, and other specific infections when ampicillin is not available (or is too costly), but should never be used for colds, flu, and common *respiratory* infections.

8. All medicines in the streptomycin group (including kanamycin and gentamicin) are quite toxic (poisonous). Too often they are prescribed for mild infections where they may do more harm than good. Use only for certain very serious infections for which these medicines are recommended.

9. Eating yogurt or curdled milk helps to replace necessary bacteria killed by antibiotics like ampicillin and to return the body's natural balance to normal (see next page).

WHAT TO DO IF AN ANTIBIOTIC DOES NOT SEEM TO HELP

For most common infections antibiotics begin to bring improvement in a day or two. **If the antibiotic you are using does not seem to help, it is possible that:**

1. The illness is not what you think. You may be using the wrong medicine. Try to find out more exactly what the illness is—and use the right medicine.

2. The dose of the antibiotic is not correct. Check it.

3 . The bacteria have become *resistant* to this antibiotic (they no longer are harmed by it). Try another one of the antibiotics recommended for that illness.

4. You may not know enough to cure the illness. Get medical help, especially if the condition is serious or getting worse.

These three children had a cold . . .

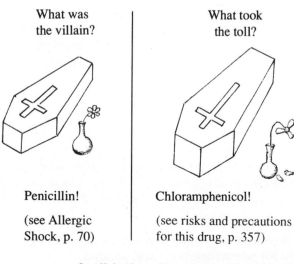

What was the villain?

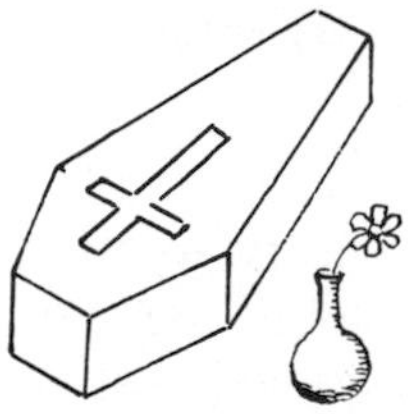

Penicillin!

(see Allergic Shock, p. 70)

What took the toll?

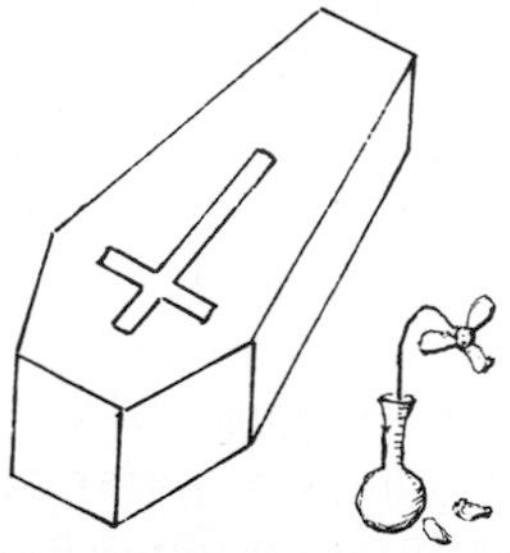

Chloramphenicol!

(see risks and precautions for this drug, p. 357)

Why did this child get well again?

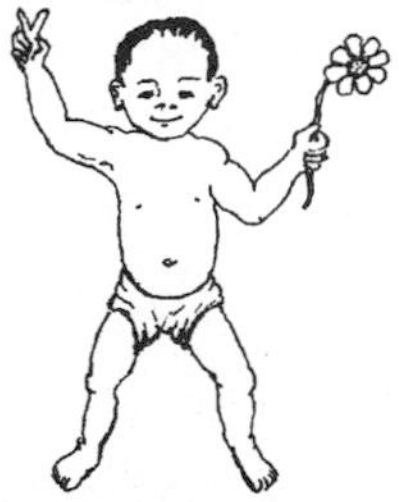

He got no risky medicine—

just fruit juice, good food, and rest.

Antibiotics do no good for the common cold.

Use antibiotics only for infections they are known to help.

IMPORTANCE OF LIMITED USE OF ANTIBIOTICS

The use of all medicines should be limited. But this is especially true of antibiotics, for the following reasons:

1. **Poisoning and reactions.** Antibiotics not only kill bacteria, they can also harm the body, either by poisoning it or by causing allergic reactions. Many people die each year because they take antibiotics they do not need.

2. **Upsetting the natural balance.** Not all bacteria in the body are harmful. Some are necessary for the body to function normally. Antibiotics often kill the good bacteria along with the harmful ones. Babies who are given antibiotics sometimes develop fungus or yeast infections of the mouth (thrush, p. 232) or skin (moniliasis, p. 242). This is because the antibiotics kill the bacteria that help keep fungus under control.

For similar reasons, persons who take ampicillin and other ***broad-spectrum*** antibiotics for several days may develop diarrhea. Antibiotics may kill some kinds of bacteria necessary for digestion, upsetting the natural balance of bacteria in the gut.

3. **Resistance to treatment.** In the long run, the most important reason the use of antibiotics should be limited, is that WHEN ANTIBIOTICS ARE USED TOO MUCH, THEY BECOME LESS EFFECTIVE.

When attacked many times by the same antibiotic, bacteria become stronger and are no longer killed by it. They become ***resistant*** to the antibiotic. For this reason, certain dangerous diseases like typhoid are becoming more difficult to treat than they were a few years ago.

In some places typhoid has become resistant to chloramphenicol, normally the best medicine for treating it. Chloramphenicol has been used far too much for minor infections, infections for which other antibiotics would be safer and work as well, or for which no antibiotic at all is needed.

Throughout the world important diseases are becoming resistant to antibiotics—largely because antibiotics are used too much for minor infections. **If antibiotics are to continue to save lives, their use must be much more limited than it is at present.** This will depend on their wise use by doctors, health workers, and the people themselves.

For most minor infections antibiotics are not needed and should not be used. Minor skin infections can usually be successfully treated with mild soap and water, or hot soaks, and perhaps painting them with gentian violet (p. 371). Minor respiratory infections are best treated by drinking lots of liquids, eating good food, and getting plenty of rest. **For most diarrheas, antibiotics are not necessary and may even be harmful.** What is most important is to drink lots of liquids (p. 155), and provide enough food as soon as the child will eat.

Do not use antibiotics for infections the body can fight successfully by itself. Save them for when they are most needed.

For more information on learning to use antibiotics sensibly, see *Helping Health Workers Learn,* Chapter 19.

CHAPTER

HOW TO MEASURE AND GIVE MEDICINE 8

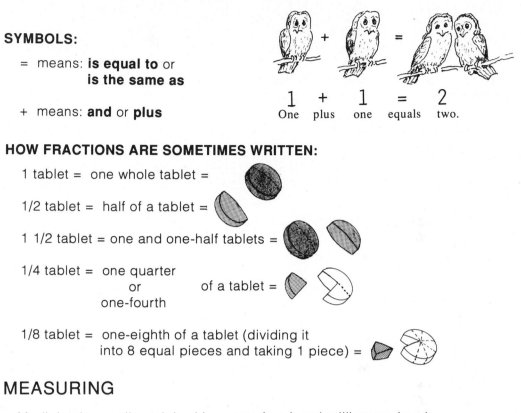

SYMBOLS:

= means: **is equal to** or **is the same as**

\+ means: **and** or **plus**

1 + 1 = 2
One plus one equals two.

HOW FRACTIONS ARE SOMETIMES WRITTEN:

1 tablet = one whole tablet = 

1/2 tablet = half of a tablet = 

1 1/2 tablet = one and one-half tablets = 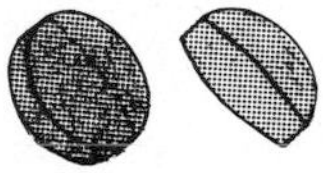

1/4 tablet = one quarter or one-fourth of a tablet = 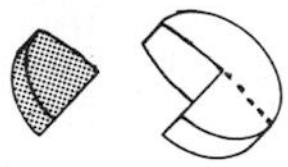

1/8 tablet = one-eighth of a tablet (dividing it into 8 equal pieces and taking 1 piece) = 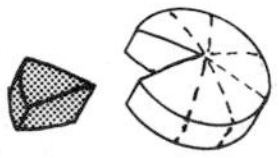

MEASURING

Medicine is usually weighed in grams (gm.) and milligrams (mg.).

1000 mg. = 1 gm. (one thousand milligrams make one gram)

1 mg. = .001 gm. (one milligram is one one-thousandth part of a gram)

Examples:

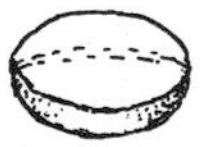	One adult aspirin tablet contains 300 milligrams of aspirin.	.3 gm. 0.3 gm. 0.300 gm. 300 mg.	All these are different ways of saying 300 milligrams.
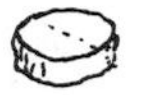	One baby aspirin contains 75 milligrams of aspirin.	.075 gm. 0.075 gm. 75.0 mg. 75 mg.	All these are different ways of saying 75 milligrams.

Note: In some countries some medicines are still weighed in grains; gr. = grain and 1 gr. = 65 mg. This means a 5 gr. aspirin tablet weighs about 300 mg.

Many times it is important to know how many grams or milligrams are in a medicine.

For example, if you want to give a small piece of adult aspirin to a child, instead of baby aspirin, but you do not know how big a piece to give . . .

read the small print on the labels of each.
It says: aspirin: acetylsalicylic acid .3 gm.
(acetylsalicylic acid = aspirin)

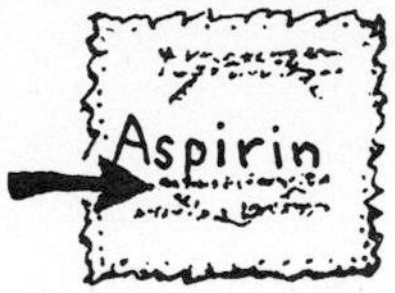

.3 gm. = 300 mg. and .075 gm. = 75 mg. So, you can see that one adult aspirin weighs 4 times as much as one baby aspirin.

75 mg.
75 mg.
75 mg.
75 mg.

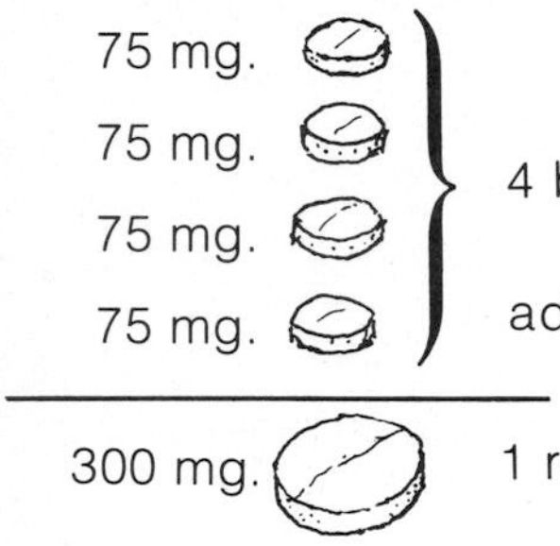

4 baby aspirin

add up to

300 mg. — 1 regular aspirin

If you cut the adult aspirin into 4 equal pieces, each quarter = one baby aspirin

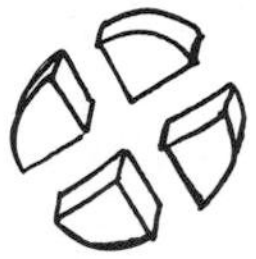

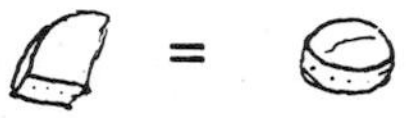

So if you cut an adult aspirin into 4 pieces, you can give the child 1 piece in place of a baby aspirin. Both are equal, and the piece of adult aspirin costs less.

CAUTION: Many medicines, especially the antibiotics, come in different weights and sizes. For example, tetracycline may come in 3 sizes of capsules:

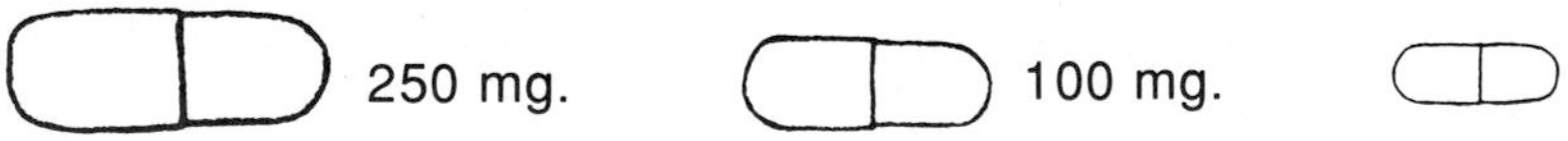

250 mg. 100 mg. 50 mg.

Be careful to only give medicine in the recommended amounts. It is very important to check how many grams or milligrams the medicine contains.

For example: if the prescription says: Take tetracycline, 1 capsule of 250 mg. 4 times a day, and you have only 50 mg. capsules, you have to take five 50 mg. capsules 4 times a day (20 capsules a day).

50 mg. + 50 mg. + 50 mg. + 50 mg. + 50 mg. = 250 mg.

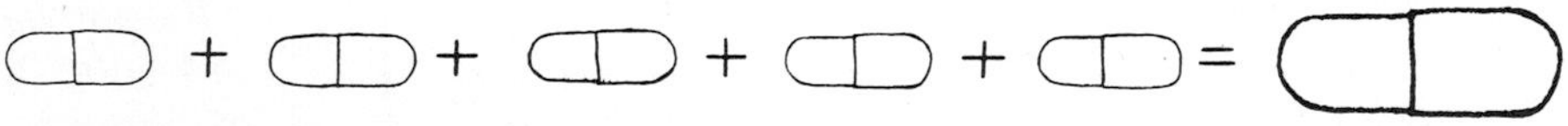

MEASURING PENICILLIN

Penicillin is often measured in units.

U. = unit 1,600,000 U. = 1 gm. or 1,000 mg.

Many forms of penicillin (pills and injections) come in doses of 400,000 U.

400,000 U. = 250 mg.

MEDICINE IN LIQUID FORM

Syrups, suspensions, tonics, and other liquid medicines are measured in milliliters:

ml. = milliliter   1 liter = 1000 ml.

Often liquid medicines are prescribed in tablespoons or teaspoons:

1 teaspoon (tsp.) = 5 ml.   1 tablespoon (Tbs.) = 15 ml.

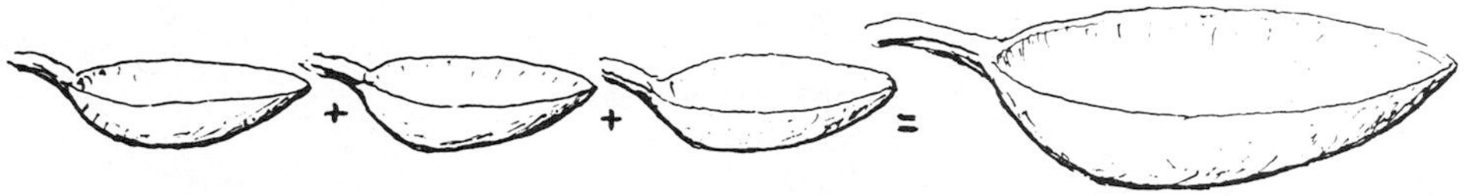

3 teaspoons = 1 tablespoon

When instructions for a medicine say: Take 1 tsp., this means take 5 ml.

Many of the 'teaspoons' people use hold as much as 8 ml. or as little as 3 ml. **When using a teaspoon to give medicine, it is important that it measure *5 ml.*— No more. No less.**

How to Make Sure that the Teaspoon Used for Medicine Measures 5 ml.

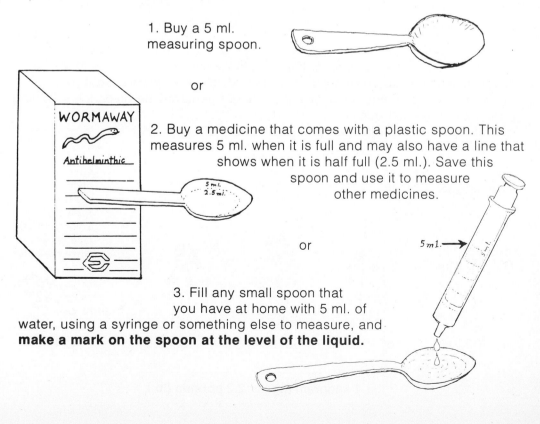

1. Buy a 5 ml. measuring spoon.

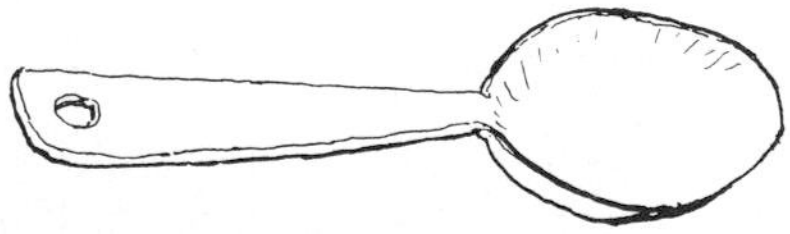

or

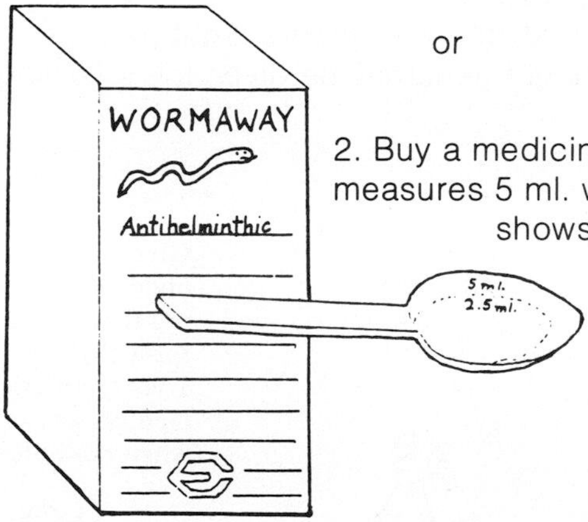

2. Buy a medicine that comes with a plastic spoon. This measures 5 ml. when it is full and may also have a line that shows when it is half full (2.5 ml.). Save this spoon and use it to measure other medicines.

or

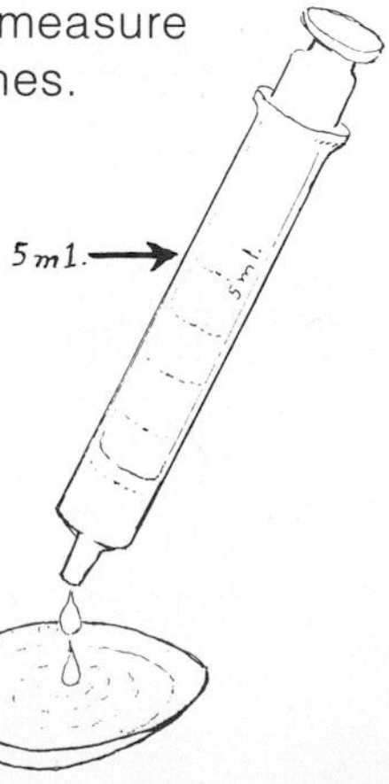

3. Fill any small spoon that you have at home with 5 ml. of water, using a syringe or something else to measure, and **make a mark on the spoon at the level of the liquid.**

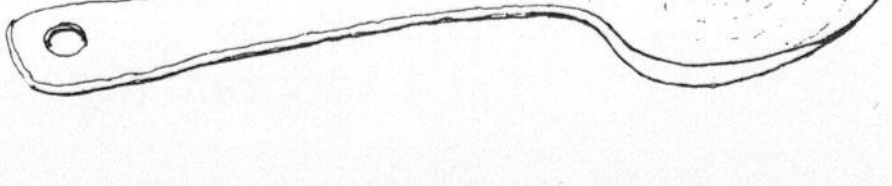

HOW TO GIVE MEDICINES TO SMALL CHILDREN

Many medicines that come as pills or capsules also come in syrups or *suspensions* (special liquid form) for children. If you compare the amount of medicine you get, the syrups are usually more expensive than pills or capsules. You can save money by making your own syrup in the following way:

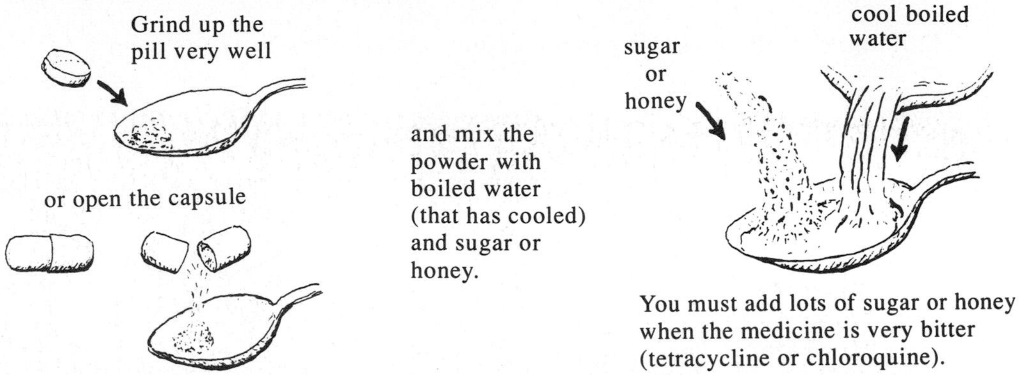

Grind up the pill very well
or open the capsule
and mix the powder with boiled water (that has cooled) and sugar or honey.
sugar or honey
cool boiled water
You must add lots of sugar or honey when the medicine is very bitter (tetracycline or chloroquine).

When making syrups for children from pills or capsules, **be very careful not to give too much medicine.** Also, **do not give honey to babies under 1 year of age.** Though it is rare, some babies can have a dangerous reaction.

CAUTION: To prevent choking, do not give medicines to a child while she is lying on her back, or if her head is pressed back. Always make sure she is sitting up or that her head is lifted forward. Never give medicines by mouth to a child while she is having a fit, or while she is asleep or unconscious.

HOW MUCH MEDICINE SHOULD YOU GIVE TO CHILDREN WHEN YOU ONLY HAVE THE INSTRUCTIONS FOR ADULTS?

Generally, the smaller the child, the less medicine he needs. Giving more than needed can be dangerous. If you have information about the doses for children, follow it carefully. If you do not know the dose, figure it out by using the weight or age of the child. Children should generally be given the following portions of the adult dose:

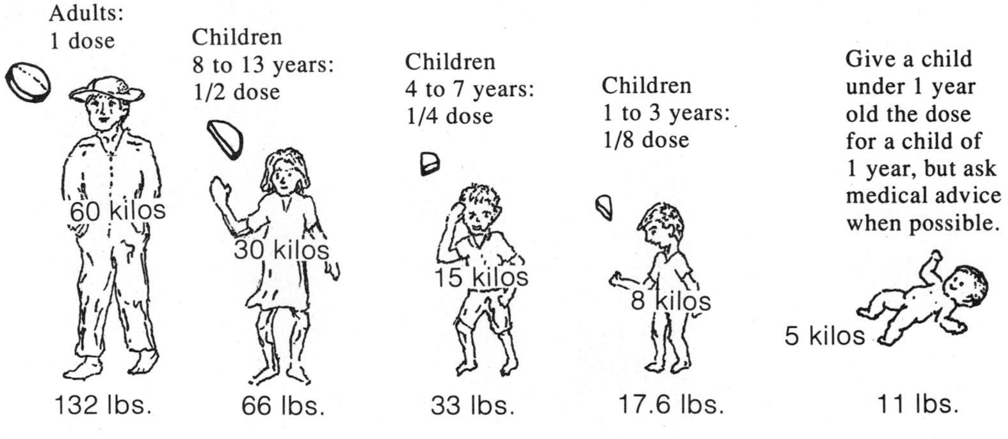

Adults: 1 dose

Children 8 to 13 years: 1/2 dose

Give a child under 1 year old the dose for a child of 1 year, but ask medical advice when possible.

1 kilogram (kg.) = 2.2 pounds (lb.)

HOW TO TAKE MEDICINES

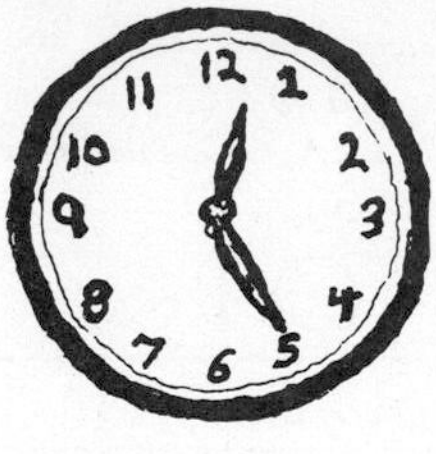

It is important to take medicines more or less at the time recommended. Some medicines should be taken only once a day, but others must be taken more often. If you do not have a clock, it does not matter. If the directions say '1 pill every 8 hours', take 3 a day: one in the morning, one in the afternoon, and one at night. If they say '1 pill every 6 hours', take 4 each day: one in the morning, one at midday, one in the afternoon, and one at night. If the directions are '1 every 4 hours', take 6 a day, allowing more or less the same time between pills.

Whenever you give a medicine to someone else, it is a good idea to write the instructions and also to have the person repeat to you how and when to take the medicine. Make very sure he understands.

To remind people who cannot read when to take their medicine, you can give them a note like this→

In the blanks at the bottom draw the amount of medicine they should take and carefully explain what it means.→

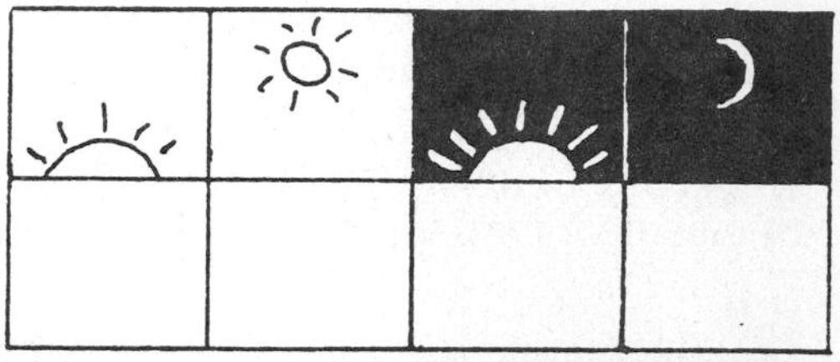

For example:

This means 1 tablet 4 times a day, 1 at sunrise, 1 at noon, 1 at sunset, and 1 in the middle of the night.

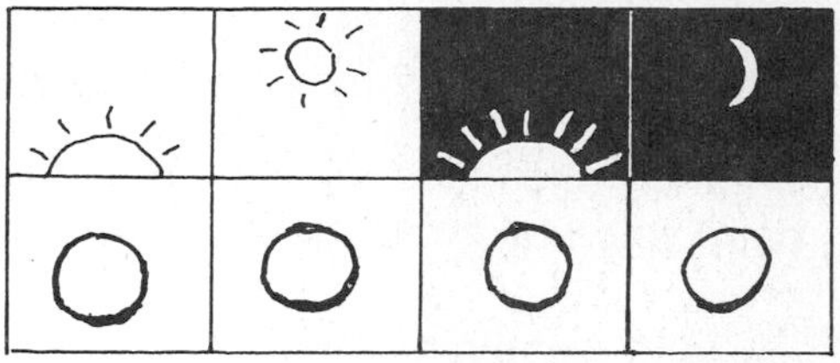

This means 1/2 tablet 4 times a day.

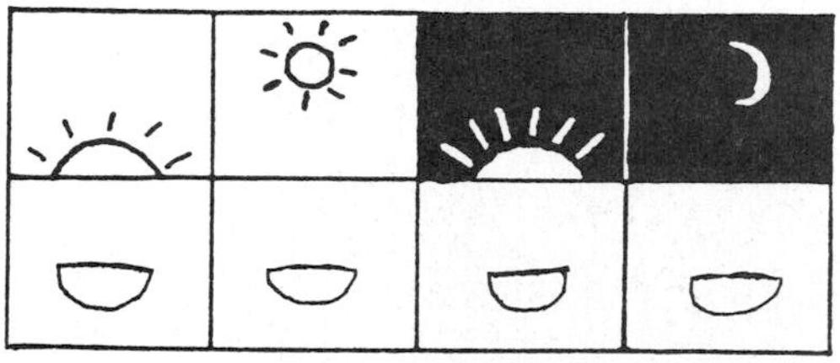

This means 1 capsule 3 times a day.

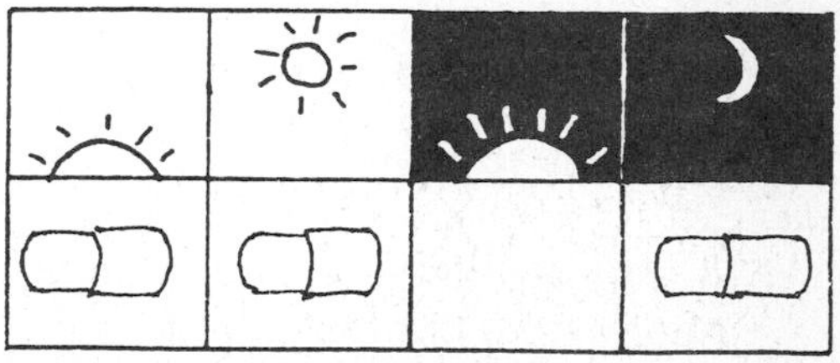

This means 1/4 tablet twice a day.

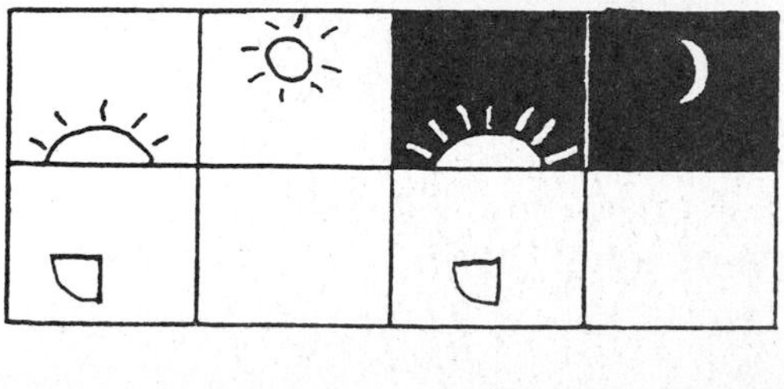

This means 2 teaspoons twice a day.

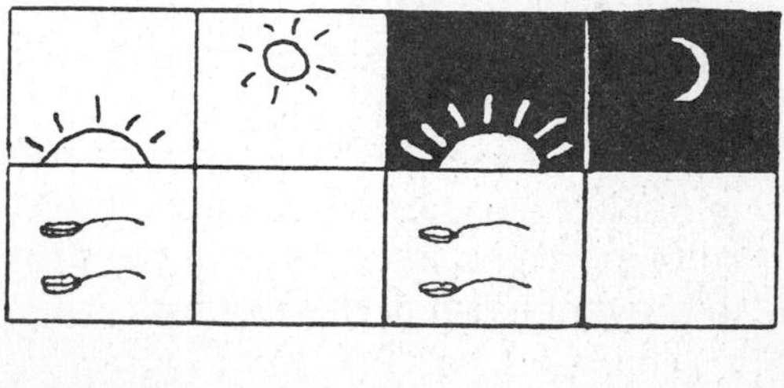

WHEN YOU GIVE MEDICINES TO ANYONE . . .

Always write all the following information on the note with the medicine—even if the person cannot read:

- the person's name
- the name of the medicine
- what it is for
- the dosage

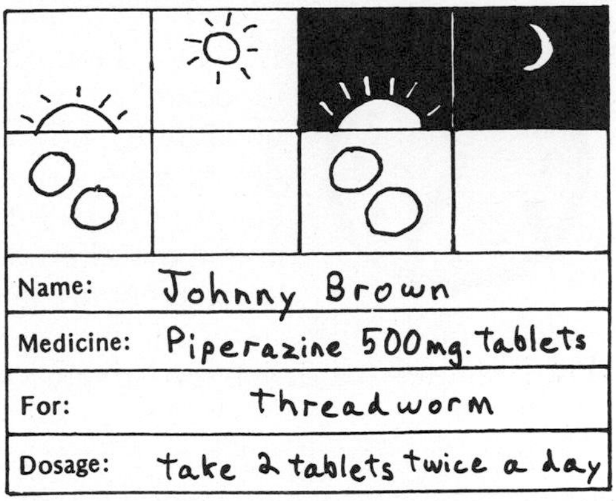

Name: Johnny Brown
Medicine: Piperazine 500 mg. tablets
For: threadworm
Dosage: take 2 tablets twice a day

This information can be put on the same note as the drawing for dosage.

A page of these dosage blanks is included at the end of the book. Cut them out and use them as needed. When you run out, you can make more yourself.

When you give medicine to someone, it is a good idea to keep a record of this same information. If possible, keep a complete Patient Report (see p. 44).

TAKING MEDICINES ON A FULL OR EMPTY STOMACH

Some medicines work best when you take them when the stomach is empty—that is, one hour before meals.

Other medicines are less likely to cause upset stomach or heartburn (chest pain) when taken along with a meal or right afterwards.

Take these medicines 1 hour before meals:

- penicillin
- ampicillin
- tetracycline

It is better not to drink milk an hour before or after taking tetracycline.

Take these medicines together with or soon after meals (or with a lot of water):

- aspirin and medicine that contains aspirin
- iron (ferrous sulfate)
- vitamins
- erythromycin

Antacids do the most good if you take them when the stomach is empty, 1 or 2 hours after meals and at bedtime.

Note: It is best to take medicines while you are standing or sitting up. Also, try to drink a glass of water each time you take a medicine. If you are taking a sulfa medicine, it is important to **drink lots of water**, at least 8 glasses a day, to prevent harm to the kidneys.

CHAPTER 9

INSTRUCTIONS AND PRECAUTIONS FOR INJECTIONS

WHEN TO INJECT AND WHEN NOT TO

Injections are not needed often. Most sicknesses that require medical treatment can be treated as well or better with medicines taken by mouth. As a general rule:

It is more dangerous to inject medicine than to take it by mouth.

Injections should be used only when absolutely necessary. Except in emergencies, they should be given only by health workers or persons trained in their use.

The only times medicines should be injected are:

1. When the recommended medicine does not come in a form that can be taken by mouth.
2. When the person vomits often, cannot swallow, or is unconscious.
3. In certain unusual emergencies and special cases (see the next page).

WHAT TO DO WHEN THE DOCTOR PRESCRIBES INJECTIONS

Doctors and other health workers sometimes prescribe injections when they are not needed. After all, they can charge more money for injections. They forget the problems and dangers of giving injections in rural areas.

1. If a health worker or healer wants to give you an injection, be sure the medicine is ***appropriate*** and that she takes all the necessary precautions.

2. If a doctor prescribes injections, explain that you live where no one is well trained to give injections and ask if it would be possible to prescribe a medicine to take by mouth.

3. If a doctor wants to prescribe injections of vitamins, liver extract, or vitamin B_{12}, but has not had your blood tested, tell him you would prefer to see another doctor.

EMERGENCIES WHEN IT IS IMPORTANT TO GIVE INJECTIONS

In case of the following sicknesses, get medical help as fast as you can. If there will be any delay in getting help or in taking the sick person to a health center, inject the appropriate medicine as soon as possible. For details of the doses, consult the pages listed below. Before injecting, know the possible side effects and take the needed precautions (see the Green Pages).

↓ **For these sicknesses**	↓ **Inject these medicines**
Severe pneumonia (p. 171) Infections after childbirth (p. 276) Gangrene (p. 213)	penicillin in high doses (p. 352)
Tetanus (p. 182)	penicillin (p. 351) and tetanus antitoxin (p. 389) and phenobarbital (p. 389) or diazepam (p. 390)
Appendicitis (p. 94) Peritonitis (p. 94) and bullet wound or other puncture wound in the belly	ampicillin in high doses (p. 353) or penicillin with streptomycin (p. 354)
Poisonous snakebite (p. 105) Scorpion sting (in children, p. 106)	snake antivenom (p. 388) scorpion antivenom (p. 388)
Meningitis (p. 185) when you do not suspect tuberculosis	ampicillin (p. 353, 354) or penicillin (p. 352) in very high doses
Meningitis (p. 185) when you suspect tuberculosis	ampicillin or penicillin together with streptomycin (p. 353, 354) and, if possible, other TB medicines (p. 361)
Vomiting (p. 161) when it cannot be controlled	antihistamines, for example, promethazine (p. 386)
Severe allergic reaction allergic shock (p. 70) and severe asthma (p. 167)	epinephrine (***Adrenalin***, p. 385) and, if possible, diphenhydramine (***Benadryl***, p. 387).

The following chronic illnesses may require injections, but they are rarely emergencies. It is best to consult a health worker for treatment.

Tuberculosis (p. 179, 180)	streptomycin (p. 363) together with other TB medicines (p. 361)
Syphilis (p. 237)	benzathine penicillin in very high doses (p. 238)
Gonorrhea (p. 236)	kanamycin or penicillin (p. 360)

WHEN NOT TO INJECT:

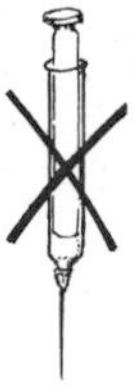

Never give injections if you can get medical help quickly.
Never give an injection for a sickness that is not serious.
Never give injections for a cold or the flu.
Never inject a medicine that is not recommended for the illness you want to treat.
Never give an injection unless your needle has been boiled or sterilized.
Never inject a medicine unless you know and take all the recommended precautions.

MEDICINES **NOT** TO INJECT

In general, it is better **never** to inject the following:

1. Vitamins. Rarely are injected vitamins any better than vitamins taken by mouth. Injections are more expensive and more dangerous. Use vitamin pills or syrups rather than injections. Better still, eat foods rich in vitamins (see p. 111).

2. Liver extract, vitamin B_{12}, and iron injections (such as *Inferon*). Injecting these can cause abscesses or dangerous reactions (shock, p. 70). Ferrous sulfate pills will do more good for almost all cases of anemia (p. 393).

3. Calcium. Injected into a vein calcium is extremely dangerous, if not given **very slowly**. An injection in the buttock may cause a large ***abscess***. Untrained people should never inject calcium.

4. Penicillin. Nearly all infections that require penicillin can be effectively treated with penicillin taken by mouth. Penicillin is more dangerous when injected. **Use injectable penicillin only for dangerous infections.**

5. Penicillin with streptomycin. As a general rule, avoid this combined medicine. Never use it for colds or the flu because it does not work. It can cause serious problems—sometimes deafness or death. Also, overuse makes it more difficult to cure tuberculosis or other serious illness.

6. Chloramphenicol or tetracycline. These medicines do as much or more good when taken by mouth. Use capsules or syrups rather than injections (p. 356 and 357).

7. Intravenous (I.V.) solutions. These should be used only for severe dehydration and given only by someone who is well trained. When not given correctly they can cause dangerous infections or death (p. 53).

8. Intravenous medicines. There is so much danger in injecting any medicine in the vein that only well-trained health workers should do it. However, never inject into a muscle (the buttock) medicine that says 'for intravenous use only'. Also, never inject in the vein medicine that says 'for intramuscular use only'.

RISKS AND PRECAUTIONS

The risks of injecting any medicines are (1) infection caused by germs entering with the needle and (2) allergic or poisonous reactions caused by the medicine.

1. To lower the chance of infection when injecting, take great care that everything is completely clean. It is very important to boil the needle and syringe before injecting. After boiling, do not touch the needle with your fingers or with anything else.

   Never use the same needle and syringe to inject more than one person without boiling it again first. Carefully follow all of the instructions for injecting (see following pages).

   Be sure to **wash your hands well** before preparing or giving injections.

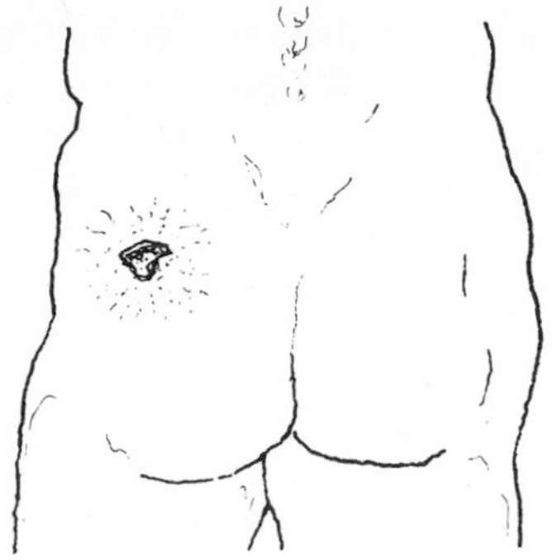

An abscess like this one comes from injecting with a needle that has not been well boiled and is not sterile (completely clean and germ-free).

2. It is very important to know what reactions a medicine can produce and to take the recommended precautions before injecting.

   If any of the following signs of allergic or poisonous reaction appear, never give the same or similar medicine again:

   - *hives* (patchy swellings on skin) or a rash with itching
   - swelling anywhere
   - difficulty breathing
   - signs of shock (see p. 70)
   - dizzy spells with nausea (wanting to vomit)
   - problems with vision
   - ringing in the ears or deafness
   - severe back pain
   - difficulty urinating

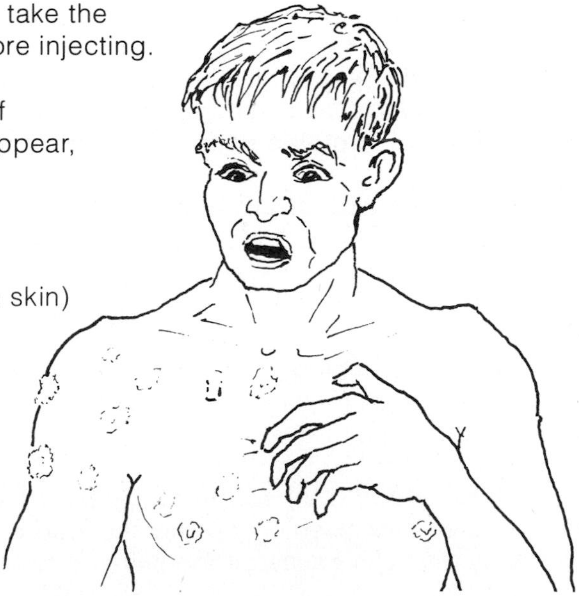

Hives, or a rash with itching, can appear a few hours or up to several days after getting an injection. If the same medicine is given to the person again, it may cause a very severe reaction or even death (see p. 70).

This child was injected with a needle that was not ***sterile*** (boiled and completely free of germs).

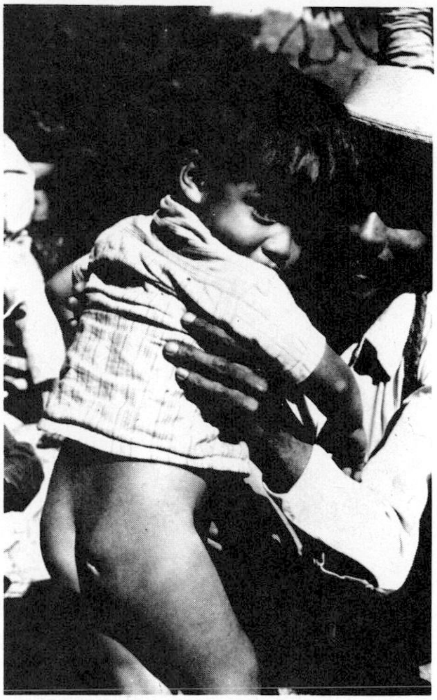

The dirty needle caused an infection that produced a large, painful abscess (pocket of pus) and gave the child a fever. Finally, the abscess burst as shown in the picture below.

This child was injected for a cold. It would have been far better to give him no medicine at all. Rather than doing good, the injection caused the child suffering and harm.

CAUTION: If possible, always give medicine by mouth instead of by injection—especially to children.

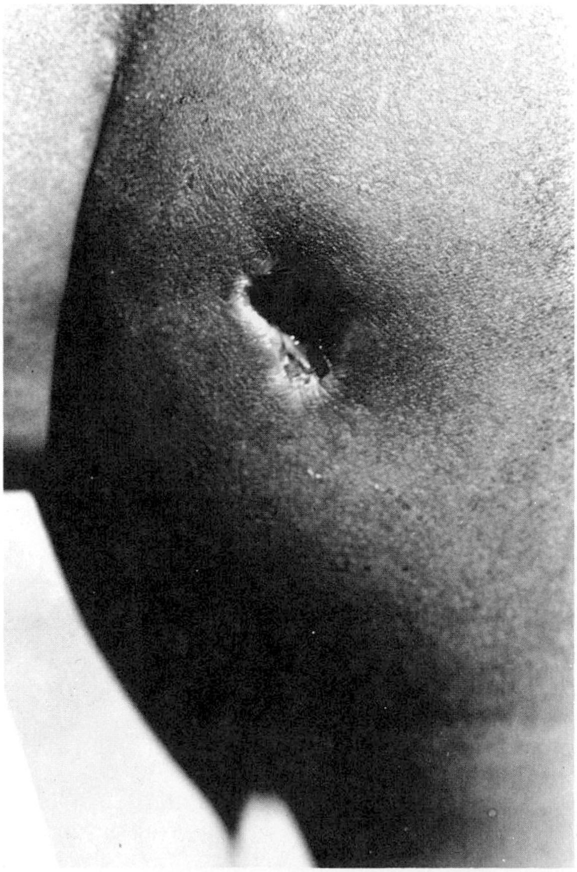

To avoid problems like these:

Inject only when absolutely necessary.

- Boil the syringe and needle just before giving the injection and be very careful to keep them completely clean.
- Use only the medicine recommended for the disease and be sure it is still in good condition and not spoiled.
- Inject in the correct place. Do not inject infants and small children in the buttock. Instead, inject them in the upper, outer part of the thigh. (Notice that this child was injected **too low** on the buttock, where it is possible to damage the nerve.)

DANGEROUS REACTIONS FROM INJECTING CERTAIN MEDICINES

The following groups of medicines sometimes produce a dangerous reaction called ALLERGIC SHOCK a short time after injection:

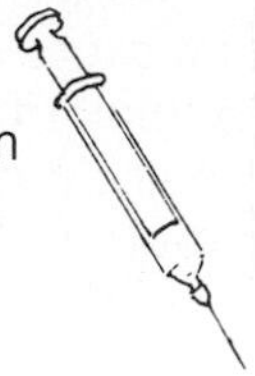

- penicillins (including ampicillin)
- antitoxins that are made from horse serum: scorpion antivenom, snake antivenom, tetanus antitoxin

The risk of a serious reaction is greater in a person who has previously been injected with one of these medicines or with another medicine of the same group. This risk is especially great if the medicine caused an allergic reaction (***hives,*** rash, itching, swelling, or trouble breathing) a few hours or days after the injection was given.

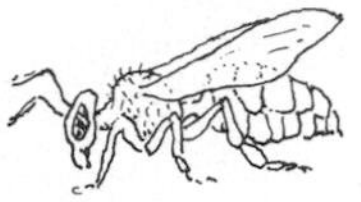

Rarely, ALLERGIC SHOCK may result from the sting of a wasp or bee or from medicine taken by mouth.

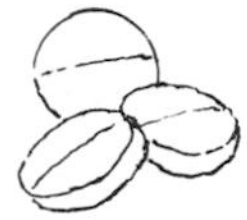

To prevent a serious reaction from an injection:

1. Use injections only when absolutely necessary.

2. Before injecting one of the medicines listed above, always have ready 2 ampules of epinephrine (***Adrenalin***, p. 385) and an ampule of an antihistamine like promethazine (***Phenergan***, p. 386) or diphenhydramine (***Benadryl,*** p. 387).

3. Before injecting, always ask if at any other time a similar injection caused itching or other reactions. If the person says yes, do not use this medicine or any other medicine of the same group, either injected or taken by mouth.

4. In very serious cases, like tetanus or snakebite, if there is a good chance that the antitoxin might produce an allergic reaction (if the person suffers from allergies or asthma or has had horse serum before), inject promethazine or diphenhydramine 15 minutes before giving the antitoxin: adults, 25 to 50 mg.; children, 10 to 25 mg., depending on their size (see p. 387).

5. After injecting any medicine, always stay with the person for 30 minutes to watch for any of the following signs of ALLERGIC SHOCK:

- cool, moist, pale, gray skin (cold sweat)
- weak, rapid pulse or heartbeat
- difficulty breathing
- loss of consciousness

6. If these signs appear, immediately inject epinephrine ***(Adrenalin)***: adults, 1/2 ml.; children, 1/4 ml. Treat the person for SHOCK (see p. 77). Follow by giving an antihistamine in double the normal dose.

How to Avoid Serious Reactions to a Penicillin Injection

1. For mild to moderate infections:

give penicillin pills

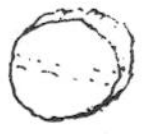

instead of injections.

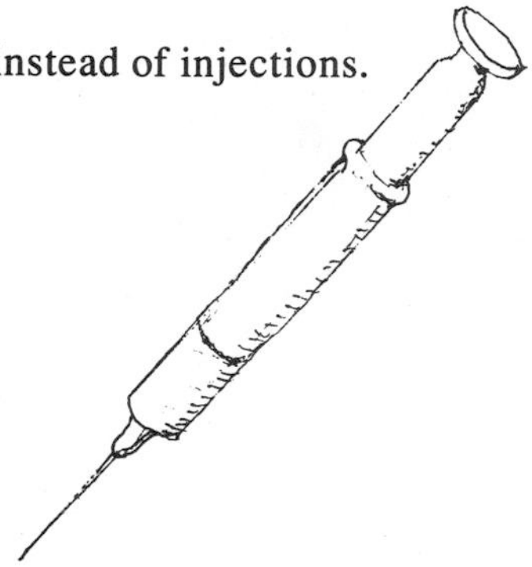

2. Before injecting ask the person:

"Have you ever had a rash, itching, swelling, or trouble breathing after getting an injection of penicillin?"

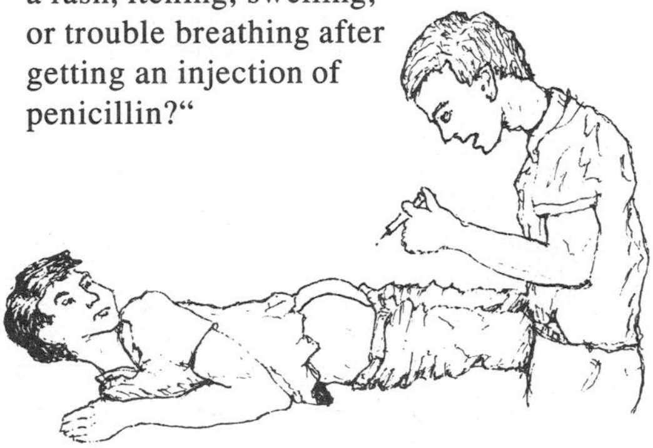

If the answer is yes, do not use penicillin, ampicillin, or amoxicillin. Use another antibiotic like erythromycin (p. 355) or a sulfonamide (p. 358).

3. Before injecting penicillin:

always have ampules of EPINEPHRINE *(Adrenalin)* ready.

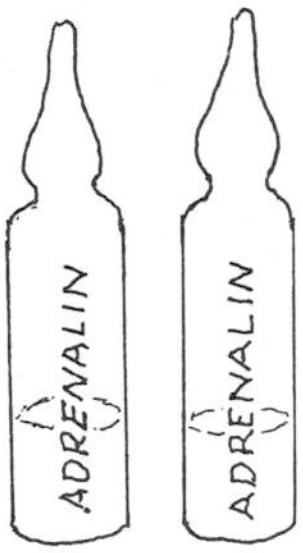

4. After injecting:

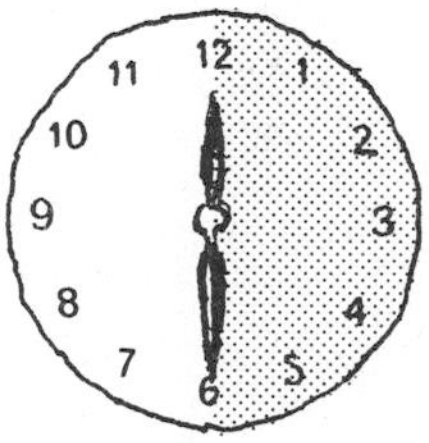

stay with the person for at least 30 minutes.

5. If the person becomes very pale, his heart beats very fast, he has difficulty breathing, or he starts to faint, immediately inject into a muscle (or just under the skin—see p. 167) half an ampule of EPINEPHRINE (*Adrenalin*, a quarter of an ampule in small children) and repeat in 10 minutes if necessary.

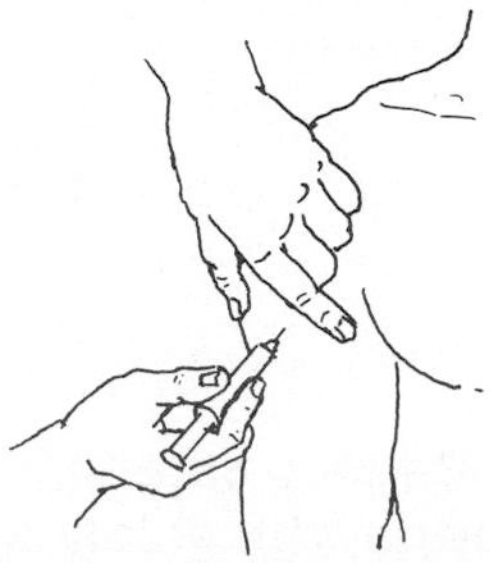

HOW TO PREPARE A SYRINGE FOR INJECTION

Before preparing a syringe, **wash hands with soap and water.**

1. Take the syringe apart and boil it and the needle for 20 minutes.

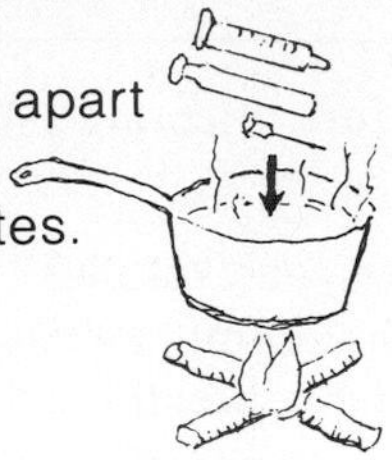

2. Pour out the boiled water without touching the syringe or the needle.

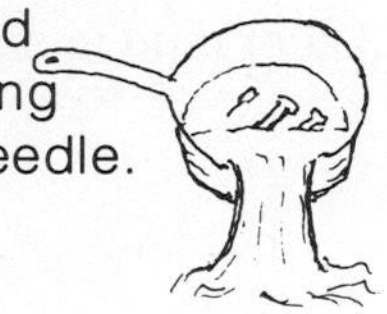

3. Put the needle and the syringe together, touching only the base of the needle and the button of the plunger.

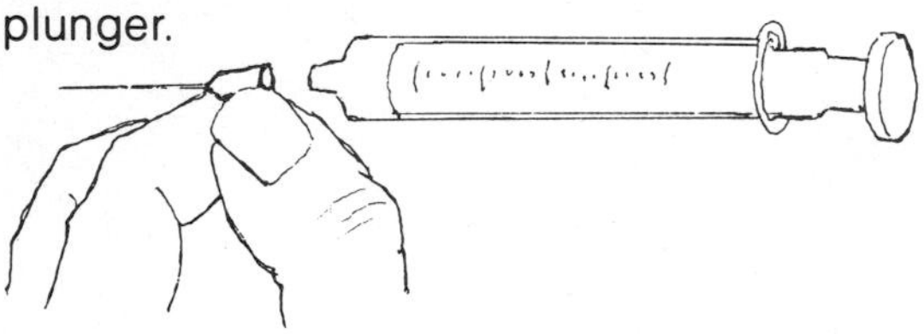

4. Clean the ampule of distilled water well, then break off the top.

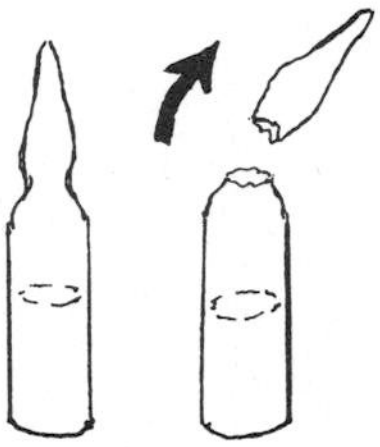

5. Fill the syringe. (Be careful that the needle does not touch the outside of the ampule.)

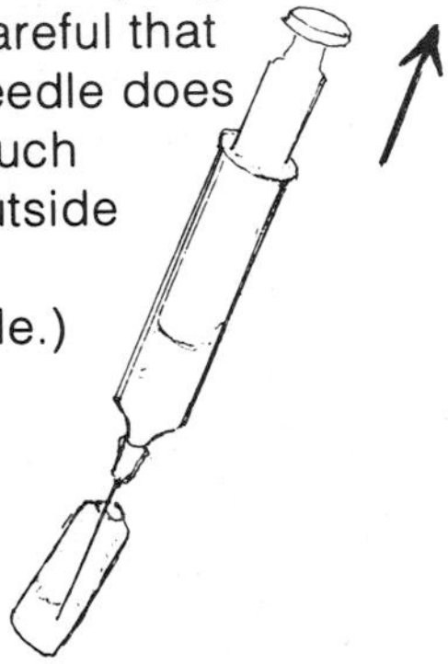

6. Rub the rubber of the bottle with clean cloth wet with alcohol or boiled water.

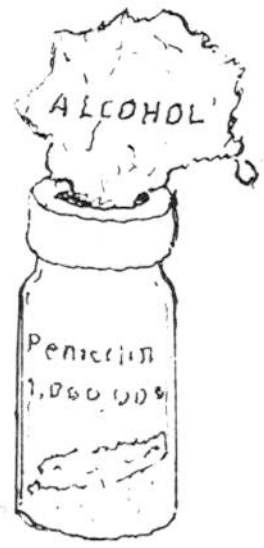

7. Inject the distilled water into the bottle with the powdered medicine.

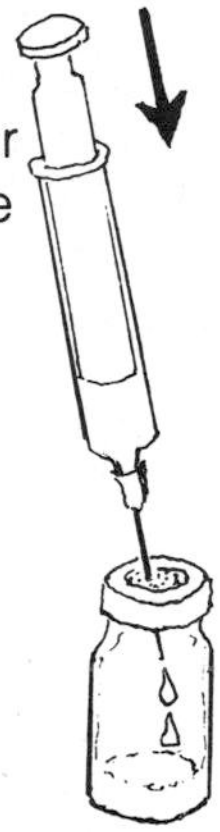

8. Shake until the medicine dissolves.

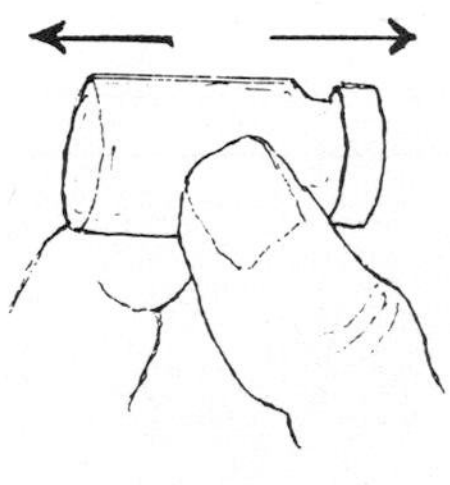

9. Fill the syringe again.

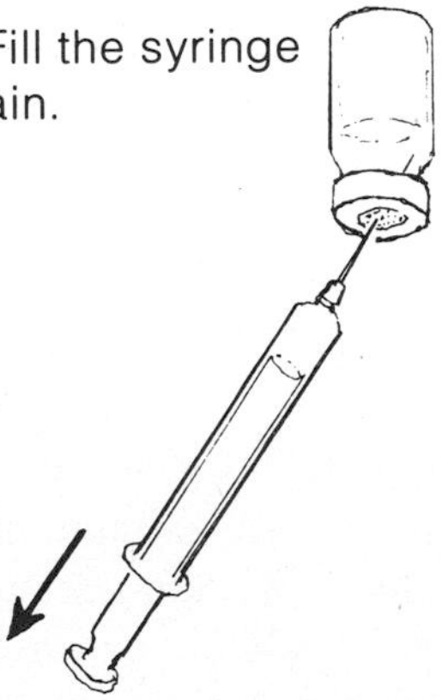

10. Remove all air from the syringe.

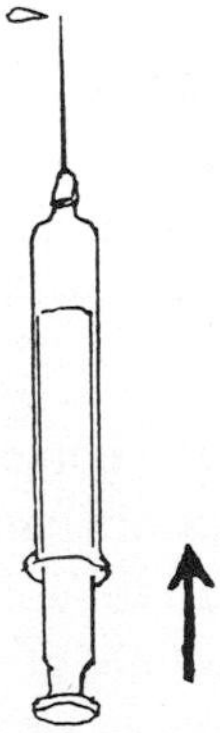

Be very careful not to touch the needle with anything—not even the cotton with alcohol. If by chance the needle touches your finger or something else, boil it again.

WHERE TO GIVE AN INJECTION

Before injecting, **wash hands with soap and water.**

It is preferable to inject in the muscle of the buttocks, always in the **upper outer** quarter.

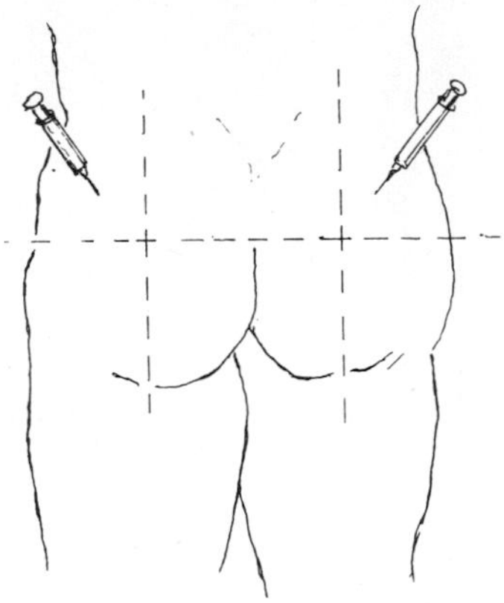

WARNING: Do not inject into an area of skin that is infected or has a rash.

Do not inject infants and small children in the buttock. Inject them in the **upper outer** part of the thigh.

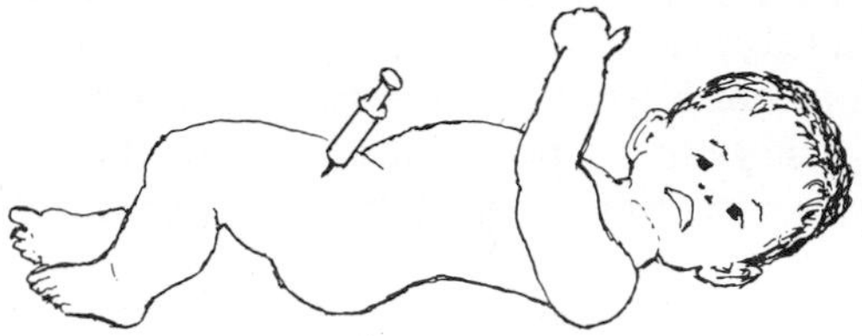

HOW TO INJECT

1. Clean the skin with soap and water (or alcohol—but to prevent severe pain, be sure the alcohol is dry before injecting).

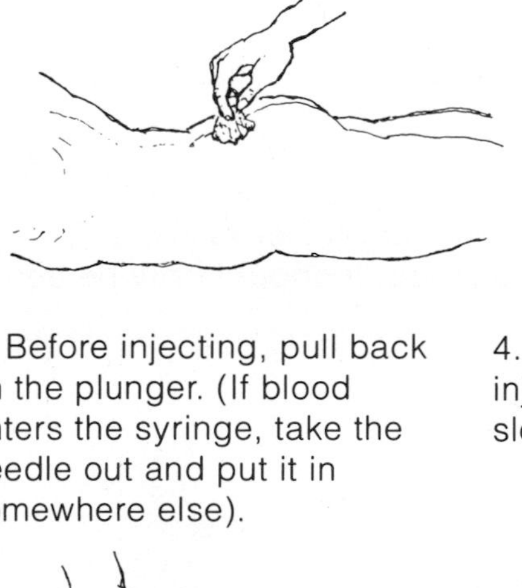

2. Put the needle straight in, all the way. (If it is done with one quick movement, it hurts less.)

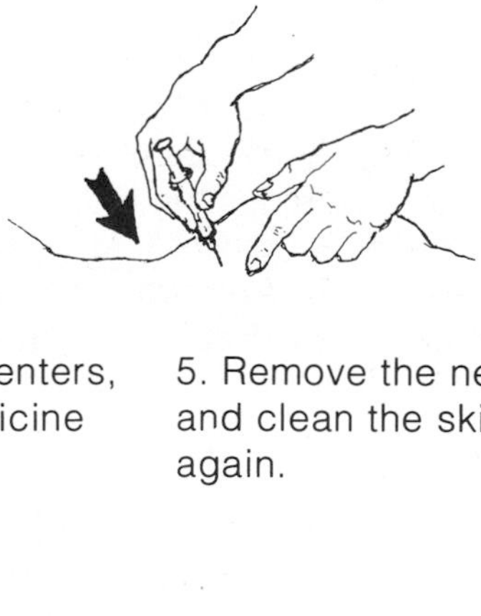

3. Before injecting, pull back on the plunger. (If blood enters the syringe, take the needle out and put it in somewhere else).

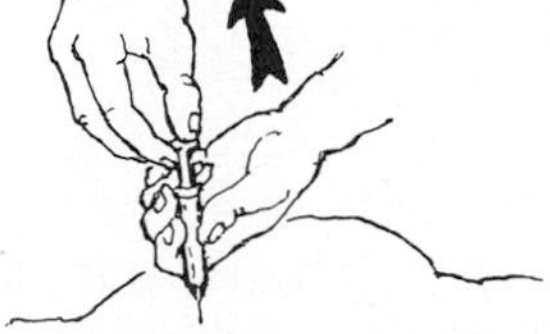

4. If no blood enters, inject the medicine slowly.

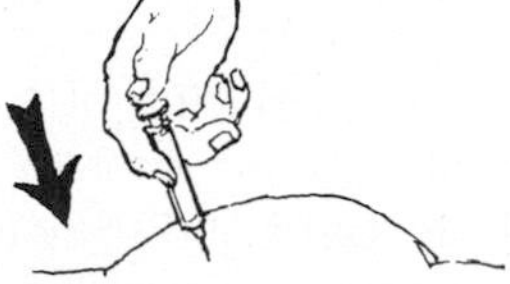

5. Remove the needle and clean the skin again.

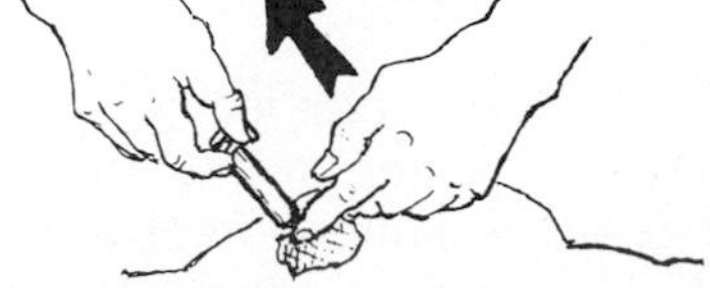

6. After injecting, rinse the syringe and needle at once. Squirt water through the needle and then take the syringe apart and wash it. Boil before using again.

HOW INJECTIONS CAN DISABLE CHILDREN

When used correctly, certain injected medicines are important to health. Vaccinations, including those that are injected, help to protect a child's health and prevent disability. However, **to reduce the chance of paralysis from polio,** it is best *not* to give vaccinations (immunizations) or any other injections when a child has a fever or signs of a cold. This could be a mild polio infection without paralysis. If so, the irritation caused by an injection could cause **permanent paralysis** from the polio. Some experts say that **each year thousands of children are paralyzed by polio because of injections. Most of these injections are not needed.**

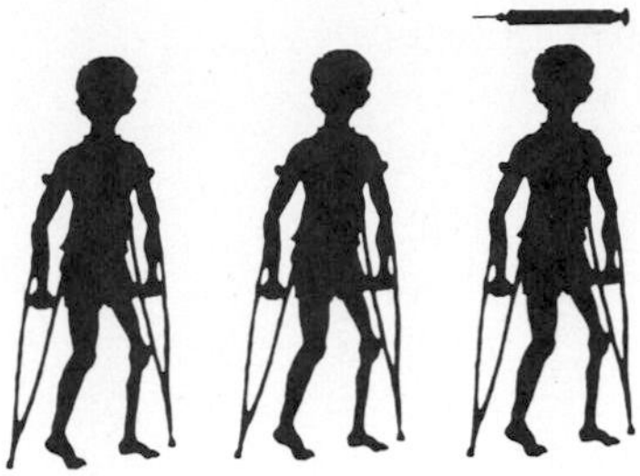

1 out of every 3 cases of paralysis from polio is caused by injections.

For more information on how injections disable children, see *Disabled Village Children,* Chapter 3.

For ideas on teaching people about the danger of unnecessary injections, see *Helping Health Workers Learn*, Chapters 18, 19, and 27.

HOW TO CLEAN (STERILIZE) EQUIPMENT

Many infectious diseases, such as AIDS (see p. 399), hepatitis (see p. 172), and tetanus (see p. 182), can be passed from a sick person to a healthy person through the use of syringes, needles, and other instruments that are not sterile (this includes the instruments used for piercing ears, acupuncture, tattoos, or circumcision). Many skin infections and abscesses also start because of this. **Any time the skin is cut or pierced, it should only be done with equipment that has been sterilized.**

Here are some ways to sterilize equipment:

- Boil for 20 minutes. (If you do not have a clock, add 1 or 2 grains of rice to the water. When the rice is cooked, the equipment will be sterile.)
- Or steam for 15 minutes in a special pot called a pressure cooker (or autoclave).
- Or soak for 20 minutes in a solution of 1 part chlorine bleach to 7 parts water, or in a solution of 70% ethanol alcohol. If possible, prepare these solutions fresh each day, because they lose their strength. (Be sure to sterilize the inside of a syringe by pulling some solution inside and then squirting it out.)

When you are helping someone who has an infectious disease, wash your hands often with soap and water.

CHAPTER

FIRST AID 10

FEVER

When a person's body temperature is too hot, we say he has a *fever.* Fever itself is not a sickness, but a sign of many different sicknesses. However, **high fever can be dangerous, especially in a small child.**

When a person has a fever:

1. Uncover him completely.

Small children should be undressed completely and left naked until the fever goes down.

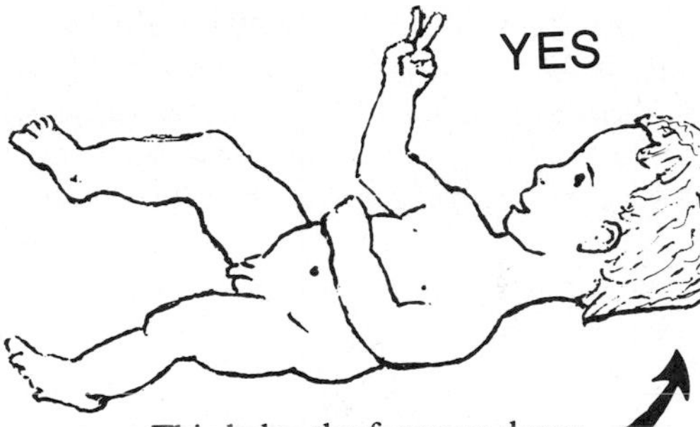

This helps the fever go down.

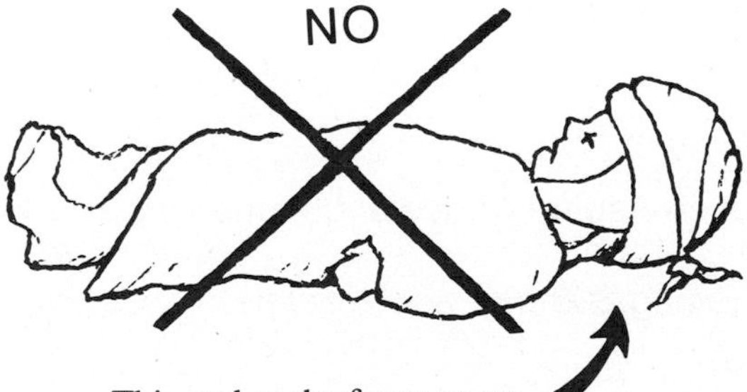

This makes the fever go up.

Never wrap the child in clothing or blankets.

To wrap up a child with fever is dangerous.

Fresh air or a breeze will not harm a person with fever. On the contrary, a fresh breeze helps lower the fever.

2. Also take aspirin to lower fever (see p. 379). For small children, it may be safer to give acetaminophen (paracetamol, p. 380). Be careful not to give too much.

3. Anyone who has a fever should **drink lots of water,** juices, or other liquids. For small children, especially babies, drinking water should be boiled first (and then cooled). Make sure the child passes urine regularly. If she does not pass much urine, or the urine is dark, give a lot more water.

4. When possible, find and treat the cause of the fever.

Very High Fevers

A very high fever can be dangerous if it is not brought down soon. It can cause fits (convulsions) or even permanent brain damage (paralysis, mental slowness, epilepsy, etc.). High fever is most dangerous for small children.

When a fever goes very high (over 40°), it must be lowered at once:

1. Put the person in a cool place.

2. Remove all clothing.

3. Fan him.

4. Pour cool (not cold) water over him, or put cloths soaked in cool water on his chest and forehead. Fan the cloths and change them often to keep them cool. Continue to do this until the fever goes down (below 38°).

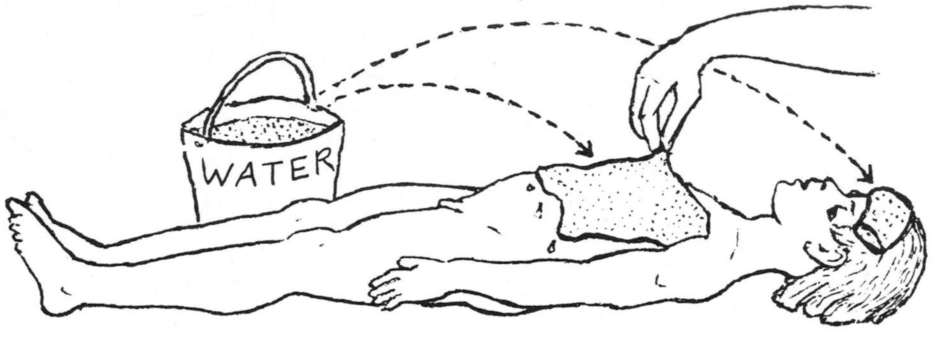

5. Give him plenty of cool (not cold) water to drink.

6. Give a medicine to bring down fever. Aspirin or acetaminophen works well.

Dosage for aspirin or acetaminophen (using 300 mg. adult tablets):

Persons over 12 years: 2 tablets every 4 hours

Children 6 to 12 years: 1 tablet every 4 hours

Children 3 to 6 years: 1/2 tablet every 4 hours

Children under 3 years: 1/4 tablet every 4 hours

Note: Acetaminophen is safer than aspirin for a child under 12 years old who has a cold, flu, or chickenpox (see p. 379).

If a person with fever cannot swallow the tablets, grind them up, mix the powder with some water, and put it up the anus as an *enema* or with a syringe without the needle.

If a high fever does not go down soon, or if fits (convulsions) begin, continue cooling with water and seek medical help at once.

SHOCK

Shock is a life-threatening condition that can result from a large burn, losing a lot of blood, severe illnesses, dehydration, or severe allergic reaction. Heavy bleeding inside the body—although not seen—can also cause shock.

Signs of SHOCK:

- weak, rapid pulse (more than 100 per minute)
- 'cold sweat'; pale, cold, damp skin
- blood pressure drops dangerously low
- mental confusion, weakness, or loss of consciousness.

What to do to prevent or treat shock:

At the first sign of shock, or if there is risk of shock . . .

- Have the person lie down with his feet a little higher than his head, like this:

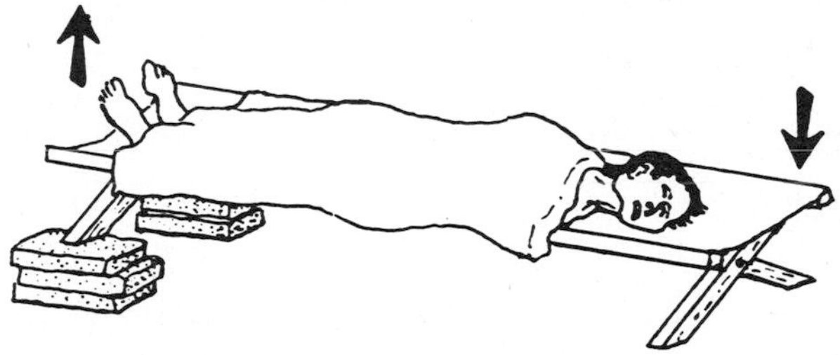

However, if he has a severe head injury, put him in a 'half-sitting' position (p. 91).

- Stop any bleeding.
- If the person feels cold, cover him with a blanket.
- If he is conscious and able to drink, give him sips of water or other drinks. If he looks dehydrated, give a lot of liquid, and Rehydration Drink (p. 152).
- Treat his wounds, if he has any.
- If he is in pain, give him aspirin or another pain medicine—but not one with a ***sedative*** such as codeine.
- Keep calm and reassure the person.

If the person is unconscious:

- Lay him on his side with his head low, tilted back and to one side (see above). If he seems to be choking, pull his tongue forward with your finger.
- If he has vomited, clear his mouth immediately. Be sure his head is low, tilted back, and to one side so he does not breathe vomit into his lungs.
- Do not give him anything by mouth until he becomes conscious.
- If you or someone nearby knows how, give intravenous solution (normal saline) at a fast drip.
- Seek medical help fast.

LOSS OF CONSCIOUSNESS

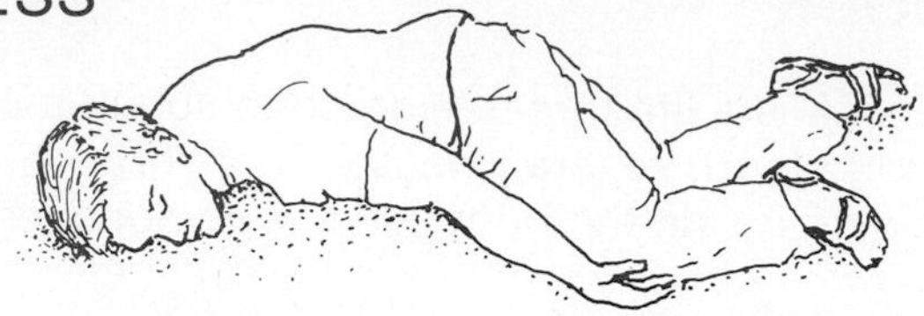

Common causes of loss of consciousness are:

- drunkenness
- a hit on the head (getting knocked out)
- shock (p. 77)
- fits (p. 178)
- poisoning (p. 103)
- fainting (from fright, weakness, etc.)
- heat stroke (p. 81)
- stroke (p. 327)
- heart attack (p. 325)

If a person is unconscious and you do not know why, **immediately check each of the following:**

1. Is he **breathing** well? If not, tilt his head way back and pull the jaw and tongue forward. If something is stuck in his throat, pull it out. If he is not breathing, use mouth-to-mouth breathing at once (see p. 80).

2. Is he **losing a lot of blood?** If so, control the bleeding (see p. 82).

3. Is he in **shock** (moist, pale skin; weak, rapid pulse)? If so, lay him with his head lower than his feet and loosen his clothing (see p. 77).

4. Could it be **heat stroke** (no sweat, high fever, hot, red skin)? If so, shade him from the sun, keep his head higher than his feet, and soak him with cold water (ice water if possible) and fan him (see p. 81).

How to position an unconscious person:

very pale skin:
(shock, fainting, etc.)

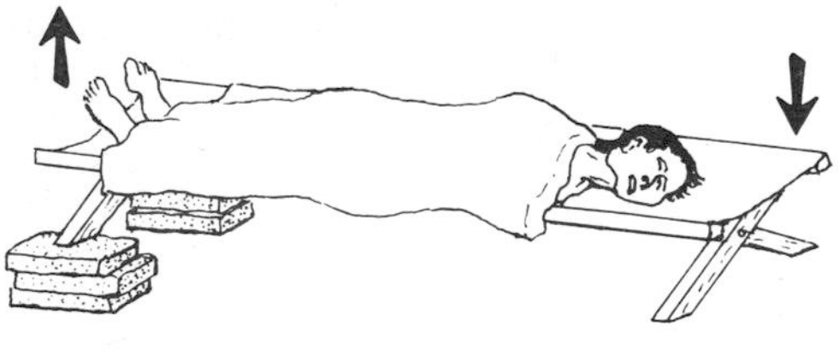

red or normal skin:
(heat stroke, stroke, heart problems, head injury)

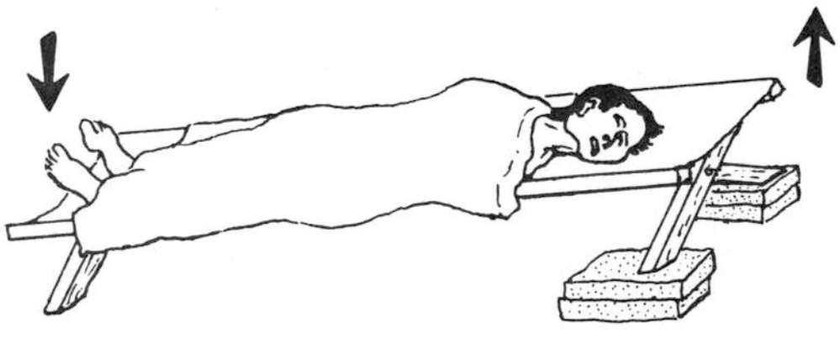

If there is any chance that the unconscious person is badly injured:

It is best not to move him until he becomes conscious. If you have to move him, do so with great care, because if his neck or back is broken, any change of position may cause greater injury (see p. 100).

Look for wounds or broken bones, but move the person as little as possible. Do not bend his back or neck.

Never give anything by mouth to a person who is unconscious.

WHEN SOMETHING GETS STUCK IN THE THROAT

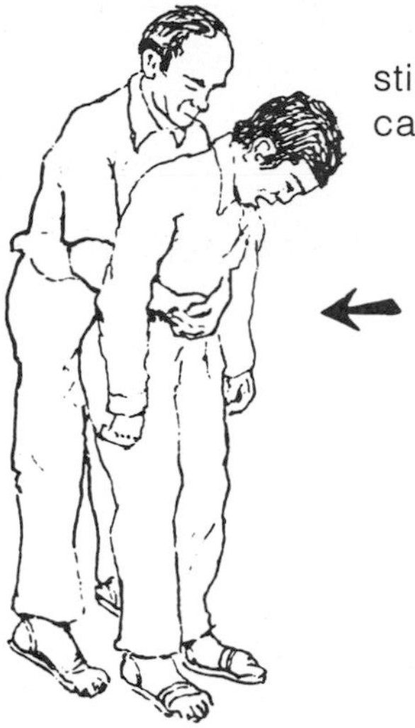

When food or something else sticks in a person's throat and he cannot breathe, **quickly** do this:

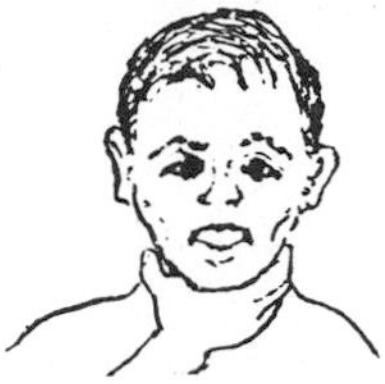

CHOKING

- Stand behind him and wrap your arms around his waist,
- put your fist against his belly above the navel and below the ribs,
- and press into his belly with a **sudden** strong upward jerk.

This forces the air from his lungs and should free his throat. Repeat several times if necessary.

If the person is a lot bigger than you, or is already unconscious, **quickly** do this:

- Lay him on his back.
- Tilt his head to one side.
- Sit over him like this, with the heel of your lower hand on his belly between his navel and ribs. (For fat persons, pregnant women, persons in wheelchairs, or small children, place hands on the chest, not the belly.)
- Make a quick, strong upward push.
- Repeat several times if necessary.
- If he still cannot breathe, try **mouth-to-mouth breathing** (see next page).

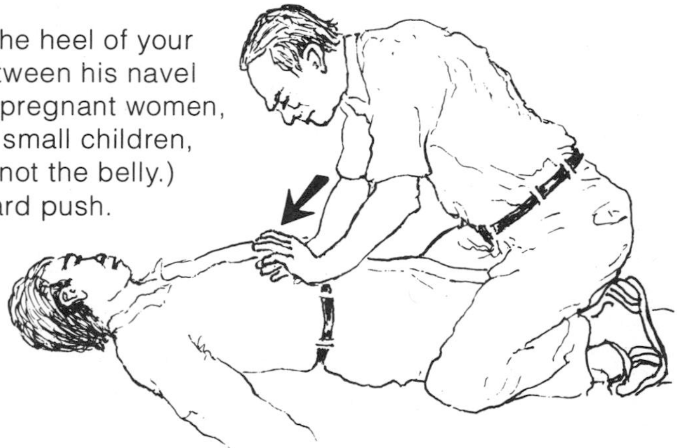

DROWNING

A person who has stopped breathing has only 4 minutes to live! You must **act fast!**

Start mouth-to-mouth breathing at once (see next page)—if possible, even before the drowning person is out of the water, as soon as it is shallow enough to stand.

If you cannot blow air into his lungs, when you reach the shore, quickly put him on his side with his head lower than his feet and push his belly as described above. Then continue mouth-to-mouth breathing at once.

ALWAYS START MOUTH-TO-MOUTH BREATHING AT ONCE before trying to get water out of the drowning person's chest.

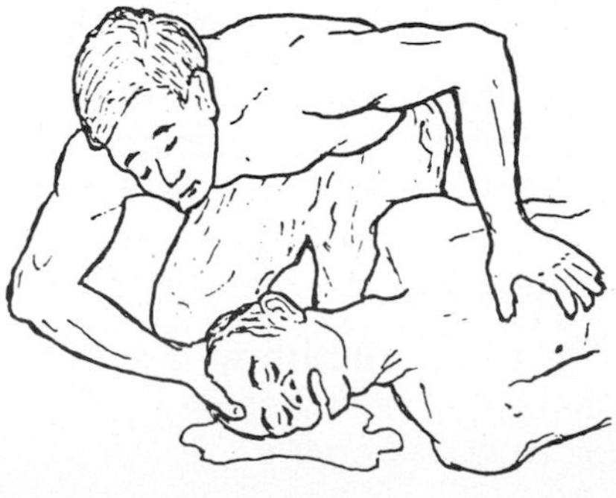

WHAT TO DO WHEN BREATHING STOPS: MOUTH-TO-MOUTH BREATHING

Common causes for breathing to stop are:

- something stuck in the throat
- the tongue or thick mucus blocking the throat of an unconscious person
- drowning, choking on smoke, or poisoning
- a strong blow to the head or chest
- a heart attack

A person can die within 4 minutes if he does not breathe.

If a person stops breathing, begin mouth-to-mouth breathing IMMEDIATELY.

Do all of the following as quickly as you can:

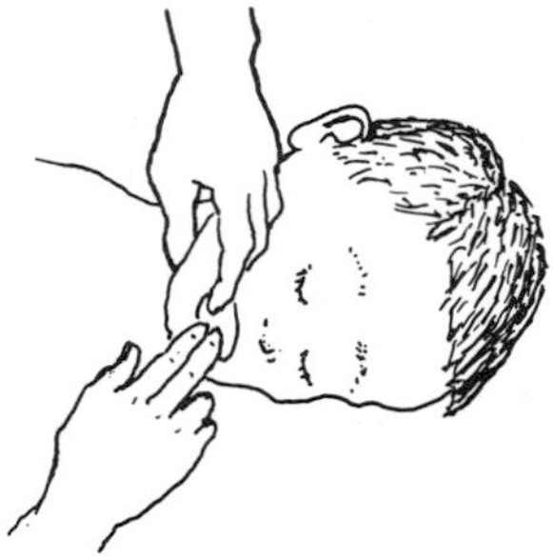

Step 1: Quickly use a finger to remove anything stuck in the mouth or throat. Pull the tongue forward. If there is mucus in the throat, quickly try to clear it out.

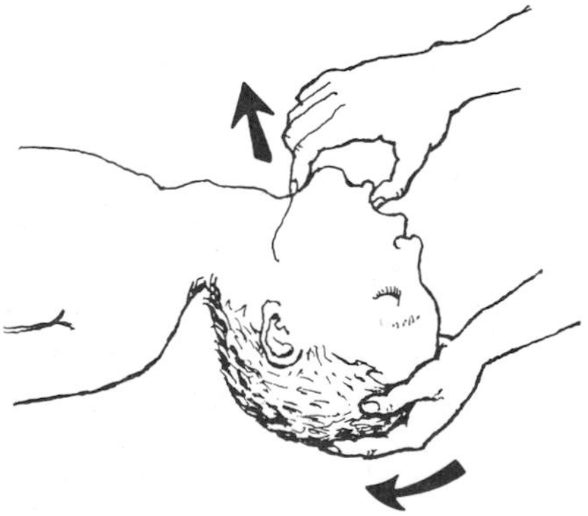

Step 2: Quickly but gently lay the person face up. Gently tilt his head back, and pull his jaw forward.

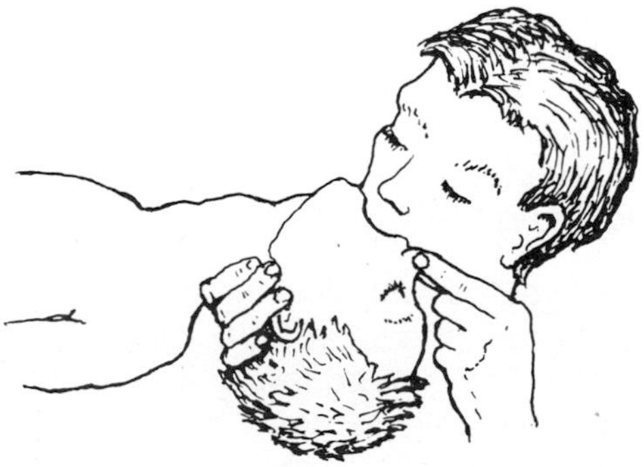

Step 3: Pinch his nostrils closed with your fingers, open his mouth wide, cover his mouth with yours, and blow strongly into his lungs so that his chest rises. Pause to let the air come back out and blow again. Repeat about once every 5 seconds. With babies and small children, cover the nose and mouth with your mouth and breathe **very gently** about once every 3 seconds.

Continue **mouth-to-mouth breathing** until the person can breathe by himself, or until there is no doubt he is dead. Sometimes you must keep trying for an hour or more.

EMERGENCIES CAUSED BY HEAT

Heat Cramps

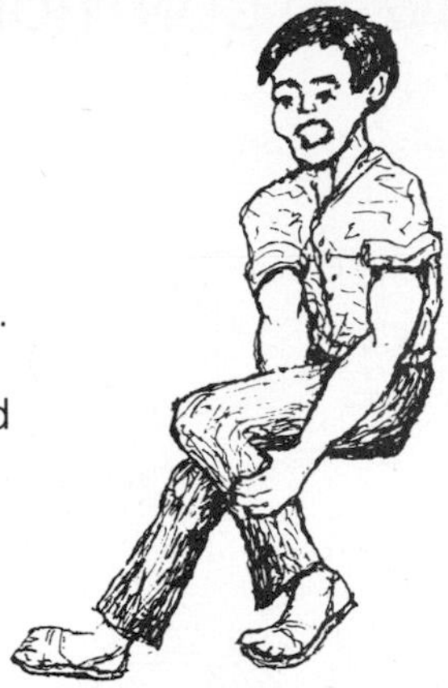

In hot weather people who work hard and sweat a lot sometimes get painful cramps in their legs, arms, or stomach. These occur because the body lacks salt.

Treatment: Put a teaspoon of salt in a liter of boiled water and drink it. Repeat once every hour until the cramps are gone. Have the person sit or lie down in a cool place and gently massage the painful areas.

Heat Exhaustion

Signs: A person who works and sweats a lot in hot weather may become very pale, weak, and nauseous, and perhaps feel faint. The skin is cool and moist. The pulse is rapid and weak. The temperature of the body is usually normal (see p. 31).

Treatment: Have the person lie down in a cool place, raise his feet, and rub his legs. Give salt water to drink: 1 teaspoon of salt in a liter of water. (Give nothing by mouth while the person is unconscious.)

Heat Stroke

Heat stroke is not common, but is very dangerous. It occurs especially in older people and ***alcoholics*** during hot weather.

Signs: The skin is red, very hot, and dry. Not even the armpits are moist. The person has a very high fever, sometimes more than 42°C. Often he is unconscious.

Treatment: **The body temperature must be lowered immediately.** Put the person in the shade. Soak him with cold water (ice water if possible) and fan him. Continue until the fever drops. Seek medical help.

DIFFERENCES BETWEEN 'HEAT EXHAUSTION' AND 'HEAT STROKE':

HEAT EXHAUSTION

- sweaty, pale, cool skin
- large pupils
- no fever
- weakness

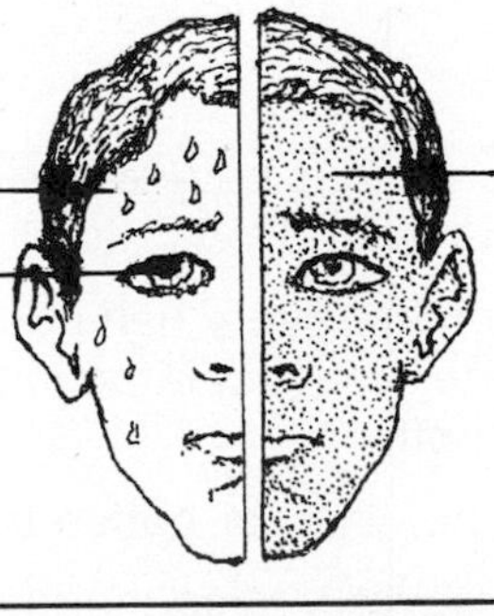

HEAT STROKE

- dry, red, hot skin
- high fever
- the person is very ill or unconscious

For emergencies caused by cold, see p. 408 and 409.

HOW TO CONTROL BLEEDING FROM A WOUND

1. Raise the injured part.

2. With a clean thick cloth (or your hand if there is no cloth) press directly on the wound. Keep pressing until the bleeding stops. This may take 15 minutes or sometimes an hour or more. This type of **direct pressure** will stop the bleeding of nearly all wounds—sometimes even when a part of the body has been cut off.

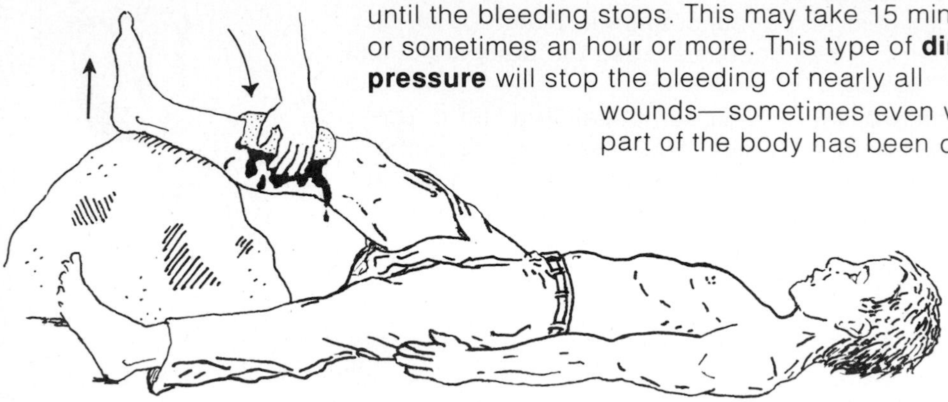

Occasionally direct pressure will not control bleedling, especially when the wound is very large or an arm or leg has been cut off. If this happens, and the person is in danger of bleeding to death, do the following:

- Keep pressing on the wound.
- Keep the wounded part as high as possible.
- Tie the arm or leg as close to the wound as possible—between the wound and the body. Tighten by twisting the stick enough to control the bleeding.
- For the tie, use a folded cloth or a wide belt; never use thin rope, string, or wire.

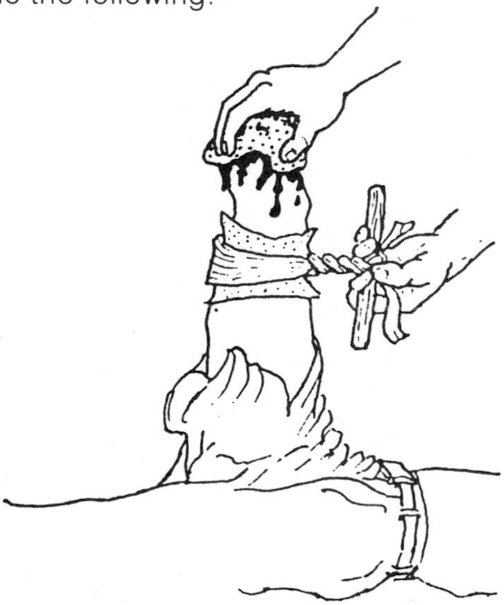

PRECAUTIONS:

- Tie the limb **only** if bleeding is severe and cannot be controlled by pressing directly on the wound.
- Loosen the tie for a moment every half hour to see if it is still needed and to let the blood circulate. Leaving it too long may damage the arm or leg so much it must be cut off.
- **Never** use dirt, kerosene, lime, or coffee to stop bleeding.
- If bleeding or injury is severe, raise the feet and lower the head to prevent shock (see p. 77).

HOW TO STOP NOSEBLEEDS

1. Sit quietly.

2. Blow the nose gently to remove mucus and blood.

3. Pinch the nose firmly for 10 minutes or until the bleeding has stopped.

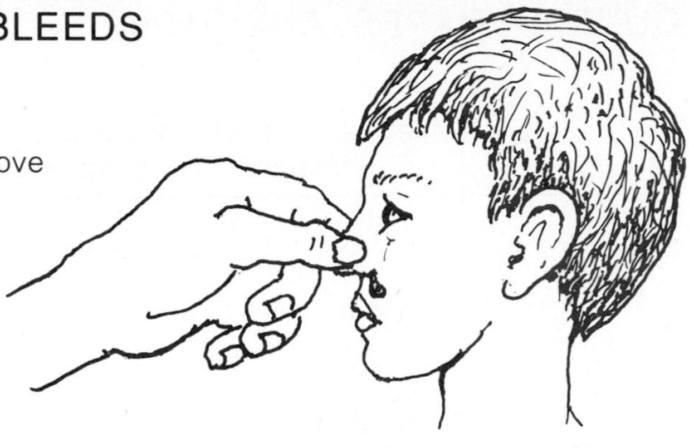

If this does not control the bleeding . . .

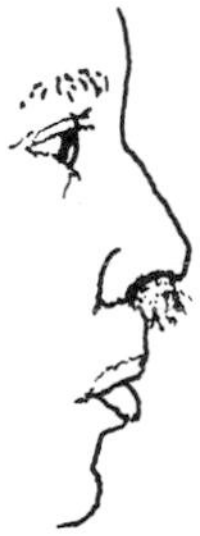

Pack the nostril with a wad of cotton, leaving part of it outside the nose. If possible, first wet the cotton with hydrogen peroxide, ***Vaseline,*** cardon cactus juice (p. 13), or lidocaine with epinephrine (p. 381).

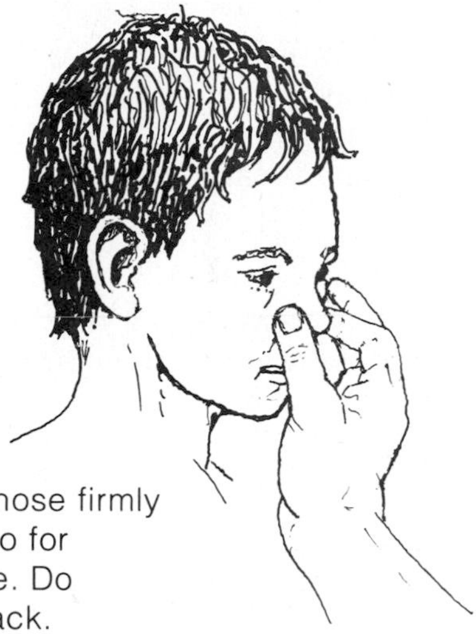

Then pinch the nose firmly again. Do not let go for 10 minutes or more. Do not tip the head back.

Leave the cotton in place for a few hours after the bleeding stops; then take it out very carefully.

In older persons especially, bleeding may come from the back part of the nose and cannot be stopped by pinching it. In this case, have the person hold a cork, corn cob, or other similar object between his teeth and, leaning forward, sit quietly and try not to swallow until the bleeding stops. (The cork helps keep him from swallowing, and that gives the blood a chance to clot.)

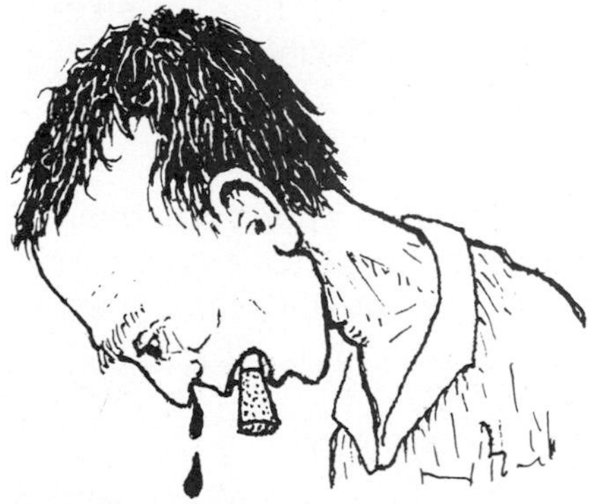

Prevention:

If a person's nose bleeds often, smear a little ***Vaseline*** inside the nostrils twice a day. Or sniff water with a little salt in it (see p. 164).

Eating oranges, tomatoes, and other fruits may help to strengthen the veins so that the nose bleeds less.

CUTS, SCRAPES, AND SMALL WOUNDS

Cleanliness is of first importance in preventing infection and helping wounds to heal.

To treat a wound . . .

First, wash your hands very well with soap and water.

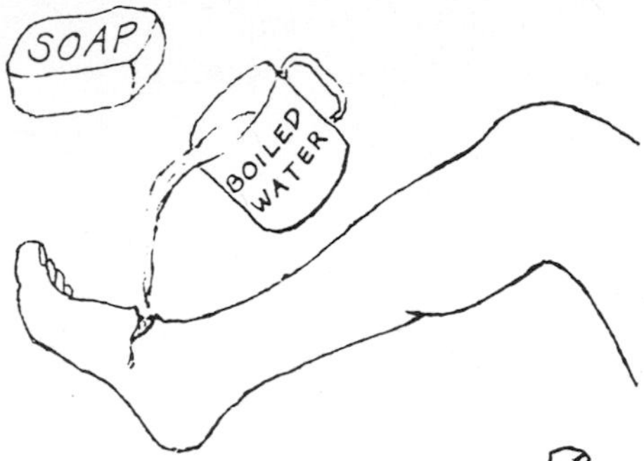

Then wash the skin around the wound with soap and cool, boiled water.

Now wash the wound well with cool, boiled water (and soap, if the wound has a lot of dirt in it. Soap helps clean but can damage the flesh).

When cleaning the wound, be careful to clean out all the dirt. Lift up and clean under any flaps of skin. You can use clean tweezers, or a clean cloth or gauze, to remove bits of dirt, but always boil them first to be sure they are sterile.

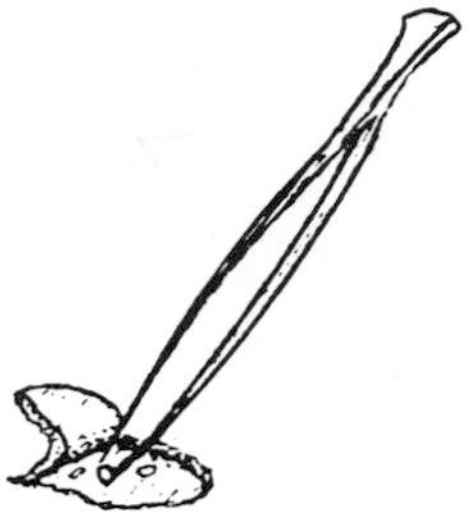

If possible, squirt out the wound with boiled water in a syringe or suction bulb.

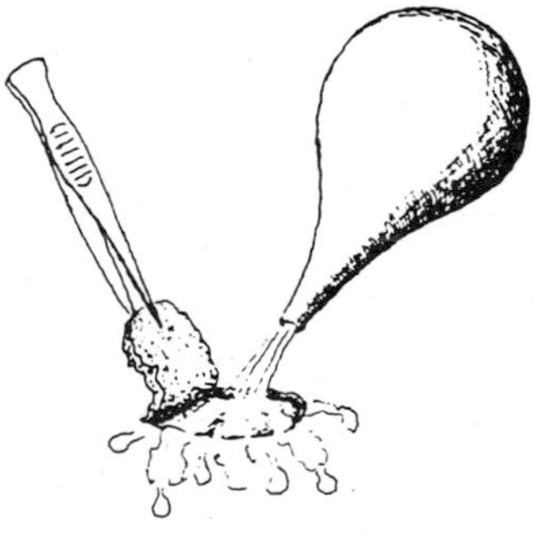

Any bit of dirt that is left in a wound can cause an infection.

After the wound has been cleaned, place a piece of clean gauze or cloth over the top. It should be light enough so that the air can get to the wound and help it to heal. Change the gauze or cloth every day and look for signs of infection (see p. 88).

NEVER put animal or human feces or mud on a wound. These can cause dangerous infections, such as tetanus.

NEVER put alcohol, tincture of iodine, or *Merthiolate* directly into a wound; doing so will damage the flesh and make healing slower.

LARGE CUTS: HOW TO CLOSE THEM

A recent cut that is very clean will heal faster if you bring the edges together so the cut stays closed.

Close a deep cut only if all of the following are true:

- the cut is less than 12 hours old,
- the cut is very clean, and
- it is impossible to get a health worker to close it the same day.

Before closing the cut, wash it very well with cool, boiled water (and soap, if the wound is dirty). If possible, squirt it out with a syringe and water. Be absolutely sure that no dirt or soap is left hidden in the cut.

There are two methods to close a cut:

'BUTTERFLY' BANDAGES OF ADHESIVE TAPE

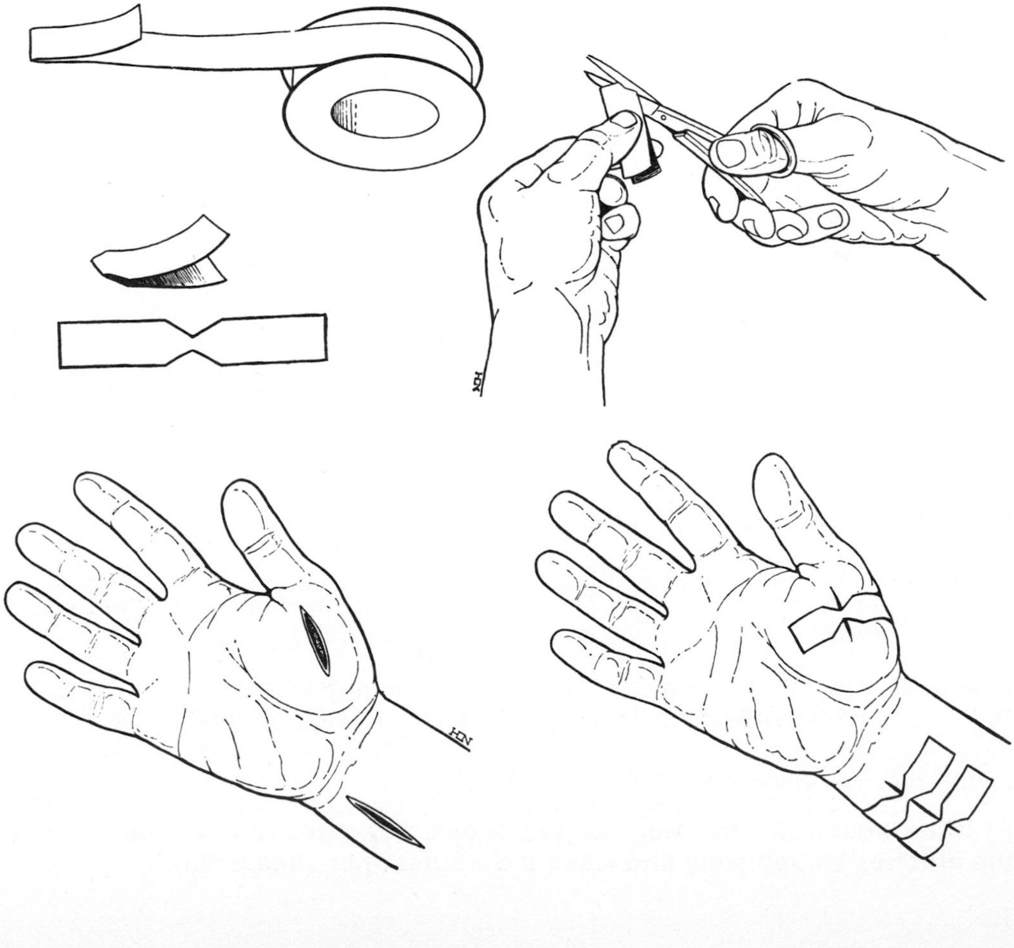

STITCHES OR SUTURES WITH THREAD

To find out if a cut needs stitches see if the edges of the skin come together by themselves. If they do, usually no stitches are needed.

To stitch a wound:

- ♦ Boil a sewing needle and a thin thread (nylon or silk is best) for 20 minutes.
- ♦ Wash the wound with cool, boiled water, as has been described.
- ♦ Wash your hands very well with boiled water and soap.
- ♦ Sew the wound like this:

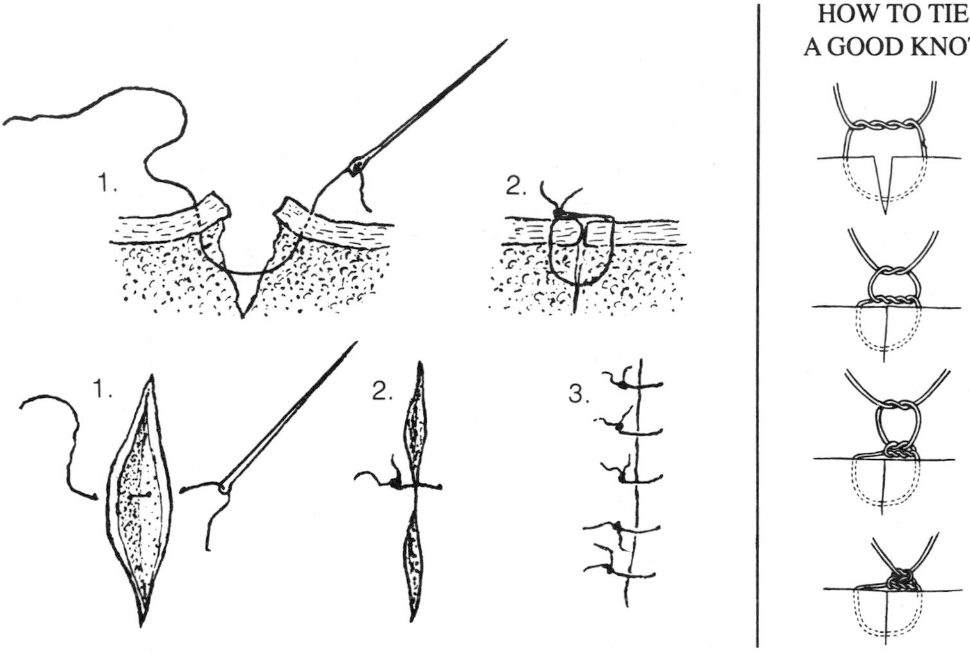

Make the first stitch in the middle of the cut, and tie it closed (1. and 2.).

If the skin is tough, hold the needle with a pair of pliers (or needle holder) that has been boiled.

Make enough other stitches to close the whole cut (3.).

Leave the stitches in place for 5 to 14 days (on the face 5 days; the body 10 days; the hand or foot 14 days). Then remove the stitches: cut the thread on one side of the knot and pull the knot until the thread comes out.

WARNING: Only close wounds that are very clean and less than 12 hours old. Old, dirty, or infected wounds must be left open. Bites from people, dogs, pigs, or other animals should also be left open. Closing these can cause dangerous infections.

If the wound that has been closed shows any signs of infection, remove the stitches immediately and leave the wound open (see p. 88).

BANDAGES

Bandages are used to help keep wounds clean. For this reason, bandages or pieces of cloth used to cover wounds must always be clean themselves. Cloth used for bandages should be washed and then dried with an iron or in the sun, in a clean, dust-free place.

Make sure the wound has first been cleaned, as shown on p. 84. If possible, cover the wound with a sterile gauze pad before bandaging. These pads are often sold in sealed envelopes in pharmacies.

Or prepare your own sterile gauze or cloth. Wrap it in thick paper, seal it with tape, and bake it for 20 minutes in an oven. Putting a pan of water in the oven under the cloth will keep it from charring.

It is better to have no bandage at all than one that is dirty or wet.

If a bandage gets wet or dirt gets under it, take the bandage off, wash the cut again, and put on a clean bandage. Change the bandage every day.

Examples of bandages:

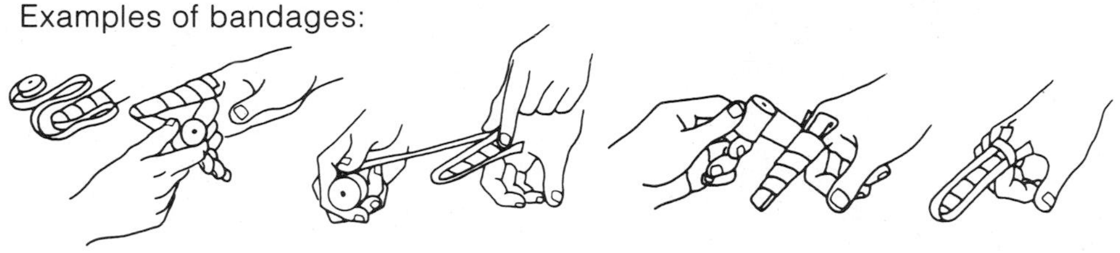

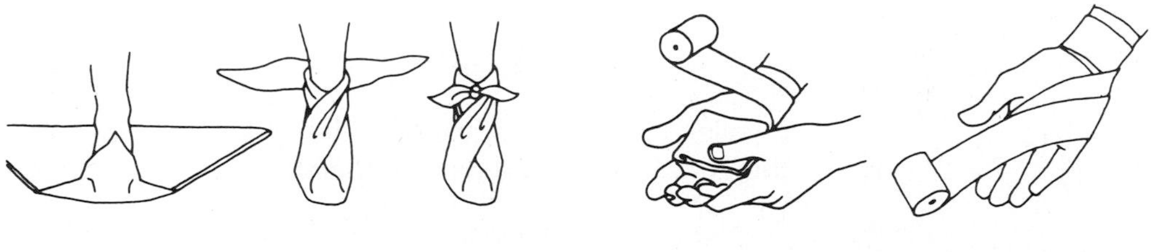

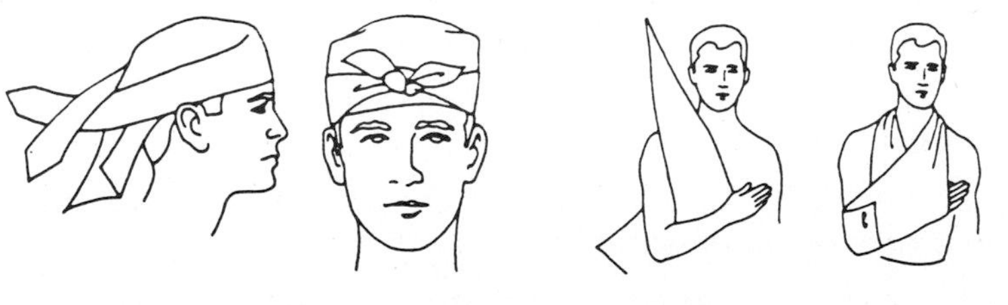

Note: For children it is often better to bandage the whole hand or foot instead of one finger or toe. The bandage will not come off as easily.

CAUTION:

Be careful that a bandage that goes around a limb is not so tight it cuts off the flow of blood.

Many small scrapes and cuts do not need bandages. They heal best if washed with soap and water and left open to the air. The most important thing is to **keep them clean.**

INFECTED WOUNDS: HOW TO RECOGNIZE AND TREAT THEM

A wound is infected if:

- it becomes **red, swollen, hot,** and **painful,**
- it has **pus,**
- or if it begins to **smell bad.**

The infection is spreading to other parts of the body if:

- it causes **fever,**
- there is a **red line above the wound,**
- or if the **lymph nodes become swollen and tender.** Lymph nodes—often called 'glands'—are little traps for germs that form small lumps under the skin when they get infected.

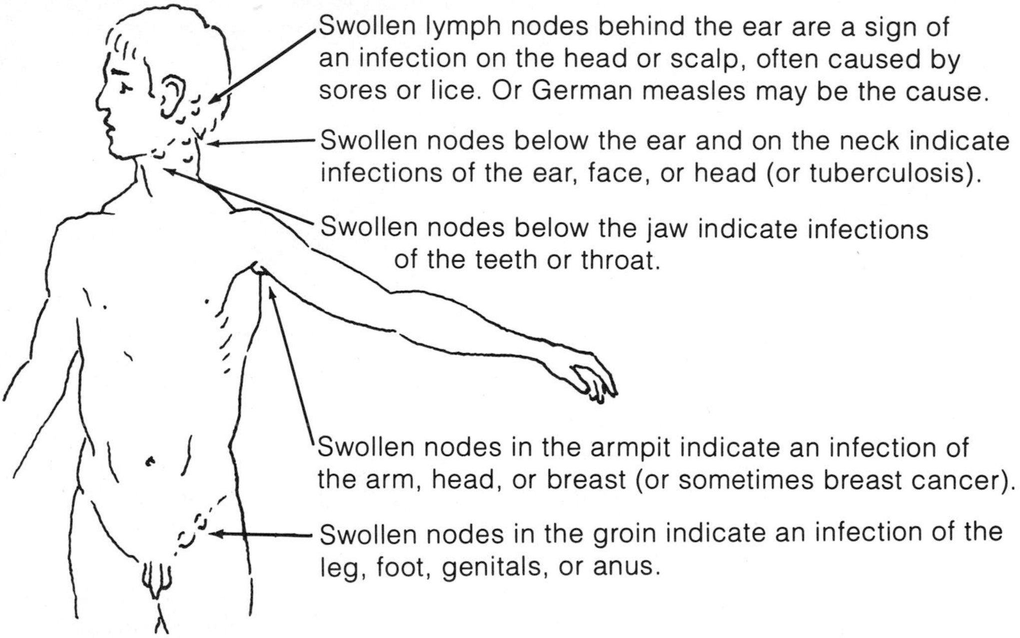

Swollen lymph nodes behind the ear are a sign of an infection on the head or scalp, often caused by sores or lice. Or German measles may be the cause.
Swollen nodes below the ear and on the neck indicate infections of the ear, face, or head (or tuberculosis).
Swollen nodes below the jaw indicate infections of the teeth or throat.
Swollen nodes in the armpit indicate an infection of the arm, head, or breast (or sometimes breast cancer).
Swollen nodes in the groin indicate an infection of the leg, foot, genitals, or anus.

Treatment of infected wounds:

- ♦ Put hot compresses over the wound for 20 minutes 4 times a day. Or hold an infected hand or foot in a bucket of hot water.
- ♦ Keep the infected part at rest and elevated (raised above the level of the heart).
- ♦ If the infection is severe or if the person has not been vaccinated against tetanus, use an antibiotic like penicillin (see p. 351, 352).

WARNING: If the wound has a bad smell, if brown or gray liquid oozes out, or if the skin around it turns black and forms air bubbles or blisters, this may be gangrene. Seek medical help fast. Meanwhile, follow the instructions for gangrene on p. 213.

WOUNDS THAT ARE LIKELY TO BECOME DANGEROUSLY INFECTED

These wounds are most likely to become dangerously infected:

- dirty wounds, or wounds made with dirty objects
- puncture wounds and other deep wounds that do not bleed much
- wounds made where animals are kept: in corrals, pig pens, etc.
- large wounds with severe mashing or bruising
- bites, especially from pigs, dogs, or people
- bullet wounds

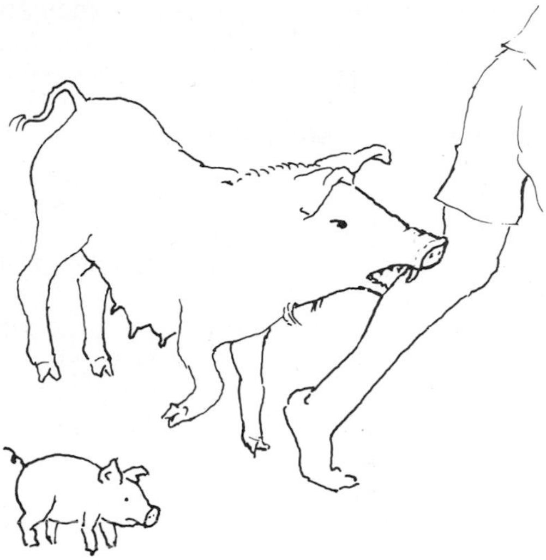

Special care for this type of 'high risk' wound:

1. Wash the wound well with boiled water and soap. **Remove all pieces of dirt, blood clots, and dead or badly damaged flesh.** Squirt out the dirt using a syringe or suction bulb.

2. If the wound is very deep, if it is a bite, or if there is a chance that it still has dirt in it, use an antibiotic. The best is penicillin. If you do not have penicillin, use ampicillin, erythromycin, tetracycline, co-trimoxazole, or a sulfa. For dosages, see the GREEN PAGES.

3. **Never** close this type of wound with stitches or 'butterfly' bandages. **Leave the wound open.** If it is very large, a skilled health worker or a doctor may be able to close it later.

The danger of tetanus is very great in people who have not been vaccinated against this deadly disease. To lower the risk, a person who has not been vaccinated against tetanus should use penicillin or ampicillin immediately after receiving a wound of this type, even if the injury is small.

If the wound of this type is very severe, a person who has not been vaccinated against tetanus should take large doses of penicillin or ampicillin for a week or more. An antitoxin for tetanus (p. 389) should also be considered—but be sure to take precautions on p. 70 if using tetanus antitoxin made from horse serum.

BULLET, KNIFE, AND OTHER SERIOUS WOUNDS

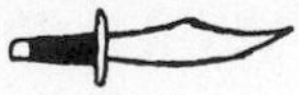

Danger of infection: Any deep bullet or knife wound runs a high risk of dangerous infection. For this reason an antibiotic, preferably penicillin (p. 351) or ampicillin (p. 353) should be used at once.

Persons who have not been vaccinated against tetanus should, if possible, be given an injection of an antitoxin for tetanus (p. 389), and also be vaccinated against tetanus.

If possible, seek medical help.

Bullet Wounds in the Arms or Legs

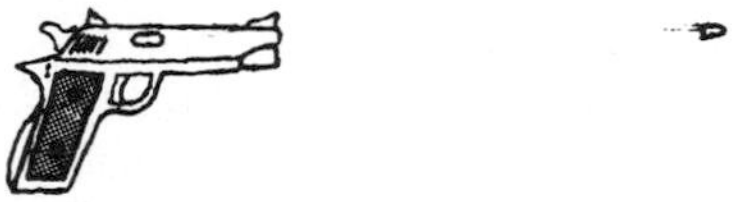

- If the wound is bleeding a lot, control the bleeding as shown on page 82.
- If the bleeding is not serious, let the wound bleed for a short while. This will help clean it out.
- Wash the wound with cool, boiled water and apply a clean bandage. In the case of a gunshot wound, wash the surface (outside) only. It is usually better not to poke anything into the hole.
- Give antibiotics.

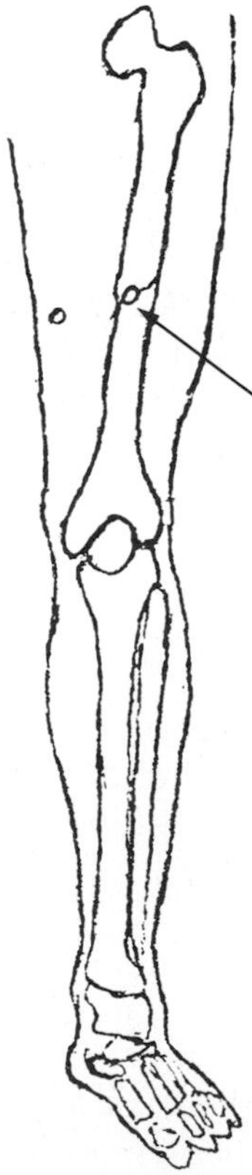

CAUTION:

If there is any possibility that the bullet has hit a bone, the bone may be broken.

Using or putting weight on the wounded limb (standing, for example) might cause a more serious break, like this:

If a break is suspected, it is best to splint the limb and not to use it for several weeks.

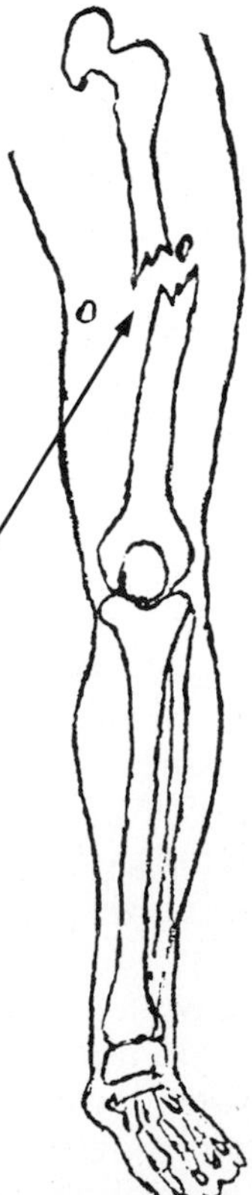

When the wound is serious, raise the wounded part a little higher than the heart and keep the injured person completely still.

This way the wound will heal faster and is less likely to become infected.

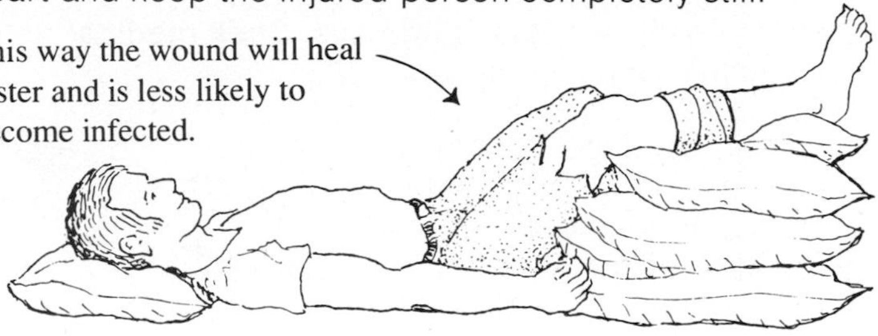

YES

Walking on an injured leg or sitting with the leg hanging down will slow healing and encourage infection.

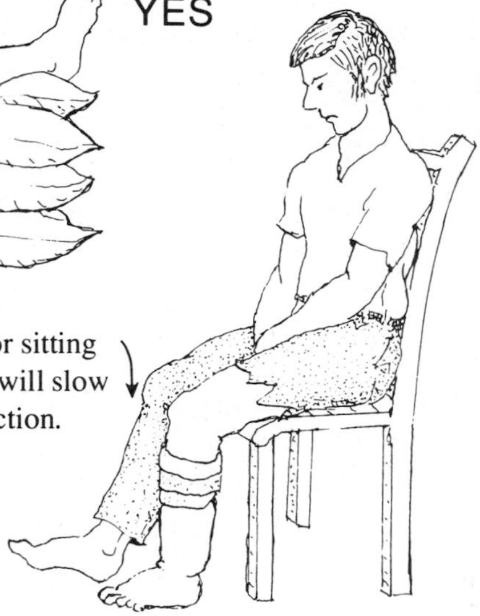

NO

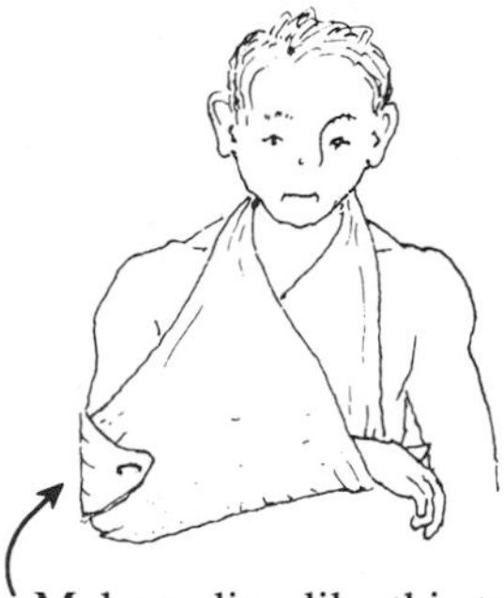

Make a sling like this to support an arm with a gunshot wound or other serious injury.

Deep Chest Wounds

Chest wounds can be very dangerous. Seek medical help at once.

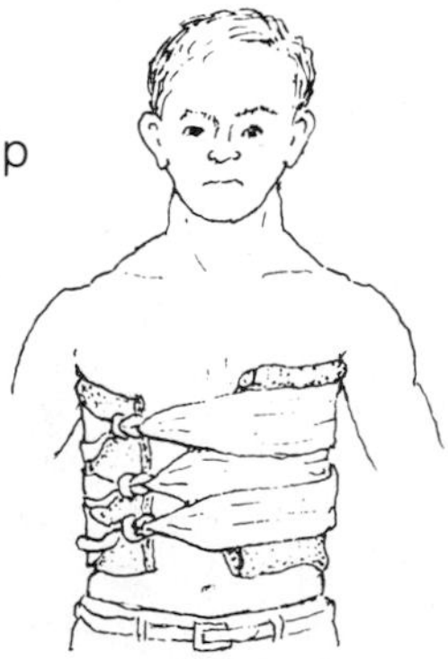

- If the wound has reached the lungs and air is being sucked through the hole when the person breathes, cover the wound at once so that no more air enters. Spread *Vaseline* or vegetable fat on a gauze pad or clean bandage and wrap it tightly over the hole like this: (*CAUTION:* If this tight bandage makes breathing more difficult, try loosening or removing it.)
- Put the injured person in the position in which he feels most comfortable.
- If there are signs of shock, give proper treatment (see p. 77).
- Give antibiotics and painkillers.

Bullet Wounds in the Head

- Place the injured person in a 'half-sitting' position.
- Cover the wound with a clean bandage.
- Give antibiotics (penicillin).
- Seek medical help.

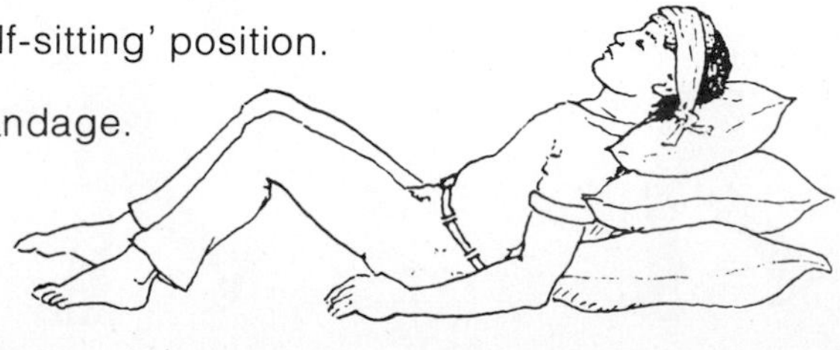

Deep Wounds in the Abdomen

Any wound that goes into the belly or gut is dangerous. **Seek medical help immediately.** But in the meantime:

Cover the wound with a clean bandage.

If the guts are partly outside the wound, cover them with a clean cloth soaked in lightly salted, cool, boiled water. Do not try to push the guts back in. Make sure the cloth stays wet.

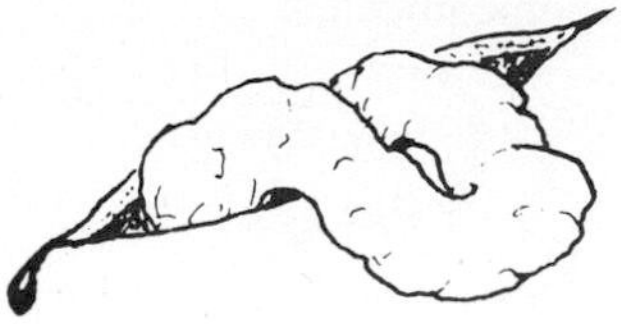

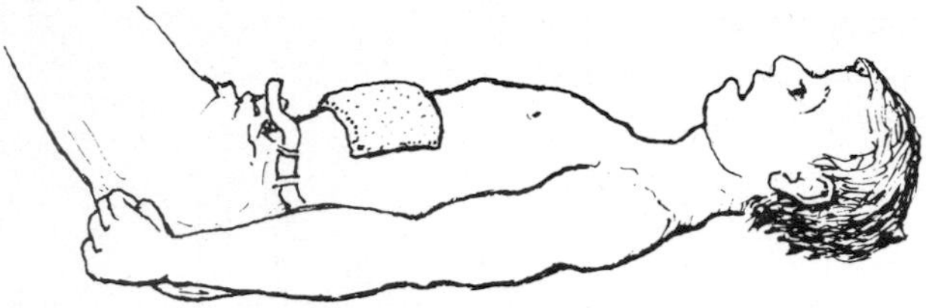

If the wounded person is in shock, raise his feet higher than his head.

Give absolutely nothing by mouth: no food, no drink, not even water—unless it will take more than 2 days to get to a health center. Then give water only, in small sips.

If the wounded person is awake and thirsty, let him suck on a piece of cloth soaked in water.

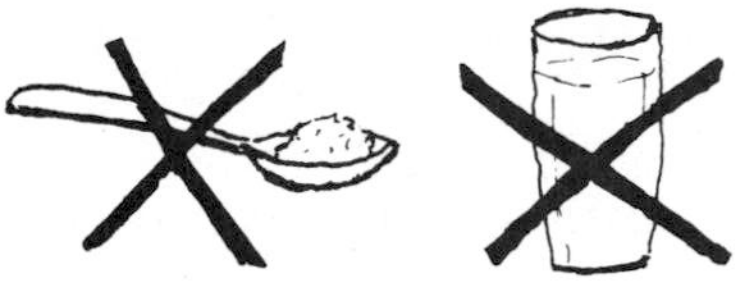

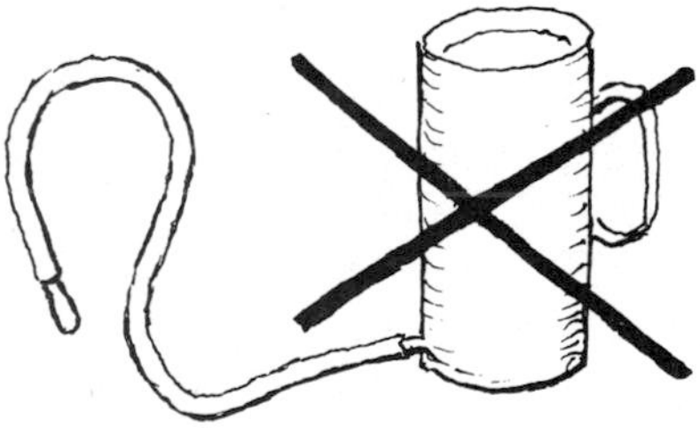

Never give an enema, even if the stomach swells up or the injured person does not move his bowels for days. If the gut is torn, an enema or purge can kill him.

Inject antibiotics (see the following page for instructions).

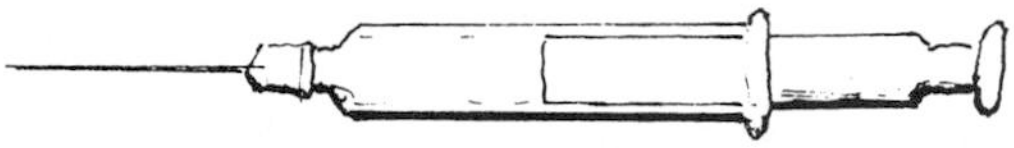

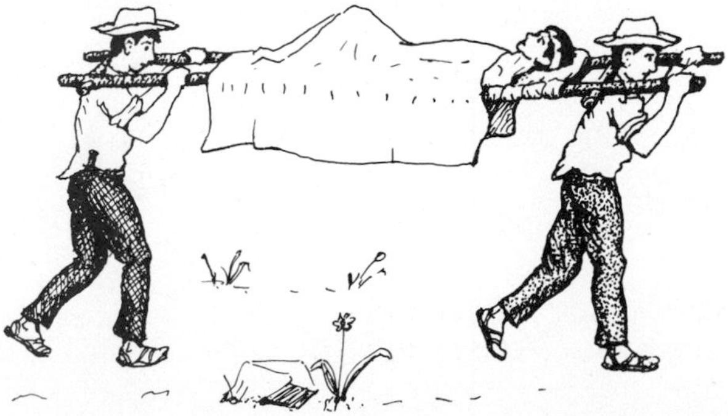

DO NOT WAIT FOR A HEALTH WORKER.

IMMEDIATELY TAKE THE INJURED PERSON TO THE CLOSEST HEALTH CENTER OR HOSPITAL. He will need an operation.

MEDICINE FOR A WOUND THAT GOES INTO THE GUT
(Also for appendicitis or peritonitis)

Until you can get medical help, do the following:

Inject ampicillin (p. 353), 1 gm. (four 250 mg. ampules) every 4 hours.

If there is no ampicillin:

Inject penicillin (crystalline, if possible, p. 353), 5 million units immediately; after that, 1 million units every 4 hours.

Together with the penicillin, give an injection of either:
streptomycin (p. 363), 2 ml. (1 gm.), 2 times a day or
chloramphenicol (p. 357), 2 ampules of 250 mg. every 4 hours.

If you cannot obtain these antibiotics in injectable form, give ampicillin or penicillin by mouth together with chloramphenicol or tetracycline, and very little water.

EMERGENCY PROBLEMS OF THE GUT (ACUTE ABDOMEN)

Acute abdomen is a name given to a number of sudden, severe conditions of the gut for which prompt surgery is often needed to prevent death. Appendicitis, peritonitis, and gut obstruction are examples (see following pages). In women, pelvic inflammatory disease, or an out-of-place pregnancy can also cause an acute abdomen. Often the exact cause of acute abdomen will be uncertain until a surgeon cuts open the belly and looks inside.

If a person has continuous severe gut pain with vomiting, but does not have diarrhea, suspect an acute abdomen.

ACUTE ABDOMEN:

Take to a hospital—surgery may be needed

- continuous severe pain that keeps getting worse
- constipation and vomiting
- belly swollen, hard, person protects it
- severely ill

LESS SERIOUS ILLNESS:

Probably can be treated in the home or health center

- pain that comes and goes (cramps)
- moderate or severe diarrhea
- sometimes signs of an infection, perhaps a cold or sore throat
- he has had pains like this before
- only moderately ill

If a person shows signs of acute abdomen, get him to a hospital as fast as you can.

Obstructed Gut

An acute abdomen may be caused by something that blocks or 'obstructs' a part of the gut, so that food and stools cannot pass. More common causes are:

- a ball or knot of roundworms (Ascaris, p. 140)
- a loop of gut that is pinched in a hernia (p. 177)
- a part of the gut that slips inside the part below it (intussusception)

Almost any kind of acute abdomen may show some signs of obstruction. Because it hurts the damaged gut to move, it stops moving.

Signs of an obstructed gut:

Steady, severe pain in the belly.

This child's belly is swollen, hard, and very tender. It hurts more when you touch it. He tries to protect his belly and keeps his legs doubled up. His belly is often 'silent'. (When you put your ear to it, you hear no sound of normal gurgles.)

Sudden vomiting with great force! The vomit may shoot out a meter or more. It may have green bile in it or smell and look like feces.

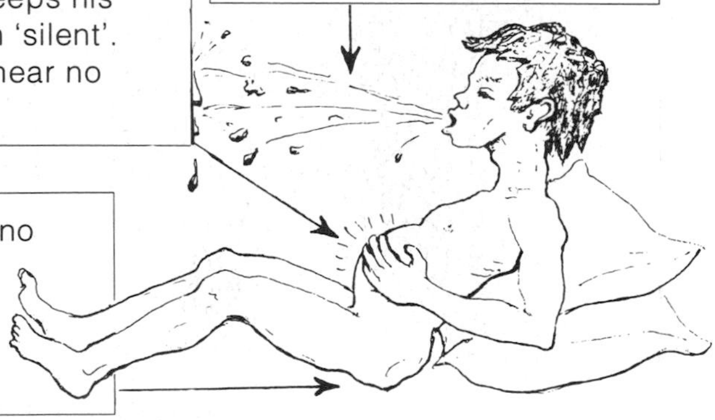

He is usually constipated (little or no bowel movements). If there is diarrhea, it is only a little bit. Sometimes all that comes out is some bloody mucus.

Get this person to a hospital **as fast as possible.** His life is in danger and surgery may be needed.

Appendicitis, Peritonitis

These dangerous conditions often require surgery. Seek medical help fast.

Appendicitis is an infection of the *appendix,* a finger-shaped sac attached to the large intestine in the lower right-hand part of the belly. An infected appendix sometimes bursts open, causing *peritonitis.*

Peritonitis is an acute, serious infection of the lining of the cavity or bag that holds the gut. It results when the appendix or another part of the gut bursts or is torn.

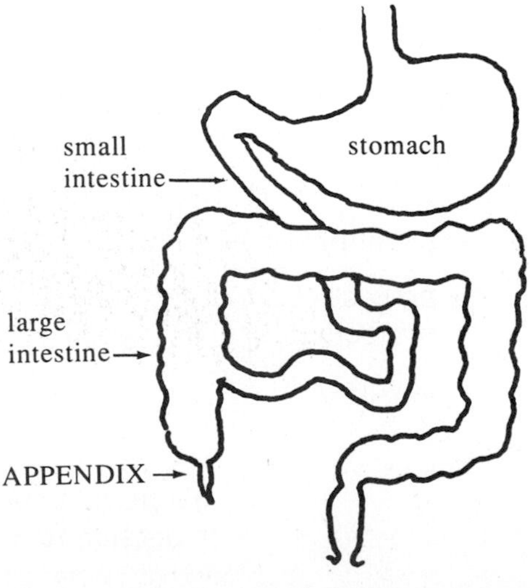

Signs of appendicitis:

- The main sign is a steady pain in the belly that gets worse and worse.
- The pain often begins around the navel ('bellybutton'),

  but it soon moves to the lower right side.
- There may be loss of appetite, vomiting, constipation, or a mild fever.

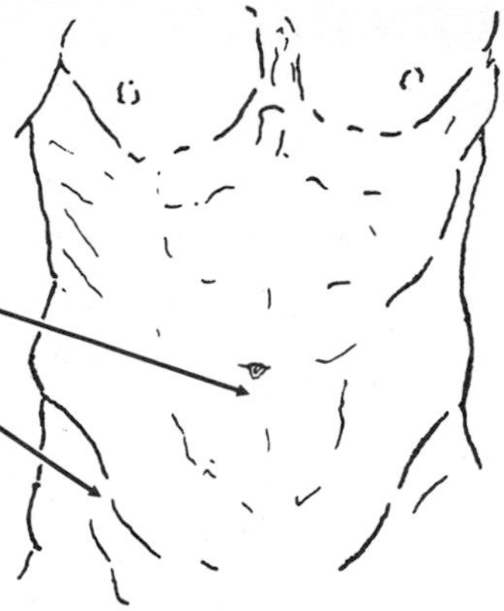

TESTS FOR APPENDICITIS OR PERITONITIS:

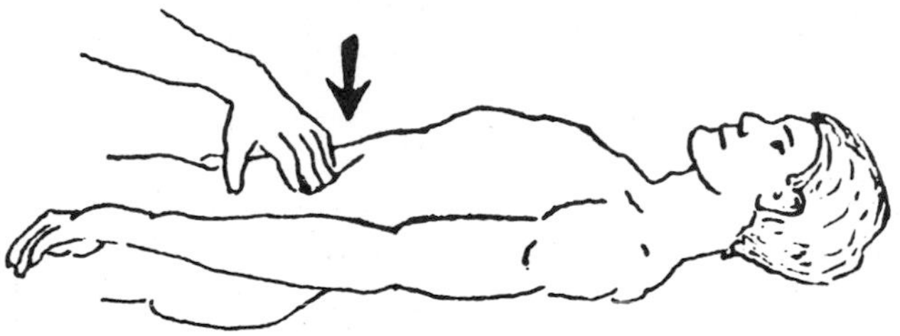

Have the person cough and see if this causes sharp pain in the belly.

Or, slowly but forcefully, press on the abdomen a little above the left groin until it hurts a little.

Then quickly remove the hand.

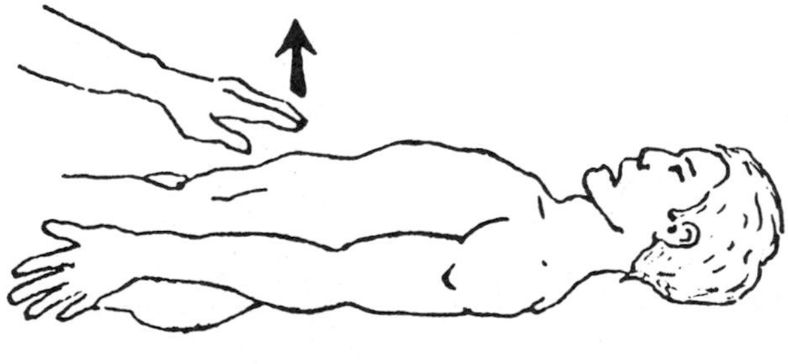

If a very sharp pain ***(rebound pain)*** occurs when the hand is removed, appendicitis or peritonitis is likely.

If no rebound pain occurs above the left groin, try the same test above the right groin.

IF IT SEEMS THAT A PERSON HAS APPENDICITIS OR PERITONITIS:

- ♦ **Seek medical help immediately.** If possible, take the person where he can have surgery.

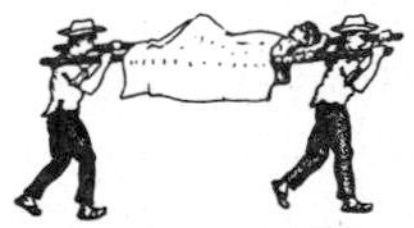

- ♦ **Do not give anything by mouth** and do not give an enema. Only if the person begins to show signs of dehydration, give sips of water or Rehydration Drink (p. 152) made with sugar and salt—but nothing more.
- ♦ The person should rest very quietly in a half-sitting position.

Note: When peritonitis is advanced, the belly becomes hard like a board, and the person feels great pain when his belly is touched even lightly. His life is in danger. Take him to a medical center immediately and on the way give him the medicines indicated at the top of page 93.

BURNS

Prevention:

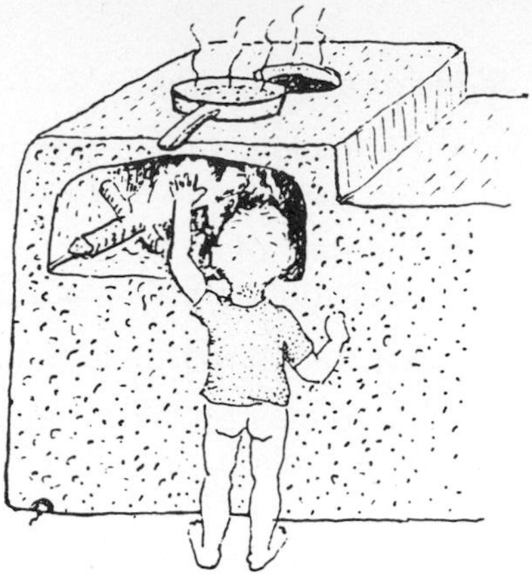

Most burns can be prevented. Take special care with children:

- Do not let small babies go near a fire.
- Keep lamps and matches out of reach.
- Turn handles of pans on the stove so children cannot reach them.

Minor Burns that Do Not Form Blisters (1st degree)

To help ease the pain and lessen the damage caused by a minor burn, put the burned part in cold water **at once.** No other treatment is needed. Take aspirin for pain.

Burns that Cause Blisters (2nd degree)

Do not break blisters.

If the blisters are broken, wash gently with soap and boiled water that has been cooled. Sterilize a little *Vaseline* by heating it until it boils and spread it on a piece of sterile gauze. Then put the gauze on the burn.

If there is no *Vaseline,* leave the burn uncovered. Never smear on grease or butter.

It is very important to keep the burn as clean as possible. Protect it from dirt, dust, and flies.

If signs of infection appear—pus, bad smell, fever, or swollen lymph nodes—apply compresses of warm salt water (1 teaspoon salt to 1 liter water) 3 times a day. (If possible, add 2 tablespoons of bleach to the salt water.) Boil both the water and cloth before use. With great care, remove the dead skin and flesh. You can spread on a little antibiotic ointment such as *Neosporin* (p. 371). In severe cases, consider taking an antibiotic such as penicillin or ampicillin.

Deep Burns (3rd degree) that destroy the skin and expose raw or charred flesh are always serious, as are any burns that cover large areas of the body. Take the person to a health center at once. In the meantime wrap the burned part with a very clean cloth or towel.

If it is impossible to get medical help, treat the burn as described above. If you do not have *Vaseline,* leave the burn in the open air, covering it only with a loose cotton cloth or sheet to protect it from dust and flies. Keep the cloth very clean and change it each time it gets dirty with liquid or blood from the burn. Give penicillin.

Never put grease, fat, hides, coffee, herbs, or feces on a burn.

Covering the burn with **honey** helps prevent and control infection and speed healing. Gently wash off the old honey and put on new at least twice a day.

Special Precautions for Very Serious Burns

Any person who has been badly burned can easily go into *shock* (see p. 77) because of combined pain, fear, and the loss of body fluids from the oozing burn.

Comfort and reassure the burned person. Give him aspirin for the pain and codeine if you can get it. Bathing open wounds in slightly salty water also helps calm pain. Put 1 teaspoon of salt for each liter of cool, boiled water.

Give the burned person plenty of liquid. If the burned area is large (more than twice the size of his hand), make up the following drink:

To a liter of water add:

half a teaspoon of salt

and half a teaspoon of bicarbonate of soda.

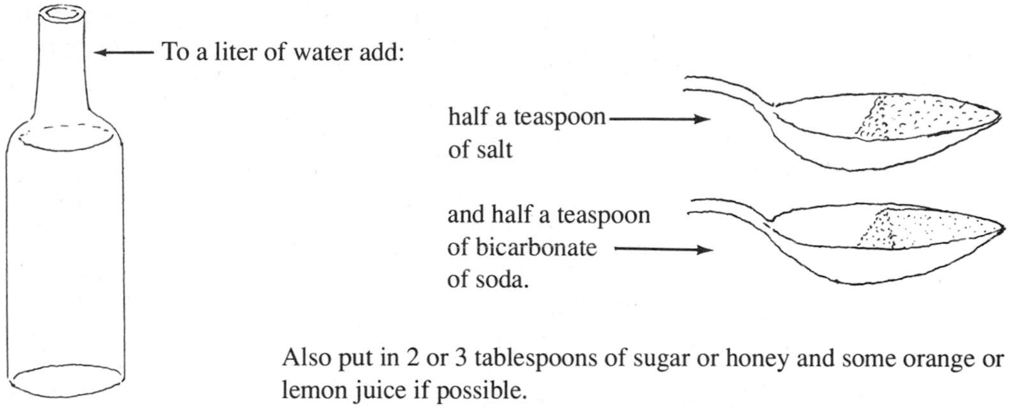

Also put in 2 or 3 tablespoons of sugar or honey and some orange or lemon juice if possible.

The burned person should drink this as often as possible, especially until he urinates frequently. He should try to drink 4 liters a day for a large burn, and 12 liters a day for a very large burn.

It is important for persons who are badly burned to eat foods rich in protein (see p. 110). No type of food needs to be avoided.

Burns around the Joints

When someone is badly burned between the fingers, in the armpit, or at other joints, gauze pads with *Vaseline* on them should be put between the burned surfaces to prevent them from growing together as they heal. Also, fingers, arms, and legs should be straightened completely several times a day while healing. This is painful but helps prevent stiff scars that limit movement. While the burned hand is healing, the fingers should be kept in a slightly bent position.

sterile gauze pads with *Vaseline*

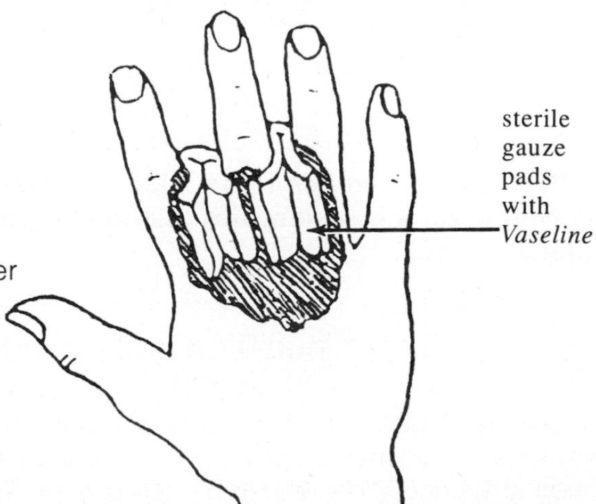

BROKEN BONES (FRACTURES)

When a bone is broken, the most important thing to do is **keep the bone in a fixed position.** This prevents further damage and lets it mend.

Before trying to move or carry a person with a broken bone, keep the bones from moving with splints, strips of bark, or a sleeve of cardboard. Later a plaster cast can be put on the limb at a health center, or perhaps you can make a 'cast' according to local tradition (see p. 14).

Setting broken bones: If the bones seem more or less in the right position, it is better not to move them—this could do more harm than good.

If the bones are far out of position and the break is recent, you can try to 'set' or straighten them before putting on a cast. The sooner the bones are set, the easier it will be. Before setting, if possible inject or give diazepam to relax the muscles and calm pain (see p. 390). Or give codeine (p. 384).

HOW TO SET A BROKEN WRIST

Pull the hand with a slow, steady force for 5 to 10 minutes, increasing the force, to separate the bones.

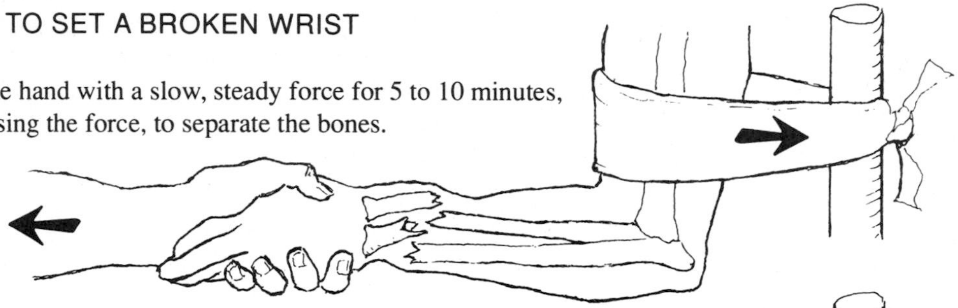

With one person still pulling the hand, have another gently line up and straighten the bones.

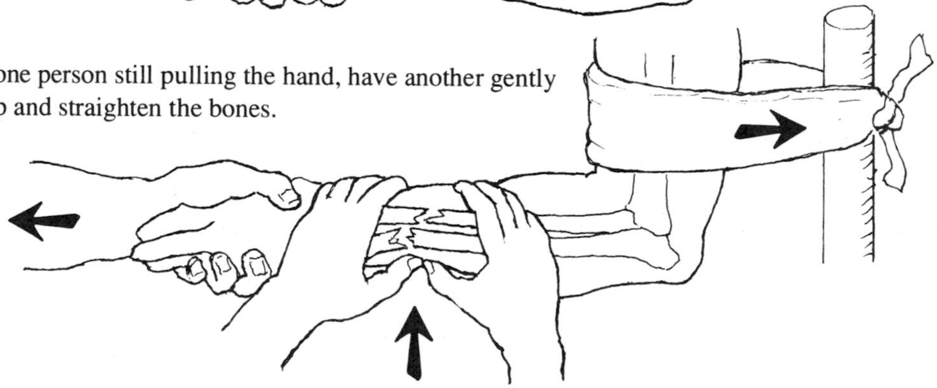

WARNING: **It is possible to do a lot of damage while trying to set a bone. Ideally, it should be done with the help of someone with experience. Do not jerk or force.**

HOW LONG DOES IT TAKE FOR BROKEN BONES TO HEAL?

The worse the break or the older the person, the longer healing takes. Children's bones mend rapidly. Those of old people sometimes never join. A broken arm should be kept in a cast for about a month, and no force put on it for another month. A broken leg should remain in a cast for about 2 months.

BROKEN THIGH OR HIP BONE

A broken upper leg or hip often needs special attention. It is best to splint the whole body like this:

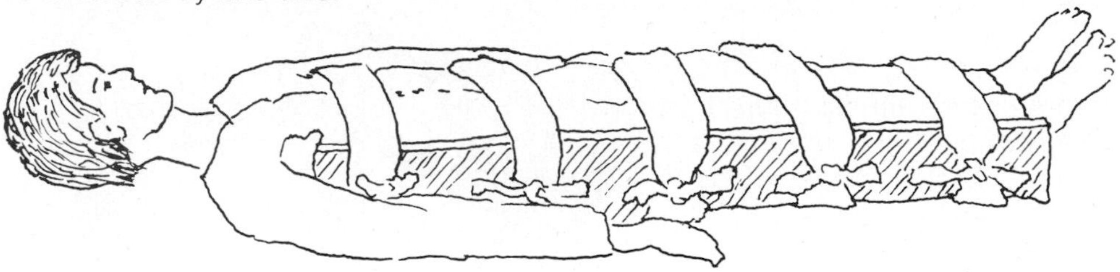

and to take the injured person to a health center at once.

BROKEN NECKS AND BACKS

If there is any chance a person's back or neck has been broken, **be very careful when moving him.** Try not to change his position. If possible, bring a health worker before moving him. If you must move him, do so without bending his back or neck. For instructions on how to move the injured person, see the next page.

BROKEN RIBS

These are very painful, but almost always heal on their own. It is better not to splint or bind the chest. The best treatment is to take aspirin—and rest. To keep the lungs healthy, take 4 to 5 deep breaths in a row, every 2 hours. Do this daily until you can breathe normally. At first, this will be very painful. It may take months before the pain is gone completely.

A broken rib does not often puncture a lung. But if a rib breaks through the skin, or if the person coughs blood or develops breathing difficulties (other than pain), use antibiotics (penicillin or ampicillin) and seek medical help.

BROKEN BONES THAT BREAK THROUGH THE SKIN (OPEN FRACTURES)

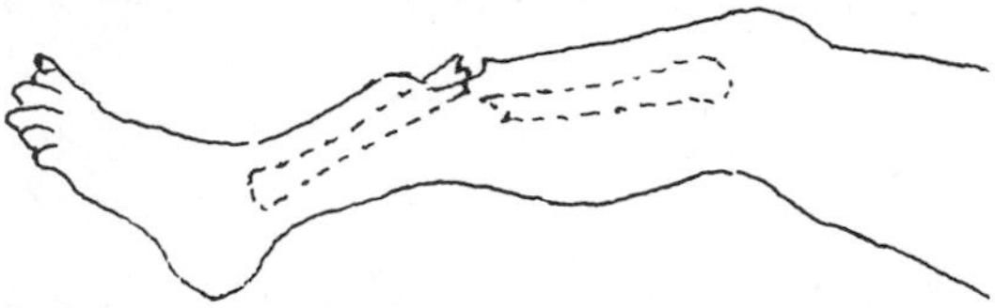

Since the danger of infection is very great in these cases, it is always better to get help from a health worker or doctor in caring for the injury. Clean the wound and the exposed bone very gently but thoroughly with cool, boiled water. Cover with a clean cloth. **Never put the bone back into the wound until the wound and the bone are absolutely clean.**

Splint the limb to prevent more injury.

If the bone has broken the skin, use an antibiotic immediately to help prevent infection: penicillin, ampicillin, or tetracycline (p. 351, 353, and 356).

CAUTION: **Never rub or massage a broken limb or a limb that may possibly be broken.**

HOW TO MOVE A BADLY INJURED PERSON

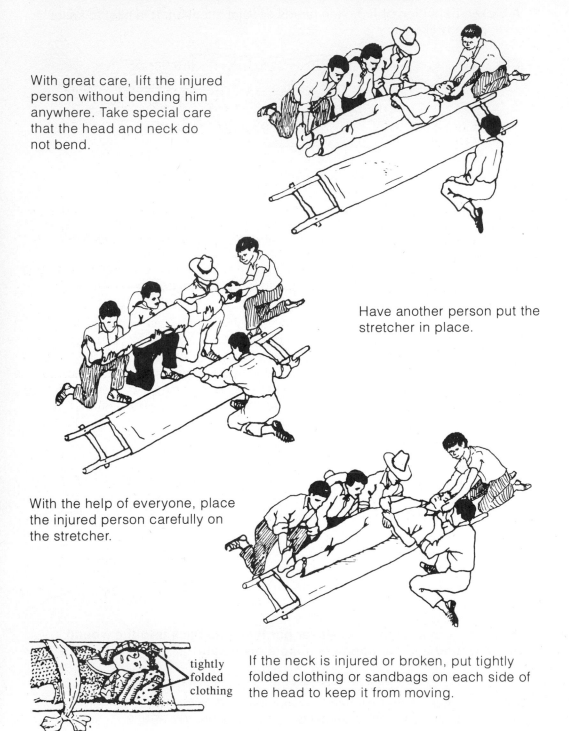

With great care, lift the injured person without bending him anywhere. Take special care that the head and neck do not bend.

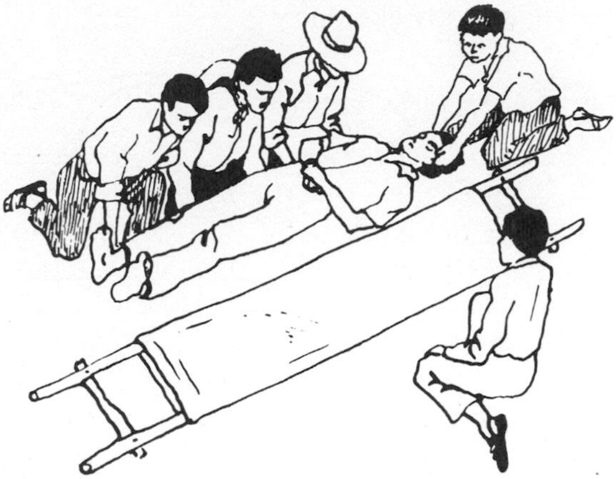

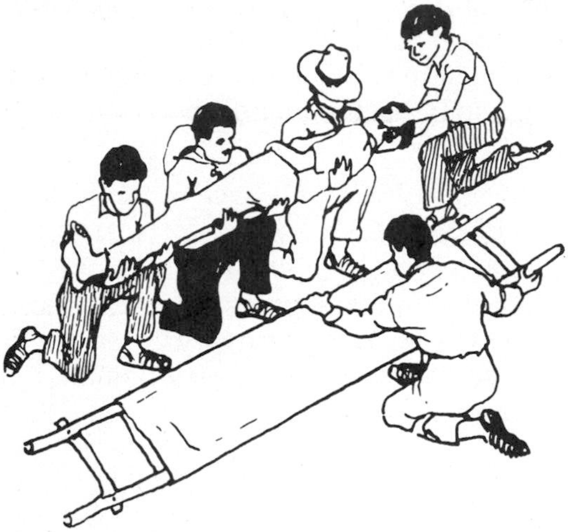

Have another person put the stretcher in place.

With the help of everyone, place the injured person carefully on the stretcher.

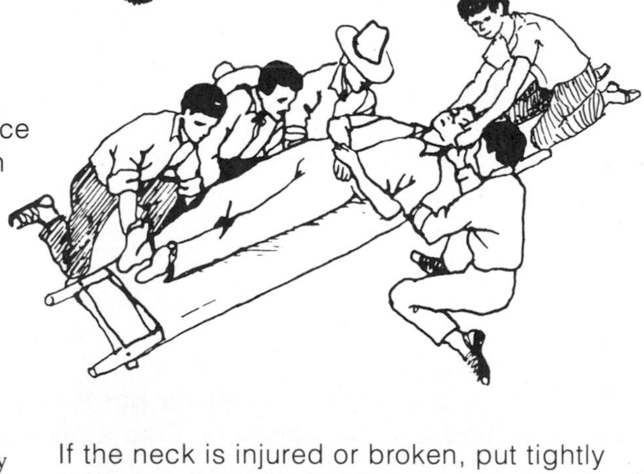

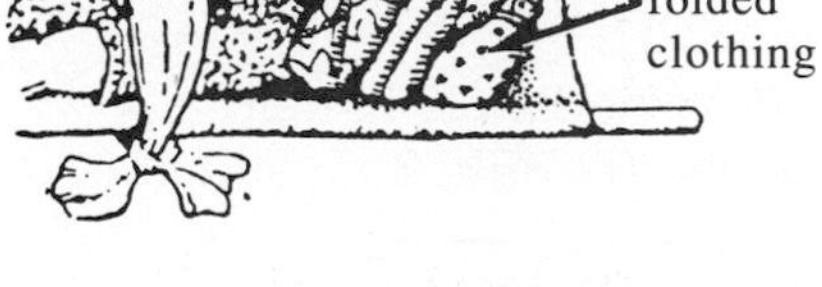

If the neck is injured or broken, put tightly folded clothing or sandbags on each side of the head to keep it from moving.

When carrying, try to keep the feet up, even on hills.

DISLOCATIONS
(BONES THAT HAVE COME OUT OF PLACE AT A JOINT)

Three important points of treatment:

- Try to put the bone back into place. **The sooner the better!**
- Keep it bandaged firmly in place so it does not slip out again (about a month).
- Avoid forceful use of the limb long enough for the joint to heal completely (2 or 3 months).

HOW TO SET A DISLOCATED SHOULDER:

Have the injured person lie face down on a table or other firm surface with his arm hanging over the side. Pull down on the arm toward the floor, using a strong, steady force, for 15 to 20 minutes. Then gently let go. The shoulder should 'pop' back into place.

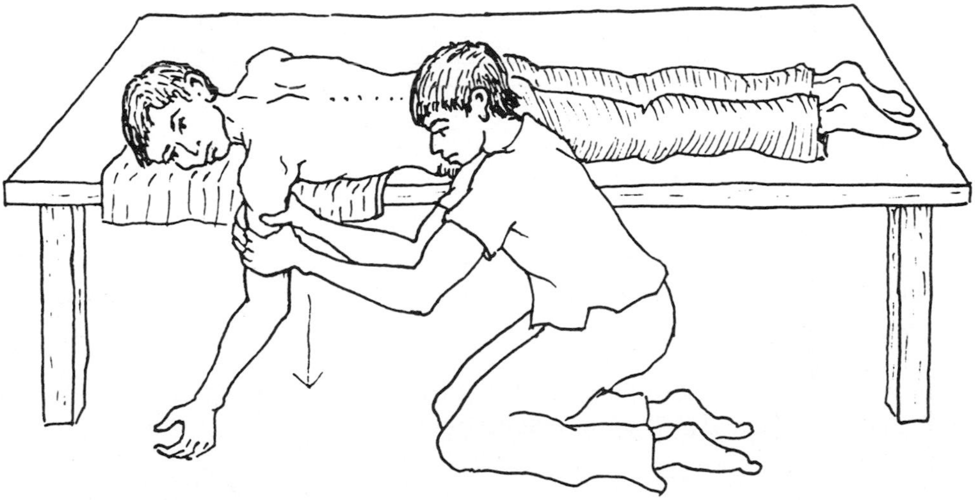

Or attach something to the arm that weighs 10 to 20 lbs. (start with 10 lbs., but do not go higher than 20 lbs.) and leave it there for 15 to 20 minutes.

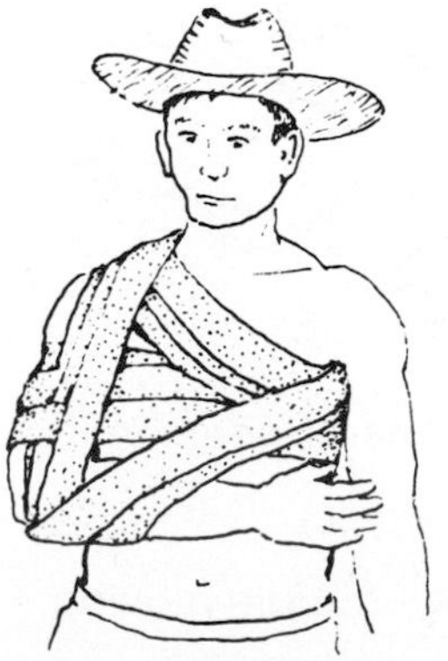

After the shoulder is in place, bandage the arm firmly against the body. Keep it bandaged for a month. To prevent the shoulder from becoming completely stiff, older persons should unbandage the arm for a few minutes 3 times a day and, with the arm hanging at the side, move it gently in narrow circles.

If you cannot put the dislocated limb back in place, look for medical help at once. The longer you wait, the harder it will be to correct.

STRAINS AND SPRAINS (BRUISING OR TEARING IN A TWISTED JOINT)

Many times it is impossible to know whether a hand or foot is bruised, sprained, or broken. It helps to have an X-ray taken.

But usually, breaks and sprains are treated more or less the same. Keep the joint motionless. Wrap it with something that gives firm support. Serious sprains need at least 3 or 4 weeks to heal. Broken bones take longer.

To relieve pain and swelling, keep the sprained part raised high. During the first day or two, put ice wrapped in cloth or plastic, or cold, wet cloths over the swollen joint for 20 to 30 minutes once every hour. This helps reduce swelling and pain. After 24 to 48 hours (when the swelling is no longer getting worse), soak the sprain in hot water several times a day.

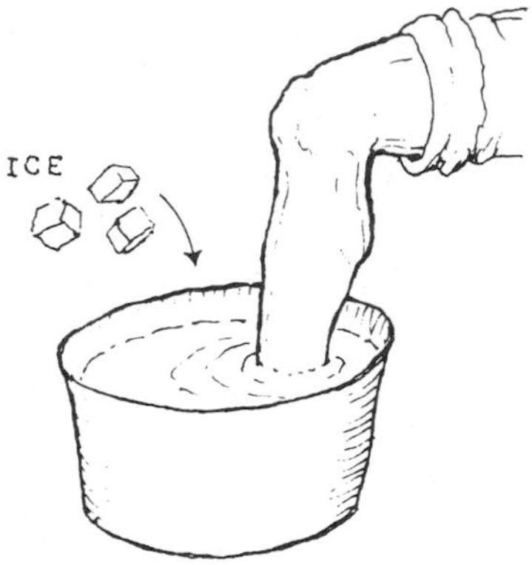

For the first day soak the sprained joint in cold water.

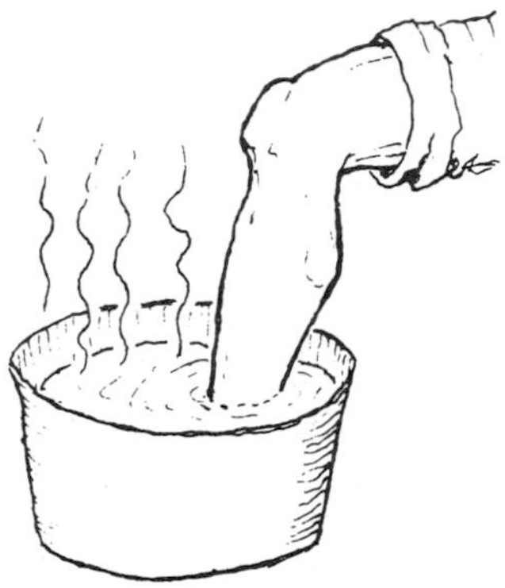

After one or two days use hot soaks.

You can keep the twisted joint in the correct position for healing by using a homemade cast (see p. 14) or an elastic bandage.

Wrapping the foot and ankle with an elastic bandage will also prevent or reduce swelling. Start from the toes and wrap upward, as shown here. Be careful not to make the bandage too tight, and remove it briefly every hour or two. Also take aspirin.

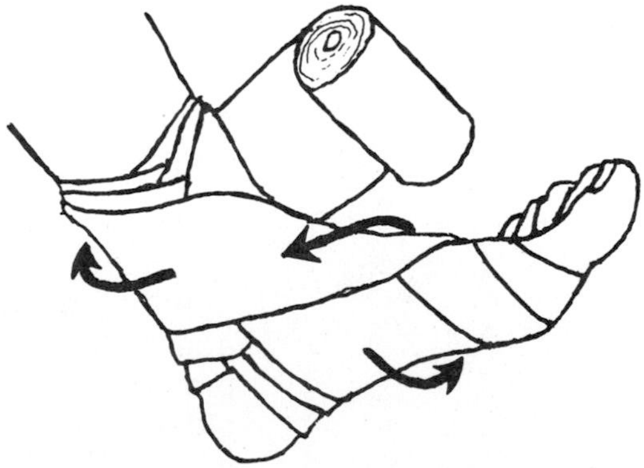

If the pain and swelling do not start to go down after 48 hours, seek medical help.

CAUTION: **Never rub or massage a sprain or broken bone.** It does no good and can do more harm.

If the foot seems very loose or 'floppy' or if the person has trouble moving his toes, look for medical help. Surgery may be needed.

POISONING

Many children die from swallowing things that are poisonous. To protect your children, take the following precautions:

Keep all poisons out of reach of children:

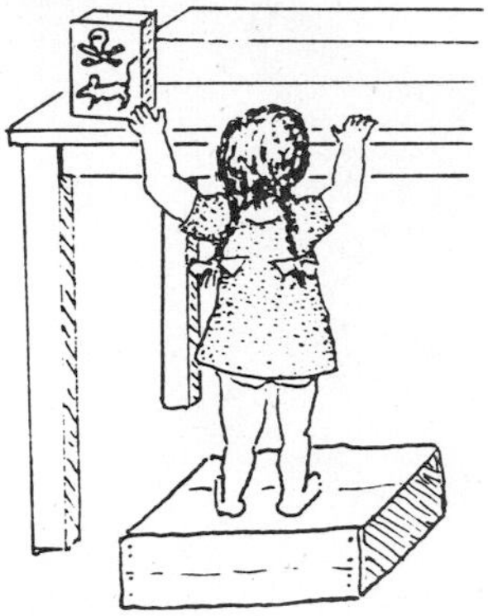

Never keep kerosene, gasoline, or other poisons in cola or soft drink bottles, because children may try to drink them.

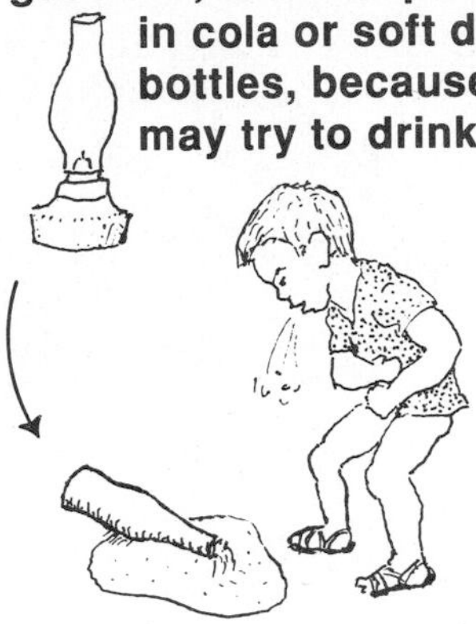

SOME COMMON POISONS TO WATCH OUT FOR:

- rat poison
- DDT, lindane, sheep dip, and other insecticides or plant poisons
- medicine (any kind when much is swallowed; take special care with **iron pills)**
- tincture of iodine
- bleach
- cigarettes
- rubbing or wood alcohol
- poisonous leaves, seeds, berries, or mushrooms
- castor beans
- matches
- kerosene, paint thinner, gasoline, petrol, lighter fluid
- lye or caustic soda
- salt—if too much is given to babies and small children
- spoiled food (see p. 135)

Treatment:

If you suspect poisoning, do the following **immediately:**

- ♦ If the child is awake and alert, make him vomit. Put your finger in his throat or give him a tablespoon of syrup of ipecac (p. 389) followed by 1 glass of water. Or make him drink water with mild soap or salt in it (6 teaspoons salt to 1 cup water).
- ♦ If you have it, give him a cup of activated charcoal (p. 389), or a tablespoon of powdered charcoal mixed into a glass of water. (For an adult, give 2 glasses of this mixture.)

CAUTION: Do not make a person vomit if he has swallowed kerosene, gasoline (petrol), or strong acids or corrosive substances (lye), or if he is unconscious. If he is awake and alert, give him plenty of water or milk to dilute the poison. (For a child, give 1 glass of water every 15 minutes.)

Cover the person if he feels cold, but avoid too much heat. **If poisoning is severe, look for medical help.**

SNAKEBITE

Note: Try to get information on the kinds of snakes in your area and put it on this page.

RATTLESNAKE—
North America,
Mexico, and
Central America

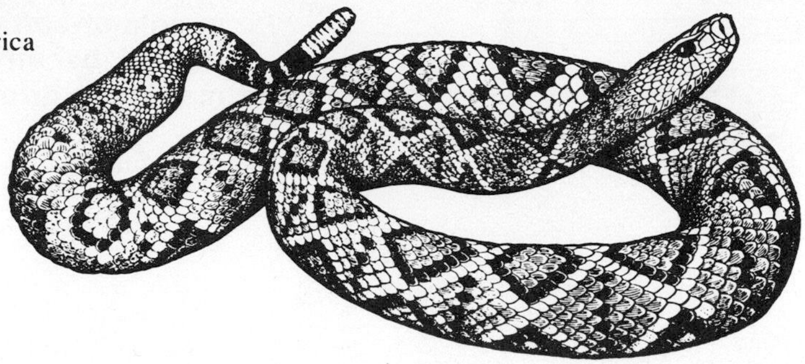

When someone has been bitten by a snake, try to find out if the snake was poisonous or harmless. Their bite marks are different:

POISONOUS
SNAKE

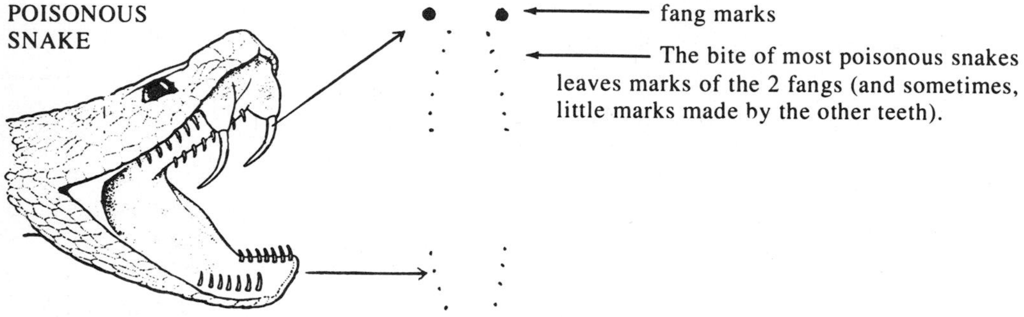

The bite of most poisonous snakes leaves marks of the 2 fangs (and sometimes, little marks made by the other teeth).

NON-POISONOUS
SNAKE

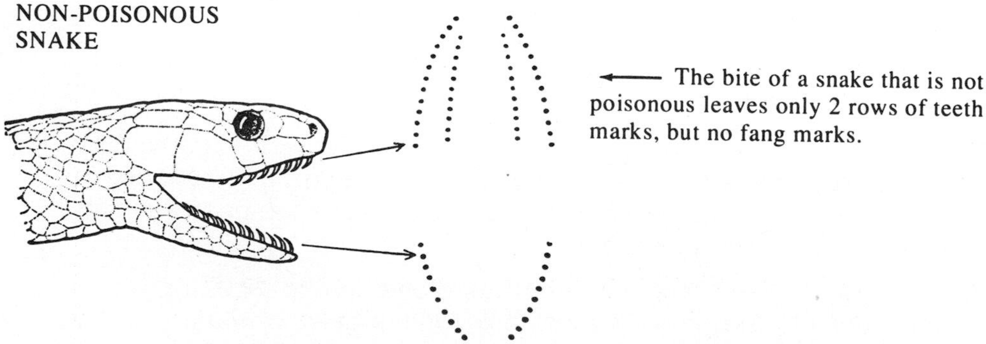

The bite of a snake that is not poisonous leaves only 2 rows of teeth marks, but no fang marks.

People often believe that certain harmless snakes are poisonous. Try to find out which of the snakes in your area are truly poisonous and which are not. Contrary to popular opinion, boa constrictors and pythons are not poisonous. Please do not kill non-poisonous snakes, because they do no harm. On the contrary, they kill mice and other pests that do lots of damage. Some even kill poisonous snakes.

Treatment for poisonous snakebite:

1. **Stay quiet; do not move the bitten part.** The more it is moved, the faster the poison will spread through the body. If the bite is on the foot, the person **should not walk at all. Send for medical help.**

2. Wrap the bitten area with a wide elastic bandage or clean cloth to slow the spread of poison. Keeping the arm or leg very still, wrap it tightly, but not so tight it stops the pulse at the wrist or on top of the foot. If you cannot feel the pulse, loosen the bandage a little.

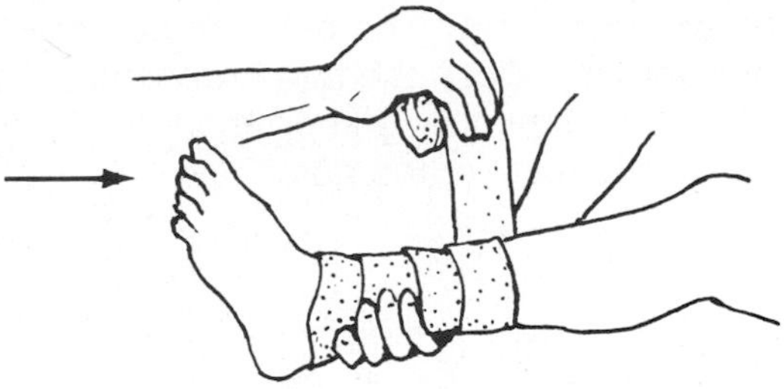

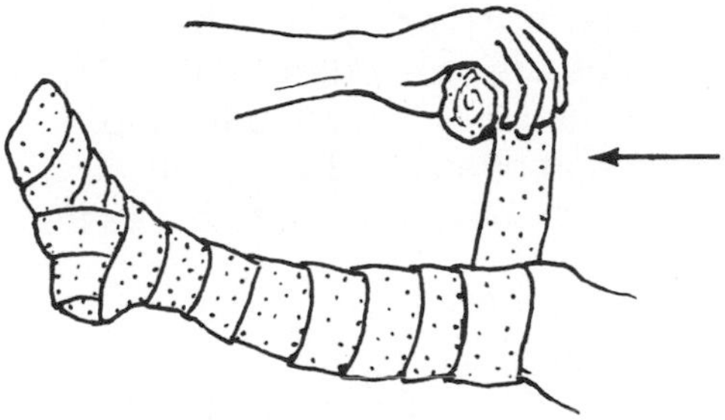

3. Wind the bandage over the hand or foot, and up the whole arm or leg. Make sure you can still feel the pulse.

4. Then, put on a splint to prevent the limb from moving (see p. 14).

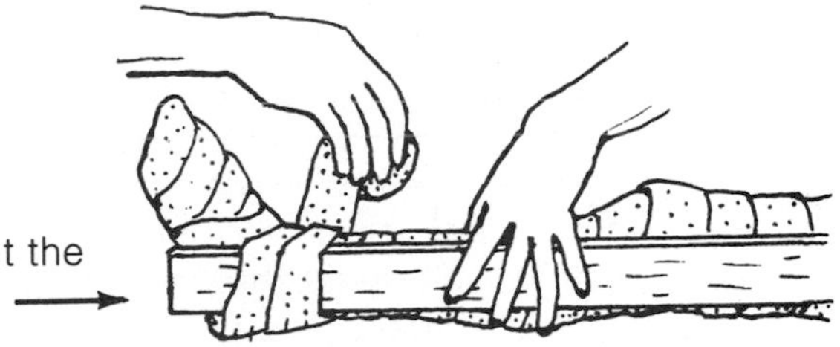

5. Carry the person, on a stretcher if possible, to the nearest health center. If you can, also take the snake, because different snakes may require different antivenoms (antitoxins, see p. 388). If an antivenom is needed, leave the bandage on until the injection is ready, and take all precautions for ALLERGIC SHOCK (see p. 70). If there is no antivenom, remove the bandage.

6. Give acetaminophen, not aspirin, for pain. If possible, give tetanus vaccine. If the bite becomes infected, give penicillin.

7. Also, **ice** helps to reduce pain and slow the poison. Wrap the arm or leg with a plastic sheet and a thick cloth. Then pack crushed ice around it. (*Caution:* Too much cold can damage skin and flesh. When it is getting too cold it begins to ache. So let the person decide when to remove the ice for a few minutes.)

Have antivenoms for snakes in your area ready and know how to use them—before someone is bitten!

Poisonous snakebite is dangerous. Send for medical help—but always do the things explained above **at once.**

Most folk remedies for snakebite do little if any good (see p. 3).

Never drink alcohol after a snakebite. It makes things worse!

BITE OF THE BEADED LIZARD (GILA MONSTER)

The bite of the beaded lizard is treated just like a poisonous snakebite, except that there are no good antivenoms for it. The bite can be very dangerous. Wash the bite area well. Avoid movement and keep the bite below the level of the heart.

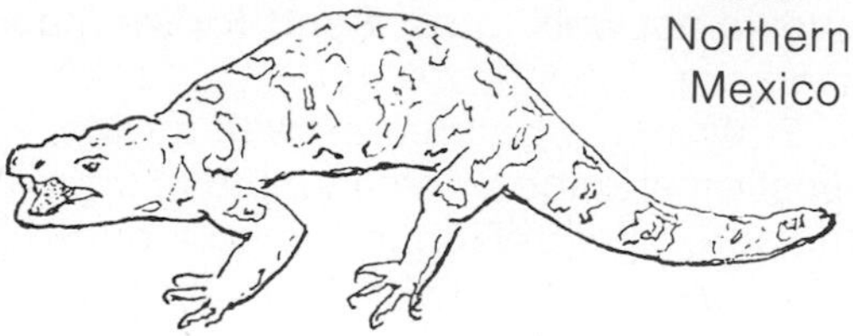

Southern U.S.A. and Northern Mexico

SCORPION STING

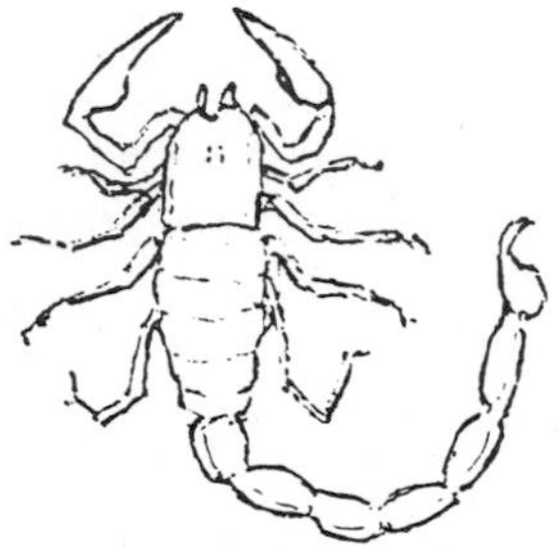

Some scorpions are far more poisonous than others. To adults, scorpion stings are rarely dangerous. Take aspirin and if possible put ice on the sting to help calm the pain. For the numbness and pain that sometimes last weeks or months, hot compresses may be helpful (see p. 193).

To children under 5 years old, scorpion stings can be dangerous, especially if the sting is on the head or body. In some countries scorpion antitoxin is available (p. 388). To do much good it must be injected within 2 hours after the child has been stung. Give acetaminophen or aspirin for the pain. If the child stops breathing, use mouth-to-mouth breathing (see p. 80). If the child who was stung is very young or has been stung on the main part of the body, or if you know the scorpion was of a deadly type—seek medical help fast.

BLACK WIDOW AND OTHER SPIDER BITES

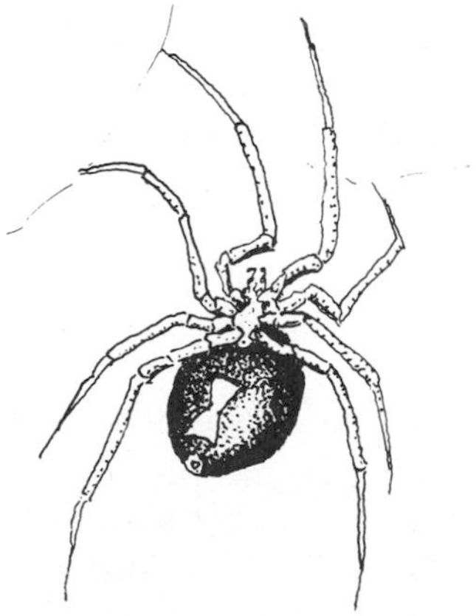

The majority of spider bites, including that of the tarantula, are painful but not dangerous. The bite of a few kinds of spiders—such as the 'black widow' and related species—can make an adult quite ill. They can be dangerous for a small child. A black widow bite often causes painful muscle cramps all over the body, and extreme pain in the stomach muscles which become rigid. (Sometimes this is confused with appendicitis!)

Give acetaminophen or aspirin and look for medical help. The most useful medicines are not found in village stores. (Injection of 10% calcium gluconate, 10 ml., injected intravenously **very slowly** over a 10-minute period, helps to reduce the muscular spasms. Also diazepam, p. 390, may be helpful. If signs of shock develop, treat for allergic shock, p. 70. Injections of cortisone may be needed in children.) A good antivenom exists but is hard to get.

CHAPTER

NUTRITION: WHAT TO EAT TO BE HEALTHY 11

SICKNESSES CAUSED BY NOT EATING WELL

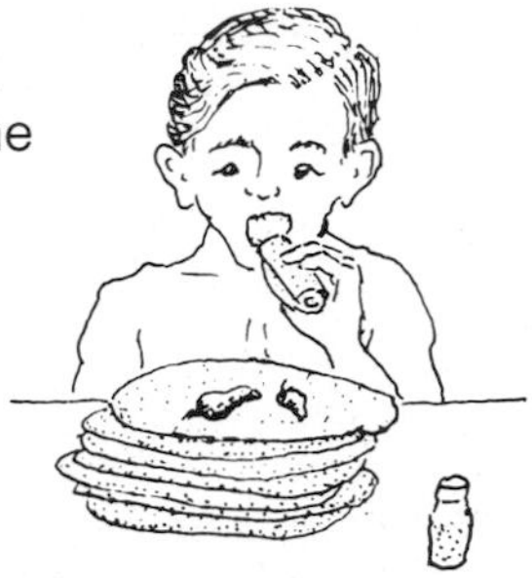

Good food is needed for a person to grow well, work hard, and stay healthy. Many common sicknesses come from not eating enough.

A person who is weak or sick because he does not eat enough, or does not eat the foods his body needs, is said to be poorly nourished—or ***malnourished.*** He suffers from ***malnutrition.***

Poor nutrition can result in the following health problems:

in children

- failure of a child to grow or gain weight normally (see p. 297)
- slowness in walking, talking, or thinking
- big bellies, thin arms and legs
- common illnesses and infections that last longer, are more severe, and more often cause death
- lack of energy, child is sad and does not play
- swelling of feet, face, and hands, often with sores or marks on the skin
- thinning, straightening, or loss of hair, or loss of its color and shine
- poor vision at night, dryness of eyes, blindness

in anyone

- weakness and tiredness
- loss of appetite
- anemia
- sores in the corners of the mouth
- painful or sore tongue
- 'burning' or numbness of the feet

Although the following problems may have other causes, they are sometimes caused and are often made worse by not eating well:

- diarrhea
- frequent infections
- ringing or buzzing in the ears
- headache
- bleeding or redness of the gums
- skin bruises easily
- nosebleeds
- stomach discomfort
- dryness and cracking of the skin
- heavy pulsing of the heart or of the 'pit' of the stomach (palpitations)
- anxiety (nervous worry) and various nerve or mental problems
- cirrhosis (liver disease)

Poor nutrition during pregnancy causes weakness and anemia in the mother and increases the risk of her dying during or after childbirth. It is also a cause of miscarriage, or of the baby being born dead, too small, or defective.

Eating right helps the body resist sickness.

Not eating well may be the direct cause of the health problems just listed. But most important, poor nutrition weakens the body's ability to resist all kinds of diseases, especially infections:

- Poorly nourished children are much more likely to get severe diarrhea, and to die from it, than are children who are well nourished.
- Measles is especially dangerous where many children are malnourished.
- Tuberculosis is more common, and gets worse more rapidly, in those who are malnourished.
- Cirrhosis of the liver, which comes in part from drinking too much alcohol, is more common and worse in persons who are poorly nourished.
- Even minor problems like the common cold are usually worse, last longer, or lead to pneumonia more often in persons who are poorly nourished.

Eating right helps the sick get well.

Not only does good food help prevent disease, it helps the sick body fight disease and become well again. So when a person is sick, eating enough nutritious food is especially important.

Unfortunately, some mothers stop feeding a child or stop giving certain nutritious foods when he is sick or has diarrhea—so the child becomes weaker, cannot fight off the illness, and may die. **Sick children need food! If a sick child will not eat, encourage him to do so.**

Feed him as much as he will eat and drink. And be patient. A sick child often does not want to eat much. So feed him something many times during the day. Also, try to make sure that he drinks a lot of liquid so that he pees (passes urine) several times a day. If the child will not take solid foods, mash them and give them as a mush or gruel.

Often the signs of poor nutrition first appear when a person has some other sickness. For example, a child who has had diarrhea for several days may develop swollen hands and feet, a swollen face, dark spots, or peeling sores on his legs. These are signs of severe malnutrition. The child needs more good food! And more often. Feed him many times during the day.

During and after any sickness, it is very important to eat well.

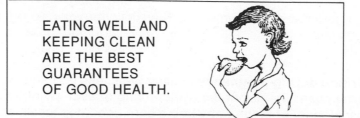

EATING WELL AND
KEEPING CLEAN
ARE THE BEST
GUARANTEES
OF GOOD HEALTH.

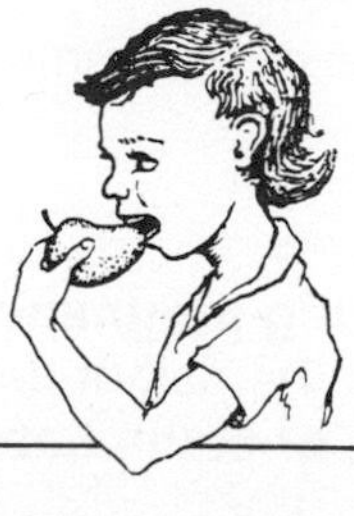

WHY IT IS IMPORTANT TO EAT RIGHT

People who do not eat right develop **malnutrition.** This can happen from not eating enough food of any kind (general malnutrition or 'undernutrition'), from not eating the right kinds of foods (specific types of malnutrition), or from eating too much of certain foods (getting too fat, see p. 126).

Anyone can develop general malnutrition, but it is especially dangerous for:

- **children,** because they need lots of food to grow well and stay healthy;
- **women** of child-bearing age, especially if they are pregnant or breast feeding, because they need extra food to stay healthy, to have healthy babies, and to do their daily work;
- **elderly persons,** because often they lose their teeth and their taste for food, so they cannot eat much at one time, even though they still need to eat well to stay healthy.

A malnourished child does not grow well. She generally is thinner and shorter than other children. Also, she is more likely to be irritable, to cry a lot, to move and play less than other children, and to get sick more often. If the child also gets diarrhea or other infections, she will lose weight. A good way to check if a child is poorly nourished is to measure the distance around her upper arm.

Checking Children for Malnutrition: The Sign of the Upper Arm

After 1 year of age, any child whose middle upper arm measures less than 13 1/2 cm. around is malnourished—no matter how 'fat' his feet, hands, and face may look. If the arm measures less than 12 1/2 cm., he is severely malnourished.

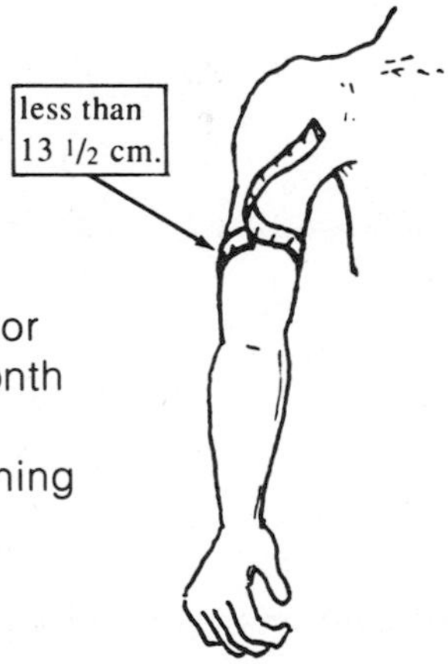

Another good way to tell if a child is well nourished or poorly nourished is to weigh him regularly: once a month in the first year, then once every 3 months. A healthy, well-nourished child gains weight regularly. The weighing of children and the use of the Child Health Chart are discussed fully in Chapter 21.

PREVENTING MALNUTRITION

To stay healthy, our bodies need plenty of good food. The food we eat has to fill many needs. First, it should provide enough **energy** to keep us active and strong. Also, it must help **build, repair,** and **protect** the different parts of our bodies. To do all this we need to eat a combination of foods every day.

MAIN FOODS AND **HELPER FOODS**

In much of the world, most people eat **one main low-cost food** with almost every meal. Depending on the region, this may be rice, maize, millet, wheat, cassava, potato, breadfruit, or banana. **This main food usually provides most of the body's daily food needs.**

However, the **main food** alone is not enough to keep a person healthy. Certain **helper foods** are needed. This is especially true for growing children, women who are pregnant or breast feeding, and older people.

Even if a child regularly gets enough of the main food to fill her, she may become thin and weak. This is because the main food often has so much water and fiber in it, that the child's belly fills up before she gets enough energy to help her grow.

We can do 2 things to help meet such children's energy needs:

1. **Feed children more often**—at least 5 times a day when a child is very young, too thin, or not growing well. Also give her snacks between meals.

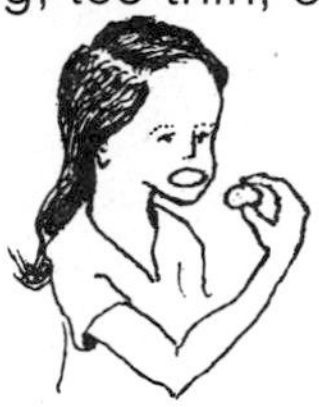

CHILDREN, LIKE CHICKENS,
SHOULD ALWAYS BE PECKING.

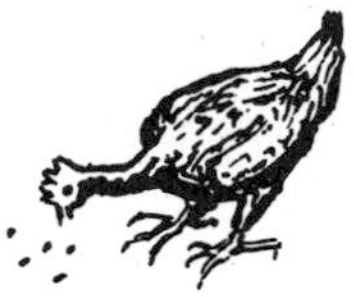

2. **Also add high energy 'helper foods'** such as oils and sugar or honey to the main food. It is best to add vegetable oil or foods containing oils—nuts, groundnuts (peanuts), or seeds, especially pumpkin or sesame seeds.

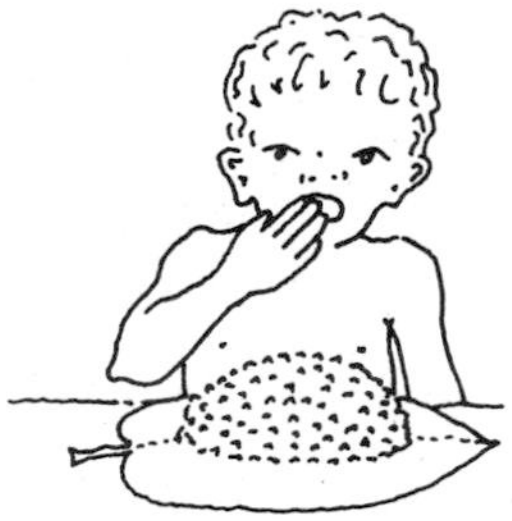

To meet her energy needs, a child would need to eat this much boiled rice.

If the child's belly fills up before her energy needs are met, the child will become thin and weak.

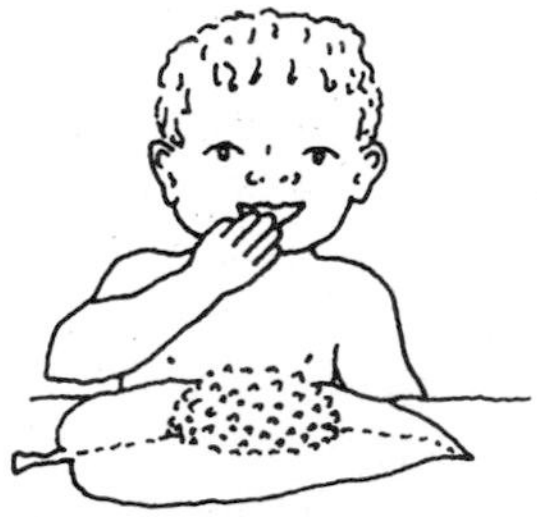

But she needs only this much rice when some vegetable oil is mixed in.

High energy foods added to the main food help to supply extra energy. Also, **2 other kinds of helper foods** should be added to the main food:

When possible, add **body-building foods** (proteins) such as beans, milk, eggs, groundnuts, fish, and meat.

Also try to add **protective foods** such as orange or yellow fruits and vegetables, and also dark green leafy vegetables. Protective foods supply important vitamins and minerals (see p. 113).

EATING RIGHT TO STAY HEALTHY

The 'main food' your family eats usually provides **most—but not all—**of the body's energy and other nutritional needs. By adding **helper foods** to the **main food** you can make low-cost nutritious meals. You do not have to eat all the foods listed here to be healthy. **Eat the main foods you are accustomed to, and add whatever 'helper foods' are available in your area.** Try to include 'helper foods' from each group, as often as possible.

GO FOODS

(energy helpers)

Examples:

Fats (vegetable oils, butter, *ghee*, lard)

Foods rich in fats (coconut, olives, fatty meat)

Nuts* (groundnuts, almonds, walnuts, cashews)

Oil seeds (pumpkin, melon, sesame, sunflower)

Sugars (sugar, honey, molasses, sugar cane, jaggery)

* *Note:* Nuts and oil seeds are also valuable as body-building helpers.

REMEMBER: Feeding children **enough** and feeding them **often** (3 to 5 times a day) is usually more important than the types of food you feed them.

MAIN FOODS

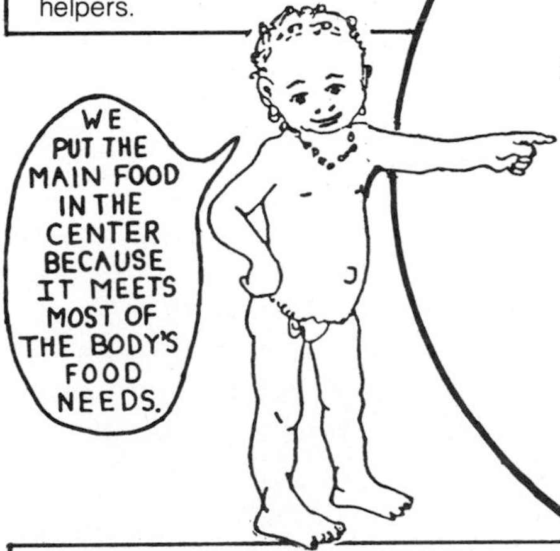
WE PUT THE MAIN FOOD IN THE CENTER BECAUSE IT MEETS MOST OF THE BODY'S FOOD NEEDS.

Examples:

Cereals and grains (wheat, maize, rice, millet, sorghum)

Starchy roots (cassava, potatoes, taro)

Starchy fruits (banana, plantain, breadfruit)

Note: Main foods are cheap sources of energy. The cereals also provide some protein, iron, and vitamins—at low cost.

GROW FOODS

(proteins or body-building helpers)

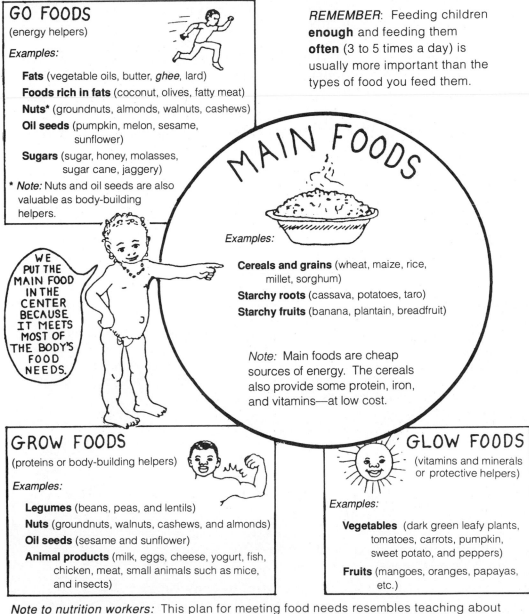

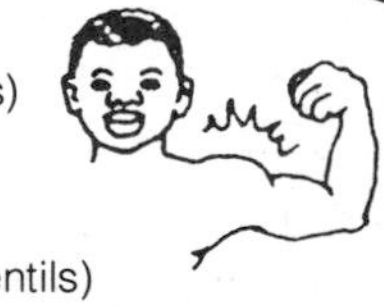

Examples:

Legumes (beans, peas, and lentils)

Nuts (groundnuts, walnuts, cashews, and almonds)

Oil seeds (sesame and sunflower)

Animal products (milk, eggs, cheese, yogurt, fish, chicken, meat, small animals such as mice, and insects)

GLOW FOODS

(vitamins and minerals or protective helpers)

Examples:

Vegetables (dark green leafy plants, tomatoes, carrots, pumpkin, sweet potato, and peppers)

Fruits (mangoes, oranges, papayas, etc.)

Note to nutrition workers: This plan for meeting food needs resembles teaching about 'food groups', but places more importance on giving enough of the traditional 'main food' and **above all, giving frequent feedings with plenty of energy-rich helpers.** This approach is more adaptable to the resources and limitations of poor families.

HOW TO RECOGNIZE MALNUTRITION

Among poor people, **malnutrition is often most severe in children, who need lots of nutritious food to grow well and stay healthy.** There are different forms of malnutrition:

MILD MALNUTRITION

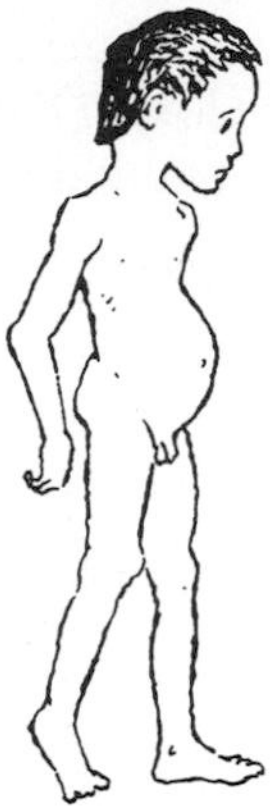

This is the most common form, but it is not always obvious. The child simply does not grow or gain weight as fast as a well-nourished child. Although he may appear rather small and thin, he usually does not look sick. However, because he is poorly nourished, he may lack strength (resistance) to fight infections. So he **becomes more seriously ill** and takes longer to get well than a well-nourished child.

Children with this form of malnutrition suffer more from diarrhea and colds. Their colds usually last longer and are more likely to turn into pneumonia. Measles, tuberculosis, and many other **infectious diseases are far more dangerous** for these malnourished children. More of them die.

It is important that children like these get special care and enough food *before* they become seriously ill. This is why regular weighing or measuring around the middle upper arm of young children is so important. It helps us to recognize mild malnutrition early and correct it.

Follow the guidelines for preventing malnutrition.

SEVERE MALNUTRITION

This occurs most often in babies who stopped breast feeding early or suddenly, and who are not given sufficient high energy foods often enough. Severe malnutrition often starts when a child has diarrhea or another infection. We can usually recognize children who are severely malnourished without taking any measurements. The 2 main examples are:

DRY MALNUTRITION—OR MARASMUS

This child does not get enough of any kind of food. He is said to have **dry malnutrition** or *marasmus.* In other words, he is starved. His body is small, very thin and wasted. He is little more than skin and bones.

This child needs more food—especially energy foods.

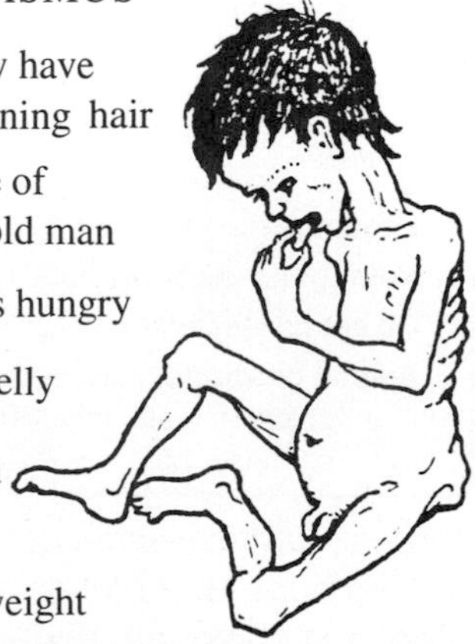

THIS CHILD IS JUST *SKIN* AND *BONES*.

WET MALNUTRITION—OR KWASHIORKOR

This child's condition is called **wet malnutrition** because **his feet, hands, and face are swollen.** This can happen when a child does not eat enough 'body-building' helper foods—or proteins. More often it happens when he does not get enough energy foods, and his body burns up whatever proteins he eats for energy.

Eating beans, lentils, or other foods that have been stored in a damp place and are a little moldy may also be part of the cause.

This child needs more food more often—a lot of foods rich in energy, and some foods rich in protein (see p. 111).

Also, try to avoid foods that are old, and may be spoiled or moldy.

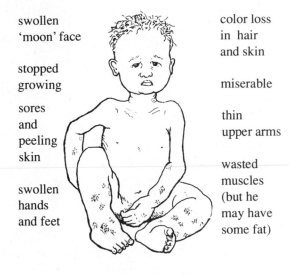

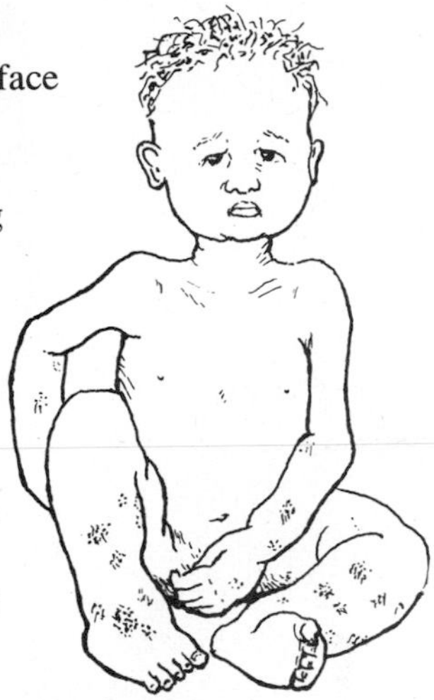

First the child becomes swollen. The other signs come later.

THIS CHILD IS *SKIN, BONES,* AND *WATER.*

OTHER FORMS OF MALNUTRITION

Among poor people the most common forms of severe malnutrition are due either to hunger (marasmus) or lack of protein (kwashiorkor). However, other forms of malnutrition may result when certain vitamins and minerals are missing from the foods people eat. Many of these specific types of malnutrition are discussed more fully later in this chapter and in other parts of this book:

- **Night blindness** in children who do not get enough vitamin A (see p. 226).
- **Rickets** from lack of vitamin D (see p. 125).
- Various **skin problems, sores on the lips and mouth,** or **bleeding gums** from not eating enough fruits, vegetables, and other foods containing certain vitamins (see p. 208 and 232).
- **Anemia** in people who do not get enough iron (see p. 124).
- **Goiter** from lack of iodine (see p. 130).

For more information about health problems related to nutrition, see *Helping Health Workers Learn,* Chapter 25, and *Disabled Village Children,* Chapters 13 and 30.

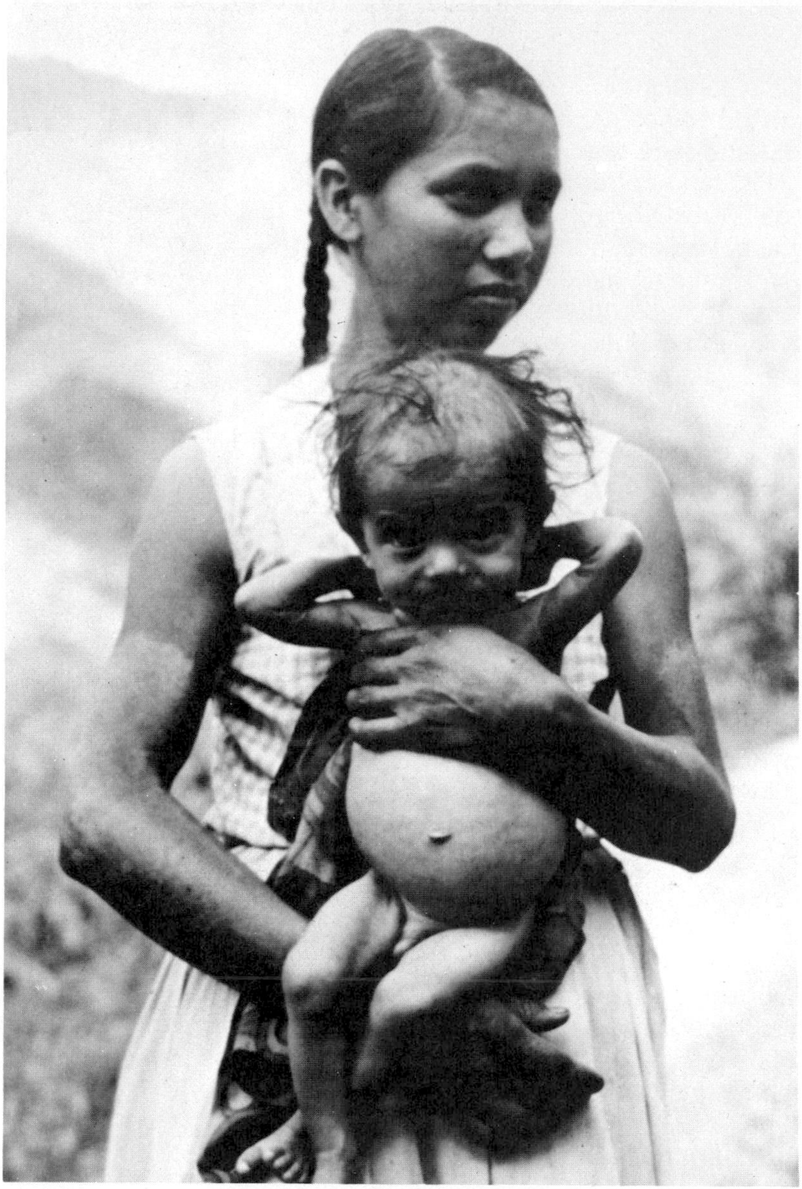

This mother and child are from a poor family and are both poorly nourished. The father works hard, but he does not earn enough to feed the family well. The patches on the mother's arms are a sign of pellagra, a type of malnutrition. She ate mostly maize and not enough nutritious foods such as beans, eggs, fruit, meat, and dark green vegetables.

The mother did not breast feed her baby. She fed him only maize porridge. Although this filled his belly, it did not provide enough nutrition for him to grow strong. As a result, this 2-year-old child is severely malnourished. He is very small and thin with a swollen belly, his hair is thin, and his physical and mental development will be slower than normal. **To prevent this, mothers and their children need to eat better.**

WAYS OF EATING BETTER WHEN YOU DO NOT HAVE MUCH MONEY OR LAND

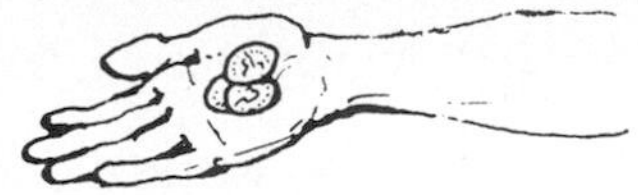

There are many reasons for hunger and poor nutrition. One main reason is poverty. In many parts of the world a few people own most of the wealth and the land. They may grow crops like coffee or tobacco, which they sell to make money, but which have no food value. Or the poor may farm small plots of borrowed land, while the owners take a big share of the harvest. **The problem of hunger and poor nutrition will never be completely solved until people learn to share with each other fairly.**

But there are many things people can do to eat better at low cost—and by eating well gain strength to stand up for their rights. On pages w13 and w14 of "Words to the Village Health Worker" are several suggestions for increasing food production. These include improved use of land through **rotating crops, contour ditches,** and **irrigation;** also ideas for **breeding fish, beekeeping, grain storage,** and **family gardens.** If the whole village or a group of families works together on some of these things, a lot can be done to improve nutrition.

When considering the question of food and land, it is important to remember that a given amount of land can feed only a certain number of persons. For this reason, some people argue that 'the small family lives better'. However, for many poor families, to have many children is an economic necessity. By the time they are 10 or 12 years old, children of poor families often produce more than they cost. Having a lot of children increases the chance that parents will receive the help and care they need in old age.

In short, lack of social and economic security creates the need for parents to have many children. Therefore, the answer to gaining a balance between people and land does not lie in telling poor people to have small families. It lies in redistributing the land more fairly, paying fair wages, and taking other steps to overcome poverty. Only then can people *afford* small families and hope to achieve a lasting balance between people and land. (For a discussion of health, food, and social problems, see *Helping Health Workers Learn.*)

When money is limited, it is important to use it wisely. This means cooperation and looking ahead. Too often the father of a poor family will spend the little bit of money he has on alcohol and tobacco rather than on buying nutritious food, a hen to lay eggs, or something to improve the family's health. Men who drink together would do well to get together sometime when they are sober, to discuss these problems and look for a healthy solution.

Also, some mothers buy sweets or soft drinks (fizzy drinks) for their children when they could spend the same money buying eggs, milk, nuts or other nutritious foods. This way their children could become more healthy for the same amount of money. Discuss this with the mothers and look for solutions.

NO

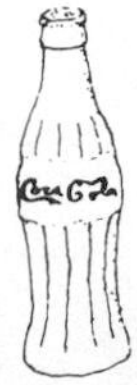

YES

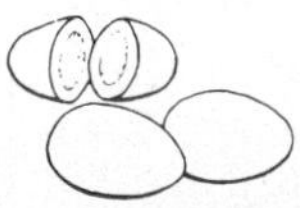

IF YOU HAVE A LITTLE MONEY
AND WANT TO HELP YOUR CHILD GROW STRONG:

DO NOT BUY HIM A SOFT DRINK OR SWEETS—
BUY HIM 2 EGGS OR A HANDFUL OF NUTS.

Better Foods at Low Cost:

Many of the world's people eat a lot of bulky, starchy foods, without adding enough helper foods to provide the extra energy, body-building, and protection they need. This is partly because many helper foods are expensive—especially those that come from animals, like milk and meat.

Most people cannot afford much food from animals. Animals require more land for the amount of food they provide. A poor family can usually be better nourished if they **grow or buy plant foods like beans, peas, lentils, and groundnuts together with a main food such as maize or rice, rather than buy costly animal foods like meat and fish.**

People can be strong and healthy when most of their proteins and other helper foods come from plants.

However, where family finances and local customs permit, it is wise to eat, when possible, some food that comes from animals. This is because even plants high in protein (body-building helpers) often do not have all of the different proteins the body needs.

Try to **eat a variety of plant foods.** Different plants supply the body with different proteins, vitamins, and minerals. For example, beans and maize together meet the body's needs much better than either beans or maize alone. And if other vegetables and fruits are added, this is even better.

Here are some suggestions for getting more vitamins, minerals, and proteins at low cost.

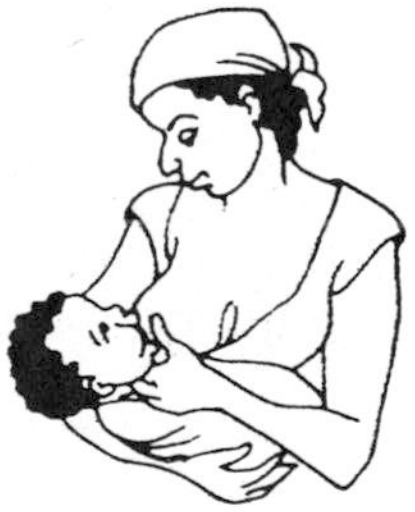

1. **Breast milk.** This is the cheapest, healthiest, and most complete food for a baby. The mother can eat plenty of plant foods and turn them into the perfect baby food—breast milk. Breast feeding is not only best for the baby, it saves money and prevents diseases!

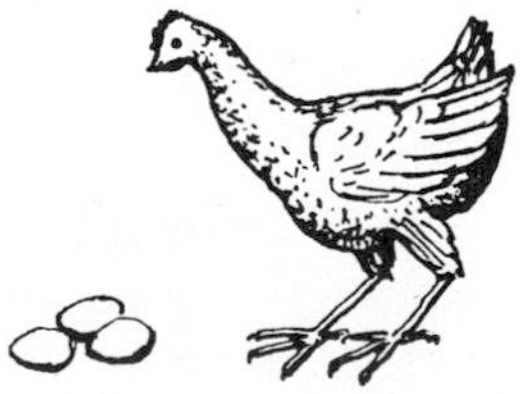

2. **Eggs and chicken.** In many places eggs are one of the cheapest and best forms of animal protein. They can be cooked and mixed with foods given to babies who cannot get breast milk. Or they can be given along with breast milk as the baby grows older.

Eggshells that are boiled, finely ground, and mixed with food can provide needed calcium for pregnant women who develop sore, loose teeth or muscle cramps.

Chicken is a good, often fairly cheap form of animal protein—especially if the family raises its own chickens.

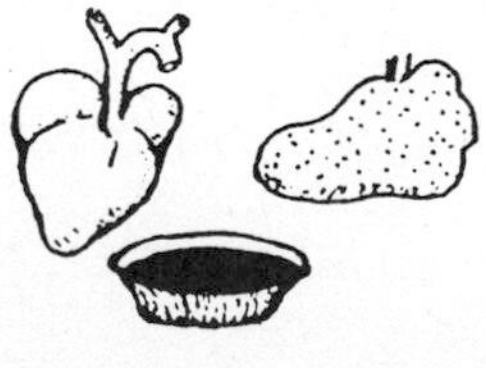

3. **Liver, heart, kidney, and blood.** These are especially high in protein, vitamins, and iron (for anemia) and are often cheaper than other meat. Also **fish** is often cheaper than other meat, and is just as nutritious.

4. **Beans, peas, lentils, and other legumes** are a good cheap source of protein. If allowed to sprout before cooking and eating, they are higher in vitamins. Baby food can be made from beans by cooking them well, and then straining them through a sieve, or by peeling off their skins, and mashing them.

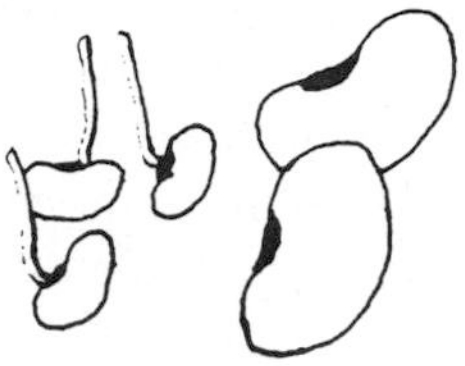

Beans, peas, and other legumes are not only a low-cost form of protein. Growing these crops makes the soil richer so that other crops will grow better afterwards. For this reason, crop rotation and mixed crops are a good idea (see p. w13).

5. **Dark green leafy vegetables** have some iron, a lot of vitamin A, and some protein. The leaves of sweet potatoes, beans and peas, pumpkins and squash, and baobab are especially nutritious. They can be dried, powdered, and mixed with babies' gruel.

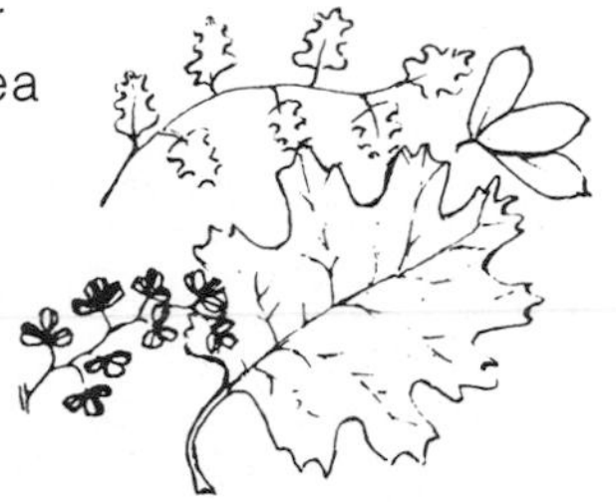

Note: Light green vegetables like cabbage and lettuce have less nutritional value. It is better to grow ones with dark-colored leaves.

6. **Cassava (manioc) leaves** contain 7 times as much protein and more vitamins than the root. If eaten together with the root, they add food value—at no additional cost. The young leaves are best.

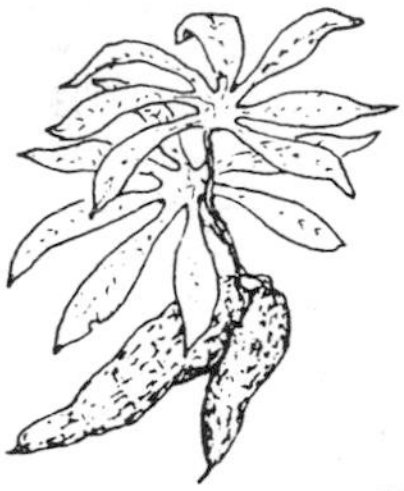

7. **Lime-soaked maize (corn).** When soaked in lime before cooking, as is the custom in much of Latin America, maize is richer in calcium. Soaking in lime also allows more of the vitamins (niacin) and protein to be used by the body.

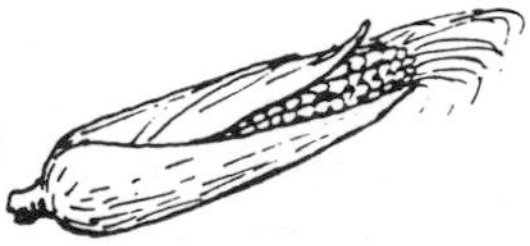

8. **Rice, wheat, and other grains** are more nutritious if their outer skins are not removed during milling. Moderately milled rice and whole wheat contain more proteins, vitamins, and minerals than the white, over-milled product.

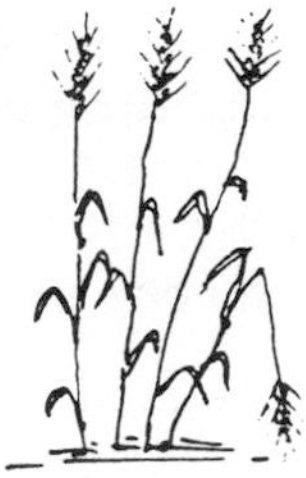

NOTE: The protein in wheat, rice, maize, and other grains can be better used by the body when they are eaten with beans or lentils.

9. **Cook vegetables, rice, and other foods in little water.** And do not overcook. This way fewer vitamins and proteins are lost. Be sure to drink the leftover water, or use it for soups or in other foods.

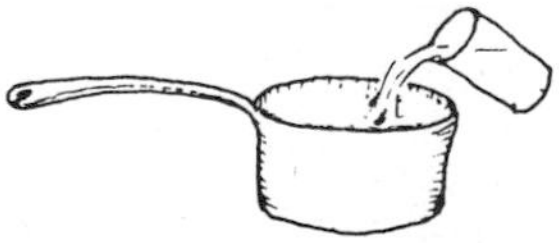

10. Many **wild fruits and berries** are rich in vitamin C as well as natural sugars. They provide extra vitamins and energy. (Be careful not to eat berries or fruit that are poisonous.)

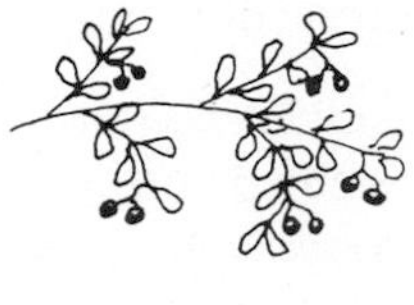

11. **Cooking in iron pots** or putting a piece of old iron or horseshoe in the pan when cooking beans and other foods adds iron to food and helps prevent anemia. More iron will be available if you also add tomatoes.

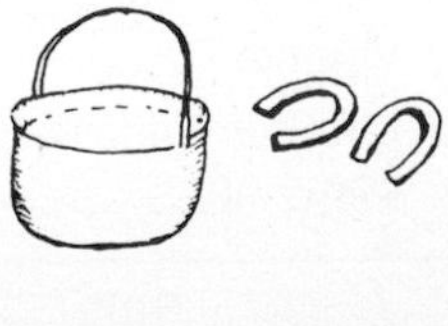

For another source of iron, put some iron nails in a little lemon juice for a few hours. Then make lemonade with the juice and drink it.

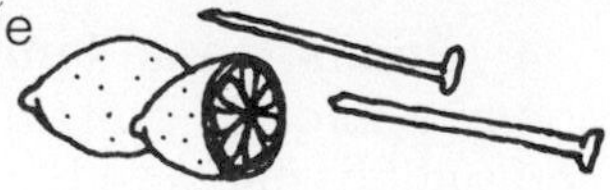

12. In some countries, **low-cost baby food preparations** are available, made from different combinations of soybean, cotton seed, skim milk, or dried fish. Some taste better than others, but most are well-balanced foods. When mixed with gruel, cooked cereal, or other baby food, they add to its nutrition content—at low cost.

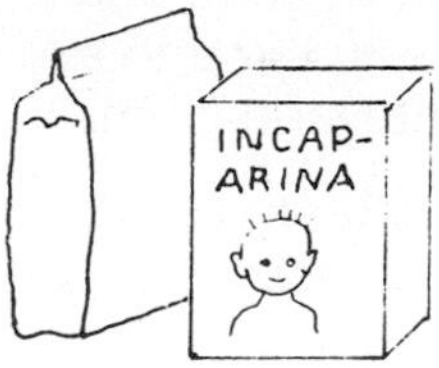

WHERE TO GET VITAMINS: IN PILLS, INJECTIONS, SYRUPS—OR IN FOODS?

Anyone who eats a good mixture of foods, including vegetables and fruits, gets all the vitamins he needs. It is always better to eat well than to buy vitamin pills, injections, syrups, or tonics.

If you want vitamins, buy eggs or other nutritious foods instead of pills or injections.

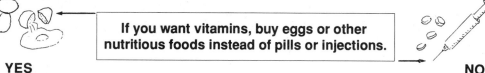

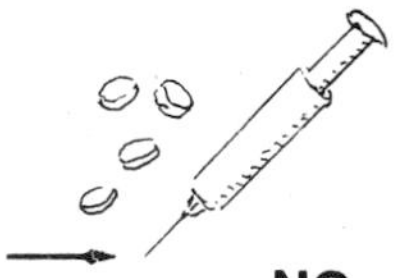

YES **NO**

Sometimes nutritious foods are scarce. If a person is already poorly nourished, he should eat as well as he can and perhaps take vitamins besides.

Vitamins taken by mouth work as well as injections, cost less, and are not as dangerous. **Do not inject vitamins! It is better to swallow them—preferably in the form of nutritious foods.**

If you buy vitamin preparations, be sure they have all these vitamins and minerals:

- Niacin (niacinamide)
- Vitamin B_1 (thiamine)
- Vitamin B_2 (riboflavin)
- Iron (ferrous sulfate, etc.)—especially for pregnant women. (For people with anemia, multi-vitamin pills do not have enough iron to help much. Iron pills are more helpful.)

In addition, certain people need extra:

- Folic Acid (folicin), for pregnant women
- Vitamin A } for small children
- Vitamin C (ascorbic acid) } for small children
- Vitamin D } for small children
- Iodine (in areas where goiter is common)
- Vitamin B_6 (pyridoxine), for small children and persons taking medicine for tuberculosis
- Calcium, for children and breast feeding mothers who do not get enough calcium in foods such as milk, cheese, or foods prepared with lime

THINGS TO AVOID IN OUR DIET

A lot of people believe that there are many kinds of foods that will hurt them, or that they should not eat when they are sick. They may think of some kinds of foods as 'hot' and others as 'cold', and not permit hot foods for 'hot' sicknesses or cold foods for 'cold' sicknesses. Or they may believe that many different foods are bad for a mother with a newborn child. Some of these beliefs are reasonable but others do more harm than good. Often the foods people think they should avoid when they are sick are the very foods they need to get well.

A sick person has even greater need for plenty of nutritious food than a healthy person. We should worry less about foods that might harm a sick person and think more about foods that help make him healthy—for example: high energy foods together with fruit, vegetables, legumes, nuts, milk, meat, eggs, and fish. As a general rule:

The same foods that are good for us when we are healthy are good for us when we are sick.

Also, the things that harm us when we are healthy do us even more harm when we are sick. Avoid these things:

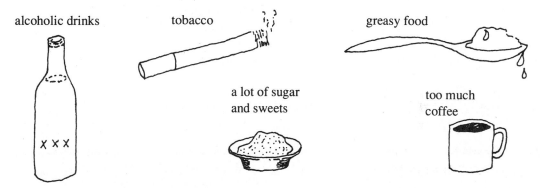

alcoholic drinks

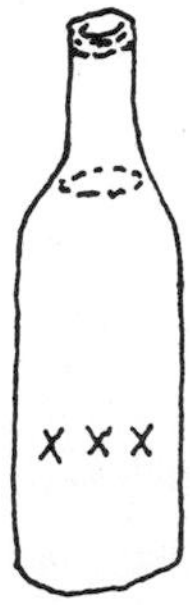

tobacco

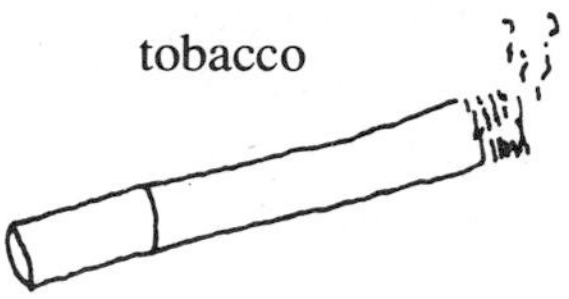

greasy food

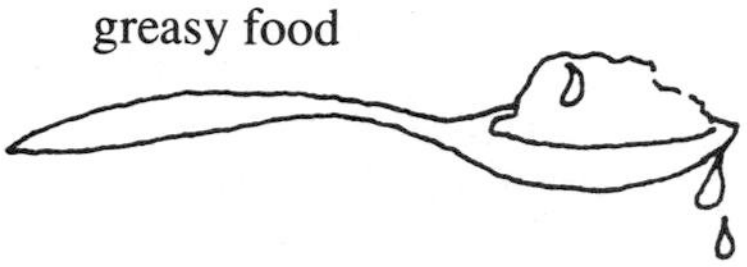

a lot of sugar and sweets

too much coffee

- Alcohol causes or makes worse diseases of the liver, stomach, heart, and nerves. It also causes social problems.
- Smoking can cause chronic (long-term) coughing or lung cancer and other problems (see p. 149). Smoking is especially bad for people with lung diseases like tuberculosis, asthma, and bronchitis.
- Too much greasy food or coffee can make stomach ulcers and other problems of the digestive tract worse.
- Too much sugar and sweets spoil the appetite and rot the teeth. However, some sugar with other foods may help give needed energy to a sick person or poorly nourished child.

A few diseases require not eating certain other foods. For example, people with high blood pressure, certain heart problems, or swollen feet should use little or no salt. Too much salt is not good for anyone. Stomach ulcers and diabetes also require special diets (see p. 127 and 128).

THE BEST DIET FOR SMALL CHILDREN

THE FIRST 6 MONTHS OF LIFE

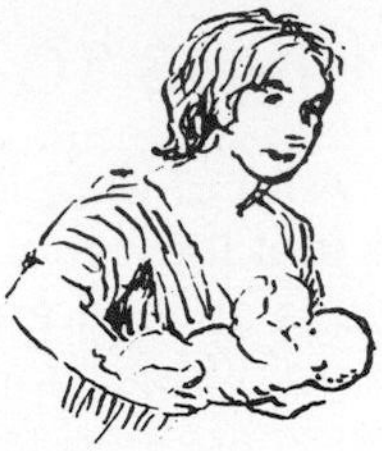

For the first 6 months give the baby breast milk and nothing else. It is better than any baby food or milks you can buy. Breast milk helps protect the baby against diarrhea and many infections. It is best not to give extra water or teas, even in hot weather.

Some mothers stop breast feeding early because they think that their milk is not good enough for their baby, or that their breasts are not making enough milk. **However, a mother's milk is always very nutritious for her baby, even if the mother herself is thin and weak.**

If a woman has HIV/AIDS, sometimes she can pass this disease to a baby in her breast milk. But if she does not have access to clean water, her baby is more likely to die from diarrhea, dehydration, and malnutrition than AIDS. Only you can evaluate the conditions in your home and community and decide what to do.

Nearly all mothers can produce all the breast milk their babies need:

- The best way for a mother to keep making enough breast milk is to **breast feed the baby often, eat well, and drink lots of liquids.**
- Do not give the baby other foods before he is 4 to 6 months old, and **always breast feed before giving the other foods.**
- If a mother's breasts produce little or no milk, she should continue to eat well, drink lots of liquids and **let the baby suck her breasts often.** After each breast feeding, give the baby, by cup (not bottle), some other type of milk—like boiled cow's or goat's milk, canned milk, or powdered milk. (Do not use condensed milk.) Add a little sugar or vegetable oil to any of these milks.

Note: Whatever type of milk is used, some cooled, boiled water should be added. Here are two examples of correct formulas:

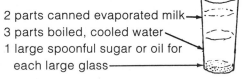

#1

2 parts boiled, cooled cow's milk
1 part boiled, cooled water
1 large spoonful sugar or oil for each large glass

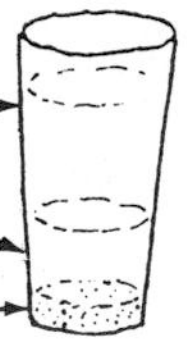

#2

2 parts canned evaporated milk
3 parts boiled, cooled water
1 large spoonful sugar or oil for each large glass

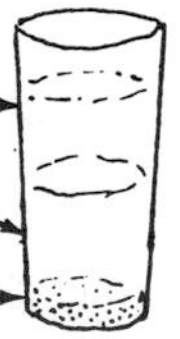

If non-fat milk is used, add another spoonful of oil.

- If possible, boil the milk and water. **It is safer to feed the baby with a cup (or cup and spoon) than to use a baby bottle.** Baby bottles and nipples are hard to keep clean and can cause infections and diarrhea (see p. 154). If a bottle is used, boil it and the nipple each time before the baby is fed.
- If you cannot buy milk for the child, make a porridge from rice, cornmeal, or other cereal. Always add to this some skinned beans, eggs, meat, chicken, or other protein. Mash these well and give them as a liquid. If possible add sugar and oil.

> *WARNING:* **Cornmeal or rice water alone is not enough for a baby. The child will not grow well. He will get sick easily and may die. The baby needs a main food with added helper foods.**

FROM 4 MONTHS TO 1 YEAR OF AGE:

1. **Keep giving breast milk,** if possible until the baby is 2 or 3 years old.

2. When the baby is between 4 and 6 months old, **start giving her other foods in addition to breast milk.** Always give the breast first, and then the other foods. It is good to start with a gruel or porridge made from the main food (p. 111) such as maize meal or rice cooked in water or milk. Then start adding a little **cooking oil** for extra energy. After a few days, start adding **other helper foods** (see p. 110). But **start with just a little of the new food,** and **add only 1 at a time** or the baby may have trouble digesting them. These **new foods need to be well cooked and mashed.** At first they can be mixed with a little breast milk to make them easier for the baby to swallow.

3. Prepare inexpensive, nutritious feedings for the baby by adding helper foods to the main food (see p. 110). Most important is to add foods that give extra energy (such as oil) and—whenever possible—extra iron (such as dark green leafy vegetables).

Remember, a young child's stomach is small and cannot hold much food at one time. So **feed her often,** and **add high-energy helpers** to the main food:

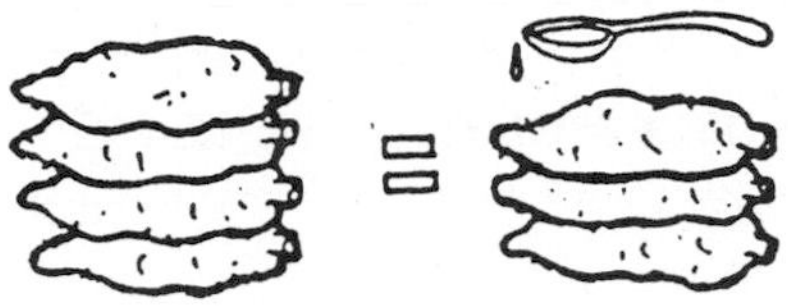

A spoonful of cooking oil added to a child's food means he has to eat only 3/4 as much of the local main food in order to meet his energy needs. The added oil helps make sure he gets enough energy (calories) by the time his belly is full.

CAUTION: The time when a child is most likely to become malnourished is from 6 months to 2 years old. This is because breast milk by itself does not provide enough energy for a baby after 6 months of age. Other foods are needed, but often the foods given do not contain enough energy either. If the mother also stops breast feeding, the child is even more likely to become malnourished.

For a child of this age to be healthy we should:

- Keep feeding her breast milk—as much as before.
- Feed her other nutritious foods also, always starting with just a little.
- Feed her at least 5 times a day and also give her snacks between meals.
- Make sure the food is clean and freshly prepared.
- Filter, boil, or purify the water she drinks.
- Keep the child and her surroundings clean.
- When she gets sick, feed her extra well and more often, and give her plenty of liquids to drink.

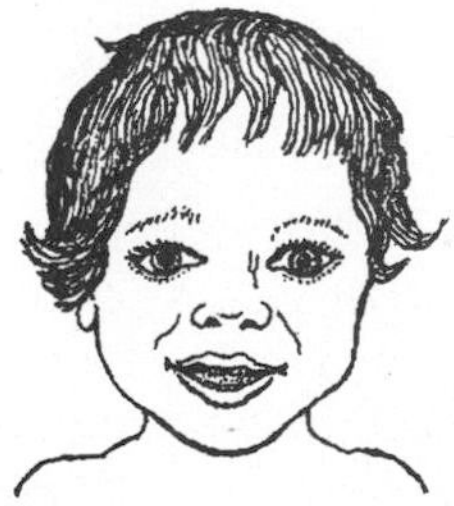

For mothers infected with the HIV/AIDS virus: After 6 months, your baby will be bigger and stronger, and will have less danger of dying from diarrhea. If you have been breast feeding her, now you should switch to other milks and feed the baby other foods. This way the baby will have less risk of getting HIV/AIDS.

ONE YEAR AND OLDER:

After a child is 1 year old, he can eat **the same foods as adults,** but should **continue to breast feed** (or drink milk whenever possible).

Every day, try to give the child plenty of the main food that people eat, together with 'helper' foods that give added high energy, proteins, vitamins, iron, and minerals (as shown on p. 111) so that he will grow up strong and healthy.

To make sure that the child gets enough to eat, **serve him in his own dish,** and let him take as long as he needs to eat his meal.

Children and candy: Do not accustom small children to eating a lot of candy and sweets or drinking soft drinks (colas). When they have too many sweets, they no longer want enough of the other foods they need. Also, sweets are bad for their teeth.

However, when food supply is limited or when the main foods have a lot of water or fiber in them, adding a little sugar and vegetable oil to the main food provides extra energy and allows children to make fuller use of the protein in the food they get.

THE BEST DIET FOR SMALL CHILDREN

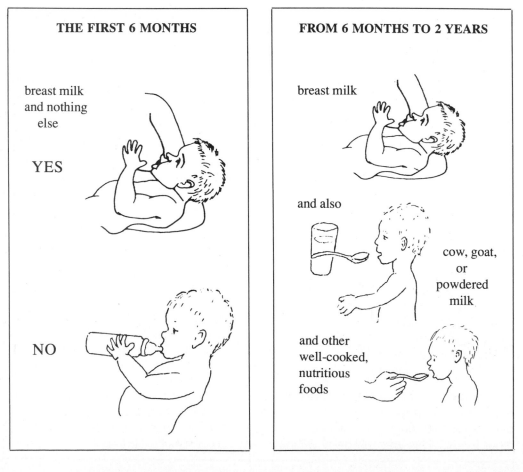

THE FIRST 6 MONTHS

breast milk and nothing else

YES

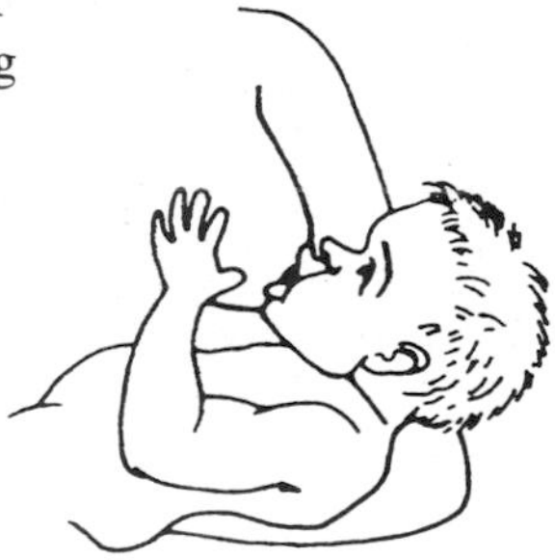

NO

FROM 6 MONTHS TO 2 YEARS

breast milk

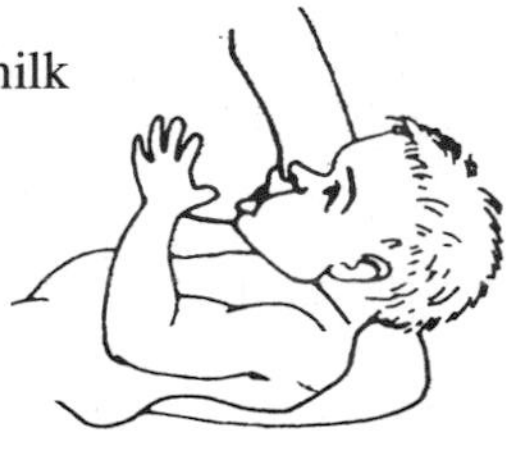

and also

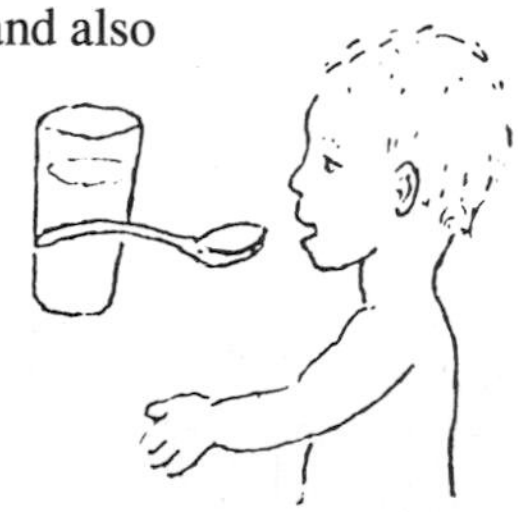

cow, goat, or powdered milk

and other well-cooked, nutritious foods

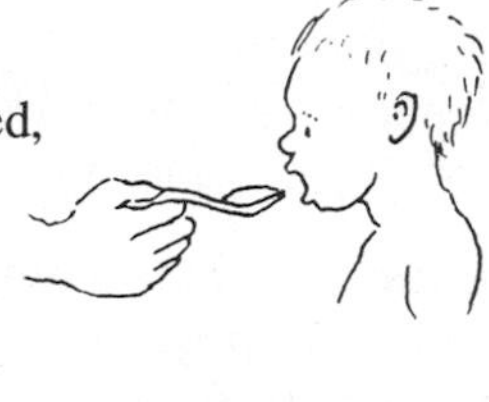

HARMFUL IDEAS ABOUT DIET

1. **The diet of mothers after giving birth:**

In many areas there is a dangerous popular belief that a woman who has just had a baby should not eat certain foods. This folk diet—which forbids some of the most nutritious foods and may only let the new mother eat things like cornmeal, noodles, or rice soup—makes her weak and anemic. It may even cause her death, by lowering her resistance to hemorrhage (bleeding) and infection.

After giving birth a mother needs to eat the most nutritious foods she can get.

In order to fight infections or bleeding and to produce enough milk for her child, **a new mother should eat the main food together with plenty of body-building foods like beans, eggs, chicken, and if possible, milk products, meat, and fish.** She also needs protective foods like fruits and vegetables, and high-energy helpers (oils and fatty foods). None of these foods will harm her; they will protect her and make her stronger.

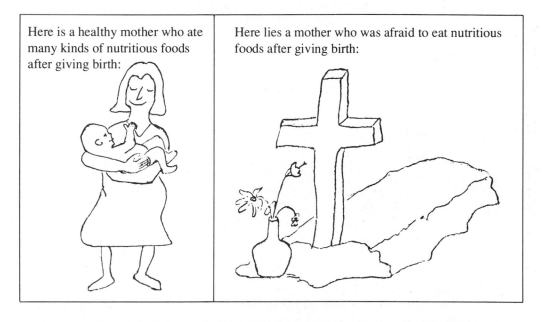

Here is a healthy mother who ate many kinds of nutritious foods after giving birth:

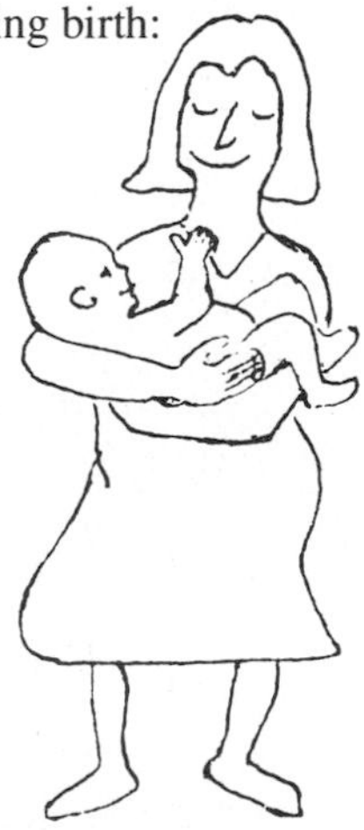

Here lies a mother who was afraid to eat nutritious foods after giving birth:

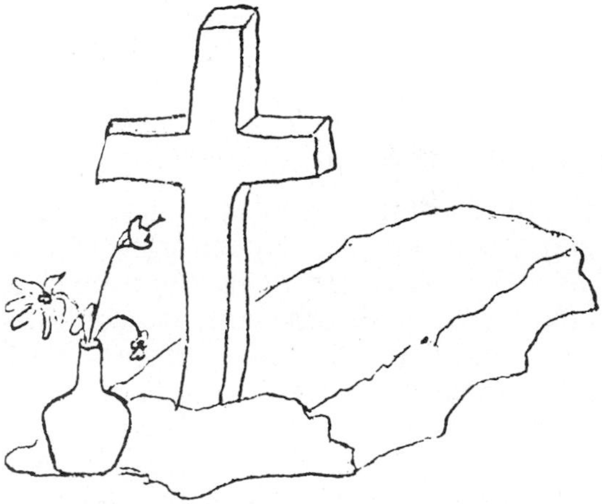

2. **It is not true that oranges, guavas, or other fruits are bad for a person who has a cold, the flu, or a cough.** In fact, fruits like oranges and tomatoes have a lot of vitamin C, which may help fight colds and other infections.

3. **It is not true that certain foods like pork, spices, or guavas cannot be eaten while taking medicine.** However, when a person has a disease of the stomach or other parts of the digestive system, eating a lot of fat or greasy foods may make this worse—whether or not one is taking medicines.

SPECIAL DIETS FOR SPECIFIC HEALTH PROBLEMS

ANEMIA

A person with anemia has thin blood. This happens when blood is lost or destroyed faster than the body can replace it. Blood loss from large wounds, bleeding ulcers, or dysentery can cause anemia. So can malaria, which destroys red blood cells. Not eating enough foods rich in iron can cause anemia or make it worse.

Women can become anemic from blood loss during monthly bleeding (menstrual periods) or childbirth if they do not eat the foods their bodies need. Pregnant women are at risk of becoming severely anemic, because they need to make extra blood for their growing babies.

In children anemia can come from not eating foods rich in iron. It can also come from not starting to give some foods in addition to breast milk, after the baby is 6 months old. Common causes of severe anemia in children are hookworm infection (see p. 142), chronic diarrhea, and dysentery.

The signs of anemia are:

- pale or transparent skin
- pale insides of eyelids
- white fingernails
- pale gums
- weakness and fatigue

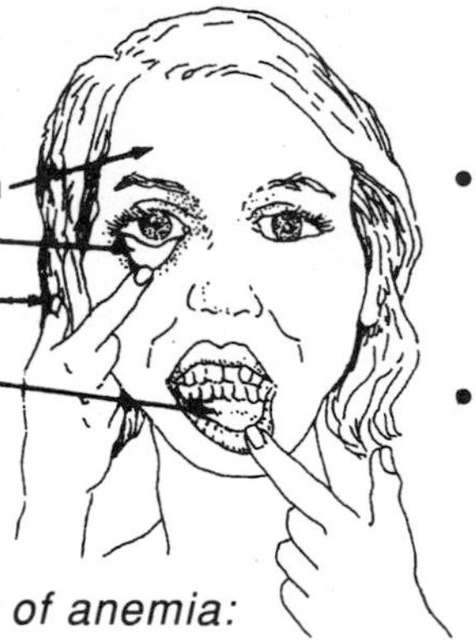

- If the anemia is very severe, face and feet may be swollen, the heartbeat rapid, and the person may have shortness of breath.
- Children and women who like to eat dirt are usually anemic.

Treatment and prevention of anemia:

- **Eat foods rich in iron.** Meat, fish, and chicken are high in iron. Liver is especially high. Dark green leafy vegetables, beans, peas, and lentils also have some iron. It also helps to cook in iron pots (see p. 117). To help the body absorb more iron, eat raw vegetables and fruit with meals, and avoid drinking coffee and tea with food.
- If the anemia is moderate or severe, the person should take iron (ferrous sulfate pills, p. 393). This is especially important for pregnant women who are anemic. For nearly all cases of anemia, ferrous sulfate tablets are much better than liver extract or vitamin B_{12}. As a general rule, **iron should be given by mouth, not injected,** because iron injections can be dangerous and are no better than pills.
- If the anemia is caused by dysentery (diarrhea with blood), hookworm, malaria, or another disease, this should also be treated.
- If the anemia is severe or does not get better, seek medical help. This is especially important for a pregnant woman.

Many women are anemic. Anemic women run a greater risk of miscarriage and of dangerous bleeding in childbirth. **It is very important that women eat as much of the foods high in iron as possible,** especially during pregnancy. Allowing 2 to 3 years between pregnancies lets the woman regain strength and make new blood (see Chapter 20).

RICKETS

Children whose skin is almost never exposed to the sunlight may become bowlegged and develop other bone deformities (rickets). This problem can be combatted by giving the child fortified milk and vitamin D (found in fish liver oil). However, **the easiest and cheapest form of prevention is to be sure direct sunlight reaches the child's skin** for at least 10 minutes a day or for longer periods more often. (Be careful not to let his skin burn.) Never give large doses of vitamin D over long periods, as it can poison the child.

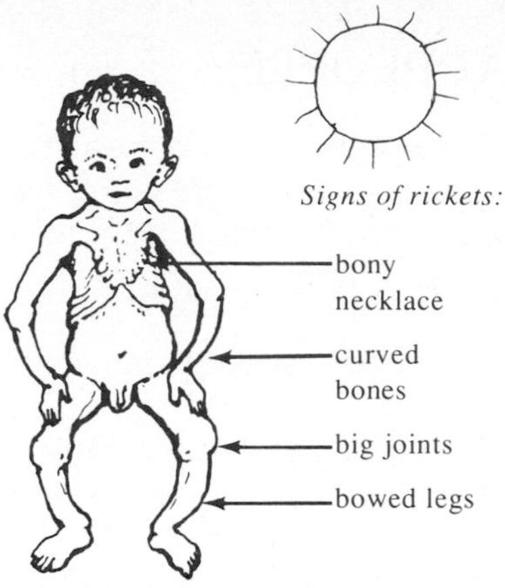

SUNLIGHT IS THE BEST PREVENTION AND TREATMENT OF RICKETS.

HIGH BLOOD PRESSURE (HYPERTENSION)

High blood pressure can cause many problems, such as heart disease, kidney disease, and stroke. Fat people are especially likely to have high blood pressure.

Signs of dangerously high blood pressure:

- frequent headaches
- pounding of the heart and shortness of breath with mild exercise
- weakness and dizziness
- occasional pain in the left shoulder and chest

All these problems may also be caused by other diseases. Therefore, if a person suspects he has high blood pressure, he should see a health worker and have his blood pressure measured.

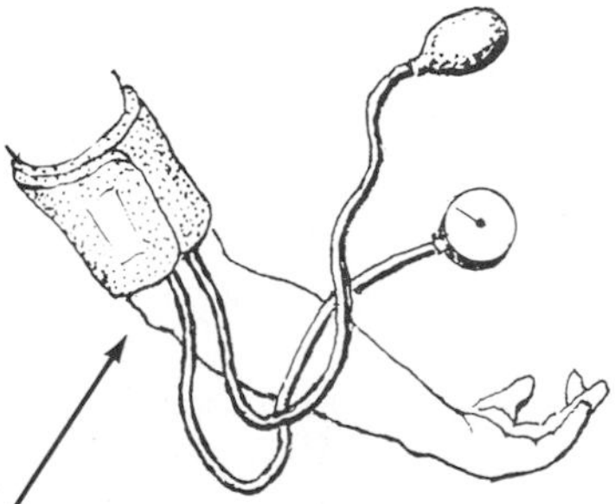

A BLOOD PRESSURE CUFF for measuring blood pressure

WARNING: High blood pressure at first causes no signs, and it should be lowered **before** danger signs develop. People who are overweight or suspect they might have high blood pressure should have their blood pressure checked regularly. For instructions on measuring blood pressure, see p. 410 and 411.

What to do to prevent or care for high blood pressure:

- If overweight, lose weight (see next page).
- Avoid fatty foods, especially pig fat, and foods with a lot of sugar or starch. Always use vegetable oil instead of pig fat.
- Prepare and eat food with little or no salt.
- Do not smoke. Do not drink much alcohol, coffee, or tea.
- When the blood pressure is very high, the health worker may give medicines to lower it. Many people can lower their blood pressure by losing weight if they are fat (next page), and by learning to relax.

FAT PEOPLE

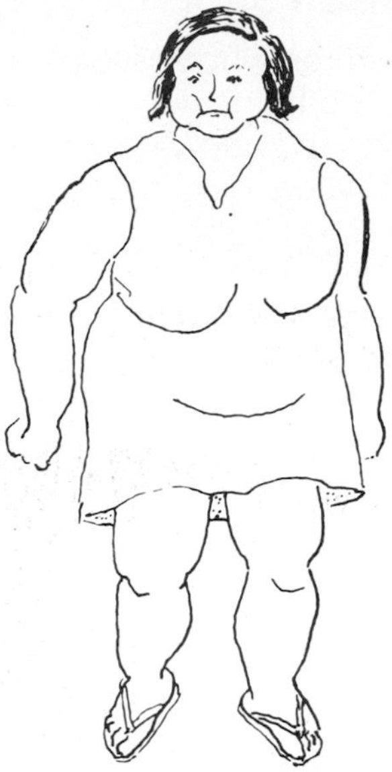

To be very fat is not healthy. Too much fat helps cause high blood pressure, heart disease, stroke, gallstones, diabetes, arthritis in legs and feet, and other problems.

Fat people should lose weight by:

- eating less greasy, fatty, or oily foods.
- eating less sugar or sweet foods.
- getting more exercise.
- **not eating so much** of anything, especially starchy foods, like corn, bread, potatoes, rice, pasta, cassava, etc. Fat people should not eat more than one piece of bread, tortilla, or chapati with each meal. However, they can eat more fruit and vegetables.

Prevention: When you begin to get overweight, start following the above guidelines.

To lose weight, eat only half of what you now eat.

CONSTIPATION

A person who has hard stools and has not had a bowel movement for 3 or more days is said to be constipated. Constipation is often caused by a poor diet (especially not eating enough fruits, green vegetables, or foods with natural fiber like whole grain bread) or by lack of exercise.

Drinking more water and eating more fruits, vegetables, and foods with natural fiber like whole grain bread, cassava, wheat bran, rye, carrots, turnips, raisins, nuts, pumpkin or sunflower seeds, is better than using laxatives. It also helps to add a little vegetable oil to food each day. Older people especially may need to walk or exercise more in order to have regular bowel movements.

A person who has not had a bowel movement for 4 or more days, if he does not have a sharp pain in his stomach, can take a mild salt laxative like milk of magnesia. **But do not take laxatives often.**

Do not give laxatives to babies or young children. If a baby is severely constipated, put a little cooking oil up the rectum (asshole). Or, if necessary, gently break up and remove the hard shit with a greased finger.

**Never use strong laxatives or purgatives—
especially if there is stomach pain.**

DIABETES

Persons with diabetes have too much sugar in their blood. This can start when a person is young (juvenile diabetes) or older (adult diabetes). It is usually more serious in young people, and they need special medicine (insulin) to control it. But it is most common in people over age 40 who eat too much and get fat.

Early signs of diabetes:

- always thirsty
- urinates (pees) often and a lot
- always tired
- always hungry
- weight loss

Later, more serious signs:

- itchy skin
- periods of blurry eyesight
- some loss of feeling in hands or feet
- frequent vaginal infections
- sores on the feet that do not heal
- loss of consciousness (in extreme cases)

All these signs may be caused by other diseases. In order to find out whether a person has diabetes, test her urine to see if there is sugar in it. One way to test the urine is to taste it. If it tastes sweet to you, have 2 other persons taste it. Have them also taste the urine of 3 other people. If everyone agrees that the same person's urine is sweeter, she is probably diabetic.

Another way of testing urine is to use special paper strips (for example, *Uristix*). If these change color when dipped in the urine, it has sugar in it.

If the person is a child or young adult, he should be seen by an experienced health worker or doctor.

When a person gets diabetes after he is 40 years old, it can often be best controlled without medicines, by eating correctly. **The diabetic person's diet is very important and must be followed carefully for life.**

The diabetic diet: Fat people with diabetes should lose weight until their weight is normal. **Diabetics must not eat any sugar or sweets, or foods that taste sweet.** It is important for them to eat lots of high-fiber foods, such as whole grain breads. But diabetics should also eat some other starchy foods, like beans, rice, and potatoes, and also foods high in protein.

Diabetes in adults can sometimes be helped by drinking the sap of the prickly pear cactus (nopal, *Opuntia*). To prepare, cut the cactus into small pieces and crush them to squeeze out the liquid. Drink 1 1/2 cups of the liquid 3 times each day before meals.

To prevent infection and injury to the skin, clean the teeth after eating, keep the skin clean, and always wear shoes to prevent foot injuries. For poor circulation in the feet (dark color, numbness), rest often with the feet up. Follow the same recommendations as for varicose veins (p. 175).

ACID INDIGESTION, HEARTBURN, AND STOMACH ULCERS

Acid indigestion and 'heartburn' often come from eating too much heavy or greasy food or from drinking too much alcohol or coffee. These make the stomach produce extra acid, which causes discomfort or a 'burning' feeling in the stomach or mid-chest. Some people mistake the chest pain, called 'heartburn', for a heart problem rather than indigestion. If the pain gets worse when lying down, it is probably heartburn.

Frequent or lasting acid indigestion is a warning sign of an ulcer.

An ulcer is a chronic sore in the stomach or small intestine, caused by too much acid. It may cause a chronic, dull (sometimes sharp) pain in the pit of the stomach. As with acid indigestion, often the pain lessens when the person eats food or drinks a lot of water. The pain usually gets worse an hour or more after eating, if the person misses a meal, or after he drinks alcohol or eats fatty or spicy foods. Pain is often worse at night. Without a special examination (endoscopy) it is often hard to know whether a person with frequent stomach pain has an ulcer or not.

An ulcer

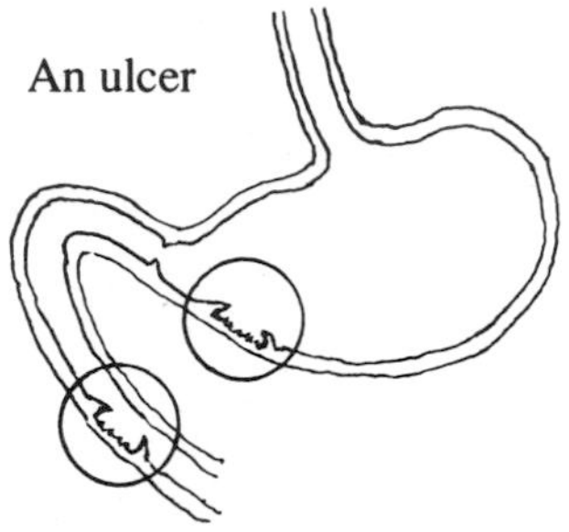

is an open sore in the stomach or gut.

If the ulcer is severe, it can cause vomiting, sometimes with fresh blood, or with digested blood that looks like coffee grounds. Stools with blood from an ulcer are usually black, like tar.

WARNING: Some ulcers are painless or 'silent', and the first sign is **blood in vomit, or black, sticky stools.** This is a medical emergency. The person can quickly bleed to death. GET MEDICAL HELP FAST.

Prevention and Treatment:

Whether stomach or chest pain is caused by heartburn, acid indigestion, or an ulcer, a few basic recommendations will probably help calm the pain and prevent it from coming back.

- **Do not eat too much.** Eat small meals and eat frequent snacks between meals. Eat mainly foods that seem to calm and not to cause the pain.
- **Notice what foods or drinks make the pain worse and avoid them.** These usually include alcoholic drinks, coffee, spices, pepper, carbonated drinks (soda, pop, colas), and fatty or greasy foods.
- If the heartburn is worse at night when lying flat, try sleeping with the upper body somewhat raised.

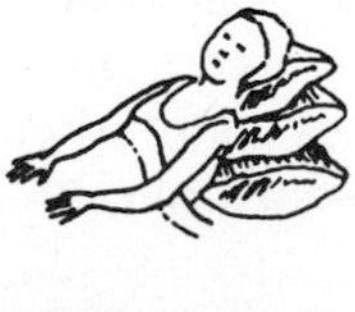

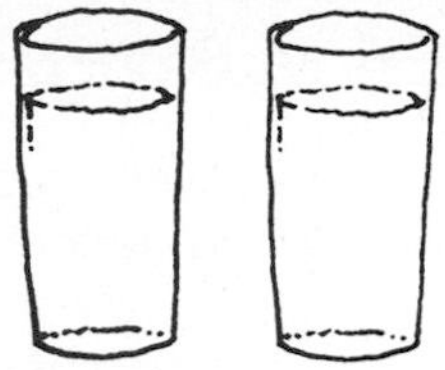

♦ **Drink a lot of water.** Try to drink 2 big glasses of water both before and after each meal. Also drink a lot of water frequently between meals. If the pain comes often, keep drinking water like this, even in those times when you have no pain.

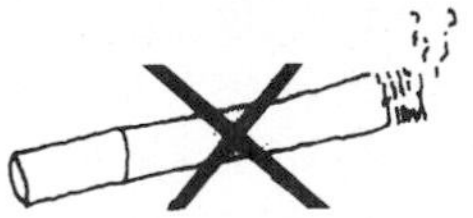

♦ **Avoid tobacco.** Smoking or chewing tobacco increases stomach acid and makes the problem worse.

♦ **Take antacids.** The best, safest antacids contain magnesium and aluminum hydroxide. (See p. 381 for information, dose, and warnings about different antacids.)

♦ For severe pain or ulcers that do not get better, try to get cimetidine (*Tagamet,* p. 382), or ranitidine (see p. 382). These are very costly but usually very effective at calming the pain and helping to heal the sore. But the ulcer may come back.

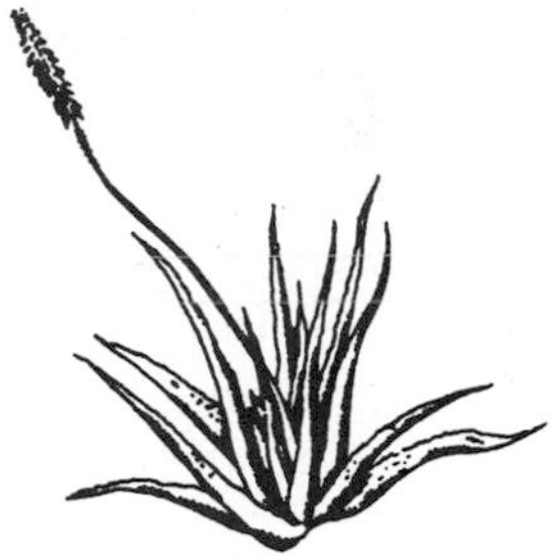

♦ **Aloe vera** is a plant found in many countries that is said to heal ulcers. Chop the spongy leaves into small pieces, soak them in water overnight, and then drink one glass of the slimy, bitter water every 2 hours.

CAUTION:

1. Many doctors used to recommend **milk** for treatment of ulcers. But although milk may calm the pain at first, it causes an increase in stomach acid which can make an ulcer worse. Most doctors now say **do not drink milk as a treatment for ulcers.**

2. Like milk, some antacids such as **sodium bicarbonate** (baking soda) and *Alka-Seltzer* may quickly calm acid indigestion, but soon cause more acid. They should be used only for occasional indigestion, never for ulcers. This is also true for antacids with calcium.

3. Some **medicines,** such as aspirin and iron salts, make ulcers worse. Persons with signs of heartburn or acid indigestion should avoid them—or take them with extra care (with meals, lots of water, and perhaps antacids). Cortico-steroids also make ulcers worse, or cause them (see p. 51).

It is important to **treat an ulcer early.** Otherwise it may lead to dangerous bleeding or peritonitis. Ulcers usually get better if the person is careful with what he eats and drinks. Anger, tension, and nervousness increase acid in the stomach. Learning to relax and keep calm will help. Continued care is necessary to prevent the ulcer from returning.

Better still, **avoid problems caused by stomach acid by not eating too much, by not drinking much alcohol or coffee, and by not smoking.**

GOITER (A SWELLING OR LUMP ON THE THROAT)

A goiter is a swelling or big lump on the throat that results from abnormal growth of a gland called the thyroid.

Most goiters are caused by a lack of iodine in the diet. Also, a lack of iodine in a pregnant woman's diet sometimes causes babies to die or to be born mentally slow and/or deaf (cretinism, p. 318). This can happen even though the mother does not have a goiter.

Goiter and cretinism are most common in mountain areas where there is little natural iodine in the soil, water, or food. In these areas, eating a lot of certain foods like cassava makes it more likely for a person to get a goiter.

How to prevent or cure a goiter and prevent cretinism:

Everyone living in areas where people get goiters should use **iodized salt.** Use of iodized salt prevents the common kind of goiter and will help many goiters go away. (Old, hard goiters can only be removed by surgery, but this is usually not necessary.)

If it is not possible to get iodized salt, use tincture of iodine. Put 1 drop in a glass of water each day and drink. BE CAREFUL: Too much tincture of iodine is poisonous. More than the recommended amount of 1 drop a day can make a goiter worse. Keep the bottle where children cannot reach it. Iodized salt is much safer.

Most home cures for goiter do not do any good. However, eating crab and other seafood can do some good because they contain iodine. Mixing a little seaweed with food also adds iodine. But the easiest way is to use **iodized salt.**

HOW TO KEEP FROM GETTING A GOITER

NEVER use regular salt.

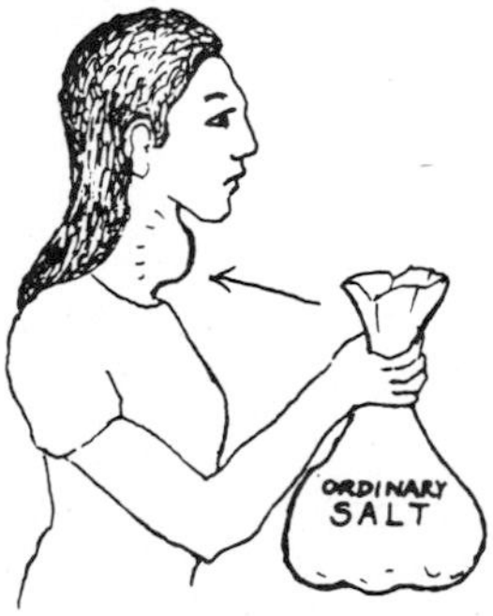

IODIZED SALT
costs only a little more than other salt and is much better.

ALWAYS use iodized salt.

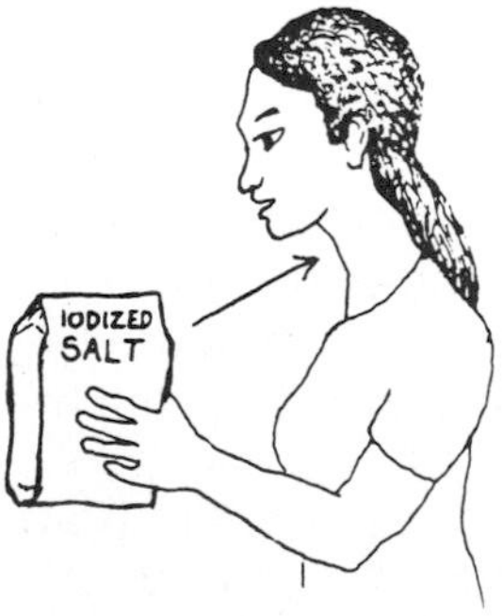

Also, if you live in an area where goiters are common, or you are beginning to develop a goiter, try to avoid eating much cassava or cabbage.

Note: If a person with a goiter trembles a lot, is very nervous, and has eyes that bulge out, this may be a different kind of goiter (toxic goiter). Seek medical advice.

CHAPTER 12

PREVENTION: HOW TO AVOID MANY SICKNESSES

An ounce of prevention is worth a pound of cure! If we all took more care to **eat well,** to **keep ourselves, our homes, and our villages clean,** and to **be sure that our children are vaccinated,** we could stop most sicknesses before they start. In Chapter 11 we discussed eating well. In this chapter we talk about cleanliness and vaccination.

CLEANLINESS—AND PROBLEMS THAT COME FROM LACK OF CLEANLINESS

Cleanliness is of great importance in the prevention of many kinds of infections—infections of the gut, the skin, the eyes, the lungs, and the whole body. Personal cleanliness (or ***hygiene***) and public cleanliness (or ***sanitation***) are both important.

Many common infections of the gut are spread from one person to another because of poor hygiene and poor sanitation. Germs and worms (or their eggs) are passed by the thousands in the ***stools*** or ***feces*** (shit) of infected persons. These are carried from the feces of one person to the mouth of another by dirty fingers or ***contaminated*** food or water. Diseases that are spread or ***transmitted*** from ***feces-to-mouth*** in this way, include:

- diarrhea and dysentery (caused by amebas and bacteria)
- intestinal worms (several types)
- hepatitis, typhoid fever, and cholera
- certain other diseases, like polio, are sometimes spread this same way

The way these infections are transmitted can be very direct.

For example: A child who has worms and who forgot to wash his hands after his last bowel movement, offers his friend a cracker. His fingers, still dirty with his own stool, are covered with hundreds of tiny worm eggs (so small they cannot be seen). Some of these worm eggs stick to the cracker. When his friend eats the cracker, he swallows the worm eggs, too.

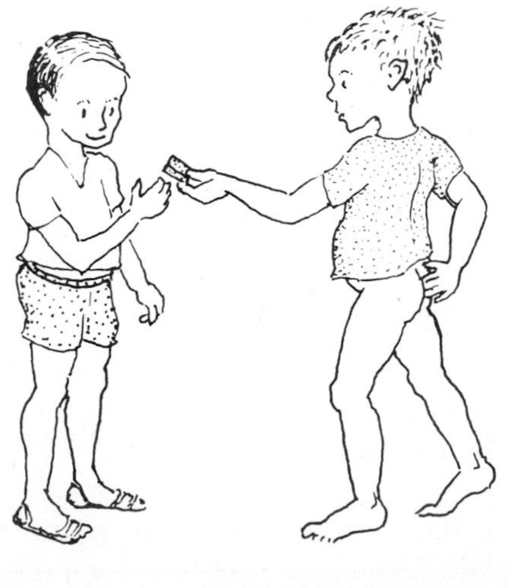

Soon the friend will also have worms. His mother may say this is because he ate sweets. But no, it is because he ate shit!

Many times pigs, dogs, chickens, and other animals spread intestinal disease and worm eggs. For example:

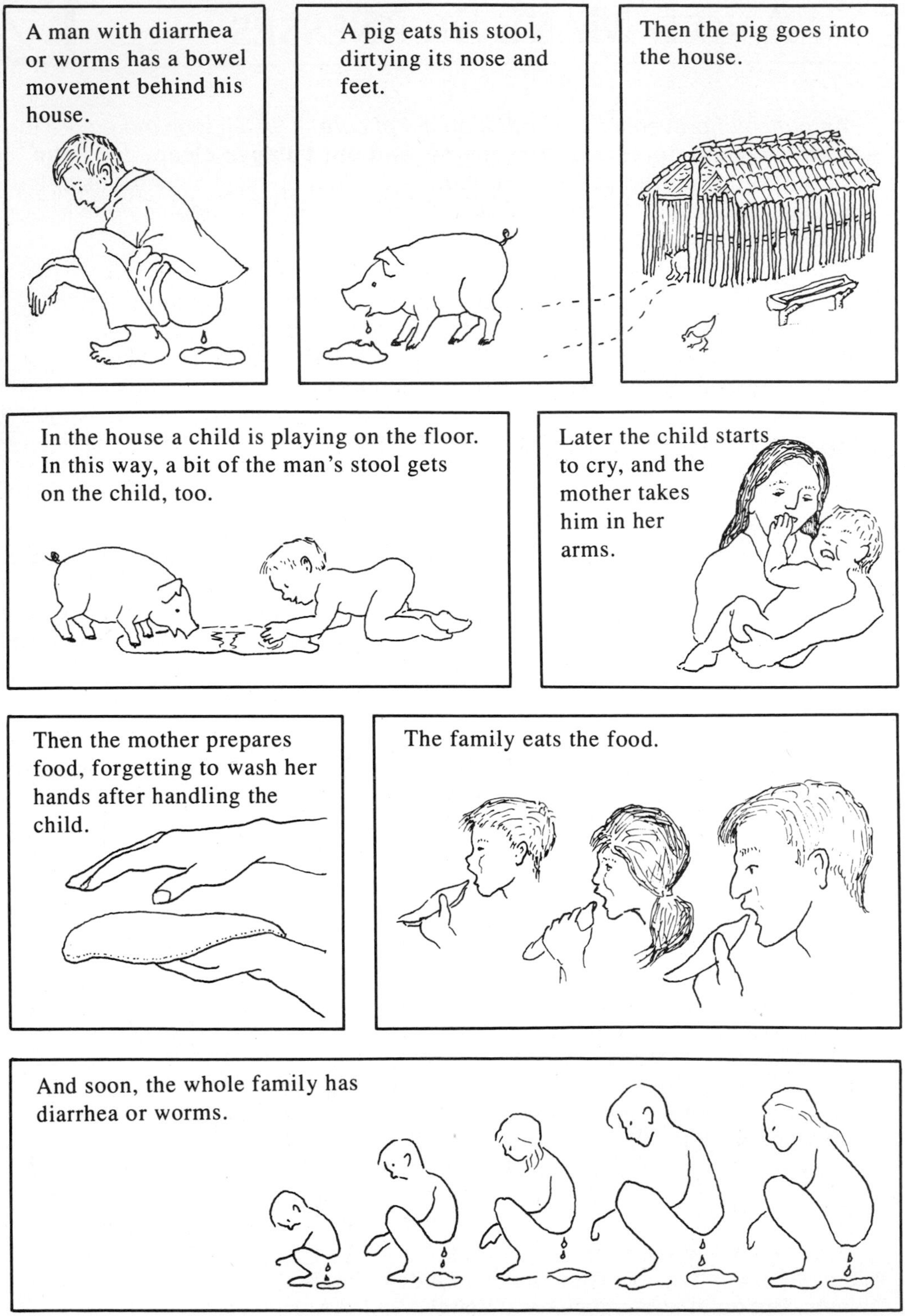
A man with diarrhea or worms has a bowel movement behind his house.
A pig eats his stool, dirtying its nose and feet.
Then the pig goes into the house.
In the house a child is playing on the floor. In this way, a bit of the man's stool gets on the child, too.
Later the child starts to cry, and the mother takes him in her arms.
Then the mother prepares food, forgetting to wash her hands after handling the child.
The family eats the food.
And soon, the whole family has diarrhea or worms.

Many kinds of infections, as well as worm eggs, are passed from one person to another in the way just shown.

If the family had taken **any** of the following precautions, the spread of the sickness could have been prevented:

- if the man had used a latrine or out-house,
- if the family had not let the pigs come into the house,
- if they had not let the child play where the pig had been,
- if the mother had washed her hands after touching the child and before preparing food.

If there are many cases of diarrhea, worms, and other intestinal parasites in your village, people are not being careful enough about cleanliness. If many children die from diarrhea, it is likely that poor nutrition is also part of the problem. **To prevent death from diarrhea, both cleanliness and good nutrition are important** (see p. 154 and Chapter 11).

BASIC GUIDELINES OF CLEANLINESS

PERSONAL CLEANLINESS (HYGIENE)

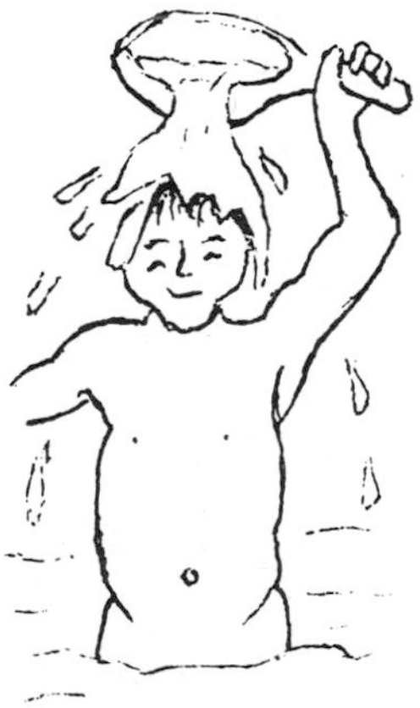

1. Always wash your hands with soap when you get up in the morning, after having a bowel movement, and before eating.

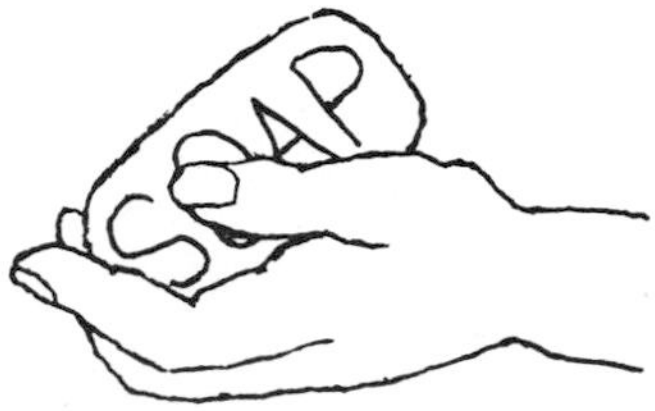

2. Bathe often—every day when the weather is hot. Bathe after working hard or sweating. Frequent bathing helps prevent skin infections, dandruff, pimples, itching, and rashes. Sick persons, including babies, should be bathed daily.

3. In areas where hookworm is common, do not go barefoot or allow children to do so. Hookworm infection causes severe anemia. These worms enter the body through the soles of the feet (see p. 142).

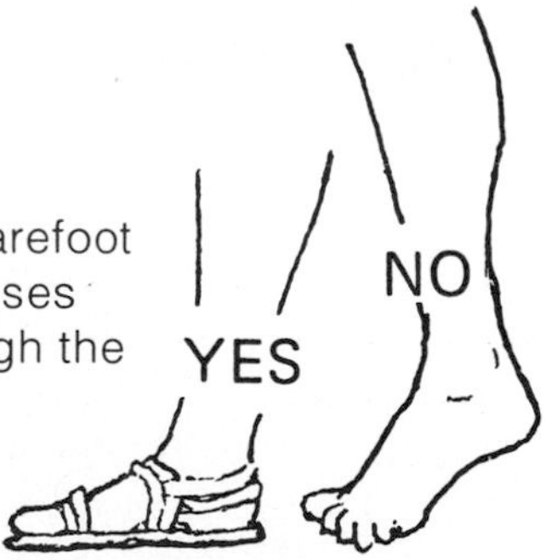

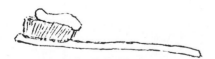

4. Brush your teeth every day and after each time you eat sweets. If you do not have a toothbrush and toothpaste, rub your teeth with salt and baking soda (see p. 230). For more information about the care of teeth, see Chapter 17.

CLEANLINESS IN THE HOME

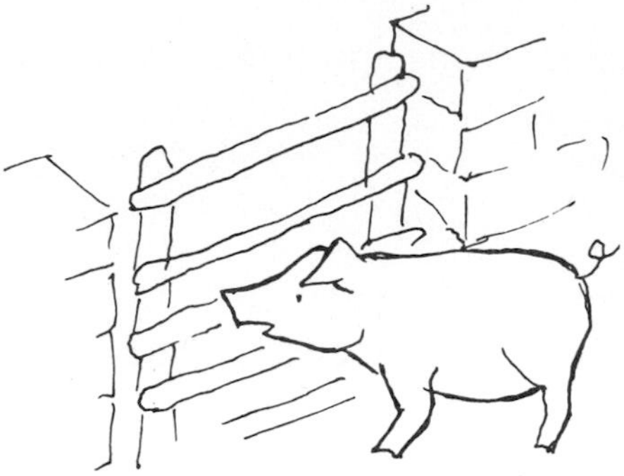

1. Do not let pigs or other animals come into the house or places where children play.

2. Do not let dogs lick children or climb up on beds. Dogs, too, can spread disease.

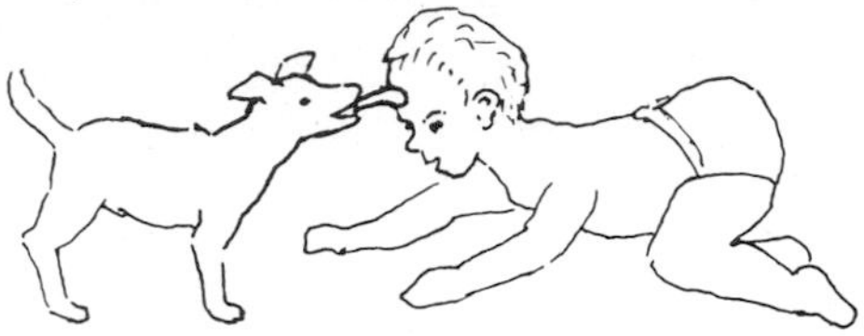

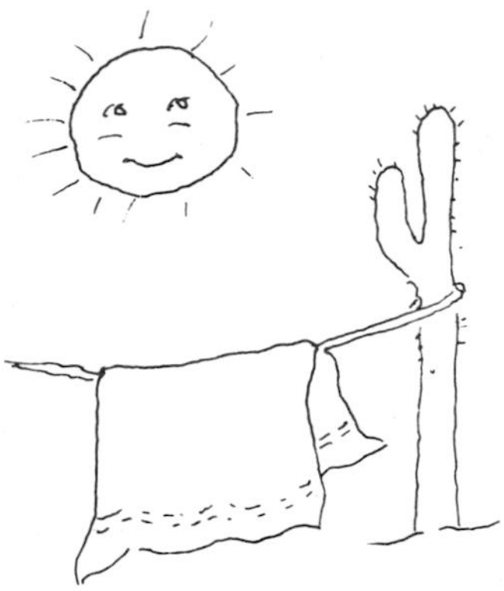

3. If children or animals have a bowel movement near the house, clean it up at once. Teach children to use a latrine or at least to go farther from the house.

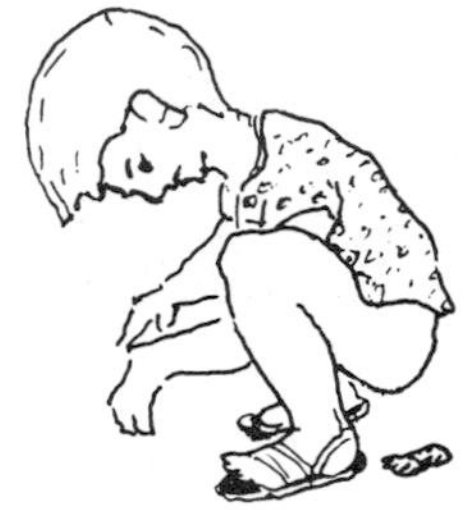

4. Hang or spread sheets and blankets in the sun often. If there are bedbugs, pour boiling water on the cots and wash the sheets and blankets—all on the same day (see p. 200).

5. De-louse the whole family often (see p. 200). Lice and fleas carry many diseases. Dogs and other animals that carry fleas should not come into the house.

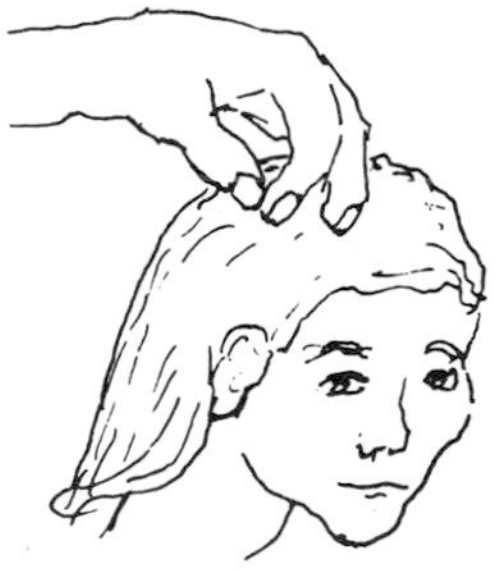

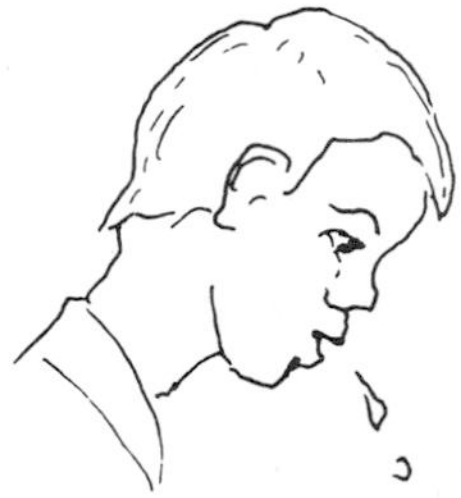

6. Do not spit on the floor. Spit can spread disease. When you cough or sneeze, cover your mouth with your hand or a cloth or handkerchief.

7. Clean house often. Sweep and wash the floors, walls, and beneath furniture. Fill in cracks and holes in the floor or walls where roaches, bedbugs, and scorpions can hide.

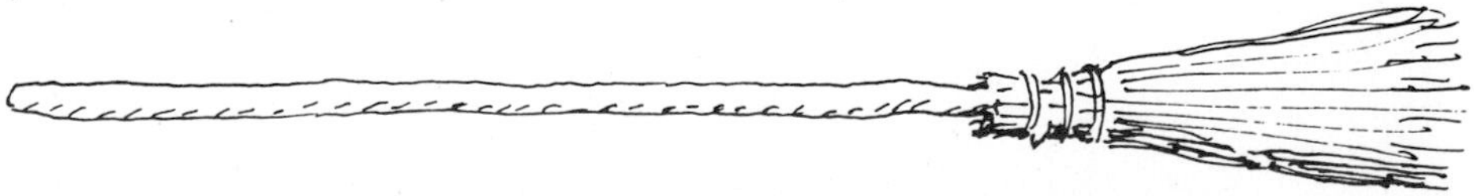

CLEANLINESS IN EATING AND DRINKING

1. Ideally all water that does not come from a pure water system should be boiled, filtered, or purified before drinking. This is especially important for small children and at times when there is a lot of diarrhea or cases of typhoid, hepatitis, or cholera. However, to prevent disease having **enough** water is more important than having **pure** water. Also, asking poor families to use a lot of time or money for fire wood to boil drinking water may do more harm than good, especially if it means less food for the children or more destruction of forests. For more information on clean water, see *Helping Health Workers Learn,* Chapter 15.

A good, low-cost way to purify water is to put it in a clear plastic bag or clear bottle and leave it in direct sunlight for a few hours. This will kill most germs in the water.

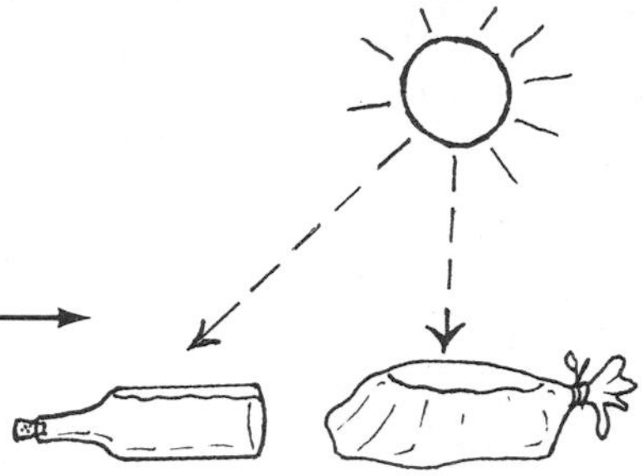

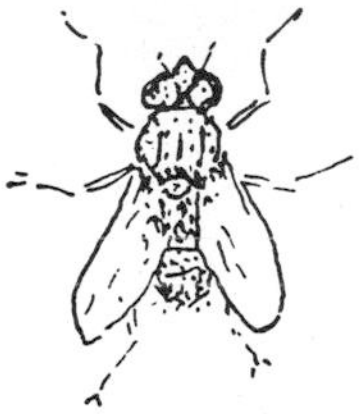

2. Do not let flies and other insects land or crawl on food. These insects carry germs and spread disease. Do not leave food scraps or dirty dishes lying around, as these attract flies and breed germs. Protect food by keeping it covered or in boxes or cabinets with wire screens.

3. Before eating fruit that has fallen to the ground, wash it well. Do not let children pick up and eat food that has been dropped —wash it first.

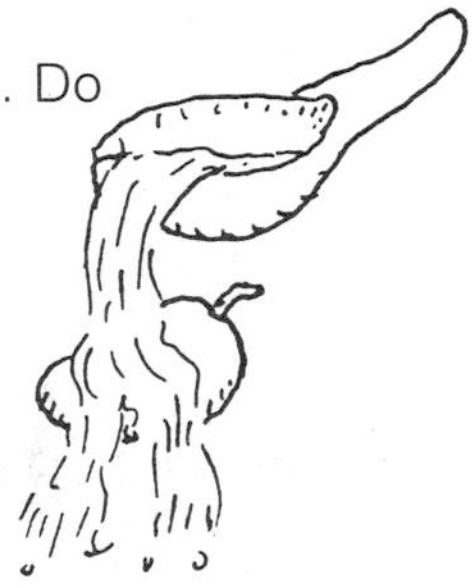

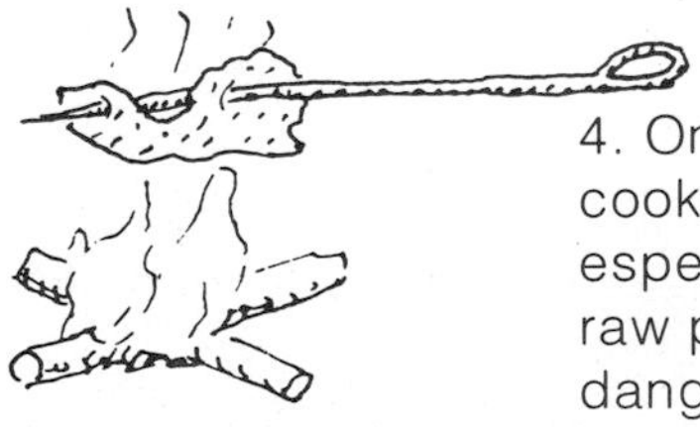

4. Only eat meat and fish that is well cooked. Be careful that roasted meat, especially pork and fish, do not have raw parts inside. Raw pork carries dangerous diseases.

5. Chickens carry germs that can cause diarrhea. Wash your hands after preparing chicken before you touch other foods.

6. Do not eat food that is old or smells bad. It may be poisonous. Do not eat canned food if the can is swollen or squirts when opened. Be especially careful with canned fish. Also, be careful with chicken that has passed several hours since it was cooked. Before eating left-over cooked foods, heat them again, very hot. If possible, give only foods that have been freshly prepared, especially to children, elderly people, and very sick people.

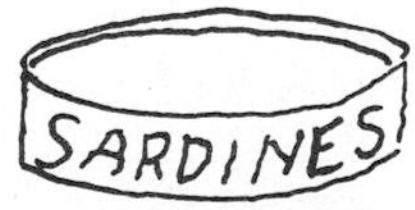

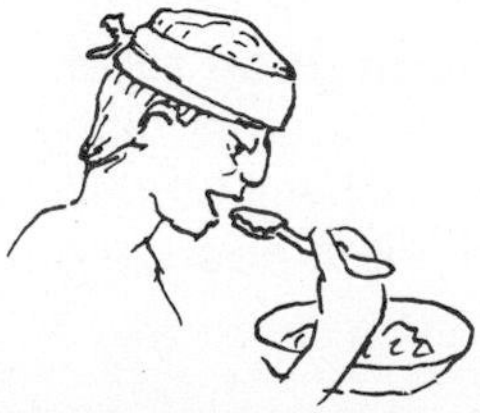

7. People with tuberculosis, flu, colds, or other infectious diseases should eat separately from others. Plates and utensils used by sick people should be boiled before being used by others.

HOW TO PROTECT YOUR CHILDREN'S HEALTH

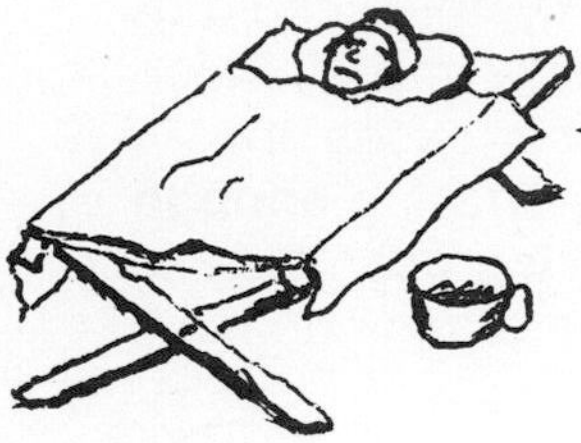

1. A sick child like this one should sleep apart from children who are well.

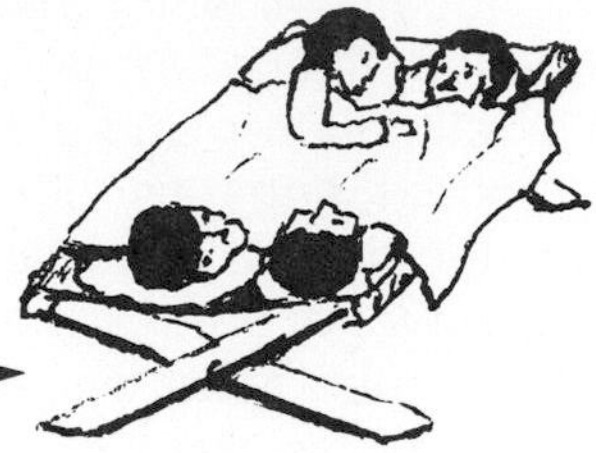

Sick children or children with sores, itchy skin, or lice should always sleep separately from those who are well. Children with infectious diseases like whooping cough, measles, or the common cold should sleep in separate rooms, if possible, and should not be allowed near babies or small children.

2. Protect children from tuberculosis. People with long-term coughing or other signs of tuberculosis should cover their mouths whenever they cough. They should **never** sleep in the same room with children. They should see a health worker and be treated as soon as possible.

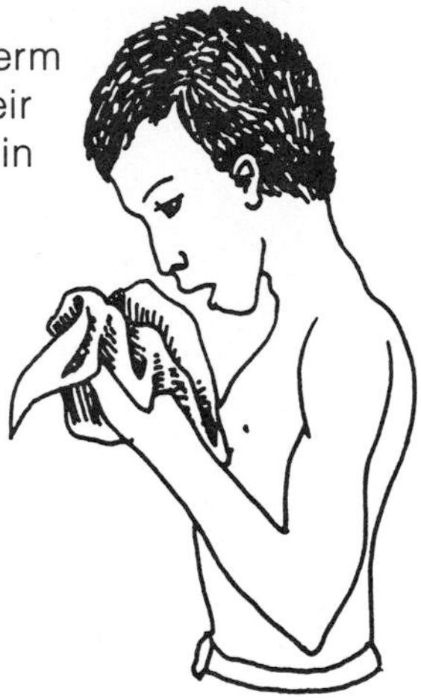

Children living with a person who has tuberculosis should be vaccinated against TB (B.C.G. Vaccine).

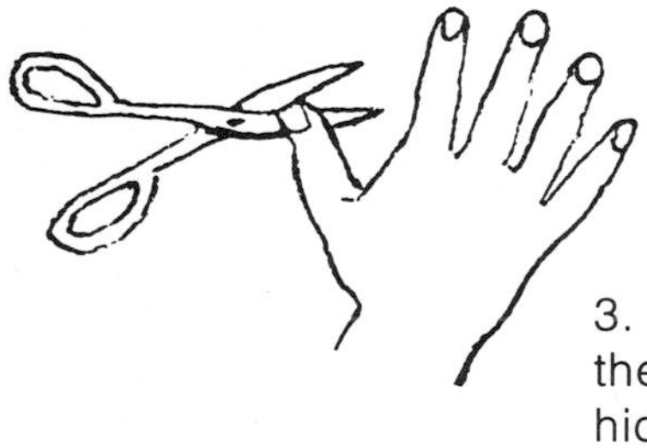

3. Bathe children, change their clothes, and cut their fingernails often. Germs and worm eggs often hide beneath long fingernails.

4. Treat children who have infectious diseases as soon as possible, so that the diseases are not spread to others.

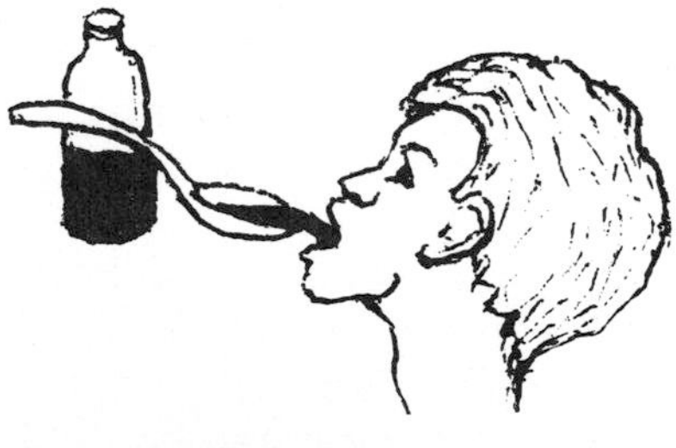

5. Follow all the guidelines of cleanliness mentioned in this chapter. Teach children to follow these guidelines and explain why they are important. Encourage children to help with projects that make the home or village a healthier place to live.

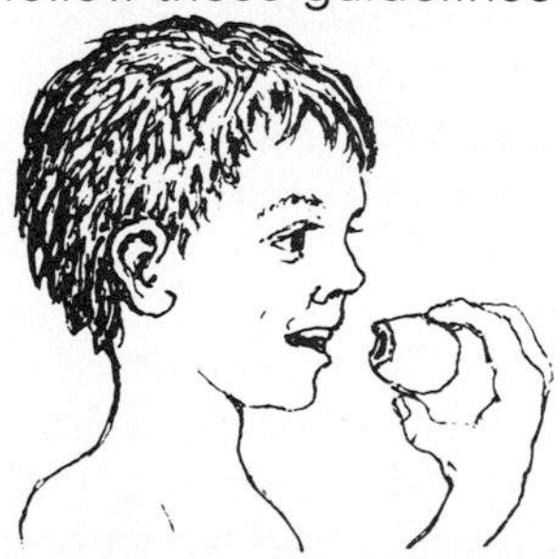

6. **Be sure children get enough good food.** Good nutrition helps protect the body against many infections. A well-nourished child will usually resist or fight off infections that can kill a poorly nourished child (read Chapter 11).

PUBLIC CLEANLINESS (SANITATION)

1. Keep wells and public water holes clean. Do not let animals go near where people get drinking water. If necessary, put a fence around the place to keep animals out.

Do not defecate (shit) or throw garbage near the water hole. Take special care to keep rivers and streams clean upstream from any place where drinking water is taken.

2. Burn all garbage that can be burned. Garbage that cannot be burned should be buried in a special pit or place far away from houses and the places where people get drinking water.

3. Build latrines (out-houses, toilets) so pigs and other animals cannot reach the human waste. A deep hole with a little house over it works well. The deeper the hole, the less problem there is with flies and smell.

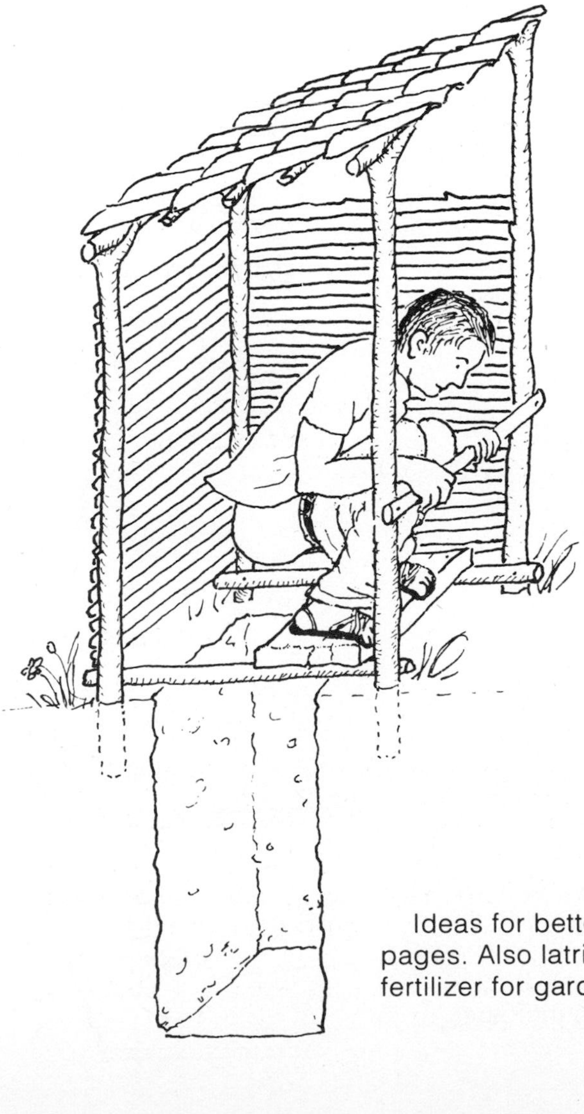

Here is a drawing of a simple out-house that is easy to build.

It helps to throw a little lime, dirt, or ashes in the hole after each use to reduce the smell and keep flies away.

Out-houses should be built at least 20 meters from homes or the source of water.

If you do not have an out-house, go far away from where people bathe or get drinking water. Teach your children to do the same.

Use of latrines helps prevent many sicknesses.

Ideas for better latrines are found on the next pages. Also latrines can be built to produce good fertilizer for gardens.

BETTER LATRINES

The latrine or out-house shown on the previous page is very simple and costs almost nothing to make. But it is open at the top and lets in flies.

Closed latrines are better because the flies stay out and the smell stays in. A closed latrine has a platform or slab with a hole in it and a lid over the hole. The slab can be made of wood or cement. Cement is better because the slab fits more tightly and will not rot.

One way to make a cement slab:

1. Dig a shallow pit, about 1 meter square and 7 cm. deep. Be sure the bottom of the pit is level and smooth.

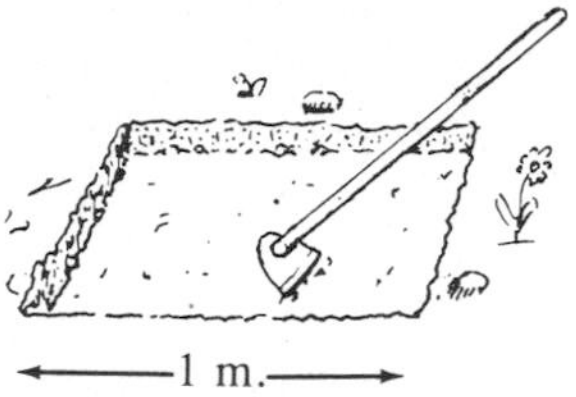

2. Make or cut a wire mesh or grid 1 meter square. The wires can be 1/4 to 1/2 cm. thick and about 10 cm. apart. Cut a hole about 25 cm. across in the middle of the grid.

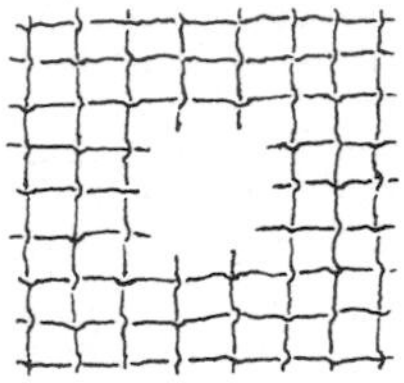

3. Put the grid in the pit. Bend the ends of the wires, or put a small stone at each corner, so that the grid stands about 3 cm. off the ground.

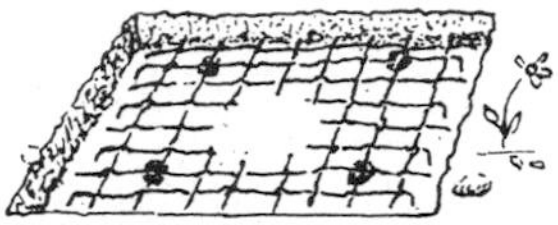

4. Put an old bucket in the hole in the grid.

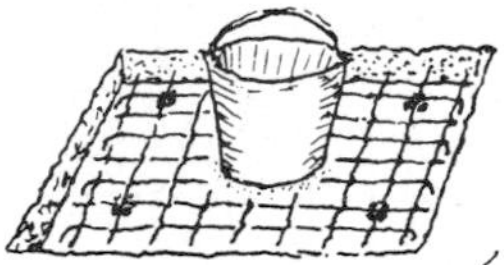

5. Mix cement with sand, gravel, and water and pour it until it is about 5 cm. thick. (With each shovel of cement mix 2 shovels of sand and 3 shovels of gravel.)

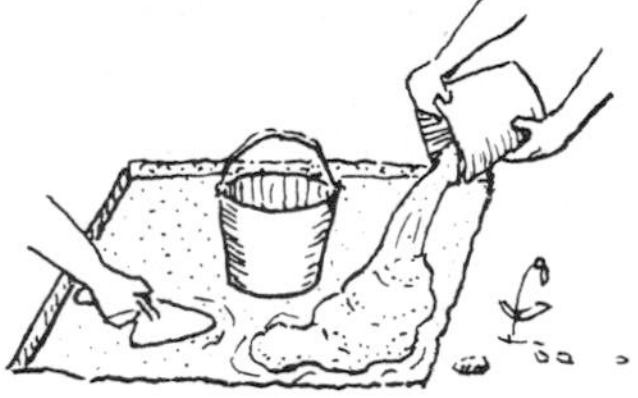

6. Remove the bucket when the cement is beginning to get hard (about 3 hours). Then cover the cement with damp cloths, sand, hay, or a sheet of plastic and keep it wet. Remove slab after 3 days.

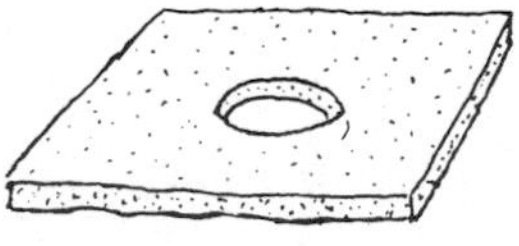

If you prefer to sit when you use the latrine, make a cement seat like this: Make a mold, or you can use 2 buckets of different sizes, one inside the other.

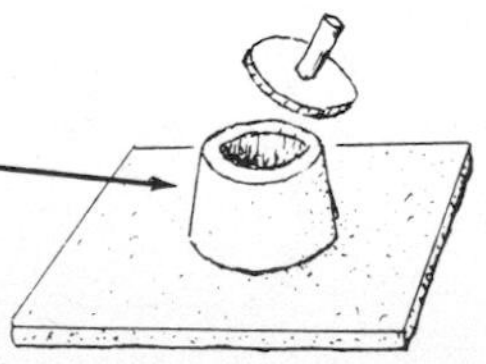

To make the **closed latrine,** the slab should be placed over a round hole in the ground. Dig the hole a little less than 1 meter across and between 1 and 2 meters deep. To be safe, the latrine should be at least 20 meters from all houses, wells, springs, rivers, or streams. If it is anywhere near where people go for water, be sure to put the latrine **downstream.**

CLOSED LATRINE:

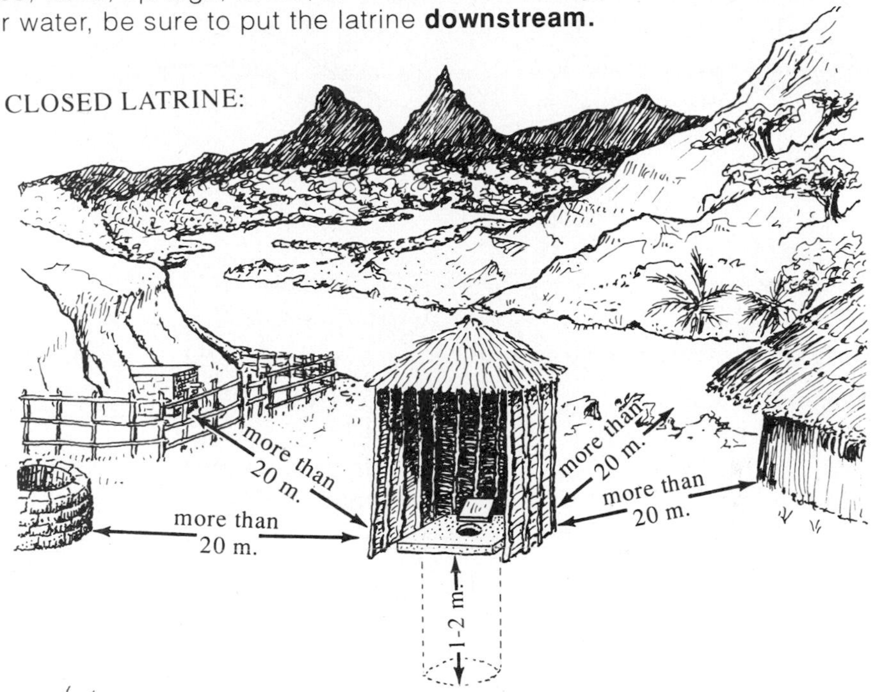

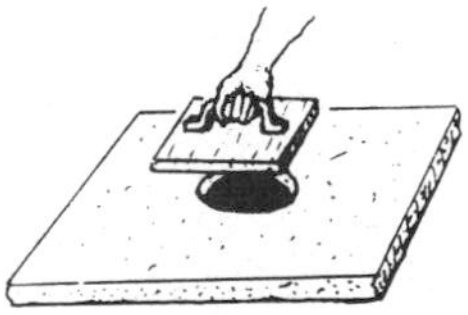

Keep your latrine clean. Wash the slab often. Be sure the hole in the slab has a cover and that the cover is kept in place. A simple cover can be made of wood.

THE FLY-TRAPPING VIP LATRINE:

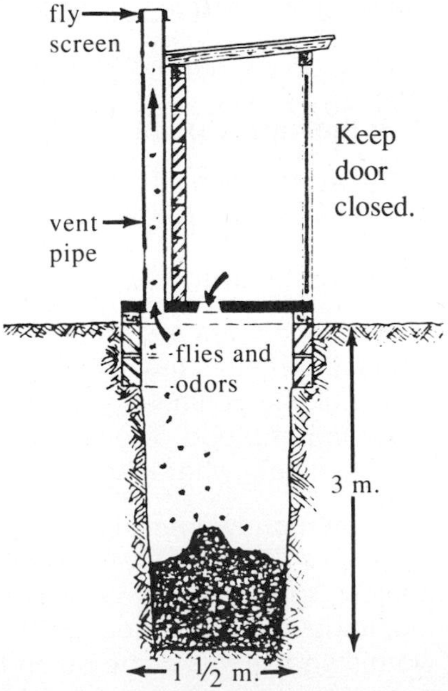

To make the ventilated improved pit (VIP) latrine, make a larger slab (2 meters square) with 2 holes in it. Over one hole put a ventilation pipe, covered with fly screen (wire screen lasts longer). Over the other hole build an out-house, which must be kept dark inside. Leave this hole uncovered.

This latrine helps get rid of odors and flies: smells escape through the pipe, and flies get trapped there and die!

WORMS AND OTHER INTESTINAL PARASITES

There are many types of worms and other tiny animals (parasites) that live in people's intestines and cause diseases. Those which are larger are sometimes seen in the stools (feces, shit):

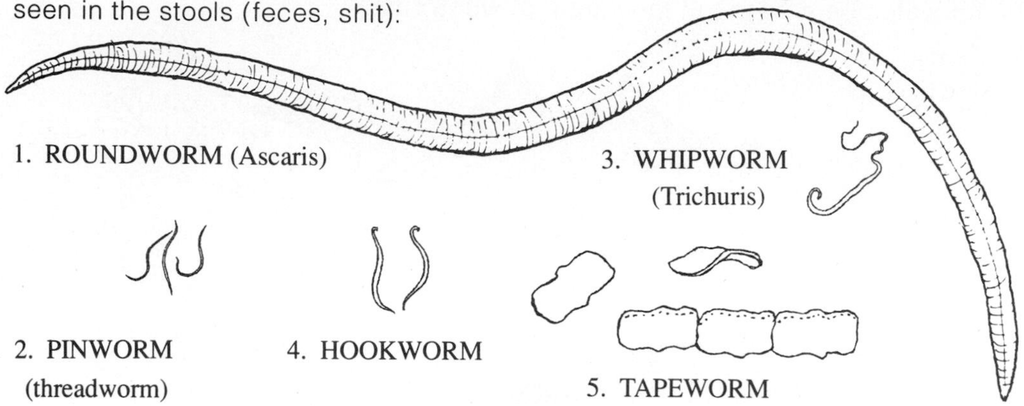

The only worms commonly seen in the stools are roundworms, pinworms, and tapeworms. Hookworms and whipworms may be present in the gut in large numbers without ever being seen in the stools.

Note on worm medicines: Many 'worm medicines' contain piperazine. These work only for roundworms and pinworms and should not be given to babies and small children. Mebendazole *(Vermox)* is safer and attacks many more kinds of worms. Albendazole and pyrantel also work for many kinds of worms, but they may be expensive. Thiabendazole attacks many kinds of worms, but causes dangerous side effects and should usually not be used. See pages 374 to 376 for more information on all these medicines.

Roundworm (Ascaris)

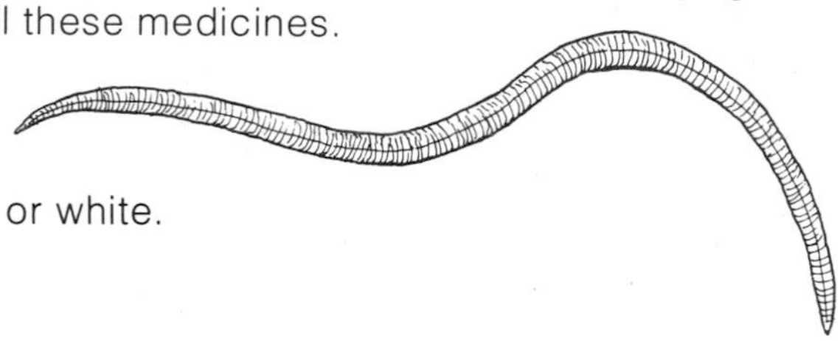

20 to 30 cm. long. Color: pink or white.

How they are spread:

Feces-to-mouth. Through lack of cleanliness, the roundworm eggs pass from one person's stools to another person's mouth.

Effect on health:

Once the eggs are swallowed, young worms hatch and enter the bloodstream; this may cause general itching. The young worms then travel to the lungs, sometimes causing a dry cough or, at worst, pneumonia with coughing of blood. The young worms are coughed up, swallowed, and reach the intestines, where they grow to full size.

Many roundworms in the intestines may cause discomfort, indigestion, and weakness. Children with many roundworms often have very large, swollen bellies. Rarely, roundworms may cause asthma, or a dangerous obstruction or blockage in the gut (see p. 94). Especially when the child has a fever, the worms sometimes come out in the stools or crawl out through the mouth or nose. Occasionally they crawl into the airway and cause gagging.

Prevention:

Use latrines, wash hands before eating or handling food, protect food from flies, and follow the guidelines of cleanliness described in the first part of this chapter.

Treatment:

Mebendazole will usually get rid of roundworms. For dosage see p. 374. Piperazine also works (see p. 375). Some home remedies work fairly well. For a home remedy using papaya see page 13.

WARNING: Do not use thiabendazole for roundworms. It often makes the worms move up to the nose or mouth and can cause gagging.

Pinworm, Threadworm, Seatworm (Enterobius)

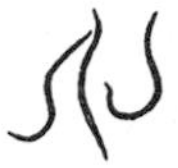

1 cm. long. Color: white. Very thin and threadlike.

How they are transmitted:

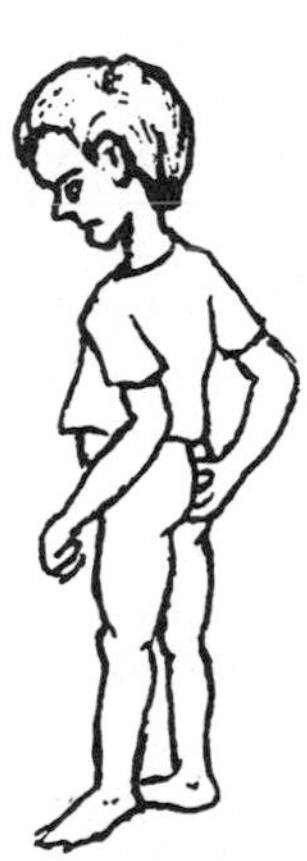

These worms lay thousands of eggs just outside the anus (ass hole). This causes itching, especially at night. When a child scratches, the eggs stick under his nails, and are carried to food and other objects. In this way they reach his own mouth or the mouths of others, causing new infections of pinworms.

Effect on health:

These worms are not dangerous. Itching may disturb the child's sleep.

Treatment and Prevention:

- A child who has pinworms should wear tight diapers or pants while sleeping to keep him from scratching his anus.
- Wash the child's hands and buttocks (anal area) when he wakes up and after he has a bowel movement. Always wash his hands before he eats.
- Cut his fingernails very short.
- Change his clothes and bathe him often—wash the buttocks and nails especially well.
- Put *Vaseline* in and around his anus at bedtime to help stop itching.
- Give mebendazole worm medicine. For dosage, see page 374. Piperazine also works, but should not be used for babies (see p. 375). When one child is treated for these worms, it is wise to treat the whole family at the same time. For a home remedy using garlic, see page 12.
- Cleanliness is the best prevention for threadworms. Even if medicine gets rid of the worms, they will be picked up again if care is not taken with personal hygiene. Pinworms only live for about 6 weeks. **By carefully following the guidelines of cleanliness, most of the worms will be gone within a few weeks, even without medicine.**

Whipworm (Trichuris, Trichocephalus)

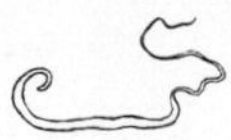

3 to 5 cm. long. Color: pink or gray.

This worm, like the roundworm, is passed from the feces of one person to the mouth of another person. Usually this worm does little harm, but it may cause diarrhea. In children it occasionally causes part of the intestines to come out of the anus (***prolapse*** of the ***rectum***).

Prevention: The same as for roundworm.

Treatment: If the worms cause a problem, give mebendazole. For dosage, see page 374. For prolapse of the rectum, turn the child upside down and pour cool water on the intestine. This should make it pull back in.

Hookworm

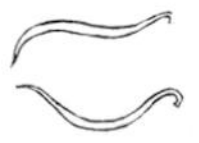

1 cm. long. Color: red.

Hookworms cannot usually be seen in the feces. A stool analysis is needed to prove that they are there.

How hookworms are spread:

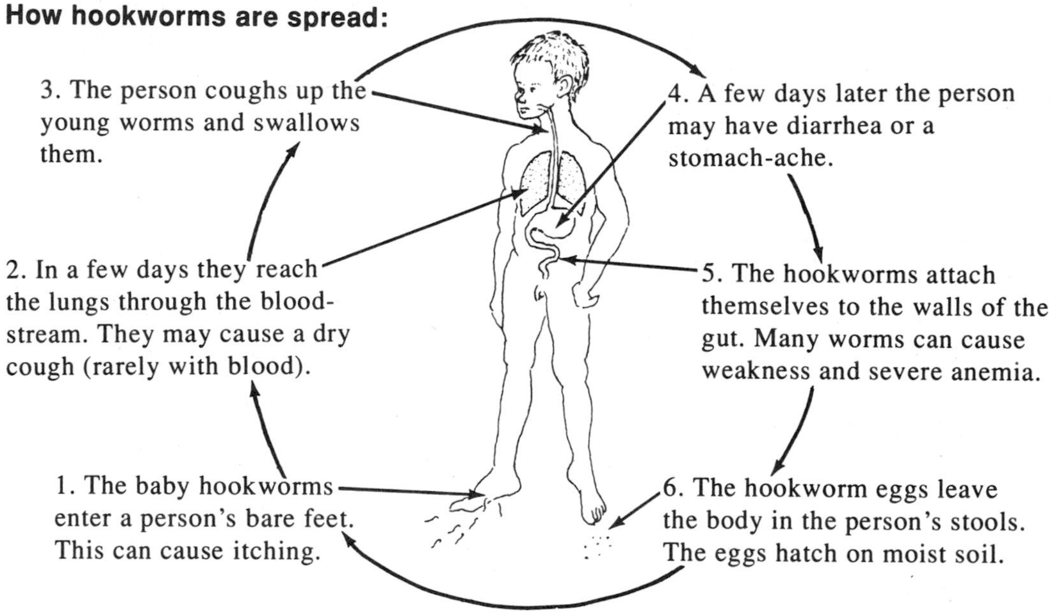

3. The person coughs up the young worms and swallows them.
4. A few days later the person may have diarrhea or a stomach-ache.
2. In a few days they reach the lungs through the blood-stream. They may cause a dry cough (rarely with blood).
5. The hookworms attach themselves to the walls of the gut. Many worms can cause weakness and severe anemia.
1. The baby hookworms enter a person's bare feet. This can cause itching.
6. The hookworm eggs leave the body in the person's stools. The eggs hatch on moist soil.

Hookworm infection can be one of the most damaging diseases of childhood. Any child who is anemic, very pale, or eats dirt may have hookworms. If possible, his stools should be analyzed.

Treatment: Use mebendazole. For dosage and precautions, see page 374. Treat anemia by eating foods rich in iron and if necessary by taking iron pills (p. 124).

Prevent hookworm: **Build and use latrines. Do not let children go barefoot.**

Tapeworm

In the intestines tapeworms grow several meters long. But the small, flat, white pieces (segments) found in the feces are usually about 1 cm. long. Occasionally a segment may crawl out by itself and be found in the underclothing.

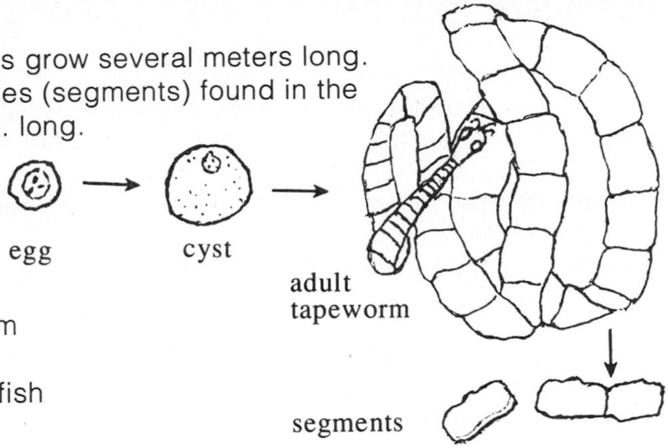

People get tapeworms from eating pork (pig meat), beef (cow meat) or other meat or fish that is not well cooked.

Prevention: **Be careful that all meat is well cooked, especially pork.** Make sure no parts in the center of roasted meat or cooked fish are still raw.

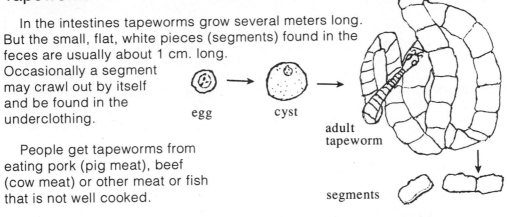

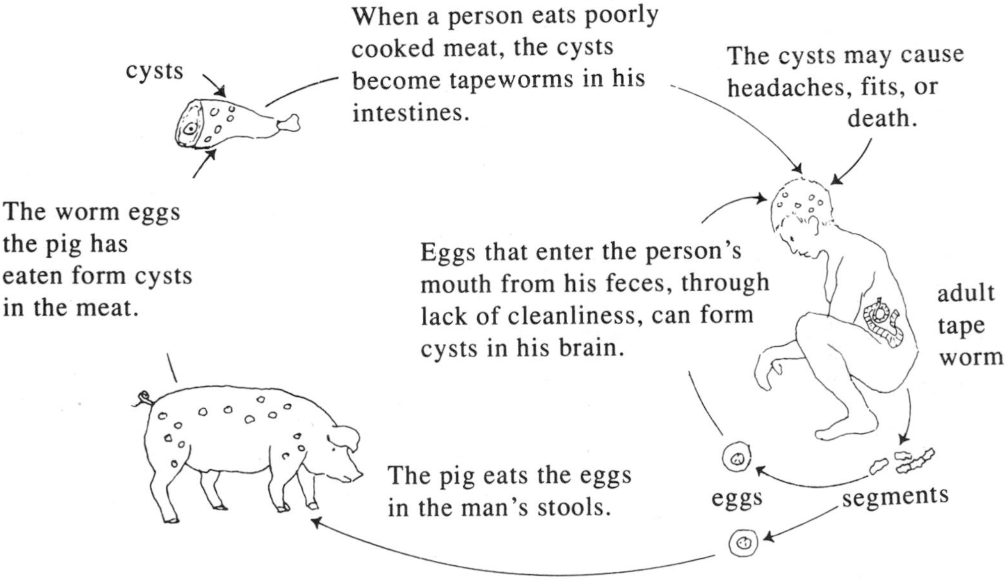

cysts
When a person eats poorly cooked meat, the cysts become tapeworms in his intestines.
The cysts may cause headaches, fits, or death.
The worm eggs the pig has eaten form cysts in the meat.
Eggs that enter the person's mouth from his feces, through lack of cleanliness, can form cysts in his brain.
adult tape worm
The pig eats the eggs in the man's stools.
eggs
segments

Effect on health: Tapeworms in the intestines sometimes cause mild stomach-aches, but few other problems.

The greatest danger exists when the *cysts* (small sacs containing baby worms) get into a person's brain. This happens when the eggs pass from his stools to his mouth. For this reason, **anyone with tapeworms must follow the guidelines of cleanliness carefully—and get treatment as soon as possible.**

Treatment: Take niclosamide (*Yomesan,* p. 376), or praziquantel (p. 376). Follow instructions carefully.

Trichinosis

These worms are never seen in the stools. They burrow through the person's intestines and get into her muscles. People get these worms, like tapeworms, from eating infected pork or other meat that is not well cooked.

Effect on health: Depending on the amount of infected meat eaten, the person may feel no effects, or she may become very sick or die. From a few hours to 5 days after eating the infected pork, the person may develop diarrhea and feel sick to her stomach.

In serious cases the person may have:

- fever with chills
- muscle pain
- swelling around the eyes and sometimes swelling of the feet
- small bruises (black or blue spots) on the skin
- bleeding in the whites of the eyes

Severe cases may last 3 or 4 weeks.

Treatment: Seek medical help at once. Thiabendazole or mebendazole may help. For dosages, see p. 374 and 375. (Cortico-steroids may help, but should be given by a health worker or doctor.)

Important: If several people who ate meat from the same pig get sick afterward, suspect trichinosis. This can be dangerous; seek medical attention.

Prevention of trichinosis:

- Only eat pork and other meat that has been well cooked.
- Do not feed scraps of meat or leftovers from butchering to pigs unless the meat has first been cooked.

Amebas

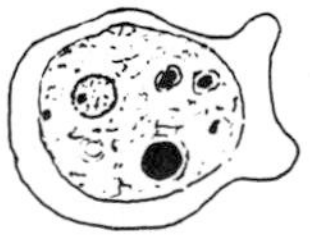
Ameba as seen under a microscope

These are not worms, but tiny animals—or parasites—that can be seen only with a ***microscope*** (an instrument that makes things look much bigger).

How they are transmitted:

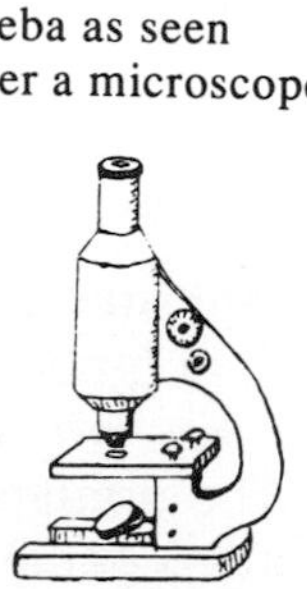
Microscope

The stools of infected people contain millions of these tiny parasites. Because of poor sanitation, they get into the source of drinking water or into food, and other people become infected.

Signs of infection with amebas:

Many healthy people have amebas without becoming sick. However, amebas are a common cause of severe diarrhea or ***dysentery*** (diarrhea with blood)—especially in persons already weakened by other sickness or poor nutrition. Less commonly, amebas cause painful, dangerous abscesses in the liver.

Typical amebic dysentery consists of:

- diarrhea that comes and goes—sometimes alternating with constipation
- cramps in the belly and a need to have frequent bowel movements, even when little or nothing—or just mucus—comes out
- many loose (but usually not watery) stools with lots of mucus, sometimes stained with blood
- in severe cases, much blood; the person may be very weak and ill
- usually there is no fever

Diarrhea with blood may be caused by either amebas or bacteria. However, bacterial dysentery (Shigella) begins more suddenly, the stools are more watery, and there is almost always fever (p. 158). As a general rule:

Diarrhea + blood + fever = bacterial infection (Shigella)
Diarrhea + blood + no fever = amebas

Occasionally bloody diarrhea has other causes. To be sure of the cause, a *stool analysis* may be necessary.

Sometimes amebas get into the liver and form an **abscess** or pocket of pus. This causes tenderness or pain in the right upper belly. Pain may extend into the right chest and is worse when the person walks. (Compare this with gallbladder pain, p. 329; hepatitis, p. 172; and cirrhosis, p. 328.) If the person with these signs begins to cough up a brown liquid, an amebic abscess is draining into his lung.

Treatment:

- ♦ If possible get medical help and a stool analysis.
- ♦ Amebic dysentery can be treated with metronidazole, if possible together with diloxanide furoate or tetracycline. For dosage, length of treatment, and precautions, see p. 369.
- ♦ For amebic abscess, treat as for amebic dysentery, and then take chloroquine for 10 days (see p. 366).

Prevention: Make and use latrines, protect the source of drinking water, and follow the guidelines of cleanliness. Eating well and avoiding fatigue and drunkenness are also important in preventing amebic dysentery.

Giardia

The giardia, like the ameba, is a microscopic parasite that lives in the gut and is a common cause of diarrhea, especially in children. The diarrhea may be *chronic* or intermittent (may come and go).

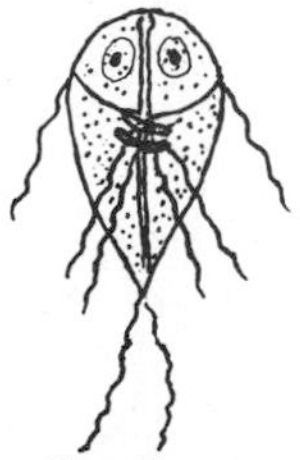
Giardia as seen under a microscope

A person who has yellow, bad-smelling diarrhea that is frothy (full of bubbles) but without blood or mucus, probably has giardia. The belly is swollen with gas and uncomfortable, there are mild intestinal cramps, and the person farts and burps a lot. The burps have a bad taste, like sulfur. There is usually no fever.

Giardia infections sometimes clear up by themselves. Good nutrition helps. Severe cases are best treated with metronidazole (see p. 369). Quinacrine (*Atabrine,* p. 370) is cheaper and often works well, but causes worse side effects.

BLOOD FLUKES (SCHISTOSOMIASIS, BILHARZIA)

This infection is caused by a kind of worm that gets into the bloodstream. Different types of blood flukes are found in different parts of the world. One kind, common in Africa and the Middle East, causes blood in the urine. Other types, which cause bloody diarrhea, occur in Africa, South America, and Asia. In areas where these diseases are known to occur, **any person who has blood in his urine or stools should have a sample of it tested for fluke eggs.**

Signs:

- **The most common sign is blood in the urine** (especially when passing the last drops)—or, for other kinds of flukes, **bloody diarrhea.**
- Pain may occur in the lower belly and between the legs; it is usually worst at the end of urinating. Low fever, weakness, and itching may occur.
- After months or years, the kidneys or liver may be badly damaged, which can eventually cause death.
- Sometimes there are no early signs. In areas where schistosomiasis is very common, persons with only mild signs or belly pain should be tested.

Treatment:

Praziquantel works for all types of blood flukes. Metrifonate and oxamniquine work for some kinds of blood flukes. For dosages see p. 377. Medicines should be given under direction of an experienced health worker.

Prevention:

Blood flukes are not spread directly from person to person. Part of their life they must live inside a certain kind of small water snail.

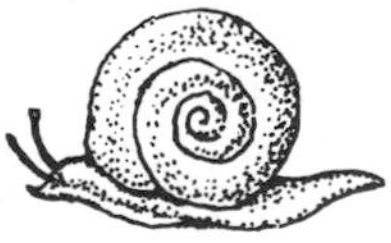

SNAIL, REAL SIZE

Blood flukes spread like this:

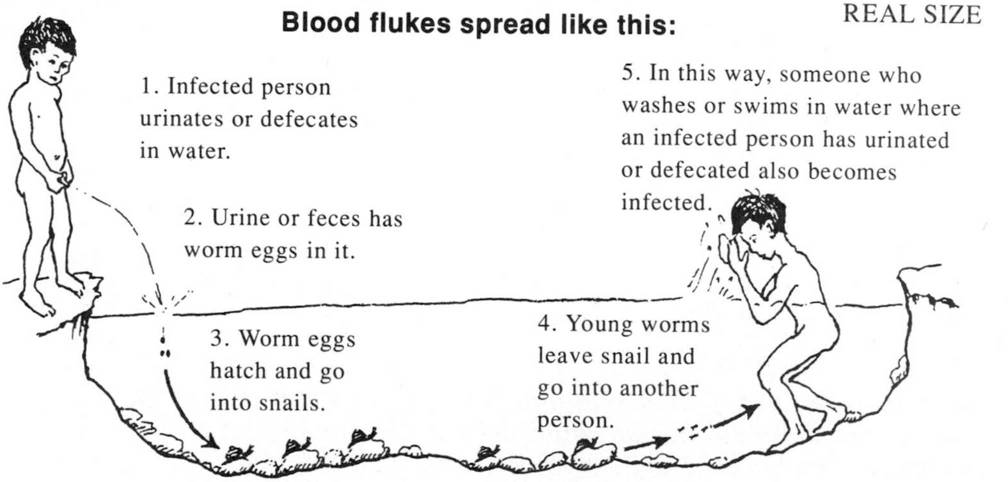

1. Infected person urinates or defecates in water.
2. Urine or feces has worm eggs in it.
3. Worm eggs hatch and go into snails.
4. Young worms leave snail and go into another person.
5. In this way, someone who washes or swims in water where an infected person has urinated or defecated also becomes infected.

To prevent schistosomiasis, cooperate with programs to kill snails and treat infected persons. But most important: **Everyone should learn to use latrines and NEVER URINATE OR DEFECATE IN OR NEAR WATER.**

For information on **guinea worm**, which is also spread in water, see p. 406 and 407.

VACCINATIONS (IMMUNIZATIONS)— SIMPLE, SURE PROTECTION

Vaccines give protection against many dangerous diseases. If health workers do not vaccinate in your village, take your children to the nearest health center to be vaccinated. It is better to take them for vaccinations while they are healthy, than to take them for treatment when they are sick or dying. Vaccinations are usually given free. (Different countries use different schedules.) The most important vaccines for children are:

1. D.P.T., for diphtheria, whooping cough (pertussis), and tetanus. For full protection, the child needs 3 injections. These are usually given at 2 months old, the second at 3 months old, and the third at 4 months old.

2. POLIO (infantile paralysis). The child needs drops in the mouth at birth, and once each month for 3 months (these are usually given with the D.P.T. injections). It is best not to breast feed the baby for 2 hours before or after giving the drops.

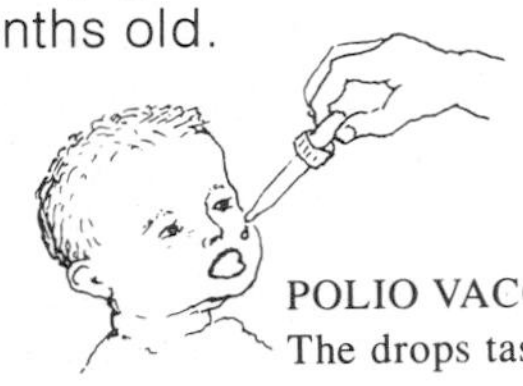

POLIO VACCINE—
The drops taste sweet.

3. B.C.G., for tuberculosis. A single injection is given into the skin of the **right** shoulder. Children can be vaccinated at birth or anytime afterwards. Early vaccination is especially important if any member of the household has tuberculosis. The vaccine makes a sore and leaves a scar.

4. MEASLES. One injection only, given no younger than 9 to 15 months of age, depending on the country.

5. TETANUS. For adults and children over 12 years old, the most important vaccine is for tetanus (lockjaw). One injection every month for 3 months, another after a year, and then one every 10 years. Everyone should be vaccinated against tetanus. Pregnant women should be vaccinated during each pregnancy so that their babies will be protected against tetanus of the newborn (see p. 182 and 250).

6. SMALL POX. This vaccination, put on the **left** shoulder, leaves a round scar. Thanks to world-wide vaccination in the past, small pox no longer exists. So vaccination against it is now not needed.

In some places there are also vaccinations for cholera, yellow fever, typhus, mumps, and German measles. The World Health Organization is also working to develop vaccines for leprosy, malaria, and meningitis.

WARNING: **Vaccines spoil easily** and then do not work. Measles vaccine must be kept **frozen.** Try to keep the polio vaccine frozen until shortly before it is used. For up to 3 months it can be thawed and refrozen. But it must be kept cold or it will spoil. D.P.T., B.C.G., and Tetanus must be kept cold (0° to 8° C.) but **never frozen.** Good D.P.T. remains cloudy at least 1 hour after shaking. If it becomes clear within 1 hour, it is spoiled. For suggestions on how to keep vaccines cold, see *Helping Health Workers Learn,* Chapter 16.

Vaccinate your children on time.
Be sure they get the complete series of each vaccine they need.

OTHER WAYS TO PREVENT SICKNESS AND INJURY

In this chapter he have talked about ways to prevent intestinal and other infections through **hygiene, sanitation,** and **vaccination.** All through this book you will find suggestions for the prevention of sickness and injury—from building healthy bodies by eating nutritious foods to the wise use of home remedies and modern medicines.

The **Introduction to the Village Health Worker** gives ideas for getting people working together to change the conditions that cause poor health.

In the remaining chapters, as specific health problems are discussed, you will find many suggestions for their prevention. By following these suggestions you can help make your home and village healthier places to live.

Keep in mind that one of the best ways to prevent serious illness and death is early and sensible treatment.

Early and sensible treatment is an important part of preventive medicine.

Before ending this chapter, I would like to mention a few aspects of prevention that are touched on in other parts of the book, but deserve special attention.

Habits that Affect Health

Some of the habits that people have not only damage their own health but in one way or another harm those around them. Many of these habits can be broken or avoided—but the first step is to understand why breaking these habits is so important.

DRINKING

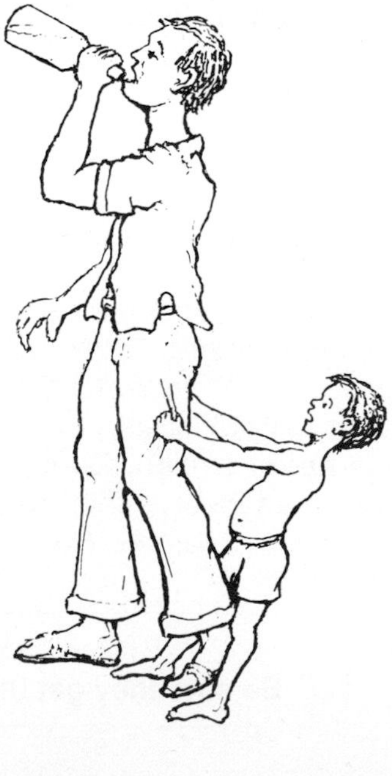

If alcohol has brought much joy to man, it has also brought much suffering—especially to the families of those who drink. A little alcohol now and then may do no harm. But too often a little leads to a lot. In much of the world, heavy or excessive drinking is one of the underlying causes of major health problems—even for those who do not drink. Not only can drunkenness harm the health of those who drink (through diseases such as cirrhosis of the liver, p. 328, and hepatitis, p. 172), but it also hurts the family and community in many ways. Through the loss of judgment when drunk—and of self-respect when sober—it leads to much unhappiness, waste, and violence, often affecting those who are loved most.

How many fathers have spent their last money on drink when their children were hungry? How many sicknesses result because a man spends the little bit of extra money he earns on drink rather than on improving his family's living conditions? How many persons, hating themselves because they have hurt those they love, take another drink—to forget?

Once a man realizes that alcohol is harming the health and happiness of those around him, what can he do? First, he must admit that his drinking is a problem. He must be honest with himself and with others. Some individuals are able to simply decide to stop drinking. More often people need help and support—from family, friends, and others who understand how hard it may be to give up this habit. People who have been heavy drinkers and have stopped are often the best persons to help others do the same. In many areas Alcoholics Anonymous (AA) groups exist where recovering alcoholics help one another to stop drinking (see p. 429).

Drinking is not so much a problem of individuals as of a whole community. A community that recognizes this can do much to encourage those who are willing to make changes. If you are concerned about the misuse of alcohol in your community, help organize a meeting to discuss these problems and decide what actions to take. For more about harm from alcohol, and community action, see *Helping Health Workers Learn,* Chapters 5 and 27.

Many problems can be resolved when people work together and give each other help and support.

SMOKING

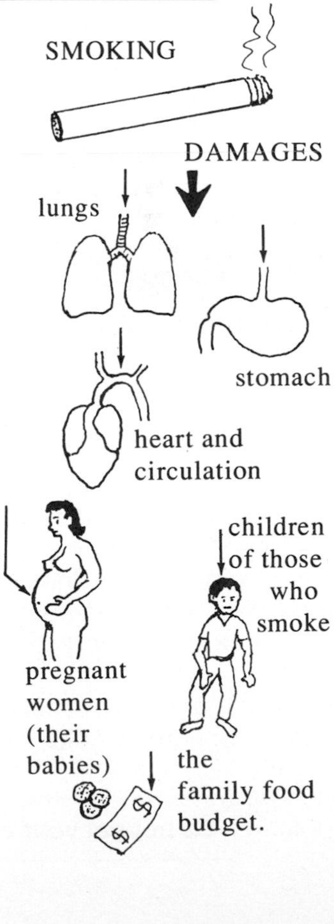
SMOKING
DAMAGES
lungs
stomach
heart and circulation
pregnant women (their babies)
children of those who smoke
the family food budget.

There are many reasons why smoking is dangerous to your own and your family's health.

1. Smoking increases the risk of cancer of the lungs, mouth, throat, and lips. (The more you smoke, the greater the chance of dying of cancer.)

2. Smoking causes serious diseases of the lungs, including chronic bronchitis and emphysema (and is deadly for persons who already have these conditions or have asthma).

3. Smoking can cause stomach ulcers or make them worse.

4. Smoking increases your chance of suffering or dying from heart disease or stroke.

5. Children whose parents smoke have more cases of pneumonia and other respiratory illness than children whose parents do not smoke.

6. Babies of mothers who smoked during pregnancy are smaller and develop more slowly than babies whose mothers did not smoke.

(turn page)

7. Parents, teachers, health workers, and others who smoke set an unhealthy example for children and young people, increasing the likelihood that they too will begin smoking.

8. Also, smoking costs money. It looks like little is spent, but it adds up to a lot. In poorer countries, many of the poorest persons spend more on tobacco than the country spends per person on its health program. **If money spent on tobacco were spent for food instead, children and whole families could be healthier.**

Anyone interested in the health of others should not smoke, and should encourage others not to smoke.

CARBONATED DRINKS (soft drinks, soda pop, Coke, fizzy drinks, colas)

In some areas these drinks have become very popular. Often a poor mother will buy carbonated drinks for a child who is poorly nourished, when the same money could be better used to buy 2 eggs or other nutritious food.

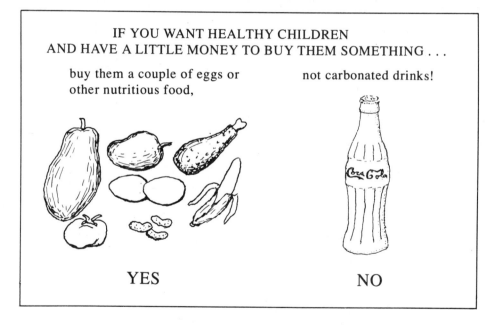

IF YOU WANT HEALTHY CHILDREN
AND HAVE A LITTLE MONEY TO BUY THEM SOMETHING . . .

buy them a couple of eggs or other nutritious food,

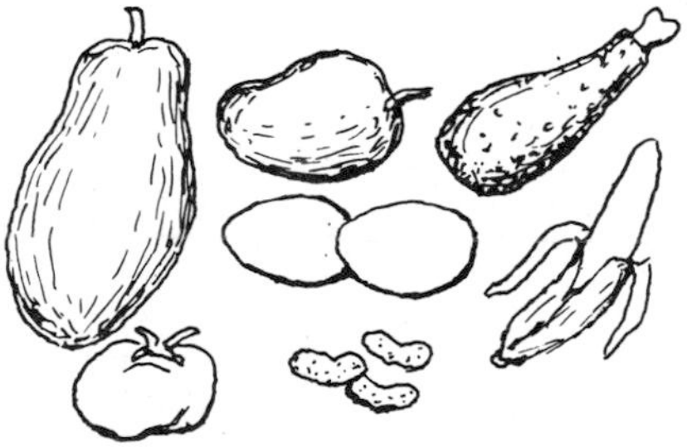

YES

not carbonated drinks!

NO

Carbonated drinks have no nutritional value apart from sugar. And for the amount of sugar they contain, they are very expensive. Children who are given a lot of carbonated drinks and other sweet things often begin to get cavities and rotten teeth at an early age. Carbonated drinks are especially bad for persons with acid indigestion or stomach ulcer.

Natural drinks you make from fruits are healthier and often much cheaper than carbonated drinks.

Do not get your children used to drinking carbonated drinks.

CHAPTER

SOME VERY COMMON SICKNESSES 13

DEHYDRATION

Most children who die from diarrhea die because they do not have enough water left in their bodies. This lack of water is called dehydration.

Dehydration results when the body loses more liquid than it takes in. This can happen with severe diarrhea, especially when there is vomiting too. It can also happen in very serious illness, when a person is too sick to take much food or liquid.

People of any age can become dehydrated, but **dehydration develops more quickly and is most dangerous in small children.**

Any child with watery diarrhea is in danger of dehydration.

It is important that everyone—especially mothers—know the signs of dehydration and how to prevent and treat it.

Signs of dehydration:

- thirst is often a first, early sign of dehydration
- little or no urine; the urine is dark yellow
- sudden weight loss
- dry mouth
- sunken, tearless eyes
- sagging in of the 'soft spot' in infants
- loss of elasticity or stretchiness of the skin

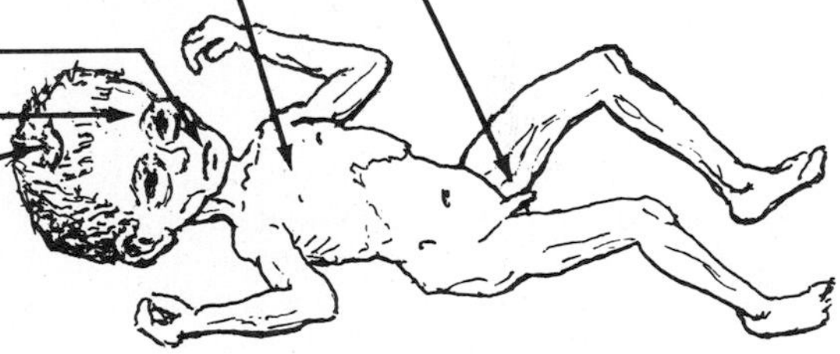

Lift the skin between two fingers, like this . . .

If the skin fold does not fall right back to normal, the child is dehydrated.

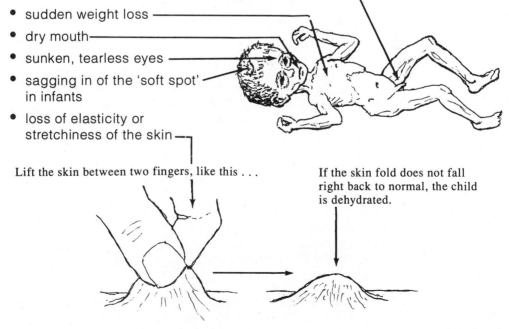

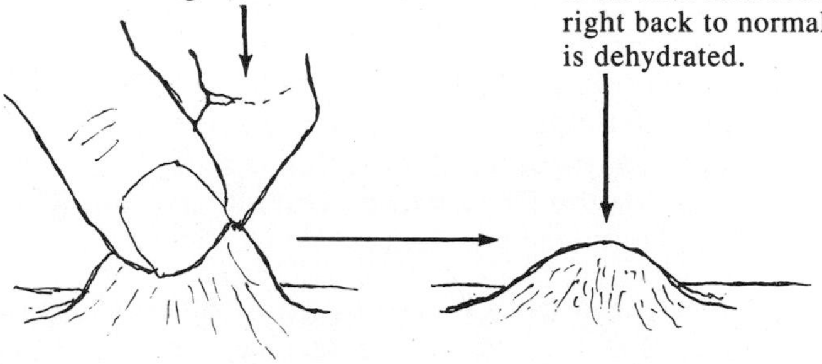

Very severe dehydration may cause rapid, weak pulse (see Shock, p. 77), fast, deep breathing, fever, or fits (convulsions, p. 178).

When a person has watery diarrhea, or diarrhea and vomiting, do not wait for signs of dehydration. **Act quickly**—see the next page.

To prevent or treat dehydration: When a person has watery diarrhea, **act quickly:**

- **Give lots of liquids to drink:** Rehydration Drink is best. Or give a thin cereal porridge or gruel, teas, soups, or even plain water.
- **Keep giving food.** As soon as the sick child (or adult) will accept food, give frequent feedings of foods he likes and accepts.
- To babies, **keep giving breast milk** often—and before other drinks.

A special **Rehydration Drink** helps to prevent or treat dehydration, especially in cases of severe watery diarrhea:

2 WAYS TO MAKE 'HOME MIX' REHYDRATION DRINK

1. **WITH SUGAR AND SALT** (Raw sugar or molasses can be used instead of sugar.)

In 1 liter of clean **WATER** put half of a level teaspoon of **SALT** and 8 level teaspoons of **SUGAR**.

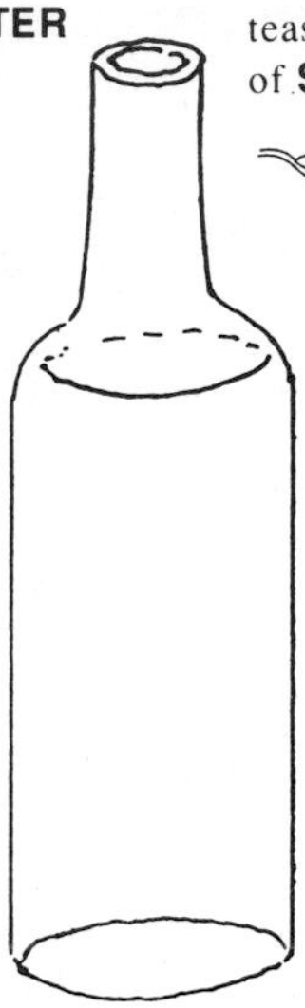

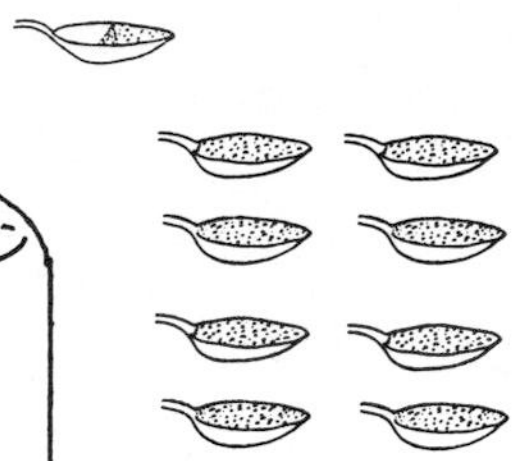

CAUTION: Before adding the sugar, taste the drink and be sure it is less salty than tears.

2. **WITH POWDERED CEREAL AND SALT** (Powdered rice is best. Or use finely ground maize, wheat flour, sorghum, or cooked and mashed potatoes.)

In 1 liter of **WATER** put half a teaspoon of **SALT** and 8 heaping teaspoons (or 2 handfuls) of powdered **CEREAL.**

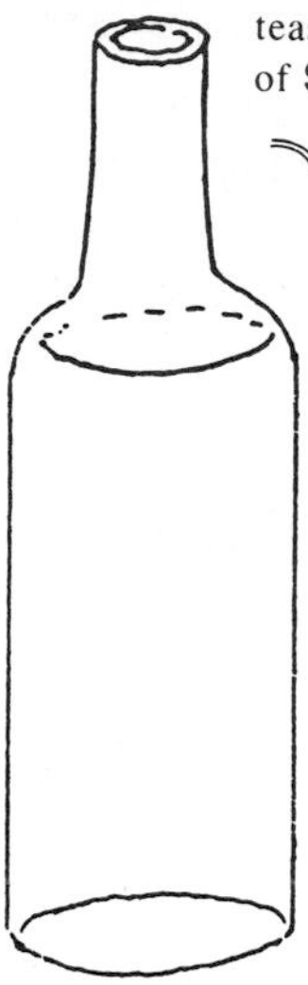

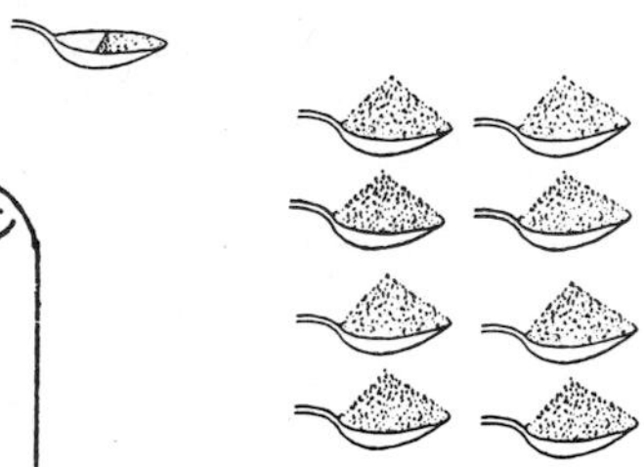

Boil for 5 to 7 minutes to form a liquid gruel or watery porridge. Cool the Drink quickly and start giving it to the child.

To either Drink add half a cup of fruit juice, coconut water, or mashed ripe banana, if available. This provides potassium which may help the child accept more food and drink.

CAUTION: Taste the Drink each time before you give it to be sure it is not spoiled. Cereal drinks can spoil in a few hours in hot weather.

IMPORTANT: Adapt the Drink to your area. If liter containers or teaspoons are not in most homes, adjust quantities to local forms of measurement. Where people traditionally give cereal gruels to young children, add enough water to make it liquid, and use that. Look for an easy and simple way.

Give the dehydrated person sips of this Drink every 5 minutes, day and night, until he begins to urinate normally. A large person needs 3 or more liters a day. A small child usually needs at least 1 liter a day, or 1 glass for each watery stool. Keep giving the Drink **often** in small sips, **even if the person vomits.** Not all of the Drink will be vomited.

WARNING: **If dehydration gets worse or other danger signs appear, go for medical help** (see p. 159). It may be necessary to give liquid in a vein (intravenous solution).

Note: In some countries packets of Oral Rehydration Salts (ORS) are available for mixing with water. These contain a simple sugar, salt, soda, and potassium (see p. 382). However, homemade drinks—especially cereal drinks—when correctly prepared are often cheaper, safer, and more effective than ORS packets.

DIARRHEA AND DYSENTERY

When a person has loose or watery stools, he has *diarrhea.* If mucus and blood can be seen in the stools, he has *dysentery.*

Diarrhea can be mild or serious. It can be *acute* (sudden and severe) or *chronic* (lasting many days).

Diarrhea is more common and more dangerous in young children, especially those who are poorly nourished.

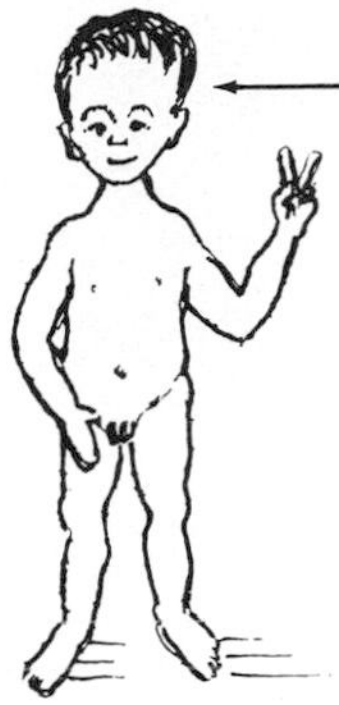

This child is well nourished. He is less likely to get diarrhea. If he gets it he usually will get well again quickly.

This child is poorly nourished. He is more likely to get diarrhea—and there is a much greater chance he will die from it.

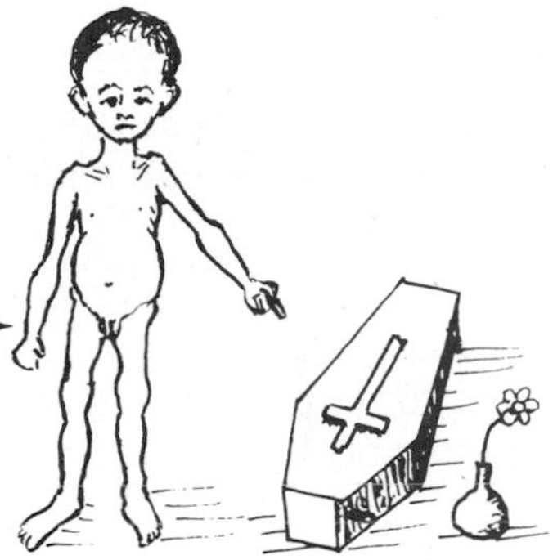

Diarrhea has many causes. **Usually no medicines are needed,** and the child gets well in a few days if you give him lots of Rehydration Drink and food. (If he does not eat much, give him a little food many times a day.) Occasionally, special treatment is needed. However, **most diarrhea can be treated successfully in the home,** even if you are not sure of the exact cause or causes.

THE MAIN CAUSES OF DIARRHEA:

poor nutrition (p. 154) This weakens the child and makes diarrhea from other causes more frequent and worse.

shortage of water and unclean conditions (no latrines) spread the germs that cause diarrhea

virus infection or 'intestinal flu'

an infection of the gut caused by bacteria (p. 131), amebas (p. 144), or giardia (p. 145)

worm infections (p. 140 to 144) (most worm infections do not cause diarrhea)

infections outside the gut (ear infections, p. 309; tonsillitis, p. 309; measles, p. 311; urinary infections, p. 234)

malaria (*falciparum* type—in parts of Africa, Asia, and the Pacific, p. 186)

food poisoning (spoiled food, p. 135)

AIDS (long-lasting diarrhea may be an early sign, p. 399)

inability to digest milk (mainly in severely malnourished children and certain adults)

difficulty babies have digesting foods that are new to them (p. 154)

allergies to certain foods (seafood, crayfish, etc., p. 166); occasionally babies are allergic to cow's milk or other milk

side effects produced by certain medicines, such as ampicillin or tetracycline (p. 58)

laxatives, purges, irritating or poisonous plants, certain poisons

eating too much unripe fruit or heavy, greasy foods

Preventing diarrhea:

Although diarrhea has many different causes, the most common are **infection** and **poor nutrition. With good hygiene and good food, most diarrhea could be prevented.** And if treated correctly by giving **lots of drink and food,** fewer children who get diarrhea would die.

Children who are poorly nourished get diarrhea and die from it far more often than those who are well nourished. Yet diarrhea itself can be part of the cause of malnutrition. And if malnutrition already exists, diarrhea rapidly makes it worse.

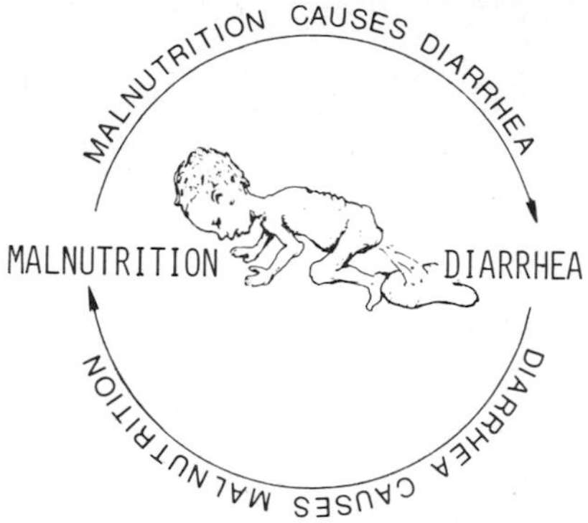

THE 'VICIOUS CIRCLE' OF MALNUTRITION AND DIARRHEA TAKES MANY CHILDREN'S LIVES.

Malnutrition causes diarrhea.
Diarrhea causes malnutrition.

This results in a vicious circle, in which each makes the other worse. For this reason, **good nutrition is important in both the prevention and treatment of diarrhea.**

Prevent diarrhea by preventing malnutrition.
Prevent malnutrition by preventing diarrhea.

To learn about the kinds of foods that help the body resist or fight off different illnesses, including diarrhea, read Chapter 11.

The prevention of diarrhea depends both on **good nutrition** and **cleanliness.** Many suggestions for personal and public cleanliness are given in Chapter 12. These include the use of **latrines,** the importance of **clean water,** and the **protection of foods** from dirt and flies.

Here are some other important suggestions for preventing diarrhea in babies:

- **Breast feed rather than bottle feed babies.** Give only breast milk for the first 4 to 6 months. Breast milk helps babies resist the infections that cause diarrhea. If it is not possible to breast feed a baby, feed her with a cup and spoon. **Do not use a baby bottle** because it is harder to keep clean and more likely to cause an infection.

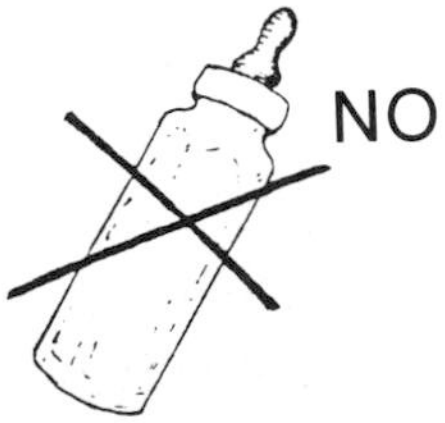

- When you begin to give the baby new or solid food, start by giving her just a little, mashing it well, and mixing it with a little breast milk. The baby has to learn how to digest new foods. If she starts with too much at one time, she may get diarrhea. **Do not stop giving breast milk suddenly. Start with other foods while the baby is still breast feeding.**

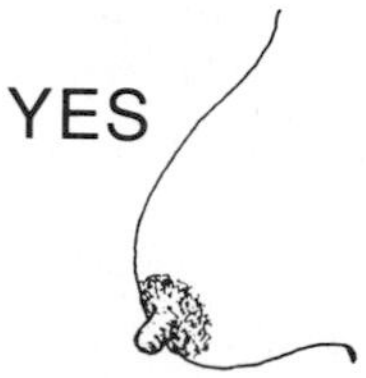

BREAST FEEDING HELPS PREVENT DIARRHEA.

- Keep the baby clean—and in a clean place. Try to keep her from putting dirty things in her mouth.
- Do not give babies unnecessary medicines.

Treatment of diarrhea:

For most cases of diarrhea no medicine is needed. If the diarrhea is severe, the biggest danger is **dehydration.** If the diarrhea lasts a long time, the biggest danger is **malnutrition.** So the most important part of treatment has to do with giving **enough liquids** and **enough food.** No matter what the cause of diarrhea, always take care with the following:

1. PREVENT OR CONTROL DEHYDRATION. A person with diarrhea must drink a lot of liquids. If diarrhea is severe or there are signs of dehydration, give him Rehydration Drink (p. 152). Even if he does not want to drink, gently insist that he do so. Have him take several swallows every few minutes.

2. MEET NUTRITIONAL NEEDS. **A person with diarrhea needs food as soon as he will eat.** This is especially important in small children or persons who are already poorly nourished. Also, when a person has diarrhea, food passes through the gut very quickly and is not all used. **So give the person food many times a day**—especially if he only takes a little at a time.

- ♦ A baby with diarrhea should **go on breast feeding.**
- ♦ An underweight child should get plenty of energy foods and some body-building foods (proteins) all the time he has diarrhea—and extra when he gets well. If he stops eating because he feels too sick or is vomiting, he should eat again as soon as he can. **Giving Rehydration Drink will help the child be able to eat.** Although giving food may cause more frequent stools at first, it can save his life.
- ♦ If a child who is underweight has diarrhea that lasts for many days or keeps coming back, give him more food more often—at least 5 or 6 meals each day. Often no other treatment is needed.

FOODS FOR A PERSON WITH DIARRHEA

When the person is vomiting or feels too sick to eat, he should drink:	As soon as the person is able to eat, in addition to giving the drinks listed at the left, he should eat a balanced selection of the following foods or similar ones:	
	energy foods	**body-building foods**
watery mush or broth of rice, maize powder, or potato	ripe or cooked bananas	chicken (boiled or roasted)
rice water (with some mashed rice)	crackers	eggs (boiled)
chicken, meat, egg, or bean broth	rice, oatmeal, or other well-cooked grain	meat (well cooked, without much fat or grease)
Kool-Aid or similar sweetened drinks	fresh maize (well cooked and mashed)	beans, lentils, or peas (well cooked and mashed)
REHYDRATION DRINK	potatoes	fish (well cooked)
Breast milk	applesauce (cooked)	milk (sometimes this causes problems, see the next page)
	papaya	
	(It helps to add a little sugar or vegetable oil to the cereal foods.)	

DO NOT EAT OR DRINK

fatty or greasy foods most raw fruits	any kind of laxative or purge	highly seasoned food alcoholic drinks

Diarrhea and milk:

Breast milk is the best food for babies. It helps prevent and combat diarrhea. **Keep giving breast milk when the baby has diarrhea.**

Cow's milk, powdered milk, or canned milk can be good sources of energy and protein. Keep on giving them to a child with diarrhea. In a very few children these milks may cause more diarrhea. If this happens, try giving less milk and mixing it with other foods. But remember: **a poorly nourished child with diarrhea must have enough energy foods and protein.** If less milk is given, well-cooked and mashed foods such as chicken, egg yolk, meat, fish, or beans should be added. Beans are easier to digest if their skins have been taken off and they are boiled and mashed.

As the child gets better, he will usually be able to drink more milk without getting diarrhea.

Medicines for diarrhea:

For most cases of diarrhea no medicines are needed. But in certain cases, using the right medicine can be important. However, many of the medicines commonly used for diarrhea do little or no good. Some are actually harmful:

GENERALLY IT IS BETTER **NOT** TO USE THE FOLLOWING MEDICINES IN THE TREATMENT OF DIARRHEA:

'Anti-diarrhea' medicines with kaolin and pectin (such as *Kaopectate,* p. 384) make diarrhea thicker and less frequent. But they do not correct dehydration or control infection. Some anti-diarrhea medicines, like loperamide *(Imodium)* or diphenoxylate *(Lomotil)* may even cause harm or make infections last longer.

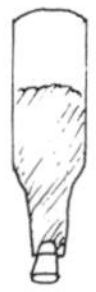

'ANTI-DIARRHEA MEDICINES' ACT LIKE PLUGS. THEY KEEP IN THE INFECTED MATERIAL THAT NEEDS TO COME OUT.

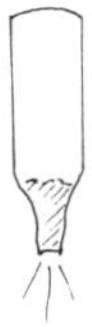

'Anti-diarrhea' mixtures containing neomycin or streptomycin should not be used. They irritate the gut and often do more harm than good.

Antibiotics like ampicillin and tetracycline are useful only in **some** cases of diarrhea (see p. 158). But they themselves sometimes cause diarrhea, especially in small children. If, after taking these antibiotics for more than 2 or 3 days, diarrhea gets worse rather than better, stop taking them—the antibiotics may be the cause.

Chloramphenicol has certain dangers in its use (see p. 357) and should never be used for mild diarrhea or given to babies less than 1 month old.

Laxatives and purges should never be given to persons with diarrhea. They will make it worse and increase the danger of dehydration.

Special treatment in different cases of diarrhea:

While most cases of diarrhea are best treated by giving plenty of **liquids** and **food,** and **no medicine,** sometimes special treatment is needed.

In considering treatment, keep in mind that some cases of diarrhea, especially in small children, are caused by **infections outside the gut.** Always check for **infections of the ears,** the **throat,** and the **urinary system.** If found, these infections should be treated. Also look for signs of **measles.**

If the child has mild diarrhea together with signs of a cold, the diarrhea is probably caused by a virus, or 'intestinal flu', and no special treatment is called for. Give lots of liquids and all the food the child will accept.

In certain difficult cases of diarrhea, analysis of the stools or other tests may be needed to know how to treat it correctly. But usually you can learn enough from asking specific questions, seeing the stools, and looking for certain signs Here are some guidelines for treatment according to signs.

1. **Sudden, mild diarrhea. No fever.** (Upset stomach? 'Intestinal flu'?)

- Drink lots of liquids. Usually no special treatment is needed. It is usually best not to use 'diarrhea plug' medicines such as kaolin with pectin (*Kaopectate,* p. 384) or diphenoxylate *(Lomotil).* They are never necessary and do not help either to correct dehydration or get rid of infection—so why waste money buying them? Never give them to persons who are very ill, or to small children.

2. **Diarrhea with vomiting.** (Many causes)

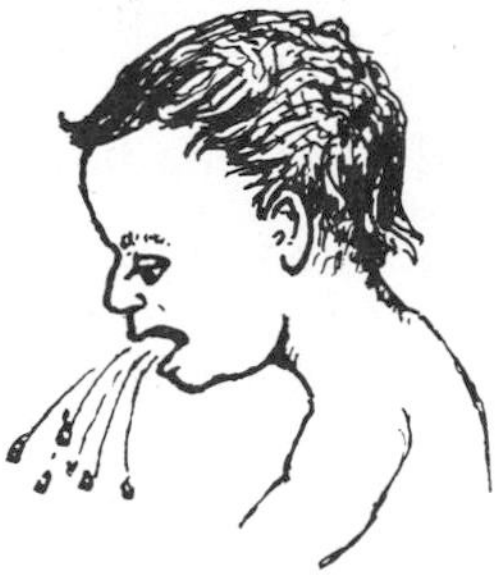

- If a person with diarrhea is also vomiting, the danger of dehydration is greater, especially in small children. It is very important to give the Rehydration Drink (p. 152), tea, soup, or whatever liquids he will take. **Keep giving the Drink, even if the person vomits it out again.** Some will stay inside. Give sips every 5 to 10 minutes. If vomiting does not stop soon, you can use medicines like promethazine (p. 386) or phenobarbital (p. 389).
- If you cannot control the vomiting or if the dehydration gets worse, seek medical help fast.

3. **Diarrhea with mucus and blood. Often chronic. No fever. There may be diarrhea some days and constipation other days.** (Possibly amebic dysentery. For more details, see page 144.)

- Use metronidazole (p. 369) or diloxanide furoate (p. 369). Take the medicine according to the recommended dose. If the diarrhea continues after treatment, seek medical advice.

4. **Severe diarrhea with blood, with fever.** (Bacterial dysentery—caused by Shigella?)

- Give co-trimoxazole (p. 358) or ampicillin (p. 353). Shigella is now often resistant to ampicillin, and sometimes to co-trimoxazole. If the first medicine you try does not bring improvement within 2 days, try another or seek medical help.

5. **Severe diarrhea with fever, usually no blood.**

- Fever may be partly caused by dehydration. Give lots of Rehydration Drink (p. 152). If the person is very ill and does not improve within 6 hours after beginning Rehydration Drink, seek medical help.
- Check for signs of typhoid fever. If present, treat for typhoid (see p. 188).
- In areas where ***falciparum*** malaria is common, it is a good idea to treat persons with diarrhea and fever for malaria (see p. 187), especially if they have a large spleen.

6. **Yellow, bad-smelling diarrhea with bubbles or froth, without blood or mucus.** Often a lot of gas in the belly, and burps that taste bad, like sulfur. (Giardia? See p. 145.)

- This may be caused by microscopic parasites called giardia or perhaps by malnutrition. In either case, plenty of liquid, nutritious food, and rest are often the only treatment needed. Severe giardia infections can be treated with metronidazole (p. 369). Quinacrine *(Atabrine)* is cheaper, but has worse side effects (p. 370).

7. **Chronic diarrhea (diarrhea that lasts a long time or keeps coming back).**

- This can be in part caused by malnutrition, or by a chronic infection such as that caused by amebas or giardia. See that the child eats more nutritious food more times a day (p. 110). If the diarrhea still continues, seek medical help.

8. **Diarrhea like rice water.** (Cholera?)

- 'Rice water' stools in very large quantities may be a sign of cholera. In countries where this dangerous disease occurs, cholera often comes in *epidemics* (striking many people at once) and is usually worse in older children and adults. Severe dehydration can develop quickly, especially if there is vomiting also. Treat the dehydration continuously (see p. 152), and give tetracycline (p. 356), co-trimoxazole (p. 358), or chloramphenicol (p. 357). Cholera should be reported to the health authorities. Seek medical help.

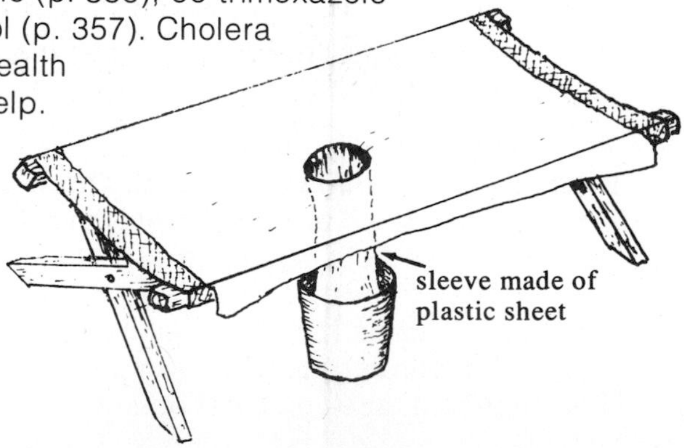

A **'cholera bed'** like this can be made for persons with very severe diarrhea. Watch how much liquid the person is losing and be sure he drinks larger amounts of Rehydration Drink. Give him the Drink almost continuously, and have him drink as much as he can.

Care of Babies with Diarrhea

Diarrhea is especially dangerous in babies and small children. Often no medicine is needed, but special care must be taken because a baby can die very quickly of dehydration.

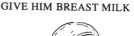

GIVE HIM BREAST MILK

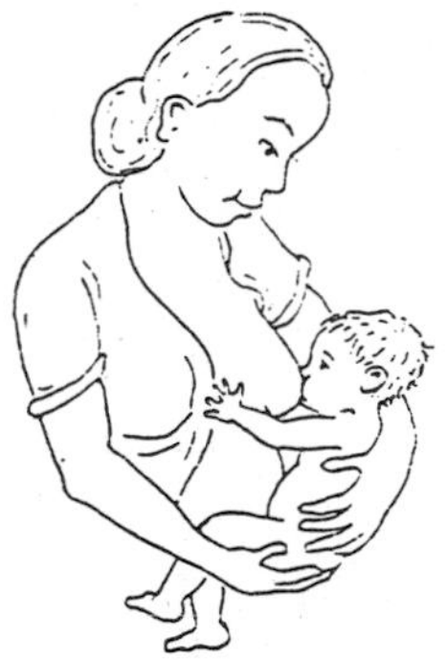

- **Continue breast feeding** and also give sips of **Rehydration Drink.**

- If vomiting is a problem, give breast milk often, but only a little at a time. Also give Rehydration Drink in small sips every 5 to 10 minutes (see Vomiting, p. 161).

AND ALSO REHYDRATION DRINK

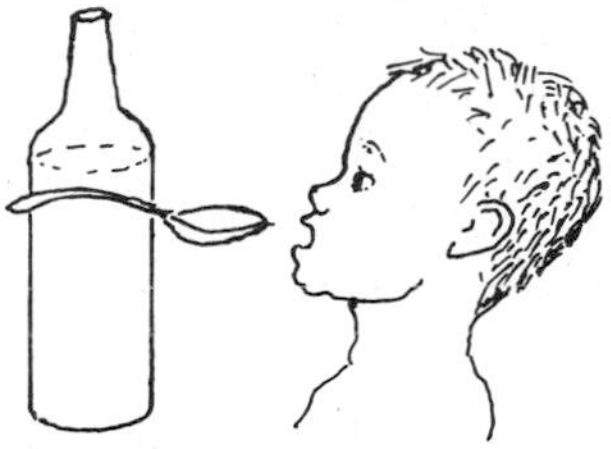

- If there is no breast milk, try giving frequent small feedings of some other milk or milk substitute (like milk made from soybeans) **mixed to half normal strength with boiled water.** If milk seems to make the diarrhea worse, give some other protein (mashed chicken, eggs, lean meat, or skinned mashed beans, mixed with sugar or well-cooked rice or another carbohydrate, and boiled water).

- If the child is younger than 1 month, try to find a health worker before giving any medicine. If there is no health worker and the child is very sick, give him an 'infant syrup' that contains ampicillin: half a teaspoon 4 times daily (see p. 353). It is better not to use other antibiotics.

When to Seek Medical Help in Cases of Diarrhea

Diarrhea and dysentery can be very dangerous—especially in small children. **In the following situations you should get medical help:**

- if diarrhea lasts more than 4 days and is not getting better—or more than 1 day in a small child with severe diarrhea

- if the person shows signs of dehydration and is getting worse

- if the child vomits everything he drinks, or drinks nothing, or if frequent vomiting continues for more than 3 hours after beginning Rehydration Drink

- if the child begins to have fits, or if the feet and face swell

- if the person was very sick, weak, or malnourished before the diarrhea began (especially a little child or a very old person)

- if there is much blood in the stools. This can be dangerous even if there is only very little diarrhea (see gut obstruction, p. 94).

THE CARE OF A PERSON WITH ACUTE DIARRHEA

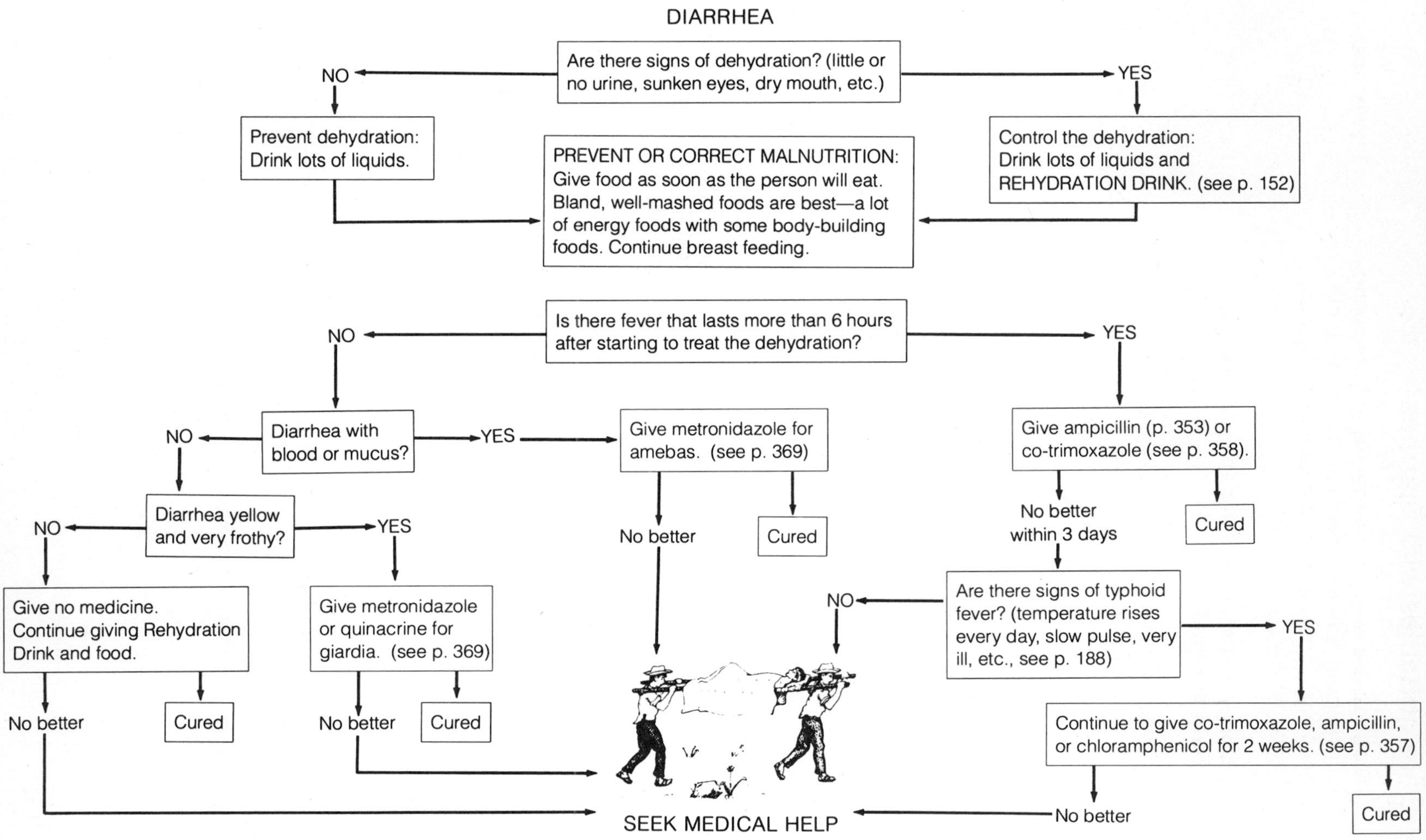
DIARRHEA
Are there signs of dehydration? (little or no urine, sunken eyes, dry mouth, etc.)
NO
Prevent dehydration: Drink lots of liquids.
YES
Control the dehydration: Drink lots of liquids and REHYDRATION DRINK. (see p. 152)
PREVENT OR CORRECT MALNUTRITION: Give food as soon as the person will eat. Bland, well-mashed foods are best—a lot of energy foods with some body-building foods. Continue breast feeding.
Is there fever that lasts more than 6 hours after starting to treat the dehydration?
NO
Diarrhea with blood or mucus?
YES
Give metronidazole for amebas. (see p. 369)
No better
Cured
NO
Diarrhea yellow and very frothy?
YES
Give metronidazole or quinacrine for giardia. (see p. 369)
No better
Cured
NO
Give no medicine. Continue giving Rehydration Drink and food.
No better
Cured
YES
Give ampicillin (p. 353) or co-trimoxazole (see p. 358).
No better within 3 days
Cured
Are there signs of typhoid fever? (temperature rises every day, slow pulse, very ill, etc., see p. 188)
NO
YES
Continue to give co-trimoxazole, ampicillin, or chloramphenicol for 2 weeks. (see p. 357)
No better
Cured
SEEK MEDICAL HELP

VOMITING

Many people, especially children, have an occasional 'stomach upset' with vomiting. Often no cause can be found. There may be mild stomach or gut ache or fever. This kind of simple vomiting usually is not serious and clears up by itself.

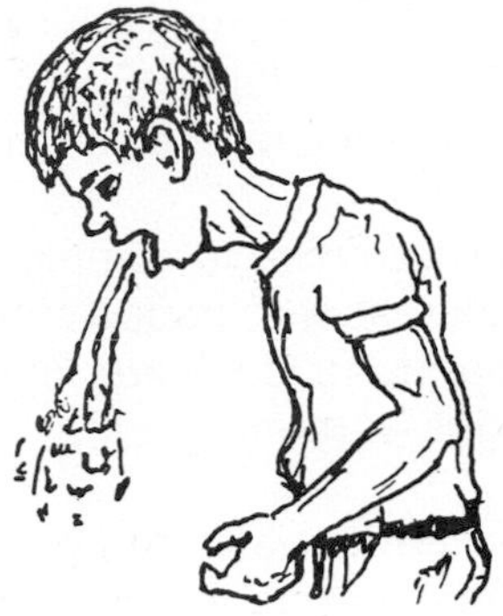

Vomiting is one of the signs of many different problems, some minor and some quite serious, so it is important to examine the person carefully. Vomiting often comes from a problem in the stomach or guts, such as: an infection (see diarrhea, p. 153), poisoning from spoiled food (p. 135), or 'acute abdomen' (for example, appendicitis or something blocking the gut, p. 94). Also, almost any sickness with high fever or severe pain may cause vomiting, especially malaria (p. 186), hepatitis (p. 172), tonsillitis (p. 309), earache (p. 309), meningitis (p. 185), urinary infection (p. 234), gallbladder pain (p. 329) or migraine headache (p. 162).

Danger signs with vomiting—seek medical help quickly!

- dehydration that increases and that you cannot control, (p. 152)
- severe vomiting that lasts more than 24 hours
- violent vomiting, especially if vomit is dark green, brown, or smells like shit (signs of obstruction, p. 94)
- constant pain in the gut, especially if the person cannot defecate (shit) or if you cannot hear gurgles when you put your ear to the belly (see acute abdomen: obstruction, appendicitis, p. 94)
- vomiting of blood (ulcer, p. 128; cirrhosis, p. 328)

To help control simple vomiting:

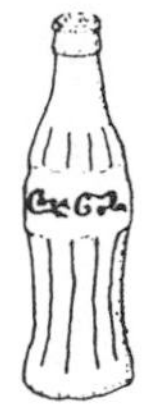

- Eat nothing while vomiting is severe,
- Sip a cola drink or ginger ale. Some herbal teas, like camomile, may also help.
- For dehydration give small frequent sips of cola, tea, or Rehydration Drink (p. 152).
- If vomiting does not stop soon, use a vomit-control medicine like promethazine (p. 386) or diphenhydramine (p. 387).

Most of these come in pills, syrups, injections, and suppositories (soft pills you push up the ***anus***). Tablets or syrup can also be put up the anus. Grind up the tablet in a little water. Put it in with an enema set or syringe without a needle.

When taken by mouth, the medicine should be swallowed with very little water and nothing else should be swallowed for 5 minutes. Never give more than the recommended dose. Do not give a second dose until dehydration has been corrected and the person has begun to urinate. If severe vomiting and diarrhea make medication by mouth or anus impossible, give an injection of one of the vomit-control medicines. Promethazine may work best. Take care not to give too much.

HEADACHES AND MIGRAINES

SIMPLE HEADACHE can be helped by rest and aspirin. It often helps to put a cloth soaked in hot water on the back of the neck and to massage (rub) the neck and shoulders gently. Some other home remedies also seem to help.

For simple or nervous headache, folk cures sometimes work as well as modern medicine.

Mexican folk cure

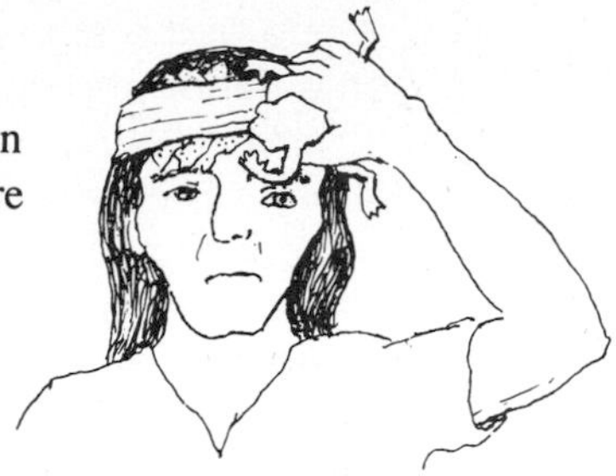

Headache is common with any sickness that causes fever. If headache is severe, check for signs of meningitis (p. 185).

aspirin

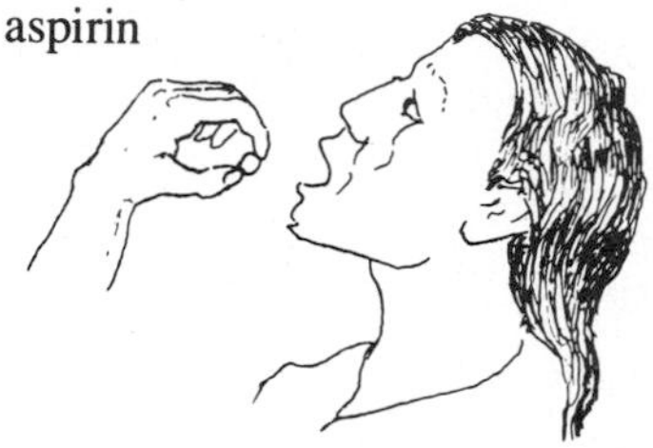

Headaches that keep coming back may be a sign of a chronic illness or poor nutrition. It is important to eat well and get enough sleep. If the headaches do not go away, seek medical help.

A **MIGRAINE** is a severe throbbing headache often on one side of the head only. Migraine attacks may come often, or months or years apart.

A typical migraine begins with blurring of vision, seeing strange spots of light, or numbness of one hand or foot. This is followed by severe headache, which may last hours or days. Often there is vomiting. Migraines are very painful, but not dangerous.

TO STOP A MIGRAINE, DO THE FOLLOWING AT THE FIRST SIGN:

- Take 2 aspirins with a cup of strong coffee or strong black tea.

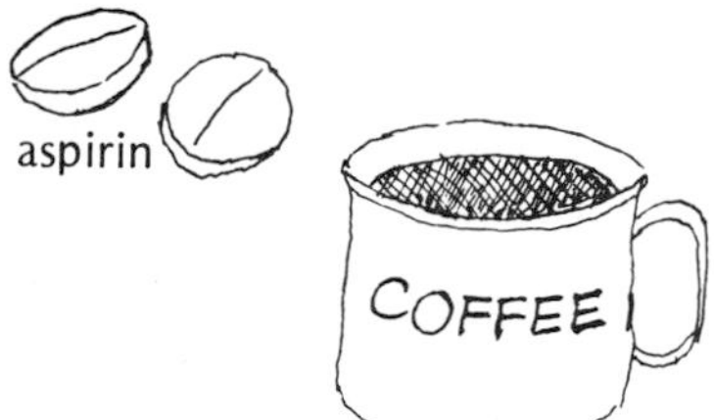

- Lie down in a dark, quiet place. Do your best to relax. Try not to think about your problems.

- For especially bad migraine headaches, take aspirin, if possible with codeine, or with another sedative. Or obtain pills of ergotamine with caffeine (***Cafergot,*** p. 380). Take 2 pills at first and 1 pill every 30 minutes until the pain goes away. Do not take more than 6 pills in 1 day.

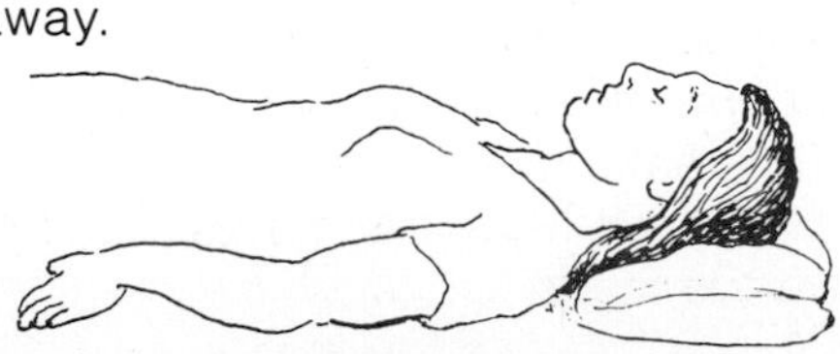

WARNING: Do not use *Cafergot* during pregnancy.

COLDS AND THE FLU

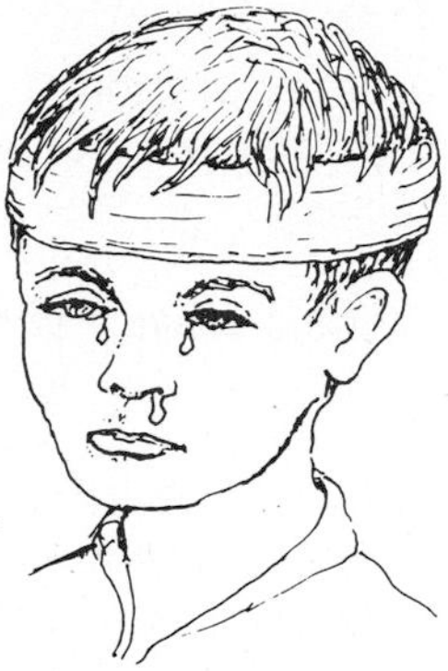

Colds and the flu are common virus infections that may cause runny nose, cough, sore throat, and sometimes fever or pain in the joints. There may be mild diarrhea, especially in young children.

Colds and the flu almost always go away without medicine. **Do not use penicillin, tetracycline, or other antibiotics,** as they will not help at all and may cause harm.

- Drink plenty of water and get enough rest.
- Aspirin (p. 379) or acetaminophen (p. 380) helps lower fever and relieve body aches and headaches. More expensive 'cold tablets' are no better than aspirin. So why waste your money?
- No special diet is needed. However, fruit juices, especially orange juice or lemonade, are helpful.

For treating coughs and stuffy noses that come with colds, see the next pages.

WARNING: Do not give any kind of antibiotic or injections to a child with a simple cold. They will not help and may cause harm. Sometimes signs of cold are caused by the polio virus, and giving the child an injection could bring on paralysis from polio (see p. 314).

If a cold or the flu lasts more than a week, or if the person has fever, coughs up a lot of ***phlegm*** (mucus with pus), has shallow fast breathing or chest pain, he could be developing bronchitis or pneumonia (see p. 170 and 171). An antibiotic may be called for. The danger of a cold turning into pneumonia is greater in old people, in those who have lung problems like chronic bronchitis, and in people who cannot move much.

Sore throat is often part of a cold. No special medicine is needed, but it may help to gargle with warm water. However, if the sore throat begins suddenly, with high fever, it could be a strep throat. Special treatment is needed (see p. 309).

Prevention of colds:

- Getting enough sleep and eating well helps prevent colds. Eating oranges, tomatoes, and other fruit containing vitamin C may also help.
- Contrary to popular belief, colds do not come from getting cold or wet (although getting very cold, wet, or tired can make a cold worse). A cold is 'caught' from others who have the infection and sneeze the virus into the air.
- To keep from giving his cold to others, the sick person should eat and sleep separately—and take special care to keep far away from small babies. He should cover his nose and mouth when he coughs or sneezes.
- To prevent a cold from leading to earache (p. 309), **try not to blow your nose—just wipe it.** Teach children to do the same.

STUFFY AND RUNNY NOSES

A stuffy or runny nose can result from a cold or allergy (see next page). A lot of mucus in the nose may cause ear infections in children or sinus problems in adults.

To help clear a stuffy nose, do the following:

1. In little children, carefully suck the mucus out of the nose with a suction bulb or syringe **without a needle,** like this:

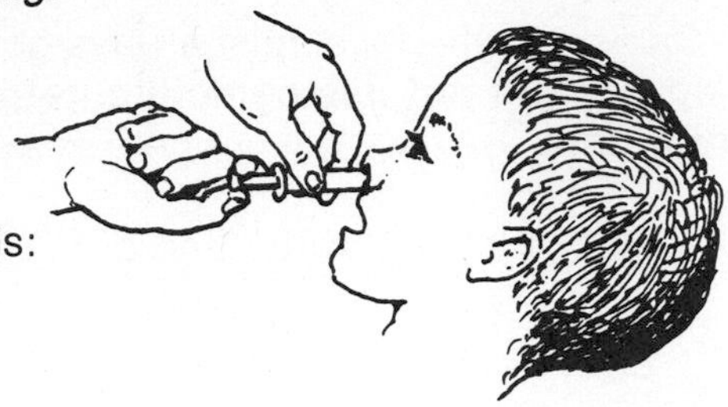

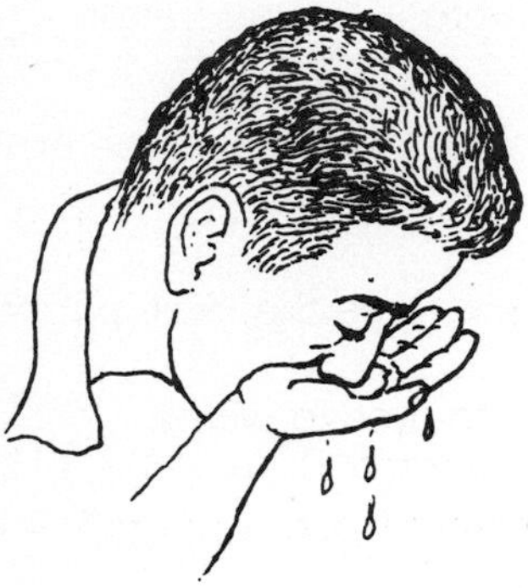

2. Older children and adults can put a little salt water into their hand and sniff it into the nose. This helps to loosen the mucus.

3. Breathing hot water vapor as described on page 168, helps clear a stuffy nose.

4. Wipe a runny or stuffy nose, but **try not to blow it.** Blowing the nose may lead to earache and sinus infections.

5. Persons who often get earaches or sinus trouble after a cold can help prevent these problems by using *decongestant* nose drops like phenylephrine (p. 384). Or make nose drops of ephedrine tablets (see p. 385). After sniffing a little salt water, put the drops in the nose like this:

With the head sideways, put 2 or 3 drops in the lower nostril. Wait a couple of minutes and then do the other side.

CAUTION: **Use decongestant drops no more than 3 times a day, for no more than 3 days.**

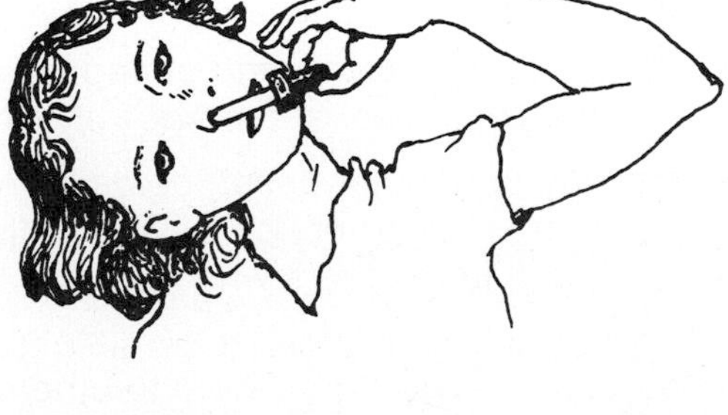

A decongestant syrup (with phenylephrine or something similar) may also help.

Prevent ear and sinus infections—try not to blow your nose, just wipe it.

SINUS TROUBLE (SINUSITIS)

Sinusitis is an acute or chronic (long-term) inflammation of the sinuses or hollows in the bone that open into the nose. It usually occurs after a person has had an infection of the ears or throat, or after a bad cold.

Signs:

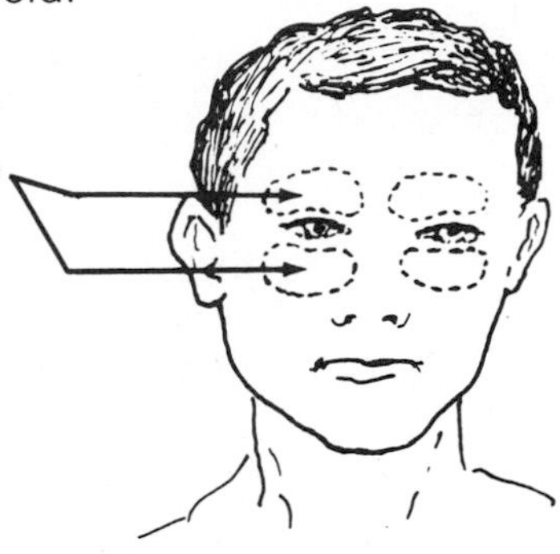

- Pain in the face above and below the eyes, here (It hurts more when you tap lightly just over the bones, or when the person bends over.)
- Thick mucus or pus in the nose, perhaps with a bad smell. The nose is often stuffy.
- Fever (sometimes).
- Certain teeth may hurt.

Treatment:

- Drink a lot of water.
- Sniff a little salt water into the nose (see p. 164), or breathe steam from hot water to clear the nose (see p. 168).
- Put hot compresses on the face.
- Use decongestant nose drops such as phenylephrine (***Neo-synephrine,*** p. 384).
- Use an antibiotic such as tetracycline (p. 356), ampicillin (p. 353), or penicillin (p. 351).
- If the person does not get better, seek medical help.

Prevention:

When you get a cold and a stuffy nose, try to keep your nose clear. Follow the instructions on page 164.

HAY FEVER (ALLERGIC RHINITIS)

Runny nose and itchy eyes can be caused by an allergic reaction to something in the air that a person has breathed in (see the next page). It is often worse at certain times of year.

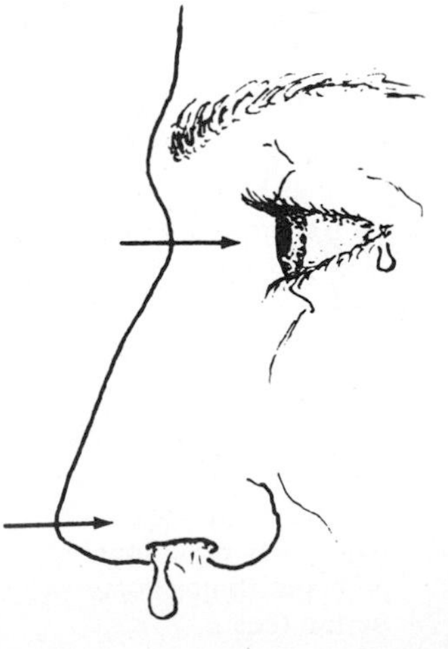

Treatment:

Use an antihistamine such as chlorpheniramine (p. 387). Dimenhydrinate (*Dramamine*, p. 387), usually sold for motion sickness, also works.

Prevention:

Find out what things cause this reaction (for example: dust, chicken feathers, *pollen,* mold) and try to avoid them.

ALLERGIC REACTIONS

An allergy is a disturbance or reaction that affects only certain persons when things they are sensitive or allergic to are . . .

- breathed in
- eaten
- injected
- or touch the skin

Allergic reactions, which can be mild or very serious, include:

- itching rashes, lumpy patches or ***hives*** (p. 203)
- runny nose and itching or burning eyes (hay fever, p. 165)
- irritation in the throat, difficulty breathing, or asthma (see next page)
- allergic shock (p. 70)
- diarrhea (in children allergic to milk—a rare cause of diarrhea, p. 156)

An allergy is not an infection and cannot be passed from one person to another. However, children of allergic parents also tend to have allergies.

Often allergic persons suffer more in certain seasons—or whenever they come in touch with the substances that bother them. Common causes of allergic reactions are:

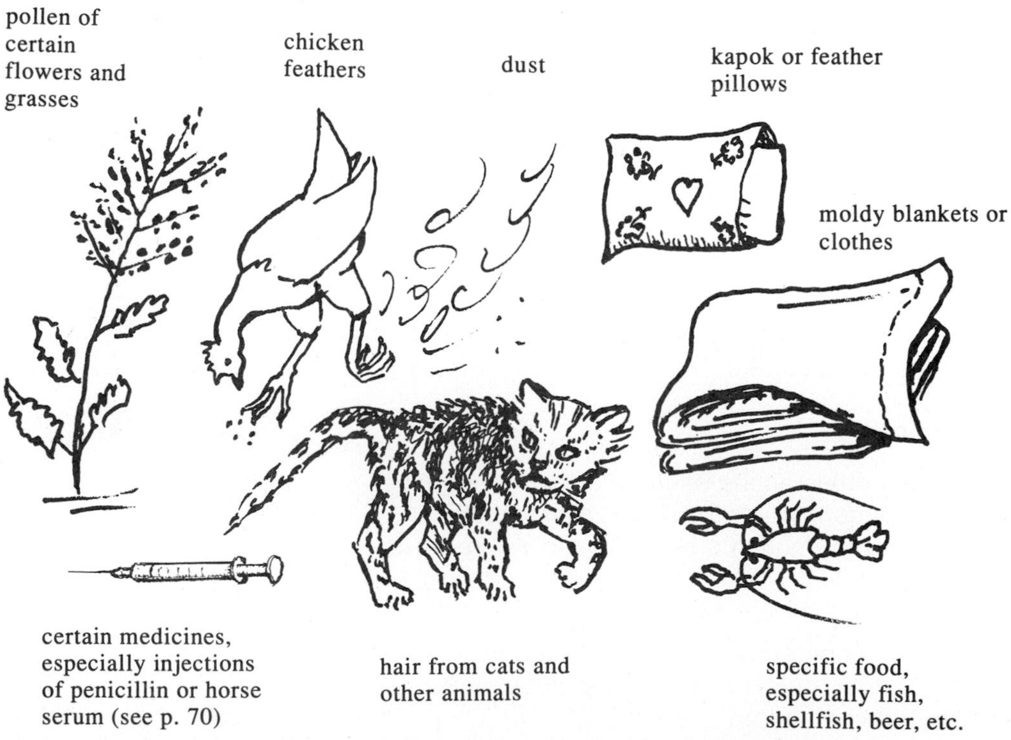

ASTHMA

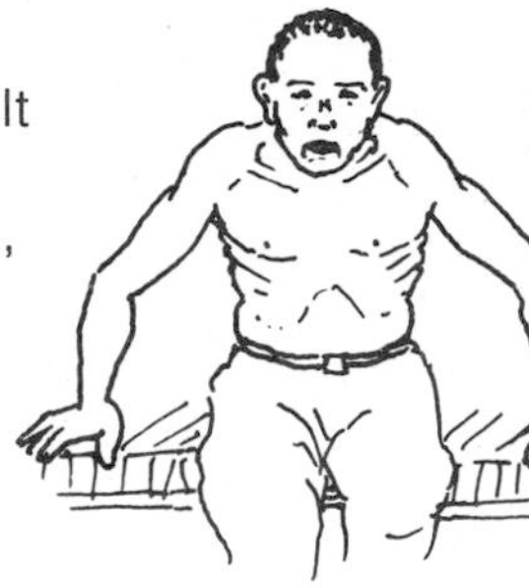
sitting
up to
breathe

A person with asthma has fits or attacks of difficult breathing. Listen for a hissing or wheezing sound, especially when breathing out. When he breathes in, the skin behind his collar bones and between his ribs may suck in as he tries to get air. If the person cannot get enough air, his nails and lips may turn blue, and his neck veins may swell. Usually there is no fever.

Asthma often begins in childhood and may be a problem for life. It is not ***contagious,*** but is more common in children with relatives who have asthma. It is generally worse during certain months of the year or at night. Persons who have had asthma for years may develop emphysema (see p. 170).

An asthma attack may be caused by eating or breathing things to which the person is allergic (see p. 166). In children asthma often starts with a cold. In some persons nervousness or worry plays a part in bringing on an asthma attack. Asthma can also be caused by unclean air (air pollution), like smoke from cigarettes or inside cooking fires, and smoke from burning fields or cars and trucks.

Treatment:

- If asthma gets worse inside the house, the person should go outside to a place where the air is cleanest. Remain calm and be gentle with the person. Reassure him.
- Give a lot of liquids. This loosens mucus and makes breathing easier. Breathing water vapor may also help (see p. 168).
- For mild attacks give ephedrine, theophylline, or salbutamol (see p. 385).
- For severe asthma, ephedrine or salbutamol can be used with theophylline.
- If the asthma attack is especially bad, inject epinephrine *(Adrenalin)*. Adults: 1/3 cc.; children ages 7 to 12: 1/5 cc. You can repeat the dose every half hour, as needed up to 3 times. For precautions, see p. 386.

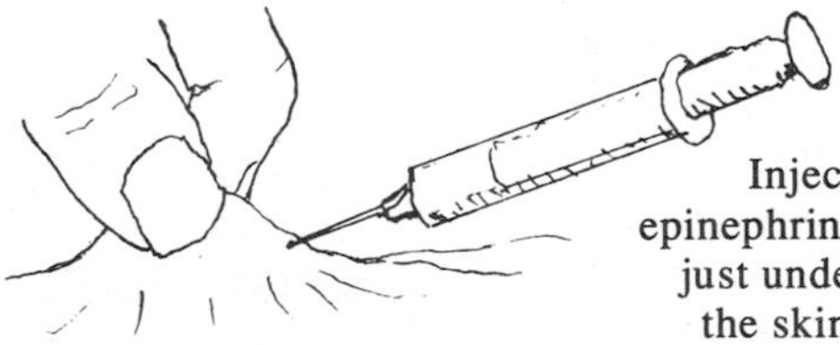
Inject
epinephrine
just under
the skin.

- If the person has a fever, or if the attack lasts more than 3 days, give tetracycline capsules (p. 356) or erythromycin (p. 355).
- In rare cases, roundworms cause asthma. Try giving piperazine (p. 375) to a child who starts having asthma if you think she has roundworms.
- **If the person does not get better, seek medical help.**

Prevention:

A person with asthma should avoid eating or breathing things that bring on attacks. The house or work place should be kept clean. Do not let chickens or other animals inside. Put bedding out to air in the sunshine. Sometimes it helps to sleep outside in the open air. Drink at least 8 glasses of water each day to keep the mucus loose. Persons with asthma may improve when they move to a different area where the air is cleaner.

If you have asthma do not smoke—smoking damages your lungs even more.

COUGH

Coughing is not a sickness in itself, but is a sign of many different sicknesses that affect the throat, lungs, or ***bronchi*** (the network of air tubes going into the lungs). Below are some of the problems that cause different kinds of coughs:

DRY COUGH WITH LITTLE OR NO PHLEGM:	COUGH WITH MUCH OR LITTLE PHLEGM:	COUGH WITH A WHEEZE OR WHOOP AND TROUBLE BREATHING:
cold or flu (p. 163) worms—when passing through the lungs (p. 140) measles (p. 311) smoker's cough (smoking, p. 149)	bronchitis (p. 170) pneumonia (p. 171) asthma (p. 167) smoker's cough, especially when getting up in the morning (p. 149)	asthma (p. 167) whooping cough (p. 313) diphtheria (p. 313) heart trouble (p. 325) something stuck in the throat (p. 79)

CHRONIC OR PERSISTENT COUGH:	COUGHING UP BLOOD:
tuberculosis (p. 179) smoker's or miner's cough (p. 149) asthma (repeated attacks, p. 167) chronic bronchitis (p. 170) emphysema (p. 170)	tuberculosis (p. 179) pneumonia (yellow, green, or blood-streaked phlegm, p. 171) severe worm infection (p. 140) cancer of the lungs or throat (p. 149)

Coughing is the body's way of cleaning the breathing system and getting rid of phlegm (mucus with pus) and germs in the throat or lungs. So when a cough produces phlegm, **do not take medicine to stop the cough, but rather do something to help loosen and bring up the phlegm.**

Treatment for cough:

1. **To loosen mucus** and ease any kind of cough, **drink lots of water.** This works better than any medicine.

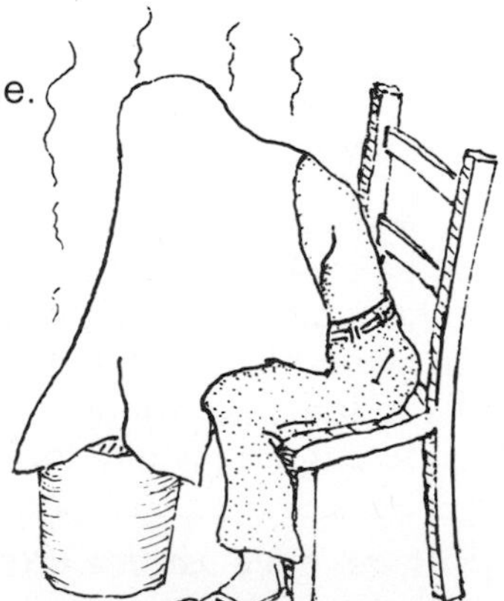

Also **breathe hot water vapors.** Sit on a chair with a bucket of very hot water at your feet. Place a sheet over your head and cover the bucket to catch the vapors as they rise. Breathe the vapors deeply for 15 minutes. Repeat several times a day. Some people like to add mint or eucalyptus leaves or *Vaporub,* but hot water works just as well alone.

CAUTION: Do not use eucalyptus or *Vaporub* if the person has asthma. They make it worse.

2. **For all kinds of cough,** especially a dry cough, the following cough syrup can be given:

Mix: 1 part honey + 1 part lemon juice

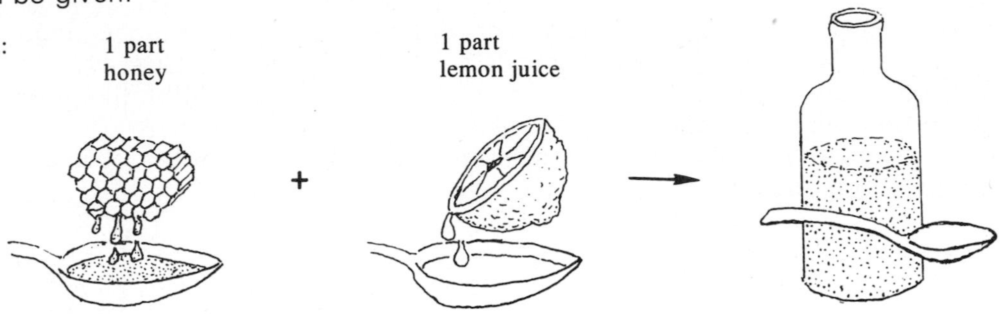

Take a teaspoonful every 2 or 3 hours.

WARNING: Do not give honey to babies under 1 year. Make the syrup with sugar instead of honey.

3. **For a severe dry cough that does not let you sleep,** you can take a syrup with codeine (p. 384). Tablets of aspirin with codeine (or even aspirin alone) also help. If there is a lot of phlegm or wheezing, do not use codeine.

4. **For a cough with wheezing** (difficult, noisy breathing), see Asthma (p. 167), Chronic Bronchitis (p. 170), and Heart Trouble (p. 325).

5. **Try to find out what sickness is causing the cough and treat that.** If the cough lasts a long time, if there is blood, pus, or smelly phlegm in it, or if the person is losing weight or has continual difficulty breathing, see a health worker.

6. **If you have any kind of a cough, do not smoke.** Smoking damages the lungs.

To prevent a cough, do not smoke.
To cure a cough, treat the illness that causes it—and do not smoke.
To calm a cough, and loosen phlegm, drink lots of water—and do not smoke.

HOW TO DRAIN MUCUS FROM THE LUNGS (POSTURAL DRAINAGE):

When a person who has a bad cough is very old or weak and cannot get rid of the sticky mucus or phlegm in his chest, it will help if he drinks a lot of water. Also do the following:

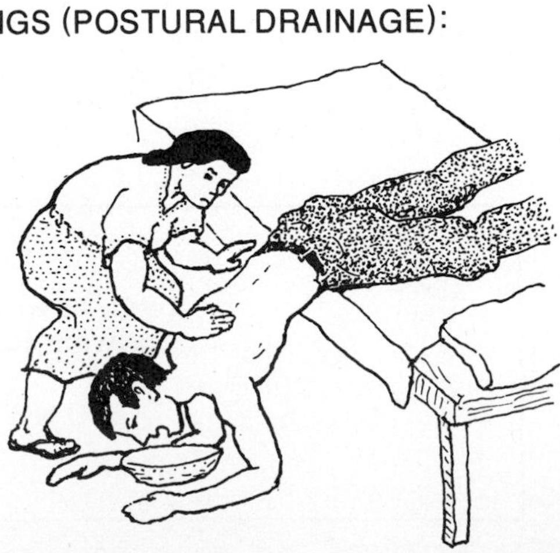

- First, have him breathe hot water vapors to loosen the mucus.
- Then have him lie partly on the bed, with his head and chest hanging over the edge. Pound him lightly on the back. This will help to bring out the mucus.

BRONCHITIS

Bronchitis is an infection of the bronchi or tubes that carry air to the lungs. It causes a noisy cough, often with mucus or phlegm. Bronchitis is usually caused by a virus, so antibiotics do not generally help. **Use antibiotics only if the bronchitis lasts more than a week** and is not getting better, if the person shows signs of **pneumonia** (see the following page), or if he already has a **chronic lung problem.**

CHRONIC BRONCHITIS:

Signs:

- A cough, with mucus that lasts for months or years. Sometimes the cough gets worse, and there may be fever. A person who has this kind of cough, but does not have another long-term illness such as tuberculosis or asthma, probably has chronic bronchitis.
- It occurs most frequently in older persons who have been heavy smokers.
- It can lead to *emphysema,* a very serious and incurable condition in which the tiny air pockets of the lungs break down. A person with emphysema has a hard time breathing, especially with exercise, and his chest becomes big 'like a barrel'.

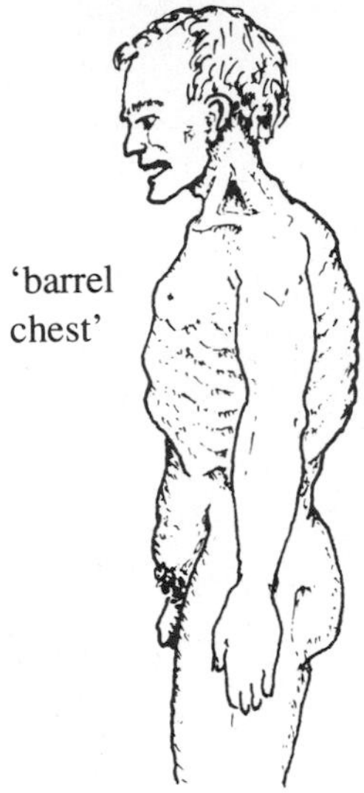

Emphysema can result from chronic asthma, chronic bronchitis, or smoking.

Treatment:

- ♦ Stop smoking.
- ♦ Take an anti-asthma medicine with ephedrine or theophylline (p. 385).
- ♦ Persons with chronic bronchitis should use ampicillin or tetracycline every time they have a cold or 'flu' with a fever.
- ♦ If the person has trouble coughing up sticky phlegm, have him breathe hot water vapors (p. 168) and then help him with postural drainage (see p. 169).

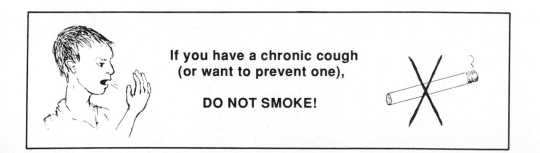

If you have a chronic cough (or want to prevent one),

DO NOT SMOKE!

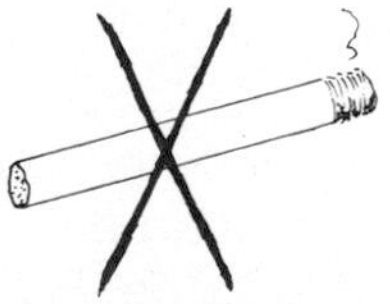

PNEUMONIA

Pneumonia is an *acute* infection of the lungs. It often occurs after another respiratory illness such as measles, whooping cough, flu, bronchitis, asthma—or any very serious illness, especially in babies and old people. Also, persons with AIDS may develop pneumonia.

Signs:

- Sudden chills and then high fever.
- Rapid, shallow breathing, with little grunts or sometimes wheezing. The nostrils may spread with each breath.
- Fever (sometimes newborns and old or very weak persons have severe pneumonia with little or no fever).
- Cough (often with yellow, greenish, rust-colored, or slightly bloody mucus).
- Chest pain (sometimes).
- The person looks very ill.
- Cold sores often appear on the face or lips (p. 232).

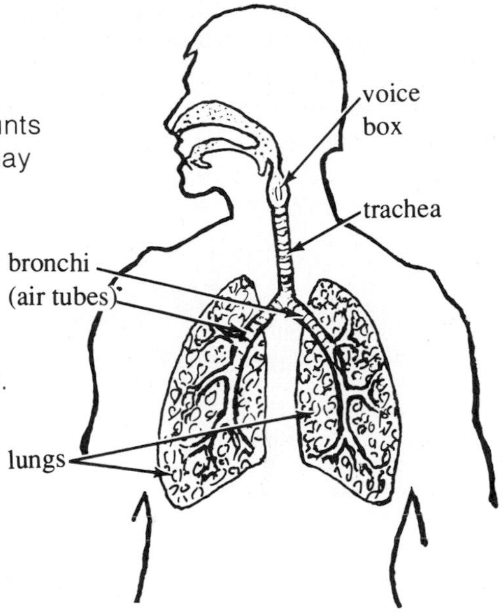

A very sick child who takes more than 50 **shallow** breaths a minute probably has pneumonia.

(If breathing is rapid and **deep,** check for dehydration, p. 151, or hyperventilation, p. 24.)

Treatment:

- For pneumonia, treatment with antibiotics can make the difference between life and death. Give penicillin (p. 351), co-trimoxazole (p. 358), or erythromycin (p. 355). In serious cases, inject procaine penicillin (p. 353), adults: 400,000 units (250 mg.) 2 or 3 times a day, or give ampicillin by mouth (p. 353), 500 mg., 4 times a day. Give small children 1/4 to 1/2 the adult dose. For children under 6, ampicillin is usually best.
- Give aspirin (p. 379) or acetaminophen (p. 380) to lower the temperature and lessen the pain.
- Give plenty of liquids. If the person will not eat, give him liquid foods or Rehydration Drink (see p. 152).
- Ease the cough and loosen the mucus by giving the person plenty of water and having him breathe hot water vapors (see p. 168). Postural drainage may also help (see p. 169).
- If the person is wheezing, an anti-asthma medicine with theophylline or ephedrine may help.

HEPATITIS

Hepatitis is the name for several virus infections (like Hepatitis A, Hepatitis B, Hepatitis C) that harm the liver. Even though in some places people call it 'the fever' (see p. 26), hepatitis often causes little or no rise in temperature.

A person with Hepatitis A or Hepatitis B is often very sick for 2 to 3 weeks, weak for 1 to 4 months after, and then usually gets better. Hepatitis can spread easily from person to person even after the signs of the disease disappear.

Hepatitis A is usually mild in small children and often more serious in older persons and in pregnant women. Hepatitis B is more serious and can lead to permanent scarring of the liver (cirrhosis), liver cancer, and even death. Hepatitis C is also very dangerous and can lead to permanent liver infections. Hepatitis C is a major cause of death for people with HIV/AIDS.

Signs:

- Feels tired. Does not want to eat or smoke. Often goes days without eating anything.
- Sometimes there is a pain on the right side near the liver. Sometimes there is pain in the muscles or joints.

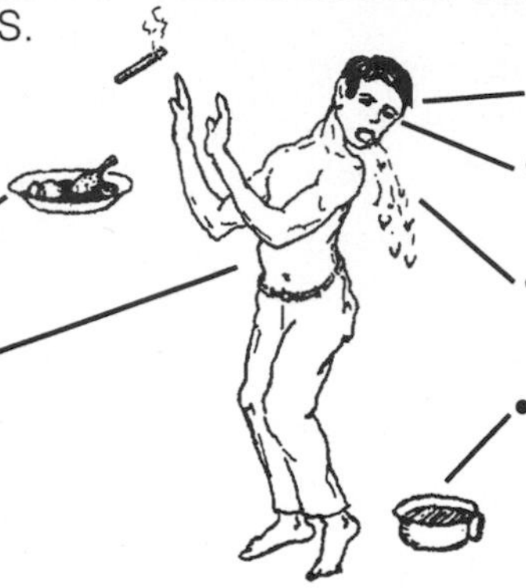

- May have a fever.
- After a few days, the eyes turn yellow.
- Sight or smell of food may cause vomiting.
- The urine may turn dark like Coca-Cola, and the stools may become whitish, or the person may have diarrhea.

Treatment:

- Antibiotics do not work against hepatitis. In fact some medicines will cause added damage to the sick liver. **Do not use medicines.**
- The sick person should rest and drink lots of liquids. If he refuses most food, give him orange juice, papaya, and other fruit plus broth or vegetable soup. It may help to take vitamins. To control vomiting, see p. 161.
- When the sick person can eat, give a balanced meal. Vegetables and fruit are good, with some protein (p. 110 to 111). But do not give a lot of protein (meat, eggs, fish, etc.) because this makes the damaged liver work too hard. Avoid lard and fatty foods. **Do not drink any alcohol** for at least 6 months.

Prevention:

- Small children often have hepatitis without any signs of sickness, but they can spread the disease to others. It is very important that everyone in the house follow all the guidelines of cleanliness with great care (see pages 133 to 139).
- The Hepatitis A virus passes from the stool of one person to the mouth of another by way of contaminated water or food. To prevent others from getting sick, bury the sick person's stools. The sick person, his family and caregivers must try to stay clean and wash their hands often.
- The Hepatitis B and Hepatitis C viruses can pass from person to person through sex, injections with unsterile needles, transfusions of infected blood, and from mother to baby at birth. Take steps to prevent passing hepatitis to others: use a condom during sex (see p. 290), follow the AIDS prevention suggestions on p. 401, and always boil needles and syringes before each use (see p. 74).
- Vaccines now exist for Hepatitis A and Hepatitis B but they may be expensive or not be available everywhere. Hepatitis B is dangerous and there is no cure, so if the vaccine is accessible all children should be vaccinated.

WARNING: Hepatitis can also be transmitted by giving injections with unsterile needles: **Always boil needles and syringes before each use** (see p. 74).

ARTHRITIS (PAINFUL, INFLAMED JOINTS)

Most chronic joint pain, or arthritis, in older people cannot be cured completely. However, the following offer some relief:

- **Rest.** If possible, avoid hard work and heavy exercise that bother the painful joints. If the arthritis causes some fever, it helps to take naps during the day.
- **Place cloths soaked in hot water** on the painful joints (see p. 195).
- **Aspirin** helps relieve pain; the dose for arthritis is higher than that for calming other pain. Adults should take 3 tablets, 4 to 6 times a day. If your ears begin to ring, take less. **To avoid stomach problems caused by aspirin,** always **take it with food, or a large glass of water.** If stomach pain continues, take the aspirin not only with food and lots of water, but also with a spoonful of an antacid such as *Maalox* or *Gelusil.*
- It is important to do simple **exercises** to help maintain or increase the range of motion in the painful joints.

If only one joint is swollen and feels hot, it may be infected—especially if there is fever. Use an antibiotic such as penicillin (see p. 351) and if possible see a health worker.

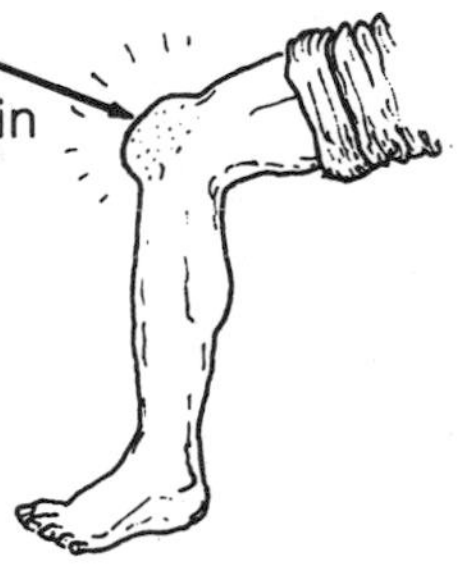

Painful joints in young people and children may be a sign of other serious illness, such as rheumatic fever (p. 310) or tuberculosis (p. 179). For more information on joint pain, see *Disabled Village Children,* Chapters 15 and 16.

BACK PAIN

Back pain has many causes. Here are some:

Chronic upper back pain with cough and weight loss may be TB of the lungs (p. 179).

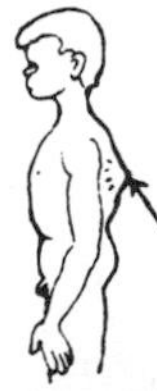

Mid back pain in a child may be TB of the spine, especially if the backbone has a hump or lump.

Low back pain that is worse the day after heavy lifting or straining may be a sprain.

Severe low back pain that first comes suddenly when lifting or twisting may be a *slipped disc,*

especially if one leg or foot becomes painful or numb and weak. This can result from a pinched nerve.

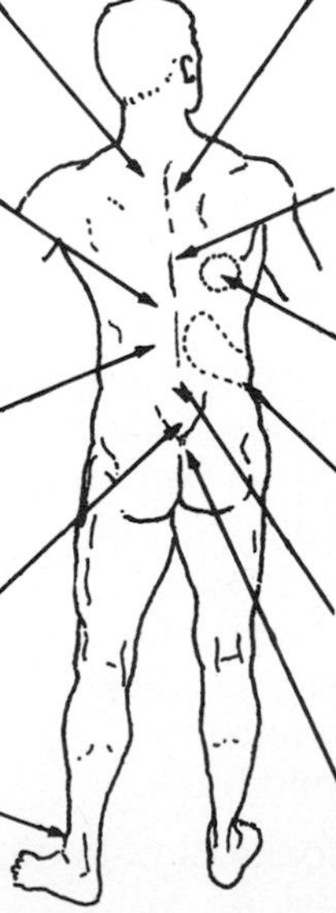

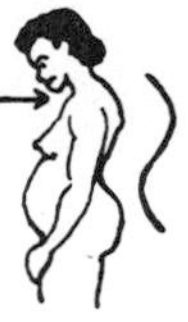

Standing or sitting wrong, with the shoulder drooped, is a common cause of backache.

In older people, chronic back pain is often arthritis.

Pain in the upper right back may be from a gallbladder problem (p. 329).

Acute (or chronic) pain here may be a urinary problem (p. 234).

Low backache is normal for some women during menstrual periods or pregnancy (p. 248).

Very low back pain sometimes comes from problems in the uterus, ovaries, or rectum.

Treatment and prevention of back pain:

- If back pain has a cause like TB, a urinary infection, or gallbladder disease, treat the cause. Seek medical help if you suspect a serious disease.
- Simple backache, including that of pregnancy, can often be prevented or made better by:

always standing straight

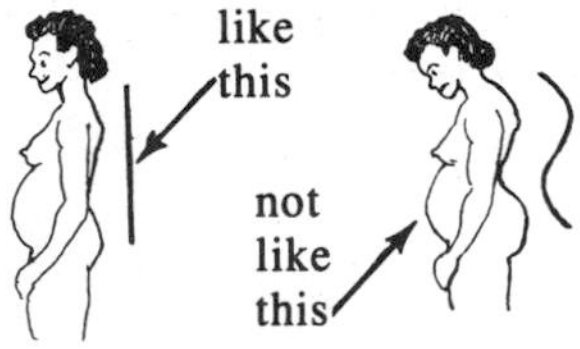

sleeping on a firm flat surface like this

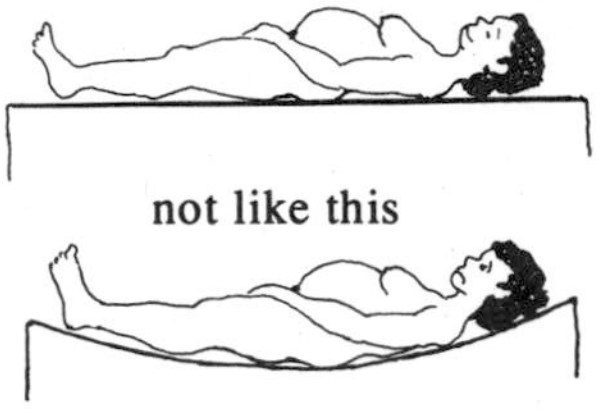

back-bending exercises (done very slowly)

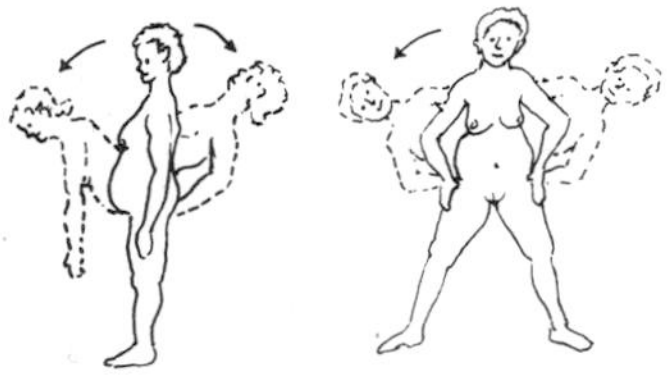

- Aspirin and hot soaks (p. 195) help calm most kinds of back pain.
- For sudden, severe, low back pain that comes from twisting, lifting, bending, or straining, quick relief can sometimes be brought like this:

Have the person lie with one foot tucked under his knee.

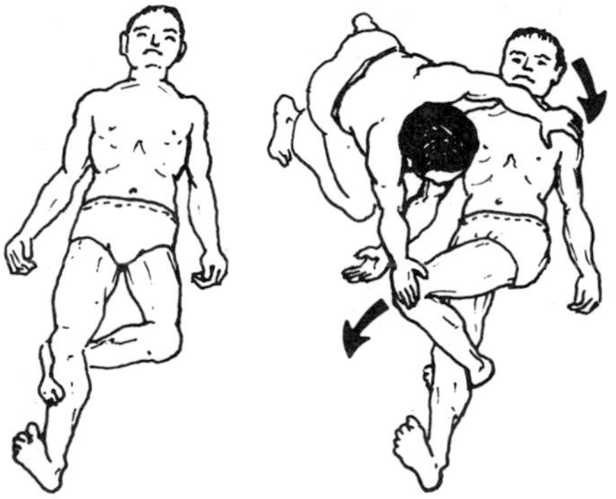

Then, holding this shoulder down,

gently but steadily push this knee over so as to twist the back.

Do this first on one side and then the other.

CAUTION: Do not try this if the back pain is from a fall or injury.

- If back pain from lifting or twisting is sudden and severe with knife-like pain when you bend over, if the pain goes into the leg(s), or if a foot becomes numb or weak, this is serious. A nerve coming from the back may be 'pinched' by a slipped disc (pad between the bones of the back). It is best to rest flat on your back for a few days. It may help to put something firm under the knees and mid back.

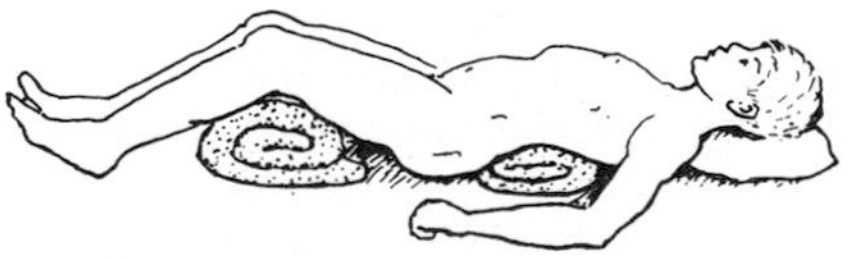

- Take aspirin and use hot soaks. If pain does not begin to get better in a few days, seek medical advice.

VARICOSE VEINS

Varicose veins are veins that are swollen, twisted, and often painful. They are often seen on the legs of older people and of women who are pregnant or who have had many children.

Treatment:

There is no medicine for varicose veins. But the following will help:

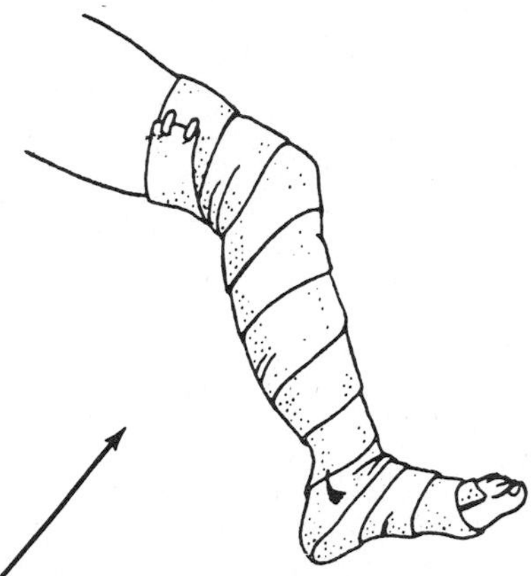

- Do not spend much time standing or sitting with your feet down. If you have no choice but to sit or stand for long periods, try to lie down with your feet up (above the level of the heart) for a few minutes every half hour. When standing, try to walk in place. Or, repeatedly lift your heels off the ground and put them back down. Also, sleep with your feet up (on pillows).
- Use elastic stockings (support hose) or elastic bandages to help hold in the veins. Be sure to take them off at night.
- Taking care of your veins in this way will help prevent chronic sores or ***varicose ulcers*** on the ankles (p. 213).

PILES (HEMORRHOIDS)

Piles or hemorrhoids are varicose veins of the anus or rectum, which feel like little lumps or balls. They may be painful, but are not dangerous. They frequently appear during pregnancy and may go away afterwards.

- Certain bitter plant juices (witch hazel, cactus, etc.) dabbed on hemorrhoids help shrink them. So do hemorrhoid ***suppositories*** (p. 392).
- Sitting in a bath of warm water can help the hemorrhoid heal.
- Piles may be caused in part by constipation. It helps to eat plenty of fruit or food with a lot of fiber, like cassava or bran.
- Very large hemorrhoids may require an operation. Get medical advice.

If a hemorrhoid begins to bleed, the bleeding can sometimes be controlled by pressing with a clean cloth directly on the hemorrhoid. If the bleeding still does not stop, seek medical advice. Or try to control the bleeding by removing the clot that is inside the swollen vein. Tweezers like these can be used after they have been sterilized by boiling.

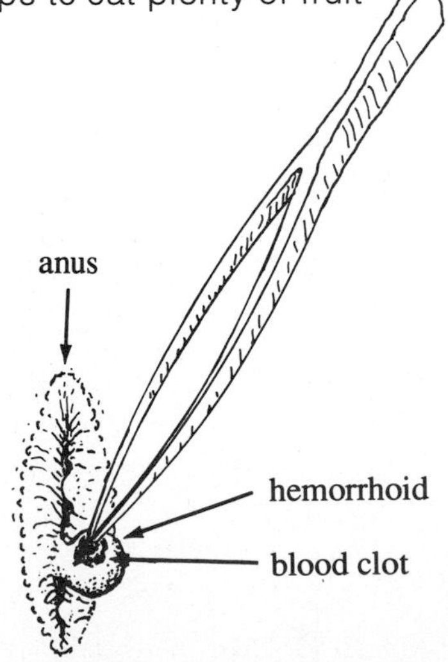

CAUTION: **Do not try to cut the hemorrhoid out.** The person can bleed to death.

SWELLING OF THE FEET AND OTHER PARTS OF THE BODY

Swelling of the feet may be caused by a number of different problems, some minor and others serious. But if the face or other parts of the body are also swollen, this is usually a sign of serious illness.

Women's feet sometimes swell during the last three months of pregnancy. This is usually not serious. It is caused by the weight of the child that presses on the veins coming from the legs in a way that limits the flow of blood. However, if the woman's hands and face also swell, she feels dizzy, has problems seeing, or does not pass much urine, she may be suffering from poisoning or ***toxemia*** of pregnancy (see p. 249). Seek medical help fast.

Old people who spend a lot of time sitting or standing in one place often get swollen feet because of poor circulation. However, swollen feet in older persons may also be due to heart trouble (p. 325) or, less commonly, kidney disease (p. 234).

Swelling of the feet in small children may result from anemia (p. 124) or malnutrition (p. 107). In severe cases the face and hands may also become swollen (see Kwashiorkor, p. 113).

Treatment:

To reduce swelling, treat the sickness that causes it. Use little or no salt in food. Herbal teas that make people urinate a lot usually help (see corn silk, p. 12). Also do the following:

WHEN YOUR FEET ARE SWOLLEN:

Do not spend time sitting with your feet down. This makes them swell more.

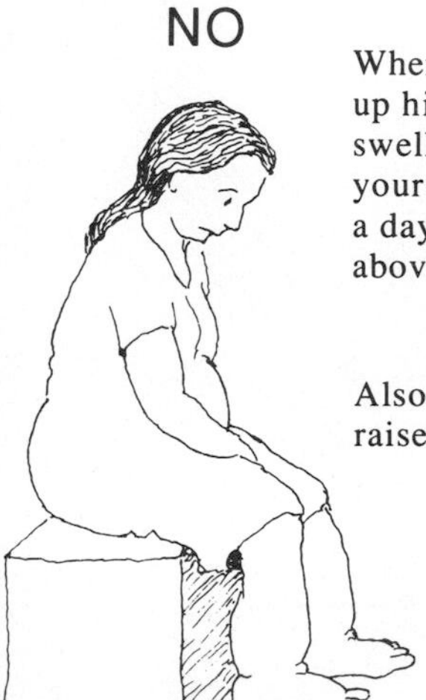

When you sit, put your feet up high. This way the swelling becomes less. Put your feet up several times a day. Your feet should be above the level of your heart.

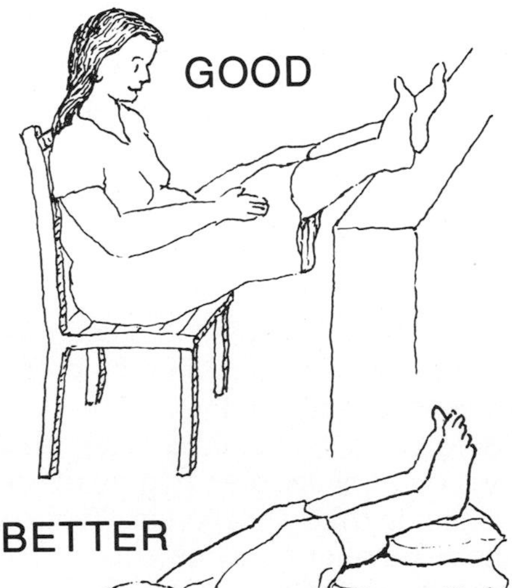

Also sleep with your feet raised.

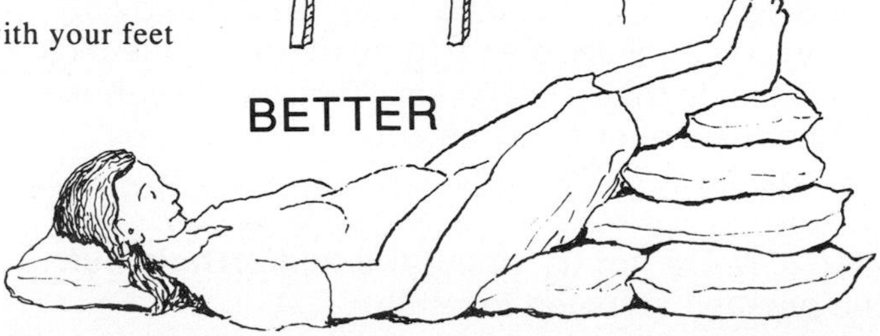

HERNIA (RUPTURE)

A hernia is an opening or tear in the muscles covering the belly. This permits a loop of gut to push through and form a lump under the skin. Hernias usually come from lifting something heavy, or straining (as during childbirth). Some babies are born with a hernia (see p. 317). In men, hernias are common in the groin. Swollen lymph nodes (p. 88) may also cause lumps in the groin. However . . .

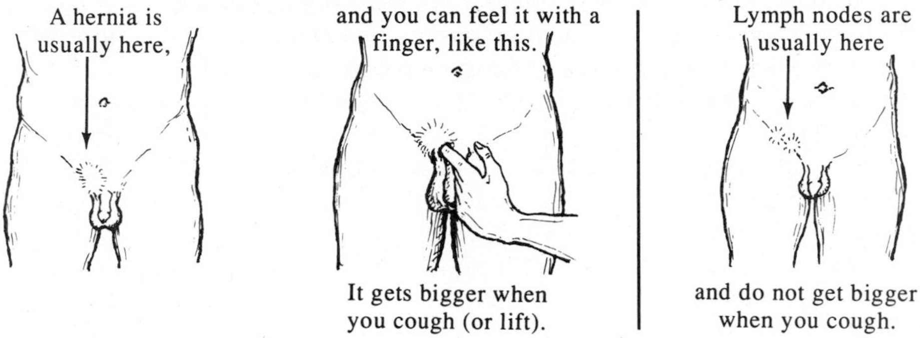

A hernia is usually here,
and you can feel it with a finger, like this.
It gets bigger when you cough (or lift).
Lymph nodes are usually here
and do not get bigger when you cough.

How to prevent a hernia:

Lift heavy things like this

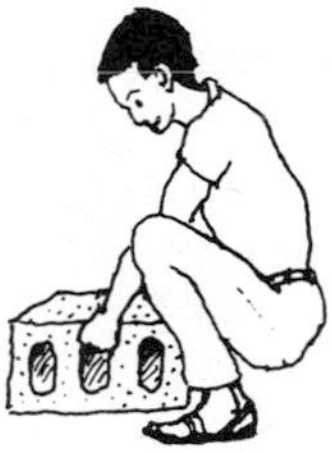

not like this.

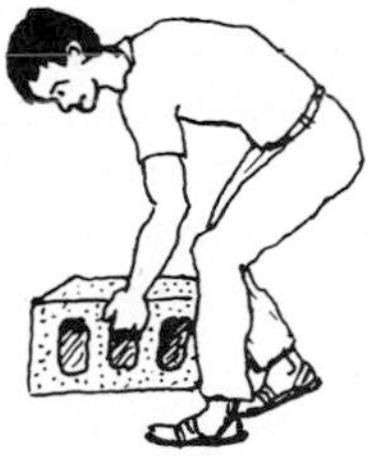

How to live with a hernia:

- Avoid lifting heavy objects.
- Make a truss to hold the hernia in.

PLAN FOR A SIMPLE TRUSS:

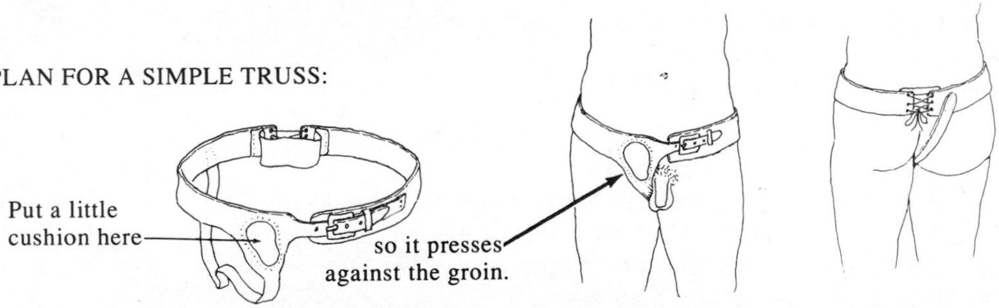

Put a little cushion here
so it presses against the groin.

CAUTION: If a hernia suddenly becomes large or painful, try to make it go back in by lying with the feet higher than the head and pressing gently on the bulge. If it will not go back, seek medical help.

If the hernia becomes very painful and causes vomiting, and the person cannot have a bowel movement, this can be very dangerous. Surgery may be necessary. Seek medical help fast. In the meantime, treat as for Appendicitis (p. 95).

FITS (CONVULSIONS)

We say a person has a fit when he suddenly loses consciousness and makes strange, jerking movements (convulsions). Fits come from a problem in the brain. In small children common causes of fits are **high fever** and **severe dehydration.** In very ill persons, the cause may be **meningitis, malaria of the brain,** or **poisoning.** A person who often has fits may have **epilepsy.**

- Try to figure out the cause of a fit and treat it, if possible.
- If the child has a high fever, lower it at once with cool water (see p. 76).
- If the child is dehydrated, give an enema of Rehydration Drink **slowly.** Send for medical help. Give nothing by mouth during a fit.
- If there are signs of meningitis (p. 185), begin treatment at once and seek medical help.
- If you suspect cerebral malaria, inject a malaria medicine (see p. 367).

EPILEPSY

Epilepsy causes fits in people who otherwise seem fairly healthy. Fits may come hours, days, weeks, or months apart. In some persons they cause loss of consciousness and violent movements. The eyes often roll back. In mild types of epilepsy the person may suddenly 'blank out' a moment, make strange movements, or behave oddly. Epilepsy is more common in some families (inherited). Or it may come from brain damage at birth, high fever in infancy, or tapeworm cysts in the brain (p. 143). Epilepsy is not an infection and cannot be 'caught'. It is often a life-long problem. However, babies sometimes get over it.

Medicines to prevent epileptic fits:

Note: These do not 'cure' epilepsy; they help prevent fits. Often the medicine must be taken for life.

- Phenobarbital often controls epilepsy. It costs little (see p. 389).
- Phenytoin may work when phenobarbital does not. Use the lowest possible dose that prevents fits (see p. 390).

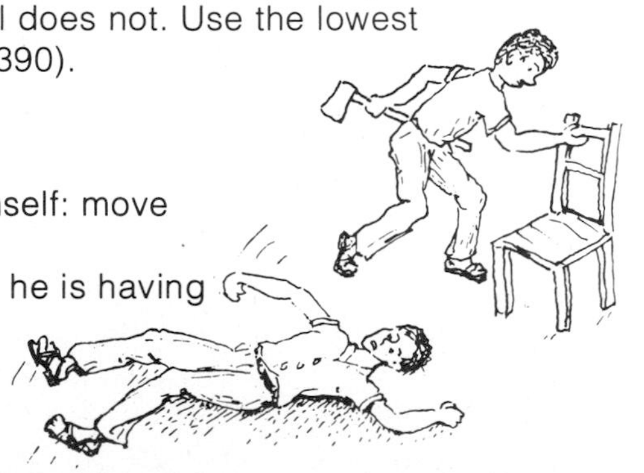

When a person is having a fit:

- Try to keep the person from hurting himself: move away all hard or sharp objects.
- Put nothing in the person's mouth while he is having a fit—no food, drink, medicine, nor any object to prevent biting the tongue.
- After the fit the person may be dull and sleepy. Let him sleep.
- If fits last a long time, inject phenobarbital or phenytoin. For dosages see p. 389 to 390. If the fit still has not stopped after 15 minutes, give a second dose. Or if someone knows how, inject IV diazepam (*Valium,* p. 391) or phenobarbital into the vein. Liquid or injectable medicine can be put up the rectum with a plastic syringe without a needle. Or grind up a pill of diazepam or phenobarbital, mix with water, and put it up the rectum.

For more information on fits, see *Disabled Village Children,* Chapter 29.

CHAPTER 14

SERIOUS ILLNESSES THAT NEED SPECIAL MEDICAL ATTENTION

The diseases covered in this chapter are often difficult or impossible to cure without medical help. Many need special medicines that are difficult to get in rural areas. Home remedies will not cure them. If a person has one of these illnesses, *THE SOONER HE GETS MEDICAL HELP, THE BETTER HIS CHANCE OF GETTING WELL.*

CAUTION: Many of the illnesses covered in other chapters may also be serious and require medical assistance. See the **Signs of Dangerous Illness**, p. 42.

TUBERCULOSIS (TB, CONSUMPTION)

Tuberculosis of the lungs is a ***chronic*** (long-lasting), ***contagious*** (easily spread) disease that anyone can get. But it often strikes persons between 15 and 35 years of age—especially those who have AIDS (p. 399), or who are weak, poorly nourished, or live with someone who has TB.

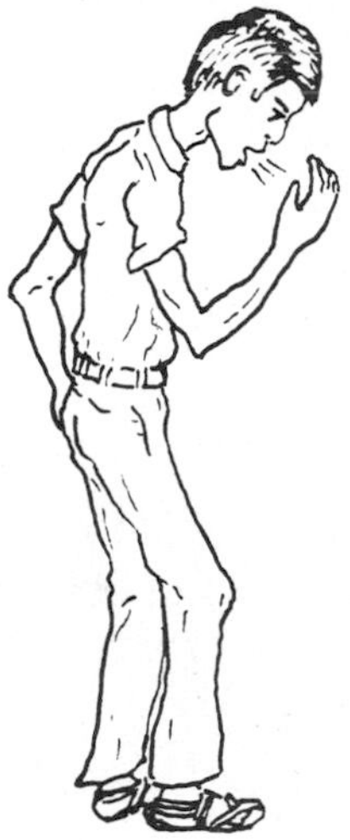

Tuberculosis is curable. Yet thousands die needlessly from this disease every year. Both for prevention and cure, it is very important to **treat tuberculosis early. Be on the lookout for the signs of tuberculosis.** A person may have some or all of them.

Most frequent signs of TB:

- A cough that lasts longer than 3 weeks, often worse just after waking up.
- There may be pain in the chest or upper back.
- Chronic loss of weight and increasing weakness.

In serious or advanced cases:

- Coughing up blood (usually a little, but in some cases a lot).
- Pale, waxy skin. The skin of a dark-skinned person tends to get lighter, especially the face.
- Voice grows hoarse (very serious).

In young children: The cough may come late. Instead, look for:

- Steady weight loss.
- Frequent fever.
- Lighter skin color.
- Swellings in the neck (lymph nodes), or the belly (p. 20).

Tuberculosis is usually only in the lungs. But it can affect any part of the body. In young children it may cause meningitis (see p. 185). For skin problems from TB, see p. 212.

If you think you might have tuberculosis: Seek medical help. At the first sign of tuberculosis, go to a health center where the workers can examine you, and test the stuff you cough up (***phlegm*** or ***sputum***) to see if you have TB or not. Many governments give TB medicines free. Ask at the nearest health center. You will probably be given some of the following medicines:

- Isoniazid (INH) pills (p. 361)
- Rifampin pills (p. 362)
- Pyrazinamide pills (p. 362)
- Ethambutol pills (p. 362)
- Streptomycin injections (p. 363)
- Thiacetazone pills (p. 363)

It is very important to take the medicines as directed. Treatments may be different in different countries, but usually the treatment has 2 parts. You will take 3 or 4 medicines for 2 months and then test your sputum. If you are getting better, you will take 2 medicines for another 4 to 6 months. Then you will be tested again to make sure you are cured. **Do not stop taking the medicines just because you feel better.** This can lead to the illness coming back, infecting other people, and drug ***resistance***. **To cure TB completely can take from 6 months to more than a year.**

Eat as well as possible: plenty of energy foods and also foods rich in proteins and vitamins (p. 110 to 111). Rest is important. If possible, stop working and take it easy until you begin to get better. From then on, try not to work so hard that you become tired or breathe with difficulty. Try to always get enough rest and sleep.

Tuberculosis in any other part of the body is treated the same as TB of the lungs. This includes TB in the glands of the neck, TB of the abdomen (see picture on p. 20), TB of the skin (see p. 212), and TB of a joint (like the knee). A child with severe TB of the backbone may also need surgery to prevent paralysis (see *Disabled Village Children,* Chapter 21).

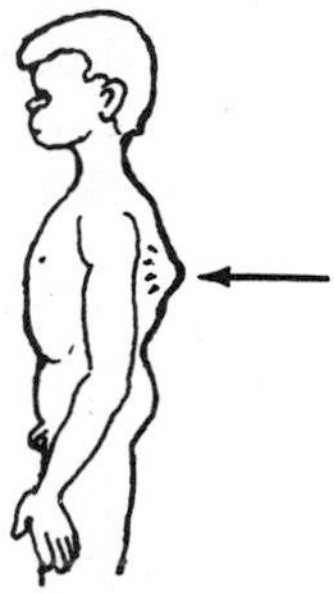

TB of
the backbone

Tuberculosis is very contagious. Persons (especially children) who live with someone who has TB, run a great risk of catching the disease.

If someone in the house has TB:

- If possible, see that the whole family is tested for TB (Tuberculin test).
- Have the children vaccinated against TB with B.C.G. vaccine.
- Everyone, especially the children, should eat plenty of nutritious food.
- The person with TB should eat and sleep separately from the children, if possible in a different room, as long as he has any cough at all.
- Also, ask him to cover his mouth when coughing and not spit on the floor.
- Watch for weight loss and other signs of TB in members of the family. If possible, weigh each person, especially the children, once a month, until the danger is past.

TB in family members often starts very slowly and quietly. If anyone in the family shows signs of TB, have tests done and **begin treatment at once.**

Early and full treatment is a key part of prevention.

RABIES

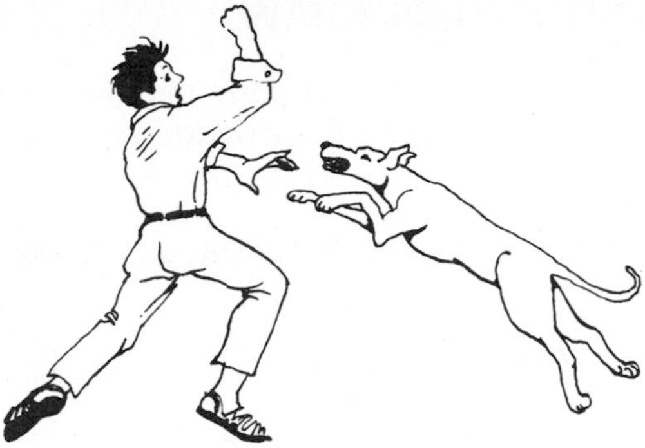

Rabies comes from the bite of a rabid or 'mad' animal, usually a rabid dog, cat, fox, wolf, skunk, or jackal. Bats and other animals may also spread rabies.

Signs of rabies:

In the animal:

- Acts strangely—sometimes sad, restless, or irritable.
- Foaming at the mouth, cannot eat or drink.
- Sometimes the animal goes wild (mad) and may bite anyone or anything nearby.
- The animal dies within 5 to 7 days.

Signs in people:

- Pain and tingling in the area of the bite.
- Irregular breathing, as if the person has just been crying.
- Pain and difficulty swallowing. A lot of thick, sticky saliva.
- The person is alert, but very nervous or excitable. Fits of anger can occur.
- As death nears, fits (convulsions) and paralysis.

If you have any reason to believe an animal that has bitten someone has rabies:

- ♦ Tie or cage the animal for a week.
- ♦ Clean the bite well with soap, water, and hydrogen peroxide. Do not close the wound; leave it open.
- ♦ If the animal dies before the week is up (or if it was killed or cannot be caught), take the bitten person at once to a health center where he can be given a series of anti-rabies injections.

The first symptoms of rabies appear from 10 days up to 2 years after the bite (usually within 3 to 7 weeks). Treatment must begin before the first signs of the sickness appear. Once the sickness begins, no treatment known to medical science can save the person's life.

Prevention:

- ♦ Kill and bury (or cage for one week) any animal suspected of having rabies.
- ♦ Cooperate with programs to vaccinate dogs.
- ♦ Keep children far away from any animal that seems sick or acts strangely.

Take great care in handling any animal that seems sick or acts strangely. Even if it does not bite anyone, its saliva can cause rabies if it gets into a cut or scratch.

TETANUS (LOCKJAW)

Tetanus results when a germ that lives in the feces of animals or people enters the body through a wound. Deep or dirty wounds are especially dangerous.

WOUNDS VERY LIKELY TO CAUSE TETANUS

animal bites, especially those of dogs and pigs

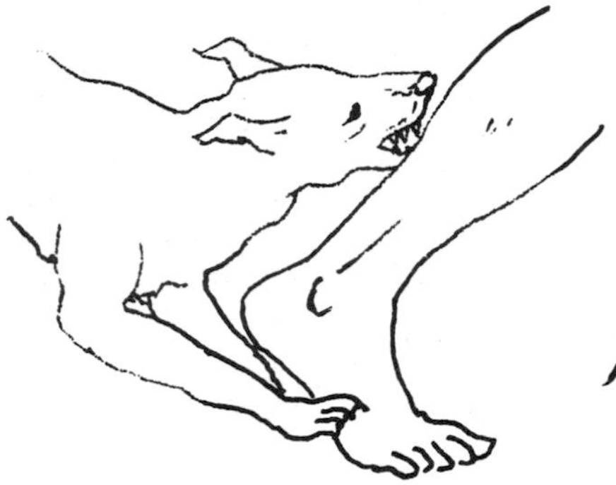

gunshot and knife wounds

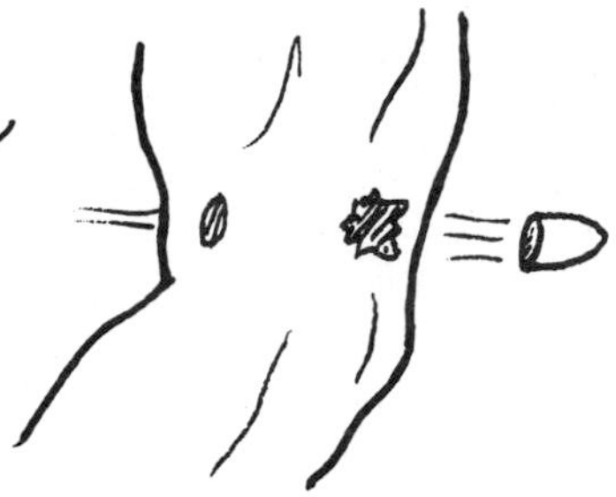

holes made with dirty needles

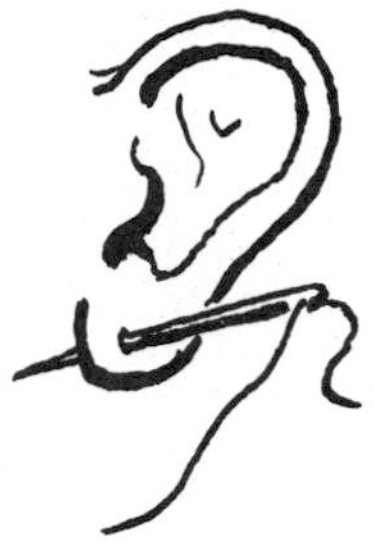

injuries caused by barbed wire

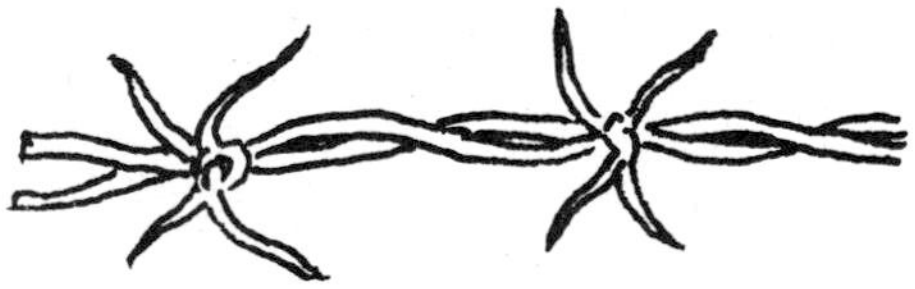

puncture wounds from thorns, splinters, or nails

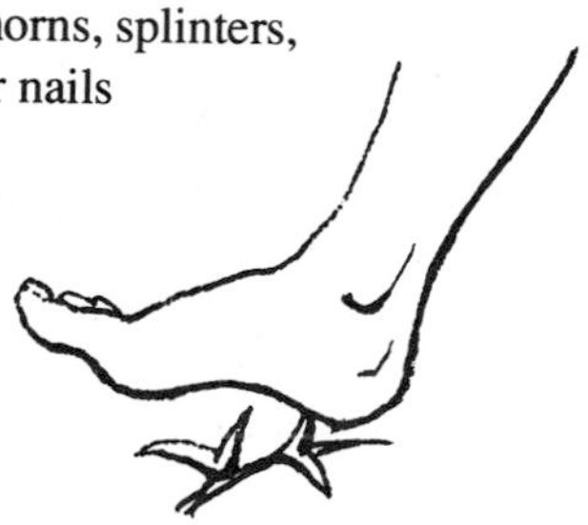

CAUSES OF TETANUS IN THE NEWBORN CHILD

Tetanus germs enter through the *umbilical cord* of a newborn baby because of lack of cleanliness or failure to take other simple precautions. The chance of tetanus is greater . . .

- when the cord has been cut with an instrument that has not been boiled and kept completely clean or
- when the cord has not been cut **close** to the body (see p. 262) or
- when the newly cut cord is tightly covered or is not kept dry.

WHEN THE CORD IS CUT A LONG WAY FROM THE BODY, LIKE THIS, THE CHANCE OF TETANUS IS GREATER.

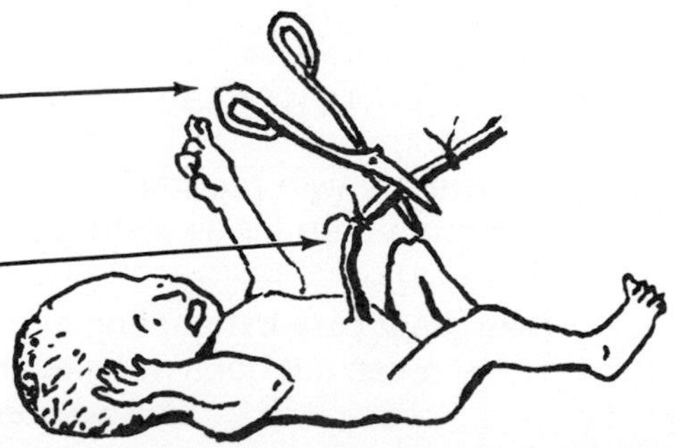

Signs of tetanus:

- An infected wound (sometimes no wound can be found).
- Discomfort and difficulty in swallowing.
- The jaw gets stiff (lockjaw), then the muscles of the neck and other parts of the body. The person has difficulty walking normally.
- Painful ***convulsions*** (sudden tightening) of the jaw and finally of the whole body. Moving or touching the person may trigger sudden ***spasms*** like this:

Sudden noise or bright light may also bring on these spasms.

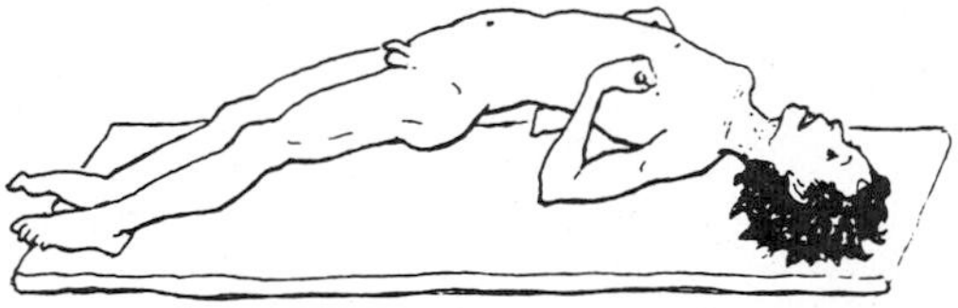

In the newborn, the first signs of tetanus generally appear 3 to 10 days after birth. The child begins to cry continuously and is **unable to suck.** Often the umbilical area is dirty or infected. After several hours or days, lockjaw and the other signs of tetanus begin.

It is very important to start treating tetanus at the first sign. If you suspect tetanus (or if a newborn child cries continuously or stops nursing), make this test:

TEST OF KNEE REFLEXES

With the leg hanging freely, tap the knee with a knuckle just below the kneecap.

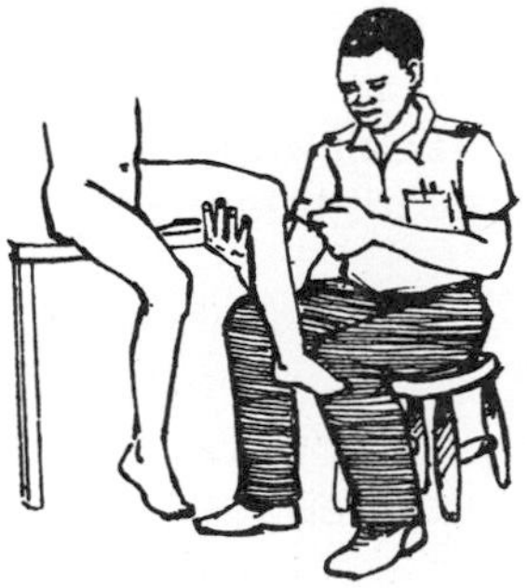

If the leg jumps just a little bit, the reaction is normal.

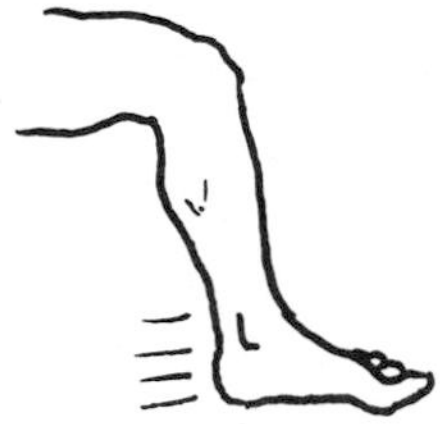

If the leg jumps high, this indicates a serious illness like tetanus (or perhaps meningitis or poisoning with certain medicines or rat poison).

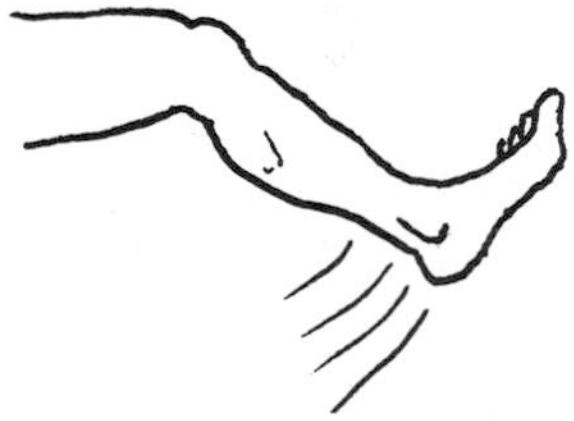

This test is especially useful when you suspect tetanus in a newborn baby.

What to do when there are signs of tetanus:

Tetanus is a deadly disease. Seek medical help at the first sign. If there is any delay in getting help, do the following things:

- Examine the whole body for infected wounds or sores. Often the wound will contain pus. Open the wound and wash it with soap and cool, boiled water; completely remove all dirt, pus, thorns, splinters, etc.; flood the wound with hydrogen peroxide if you have any.

(continued on the next page)

What to do when there are signs of tetanus: (continued)

- Inject 1 million units of procaine penicillin at once and repeat every 12 hours (p. 353). (For newborn babies crystalline penicillin is better.) If there is no penicillin, use another antibiotic, like tetracycline.
- If you can get it, inject 5,000 units of **Human Immune Globulin** or 40,000 to 50,000 units of **Tetanus Antitoxin.** Be sure to follow all the precautions (see p. 70 and 389). Human Immune Globulin has less risk of severe allergic reaction, but may be more expensive and harder to obtain.
- As long as the person can swallow, give nutritious liquids in frequent, small sips.
- To control convulsions, inject phenobarbital (for the dose, see p. 390) or diazepam (*Valium,* p. 390), adults: 10 to 20 mg. to start with, and more as necessary.
- Touch and move the person as little as possible. Avoid noise and bright light.
- If necessary, use a *catheter* (rubber tube) connected to a syringe to suck the mucus from the nose and throat. This helps clear the airway.
- For the newborn with tetanus, if possible, have a health worker or doctor put in a nose-to-stomach tube and feed the baby the mother's breast milk. This provides needed nutrition and fights infection.

How to prevent tetanus:

Even in the best hospitals, half the people with tetanus die. It is much easier to prevent tetanus than to treat it.

- **Vaccination:** This is the surest protection against tetanus. Both children and adults should be vaccinated. Vaccinate your whole family at the nearest health center (see p. 147). For complete protection, the vaccination should be repeated once every 10 years. **Vaccinating women against tetanus each time they are pregnant will prevent tetanus in newborn infants** (see p. 250).
- When you have a wound, especially a dirty or deep wound, clean and take care of it in the manner described on page 89.
- If the wound is very big, deep, or dirty, seek medical help. If you have not been vaccinated against tetanus, take penicillin. Also consider getting an injection of an antitoxin for tetanus (see p. 389).
- In newborn babies, cleanliness is very important to prevent tetanus. The instrument used to cut the umbilical cord should be sterilized (p. 262); the cord should be cut short, and the umbilical area kept clean and dry.

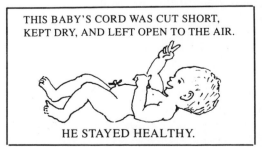

THIS BABY'S CORD WAS CUT SHORT, KEPT DRY, AND LEFT OPEN TO THE AIR.

HE STAYED HEALTHY.

THIS BABY'S CORD WAS LEFT LONG, KEPT TIGHTLY COVERED, AND NOT KEPT DRY.

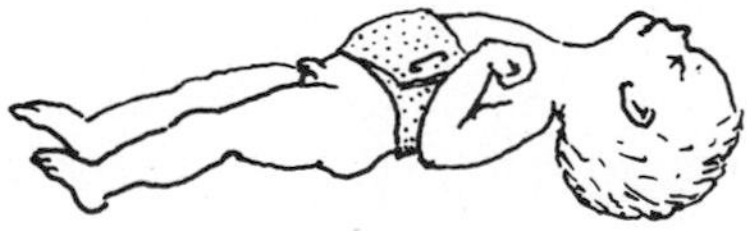

HE DIED OF TETANUS.

MENINGITIS

This is a very serious infection of the brain, more common in children. It may begin as a *complication* of another illness, such as measles, mumps, whooping cough, or an ear infection. Children of mothers who have tuberculosis sometimes get tubercular meningitis in the first few months of life.

Signs:

- Fever.
- Severe headache.
- Stiff neck. The child looks very ill, and lies with his head and neck bent back, like this:

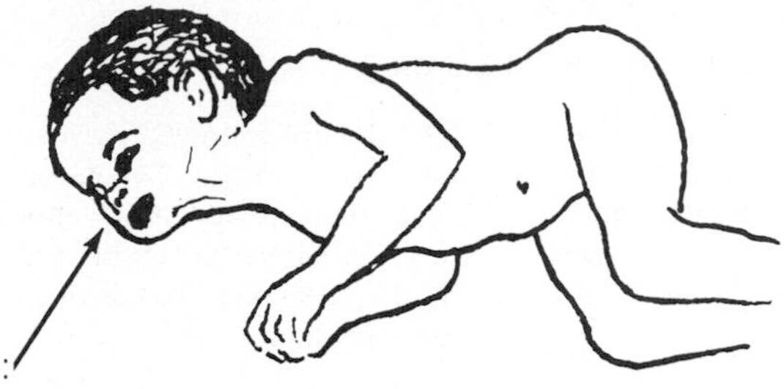

- The back is too stiff to put the head between the knees.
- In babies under a year old: the fontanel (soft spot on top of the head) bulges out.
- Vomiting is common.
- In babies and young children, early meningitis may be hard to recognize. The child may cry in a strange way (the 'meningitis cry'), even when the mother puts the child on her breast. Or the child may become very sleepy.
- Sometimes there are fits (convulsions) or strange movements.
- The child often gets worse and worse and only becomes quiet when he loses consciousness completely.
- Tubercular meningitis develops slowly, over days or weeks. Other forms of meningitis come on more quickly, in hours or days.

Treatment:

Get medical help fast—every minute counts! If possible take the person to a hospital. Meanwhile:

- ♦ Inject ampicillin, 500 mg. every 4 hours (see p. 353). Or inject crystalline penicillin, 1,000,000 U. every 4 hours (see p. 353). If possible, also give chloramphenicol (see p. 357).
- ♦ If there is high fever (more than 40°), lower it with wet cloths and acetaminophen or aspirin (see p. 379 to 380).
- ♦ If the mother has tuberculosis or if you have any other reason to suspect that the child has tubercular meningitis, inject him with 0.2 ml. of streptomycin for each 5 kilos he weighs and get medical help at once. Also, use ampicillin or penicillin in case the meningitis is not from TB.

Prevention:

For prevention of tubercular meningitis, newborn babies of mothers with tuberculosis should be vaccinated with B.C.G. at birth. Dose for the newborn is 0.05 ml. (half the normal dose of 0.1 ml.). For other suggestions on prevention of TB, see pages 179 to 180.

MALARIA

Malaria is an infection of the blood that causes chills and high fever. Malaria is spread by mosquitos. The mosquito sucks up the malaria parasites in the blood of an infected person and injects them into the next person it bites.

Signs of malaria:

- The typical attack has 3 stages:

1. It begins with chills—and often headache. The person shivers or shakes for 15 minutes to an hour.

2. Chills are followed by fever, often 40° or more. The person is weak, flushed (red skin), and at times delirious (not in his right mind). The fever lasts several hours or days.

3. Finally the person begins to sweat, and his temperature goes down. After an attack, the person feels weak, but may feel more or less OK.

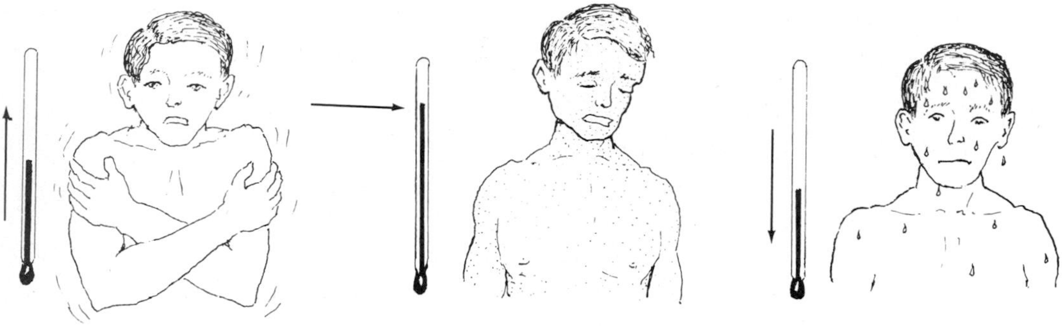

- Usually malaria causes fevers every 2 or 3 days (depending on the kind of malaria), but in the beginning it may cause fever daily. Also, the fever pattern may not be regular or typical. For this reason anyone who suffers from unexplained fevers should have his blood tested for malaria.
- Chronic malaria often causes a large ***spleen*** and anemia (see p. 124).
- In young children, anemia and paleness can begin within a day or two. In children with malaria affecting the brain (cerebral malaria), fits may be followed by periods of unconsciousness. Also, the palms may show a blue-gray color, and breathing may be rapid and deep. (***Note:*** Children who have not been breast fed are more likely to get malaria.)

Analysis and treatment:

- ♦ If you suspect malaria or have repeated fevers, if possible go to a health center for a blood test. In areas where an especially dangerous type of malaria called ***falciparum*** occurs, seek treatment immediately.
- ♦ In areas where malaria is common, treat any unexplained high fever as malaria. Take the malaria medicine known to work best in your area. (See pages 365 to 368 for dosages and information on malaria medicines.)
- ♦ If you get better with the medicine, but after several days the fevers start again, you may need another medicine. Get advice from the nearest health center.
- ♦ If a person who possibly has malaria begins to have fits or other signs of meningitis (p. 185) he may have ***cerebral*** malaria. If possible, inject malaria medicine at once (see p. 367).

HOW TO AVOID MALARIA (AND DENGUE)

Malaria occurs more often during hot, rainy seasons. If everyone cooperates, it can be controlled. All these control measures should be practiced at once.

1. Avoid mosquitos. Sleep where there are no mosquitos or underneath a bed net treated with insecticide or under a sheet. Cover the baby's cradle with treated mosquito netting or a thin cloth.

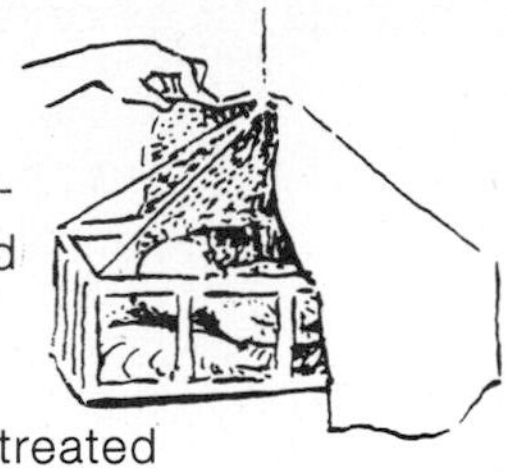

2. Cooperate with the malaria control workers when they come to your village. Tell them if anyone in the family has had fevers and let them take blood for testing.

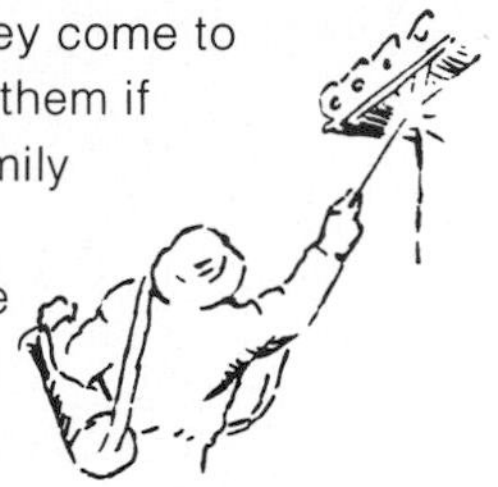

3. If you suspect malaria, get treatment quickly. After you have been treated, mosquitos that bite you will not pass malaria on to others.

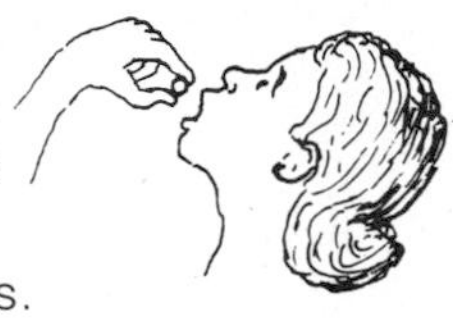

4. Destroy mosquitos and their young. Mosquitos breed in water that is not flowing. Clear ponds, pits, old cans, or broken pots that collect water. Drain or put a little oil on pools or marshes where mosquitos breed. Fill the tops of bamboo posts with sand.

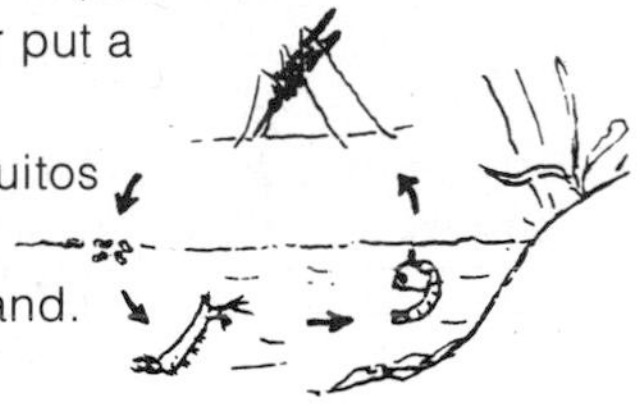

5. Malaria can also be prevented, or its effects greatly reduced, by taking anti-malaria medicines on a regular schedule. See pages 365 to 368.

DENGUE (BREAKBONE FEVER, DANDY FEVER)

This illness is sometimes confused with malaria. It is caused by a virus that is spread by mosquitos. In recent years it has become much more common in many countries. It often occurs in epidemics (many persons get it at the same time), usually during the hot, rainy season. A person can get dengue more than once. Repeat illnesses are often worse. ***To prevent dengue,*** control mosquitos and protect against their bites, as described above.

Signs:

- Sudden high fever with chills.
- Severe body aches, headache, sore throat.
- Person feels very ill, weak, miserable.
- After 3 to 4 days person feels better for a few hours to 2 days.
- Then illness returns for 1 or 2 days, often with a rash that begins on hands and feet.
- The rash then spreads to arms, legs, and finally the body (usually not the face).
- In Southeast Asia, a severe form of dengue may cause bleeding into the skin (small dark spots), or dangerous bleeding inside the body.

Treatment:

- ♦ No medicine cures it, but the illness goes away by itself in a few days.
- ♦ Rest, lots of liquids, acetaminophen (but **not** aspirin) for fever and pain.
- ♦ In case of severe bleeding, treat for shock, if necessary (see p. 77).

BRUCELLOSIS (UNDULANT FEVER, MALTA FEVER)

This is a disease that comes from drinking fresh milk from infected cows or goats. It may also enter the body through scrapes or wounds in the skin of persons who work with sick cattle, goats, or pigs, or by breathing it into the lungs.

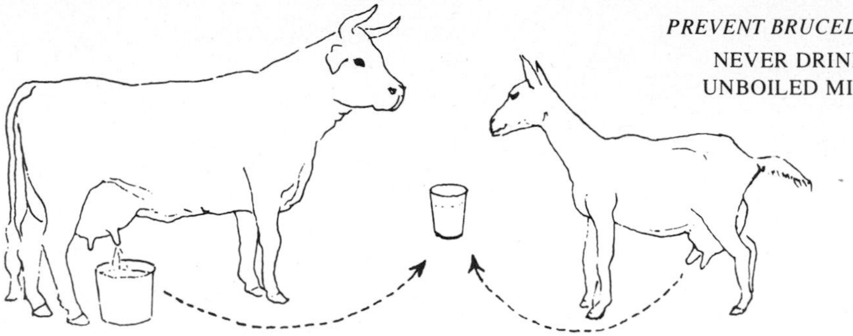
PREVENT BRUCELLOSIS:
NEVER DRINK
UNBOILED MILK

Signs:

- Brucellosis may start with fever and chills, but it often begins very gradually, with increasing tiredness, weakness, loss of appetite, headache, stomach-ache, and sometimes joint pains.
- The fevers may be mild or severe. Typically, these begin with afternoon chills and end with sweating in the early morning. In chronic brucellosis, the fevers may stop for several days and then return. Without treatment, brucellosis may last for years.
- There may be swollen lymph nodes in the neck, armpits, and groin (p. 88).

Treatment:

- If you suspect brucellosis, get medical advice, because it is easy to confuse this disease with others, and the treatment is long and expensive.
- Treat with tetracycline, adults: two 250 mg. capsules 4 times a day for 3 weeks. For precautions, see page 356. Or use co-trimoxazole. (For dosage and precautions, see p. 358.)

Prevention:

- **Drink only cow's or goat's milk that has been boiled or pasteurized.** In areas where brucellosis is a problem, it is safer not to eat cheese made from unboiled milk.
- Be careful when handling cattle, goats, and pigs, especially if you have any cuts or scrapes.
- Cooperate with livestock inspectors who check to be sure your animals are healthy.

TYPHOID FEVER

Typhoid is an infection of the gut that affects the whole body. It is spread from *feces-to-mouth* in contaminated food and water and often comes in *epidemics* (many people sick at once). Of the different infections sometimes called 'the fever' (see p. 26), typhoid is one of the most dangerous.

Signs of typhoid:

First week:

- It begins like a cold or flu.
- Headache, sore throat, and often a dry cough.
- The fever goes up and down, but rises a little more each day until it reaches 40°or more.
- Pulse is often relatively slow for the amount of fever present. Take the pulse and temperature every half hour. **If the pulse gets slower when the fever goes up, the person probably has typhoid** (see p. 26).
- Sometimes there is vomiting, diarrhea, or constipation.

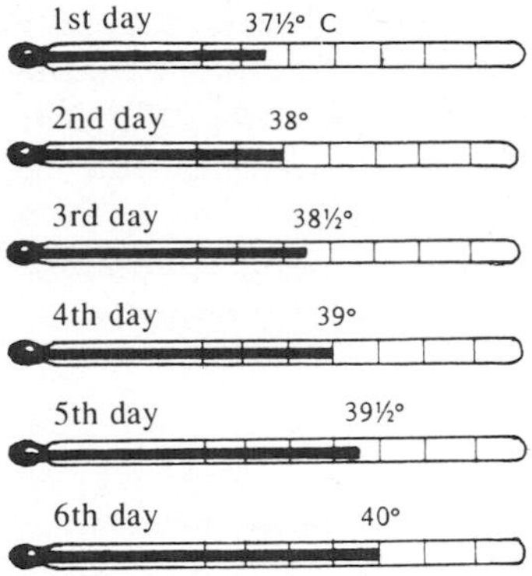

Second week:

- High fever, pulse relatively slow.
- A few pink spots may appear on the body.
- Trembling.
- Delirium (person does not think clearly or make sense).
- Weakness, weight loss, dehydration.

Third week:

- If there are no complications, the fever and other symptoms slowly go away.

Treatment:

- Seek medical help.
- In areas where typhoid has become resistant to chloramphenicol and ampicillin, give co-trimoxazole (p. 358) for at least 2 weeks.
- Or, try chloramphenicol (see p. 357), adults: 3 capsules of 250 mg. 4 times a day for at least 2 weeks. If there is no chloramphenicol, use ampicillin (p. 353) or tetracycline (p. 356).
- Lower the fever with cool wet cloths (see p. 76).
- Give plenty of liquids: soups, juices, and Rehydration Drink to avoid dehydration (see p. 152).
- Give nutritious foods, in liquid form if necessary.
- The person should stay in bed until the fever is completely gone.
- If the person shits blood or develops signs of peritonitis (p. 94) or pneumonia (p. 171), take her to a hospital at once.

Prevention:

- To prevent typhoid, care must be taken to avoid contamination of water and food by human feces. Follow the guidelines of personal and public hygiene in Chapter 12. Make and use latrines. Be sure latrines are a safe distance from where people get drinking water.
- Cases of typhoid often appear after a flood or other disaster, and special care must be taken with cleanliness at these times. Be sure drinking water is clean. If there are cases of typhoid in your village, all drinking water should be boiled. Look for the cause of contaminated water or food.

(Continued on the next page)

Prevention of typhoid: (continued)

- To avoid the spread of typhoid, a person who has the disease should stay in a separate room. No one else should eat or drink from the dishes he uses. His stools should be burned or buried in deep holes. Persons who care for him should wash their hands right afterwards.
- After recovering from typhoid, some persons still carry the disease and can spread it to others. So anyone who has had typhoid should be extra careful with personal cleanliness and should not work in restaurants or where food is handled. Sometimes ampicillin is effective in treating typhoid carriers.

TYPHUS

Typhus is an illness similar to but different from typhoid. The infection is transmitted by bites of:

lice 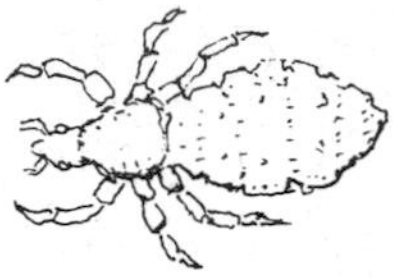

ticks 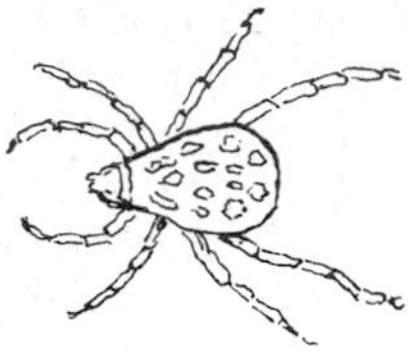

rat fleas 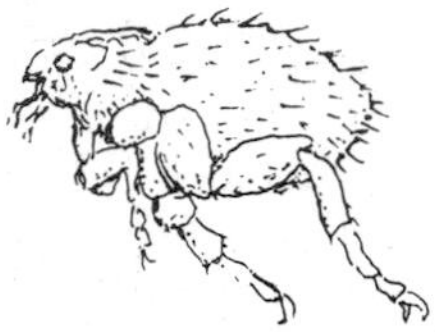

Signs:

- Typhus begins like a bad cold. After a week or more fever begins, with chills, headache, and pain in the muscles and chest.
- After a few days of fever a typical rash appears, first in the armpits and then on the body, then the arms and legs (but not on the face, palms of the hands, or soles of the feet). The rash looks like many tiny bruises.
- The fever lasts 2 weeks or more. Typhus is usually mild in children and very severe in old people. An epidemic form of typhus is especially dangerous.
- In typhus spread by ticks, there is often a large painful sore at the point of the bite, and the lymph nodes near the bite are swollen and painful.

Treatment:

- If you think someone may have typhus, get medical advice. Special tests are often needed.
- Give tetracycline, adults: 2 capsules of 250 mg., 4 times a day for 7 days (see p. 356). Chloramphenicol also works, but is riskier (p. 357).

Prevention:

- Keep clean. De-louse the whole family regularly.
- Remove ticks from your dogs and do not allow dogs in your house.
- Kill rats. Use cats or traps (not poison, which can be dangerous to other animals and children).
- Kill rat fleas. Do not handle dead rats. The fleas may jump off onto you. Drown and burn the rats and their fleas. Put insecticide into rat holes and nests.

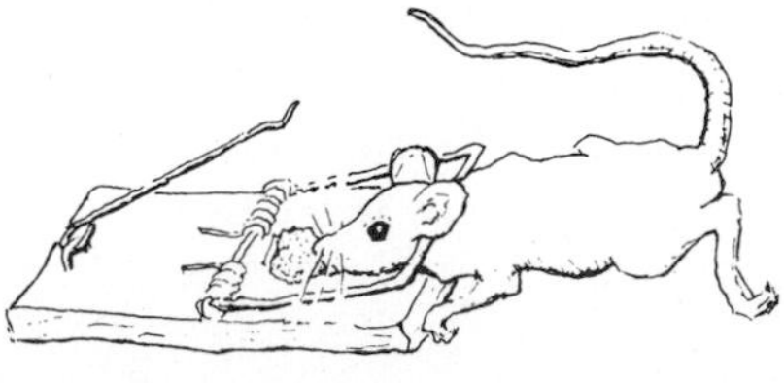

LEPROSY (HANSEN'S DISEASE)

This mildly infectious disease develops slowly, often over many years. It can only spread from persons who have untreated leprosy, to persons who have 'low resistance' to the disease. In areas where leprosy is common, children should be checked every 6 to 12 months—especially children living with persons who have leprosy.

Signs: Leprosy can cause a variety of skin problems, loss of feeling, and paralysis of the hands and feet.

The first sign of leprosy is often **a slowly growing patch on the skin that does not itch or hurt.** At first, feeling inside the patch may be normal. Keep watching it. If feeling in the patch becomes reduced or absent (see p. 38) it is probably leprosy.

Examine the whole body for skin patches, especially the face, arms, back, butt, and legs.

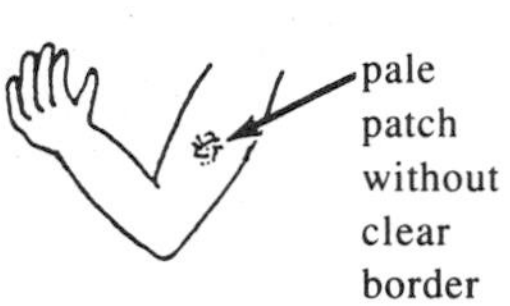
pale
patch
without
clear
border

Patches are a different color from surrounding skin, but never completely white or scaly.

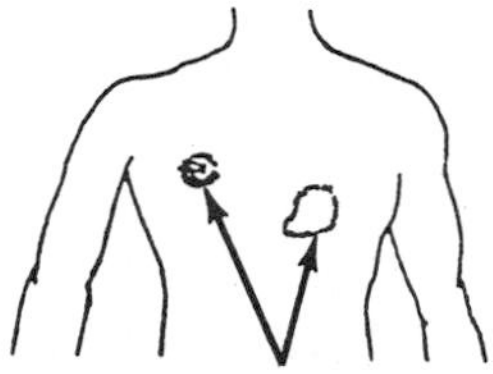

ringworm-like patch with or without raised border

Later signs differ according to the person's natural resistance to the disease. Watch out for:

- Tingling, numbness or loss of feeling in hands or feet. Or deformities or loss of feeling in skin patches.
- Slight weakness or deformities in the hands and feet.
- Swollen nerves that form thick cords under the skin. Nerves may or may not be painful when you press them.

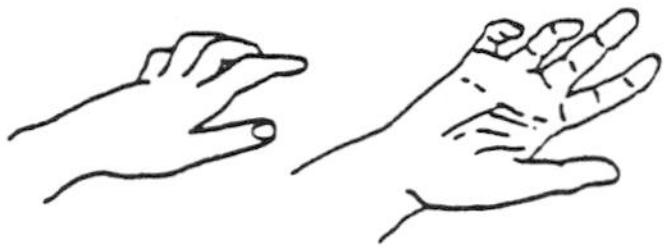

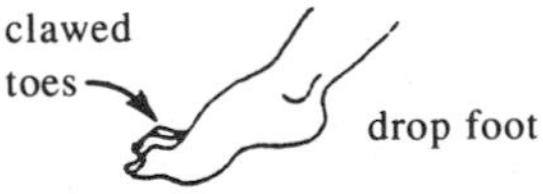
clawed
toes
drop foot

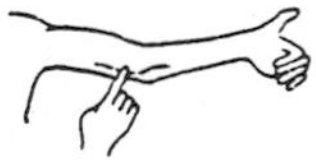

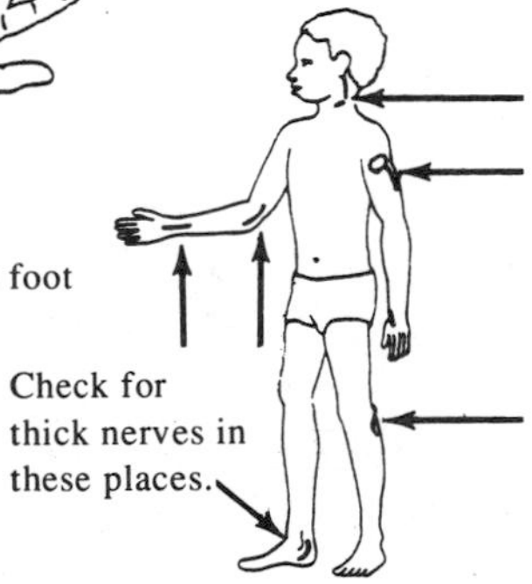
Check for
thick nerves in
these places.

Advanced signs may include:

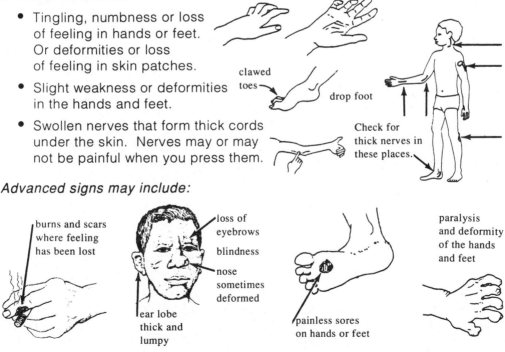

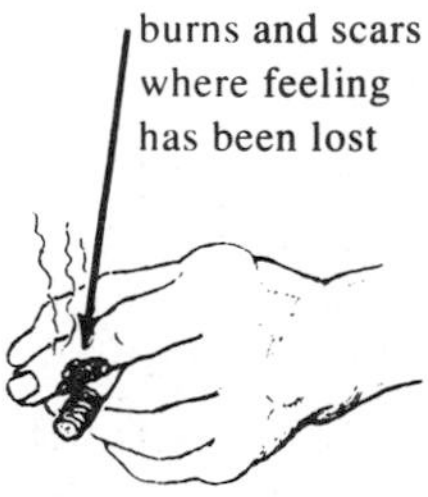
burns and scars
where feeling
has been lost

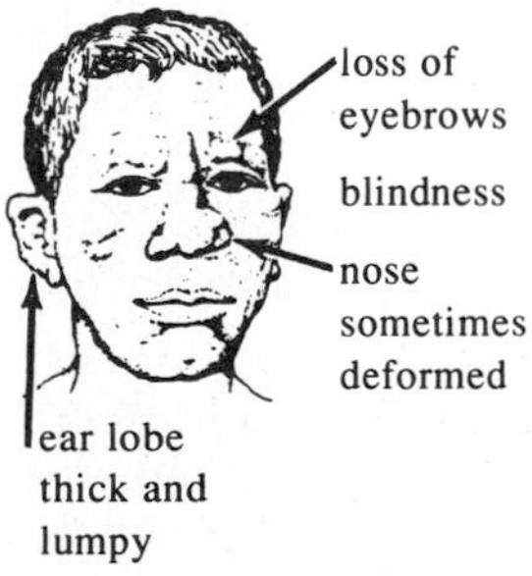
loss of
eyebrows
blindness
nose
sometimes
deformed
ear lobe
thick and
lumpy

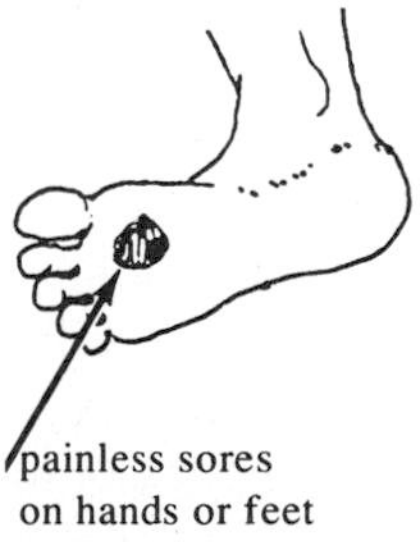
painless sores
on hands or feet

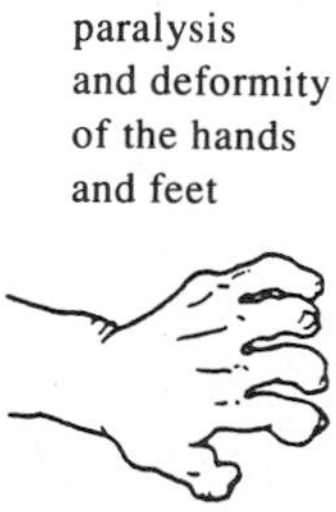
paralysis
and deformity
of the hands
and feet

Treatment of leprosy: Leprosy is usually curable, but medicine must usually be taken for years. The best medicine is dapsone, if possible combined with rifampin and clofazimine (see pages 364 to 365). If a 'lepra reaction' (fever, a rash, pain and perhaps swelling of hands and feet, or eye damage) occurs or gets worse while taking the medicine, keep taking it but get medical help.

Prevention of damage to hands, feet, and eyes: The large open sores often seen on the hands and feet of persons with leprosy are not caused by the disease itself and can be prevented. They result because, when feeling has been lost, a person no longer protects himself against injury.

For example, if a person with normal feeling walks a long way and gets a blister, it hurts, so he stops walking or limps.

But when a person with leprosy gets a blister, it does not hurt.

So he keeps walking until the blister bursts and becomes infected.

Still without pain, the infection gets deeper and attacks the bone.

In time the bone is destroyed and the foot becomes more and more deformed.

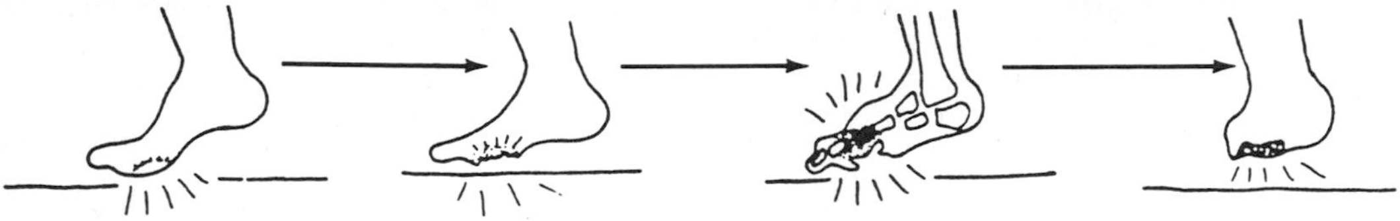

1. Protect hands and feet from things that can cut, bruise, blister, or burn them:

Do not go barefoot, especially not where there are sharp stones or thorns. Wear shoes or sandals. Put soft padding inside shoes and under straps that may rub.

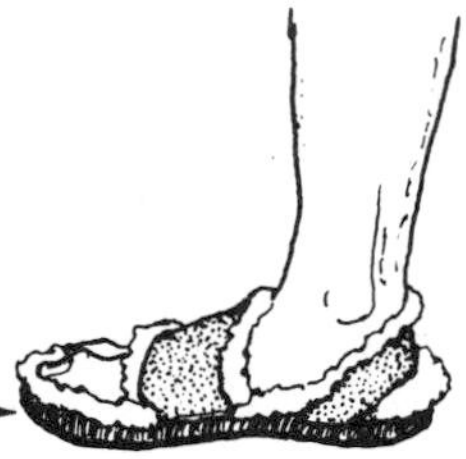

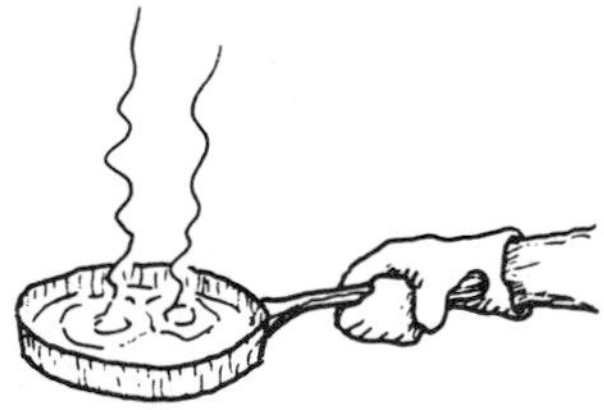

When working or cooking meals, wear gloves. Never pick up an object that **might** be hot without first protecting your hand with a thick glove or folded cloth. If possible, avoid work that involves handling sharp or hot objects. Do not smoke.

2. At the end of each day (or more often if you work hard or walk far) examine your hands and feet very carefully—or have someone else examine them. Look for cuts, bruises, or thorns. Also look for spots or areas on the hands and feet that are red, hot, swollen or show the beginnings of blisters. If you find any of these, rest the hands or feet until the skin is completely normal again. This will help callous and strengthen the skin. Sores can be prevented.

3. If you have an open sore, keep the part with the sore very clean and at rest until it has completely healed. Take great care not to injure the area again.

4. Protect your eyes. Much eye damage comes from not blinking enough, because of weakness or loss of feeling. Blink your eyes often to keep them wet and clean. If you cannot blink well, close your eyes tightly often during the day, especially when dust blows. Wear sun glasses with side shades, and maybe a sun hat. Keep eyes clean and flies away.

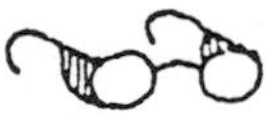

If you do these things and begin treatment early, **most deformities with leprosy can be prevented.** For more information about Hansen's disease, see *Disabled Village Children,* Chapter 26.

CHAPTER 15

Skin Problems

Some skin problems are caused by diseases or irritations that affect the skin only—such as ringworm, diaper rash, or warts. Other skin problems are signs of diseases that affect the whole body—such as the rash of measles or the sore, dry patches of pellagra (malnutrition). Certain kinds of sores or skin conditions may be signs of serious diseases—like tuberculosis, syphilis, or leprosy.

This chapter deals only with the more common skin problems in rural areas. However, there are hundreds of diseases of the skin. Some look so much alike that they are hard to tell apart—yet their causes and the specific treatments they require may be quite different.

If a skin problem is serious or gets worse in spite of treatment, seek medical help.

GENERAL RULES FOR TREATING SKIN PROBLEMS

Although many skin problems need specific treatment, there are a few general measures that often help:

RULE #1

If the affected area is **hot** and painful, or oozes pus, treat it with **heat.** Put hot, moist cloths on it *(hot compresses).*

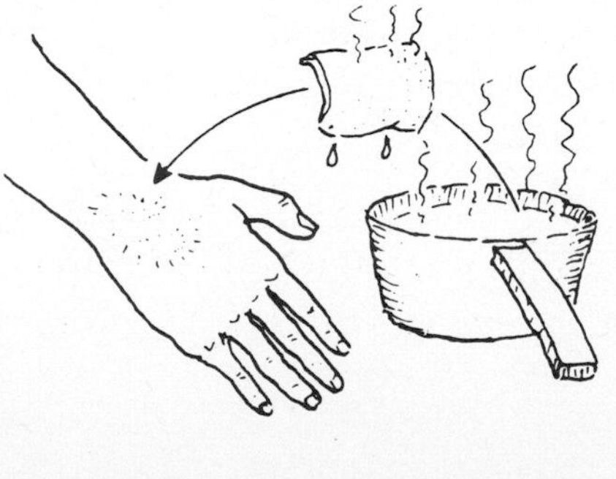

RULE #2

If the affected area itches, stings, or oozes clear fluid, treat it with **cold.** Put cool, wet cloths on it *(cold compresses).*

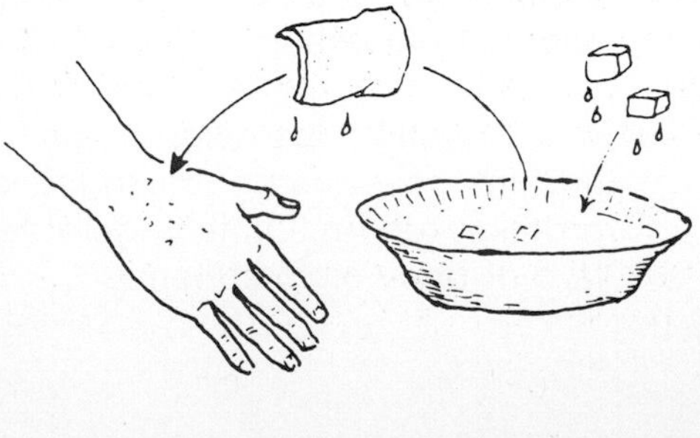

RULE #1 (in greater detail)

If the skin shows signs of serious infection such as:

- inflammation (redness or darkening of skin around the affected areas)
- swelling
- pain
- heat (it feels hot)
- pus

Do the following:

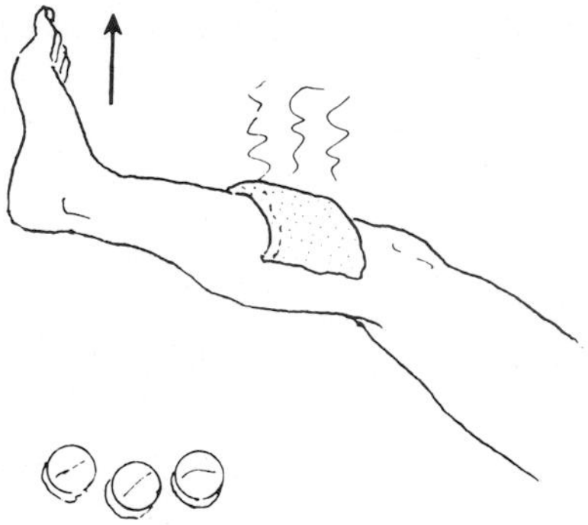

- ♦ Keep the affected part still and elevate it (put it higher than the rest of the body).
- ♦ Apply hot, moist cloths.
- ♦ If the infection is severe or the person has a fever, give antibiotics (penicillin, a sulfonamide, or erythromycin).

Danger signs include: swollen lymph nodes, a red or dark line above the infected area, or a bad smell. If these do not get better with treatment—use an antibiotic and seek medical help quickly.

RULE #2 (in greater detail)

If the affected skin forms blisters or a crust, oozes, itches, stings, or burns, do the following:

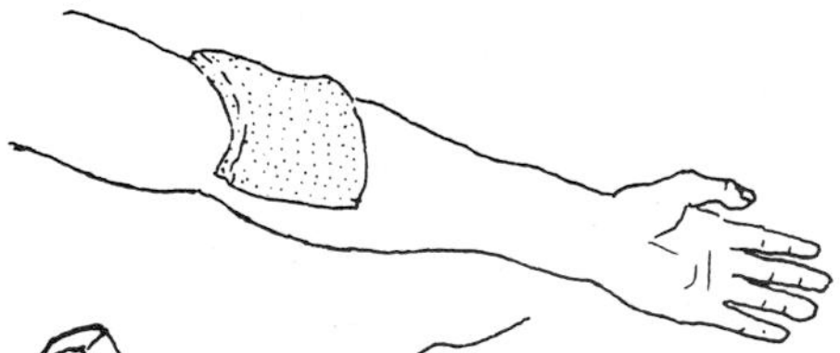

- ♦ Apply cloths soaked in cool water with white vinegar (2 tablespoons of vinegar in 1 quart of pure or boiled water).

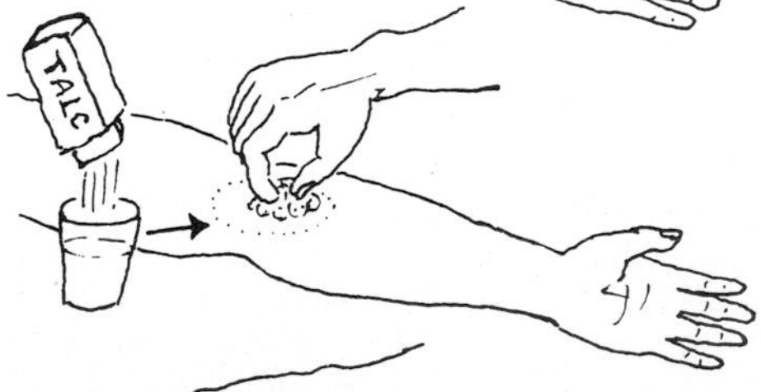

- ♦ When the affected area feels better, no longer oozes, and has formed tender new skin, lightly spread on a mixture of talc and water (1 part talc to 1 part water).

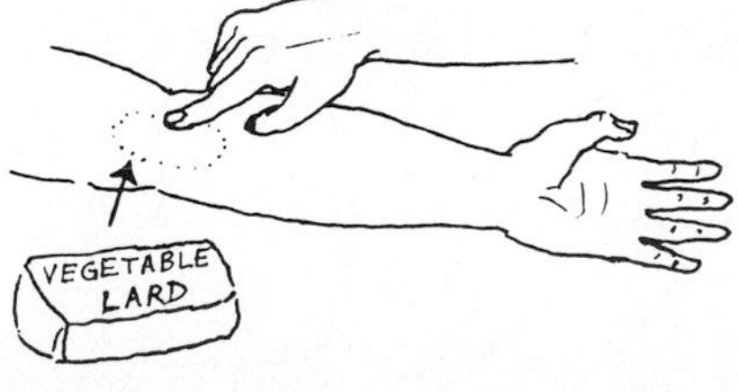

- ♦ When healing has taken place, and the new skin begins to thicken or flake, rub on a little vegetable lard or body oil to soften it.

RULE #3

If the skin areas affected are on parts of the body often exposed to sunlight, protect them from the sun.

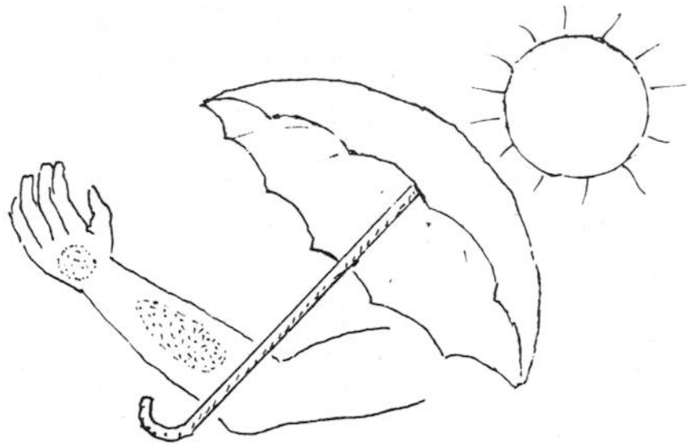

RULE #4

If the skin areas most affected are usually covered by clothing, expose them to direct sunlight for 10 to 20 minutes, 2 or 3 times a day.

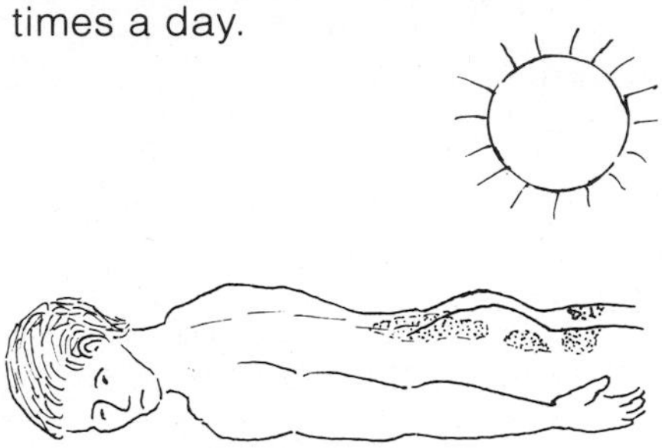

Instructions for Using Hot Compresses (Hot Soaks):

1. Boil water and allow it to cool until you can just hold your hand in it.

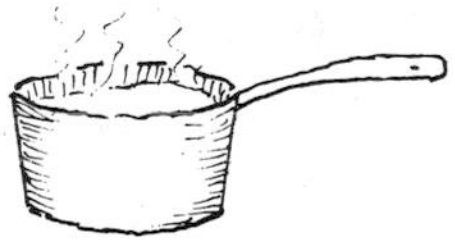

2. Fold a clean cloth so it is slightly larger than the area you want to treat, wet the cloth in the hot water, and squeeze out the extra water.

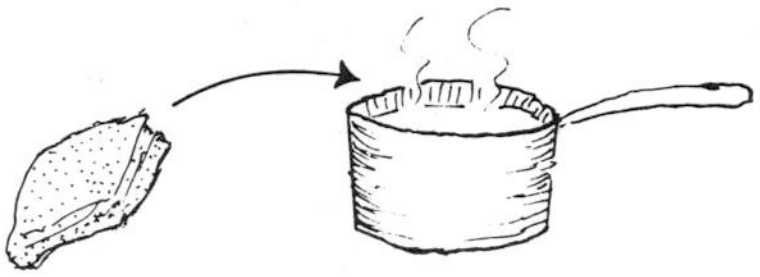

3. Put the cloth over the affected skin.

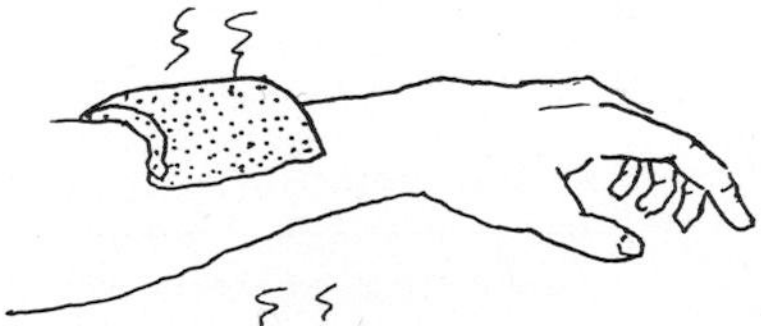

4. Cover the cloth with a sheet of thin plastic or cellophane.

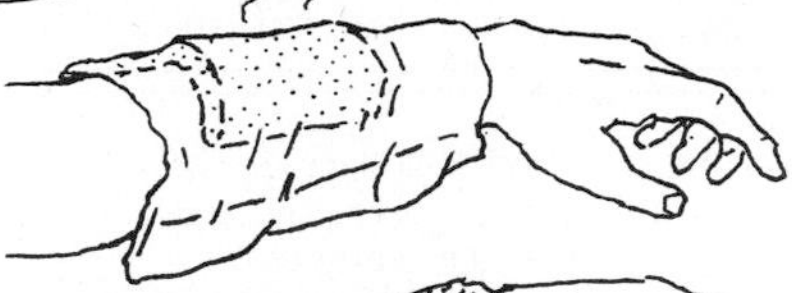

5. Wrap it with a towel to hold in the heat.

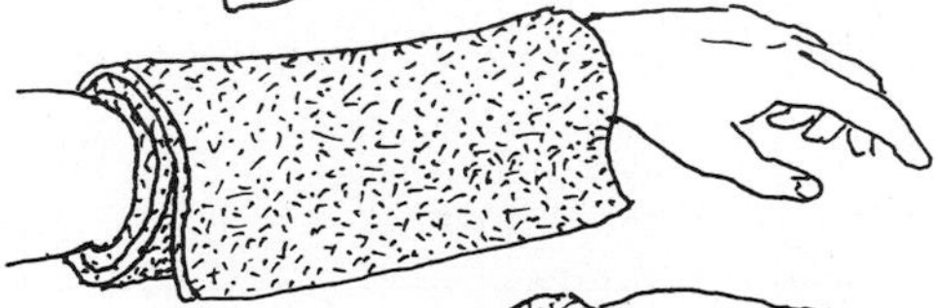

6. Keep the affected part raised.

7. When the cloth starts to cool, put it back in the hot water and repeat.

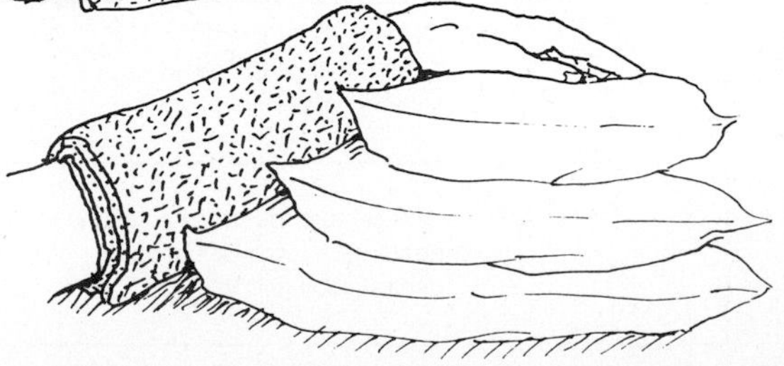

SKIN PROBLEMS—A Guide to Identification

IF THE SKIN HAS:	AND LOOKS LIKE:	YOU MAY HAVE:	SEE PAGE:
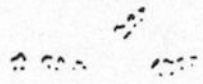 small or pimple-like sores 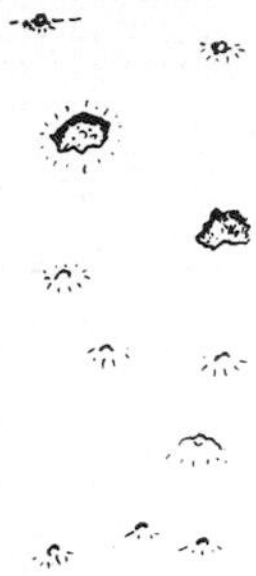	Tiny bumps or sores with much itching—first between fingers, on the wrists, or the waist. 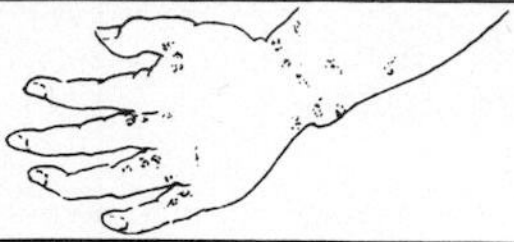	scabies	199
	Pimples or sores with pus or inflammation, often from scratching insect bites. May cause swollen lymph nodes. 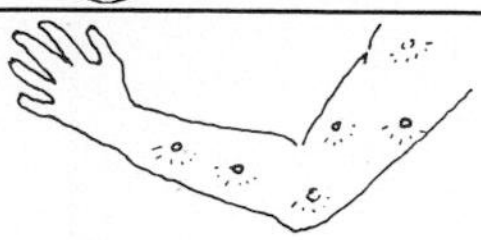	infection from bacteria	201
	Irregular, spreading sores with shiny, yellow crusts. 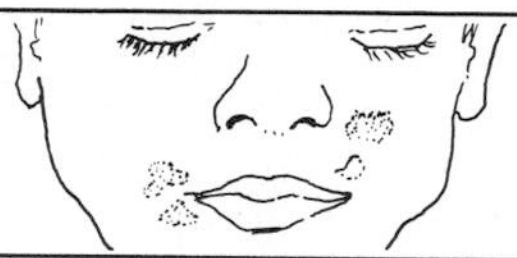	impetigo (bacterial infection)	202
	Pimples on young people's faces, sometimes chest and back, often with small heads of pus. 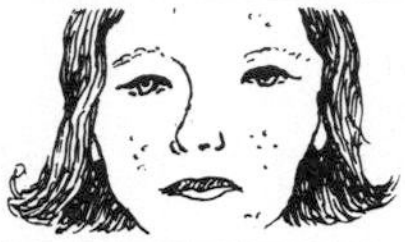	acne, pimples, blackheads	211
	A sore on the genitals, 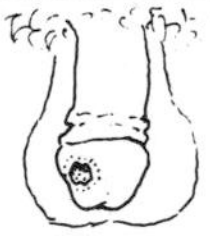 without itching or pain.	syphilis	237
		venereal lymphogranuloma	238
	with pain and pus.	chancroid	403
a large, open sore or skin ulcer 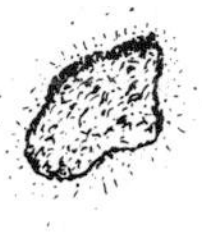	A large chronic (unhealing) sore surrounded by purplish skin—on or near the ankles of older people with varicose veins. 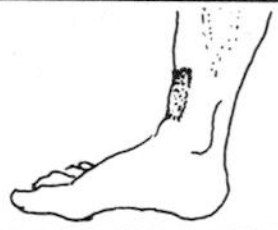	ulcers from bad circulation	213
		(possibly diabetes)	127
	Sores over the bones and joints of very sick persons who cannot get out of bed. 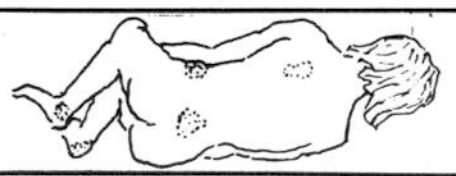	bed sores	214
	Sores with loss of feeling on the feet or hands. (They do not hurt even when pricked with a needle.) 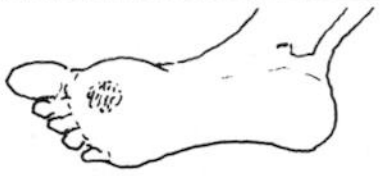	leprosy	191
	A bump and then a sore that will not heal, anywhere on the body or face. 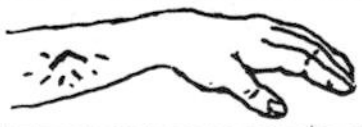	leishmaniasis	406
lumps under the skin 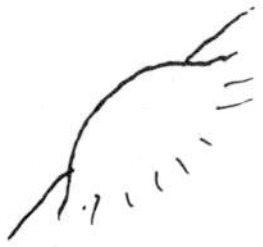	A warm, painful swelling that eventually may break open and drain pus. 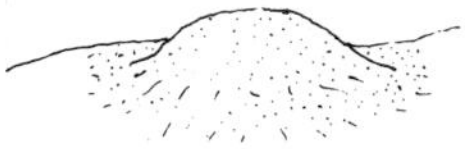	abscess or boil	202
	A warm, painful lump in the breast of a woman breast feeding. 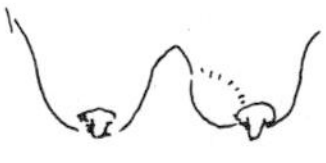	mastitis (bacterial infection),	278
		possibly cancer	279
	A lump that keeps growing. Usually not painful at first. 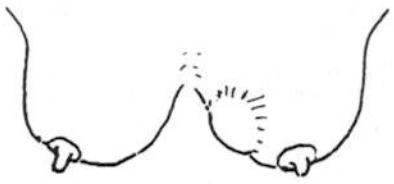	cancer	279
		(also see lymph nodes)	88
	One or more round lumps on the head, neck, or upper body (or central body and thighs). 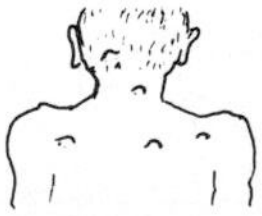	river blindness	227
		(also see lymph nodes)	88

A Guide to Identification

IF THE SKIN HAS:	AND LOOKS LIKE:	YOU MAY HAVE:	SEE PAGE:
swollen lymph nodes 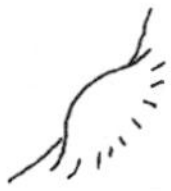	Nodes on the side of the neck that continuously break open and scar. 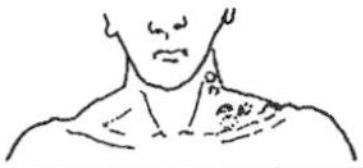	scrofula (a type of tuberculosis)	212
	Nodes in the groin that continuously break open and scar. 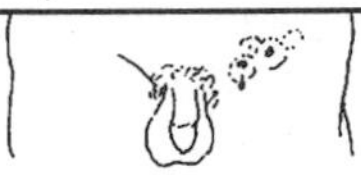	venereal lymphogranuloma chancroid	238 403
large spots or patches 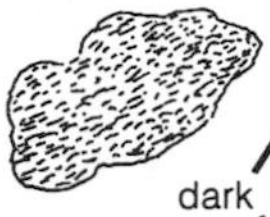 dark	Dark patches on the forehead and cheeks of pregnant women. 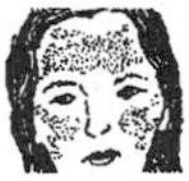	mask of pregnancy	207
dark	Scaly, cracking areas that look like sunburn on the arms, legs, neck, or face. 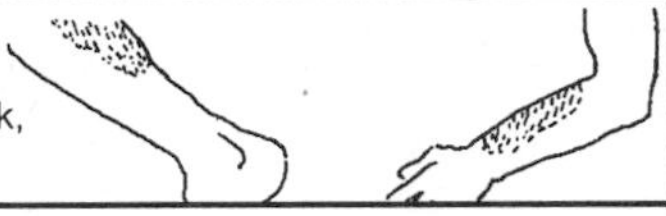	pellagra (a type of malnutrition)	208 209
dark	Dark, painless patches on the skin or mouth that start small and grow 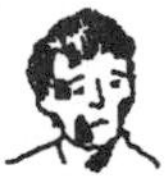	Karposi's Sarcoma (KS, cancer related to the HIV/AIDS virus).	399-401
dark	Purple spots or peeling sores on children with swollen feet. 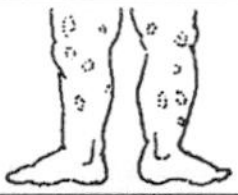	malnutrition	208 209
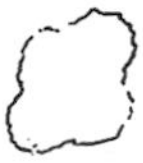 white	Round or irregular patches on the face or body, especially of children 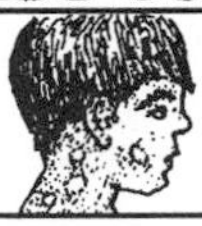	tinea versicolor (fungus infection)	206
white	White patches, especially on hands, feet, or lips 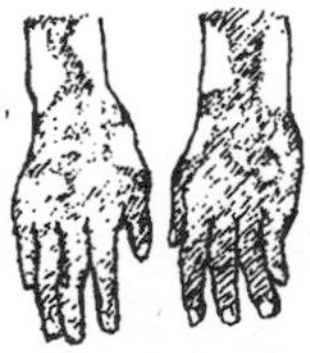 that begin with reddish or bluish pimples.	pinta (infection)	207
white	White patches, especially on hands, feet, or lips that begin without other signs.	vitiligo (loss of color, nothing more)	207
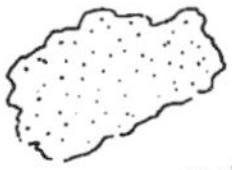 reddish	Reddish or blistering patches on the cheeks or behind the knees and elbows of young children 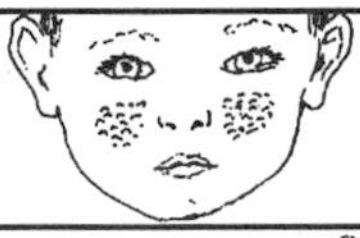	eczema	216
reddish	A reddish, hot, painful patch that spreads rapidly. 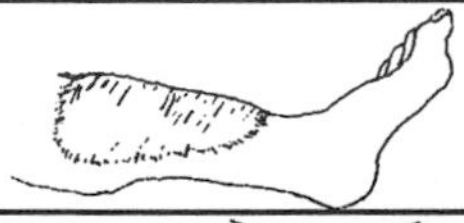	erysipelas (cellulitis or very serious bacterial infections)	212
reddish	A reddish area between the baby's legs. 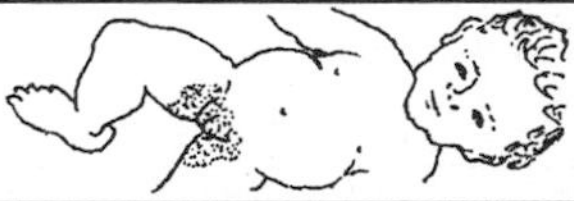	diaper rash from urine or heat	215
reddish	Beef-red patches with white, milky curds in the skin folds. 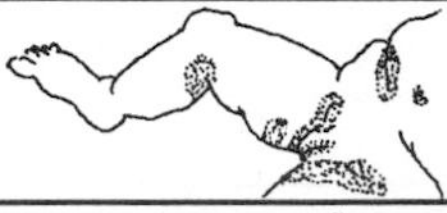	moniliasis (yeast infection)	242
reddish or gray	Raised reddish or gray patches with silvery scales; especially on elbows and knees; chronic (long-term) 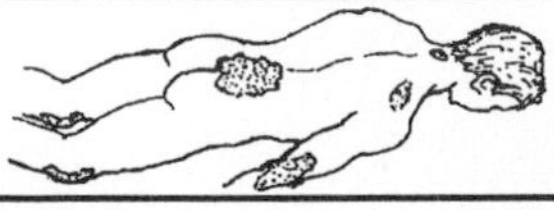	psoriasis (or sometimes tuberculosis)	216 212

A Guide to Identification

IF THE SKIN HAS:	AND LOOKS LIKE:	YOU MAY HAVE:	SEE PAGE:
warts 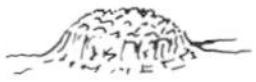	Simple warts, not very large. 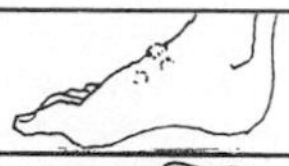	common warts (virus infection)	210
	Wart-like growths on the penis, vagina, or around the anus. 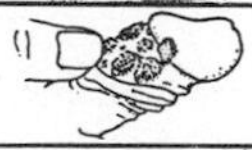	genital warts	402
	Large warts (more than 1 cm.), often on arms or feet. 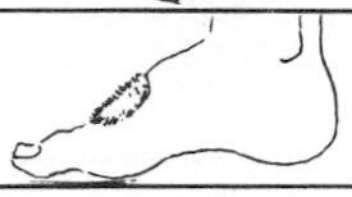	a type of tuberculosis of the skin	212
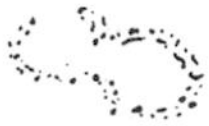 rings (spots with raised or red edges, often clear in the center) 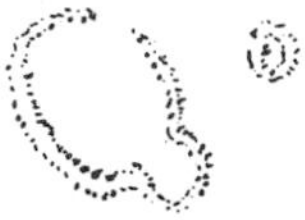	Small rings that continue to grow or spread and may itch. 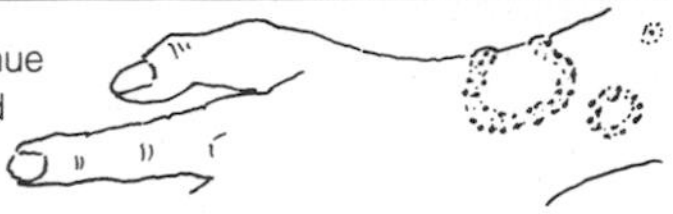	Ringworm (fungus infection)	205
	large circles with a thick border that do not itch 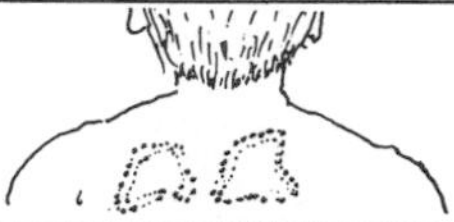	advanced stage of syphilis	237
	Large rings that are numb in the center. (A needle prick does not hurt them.) 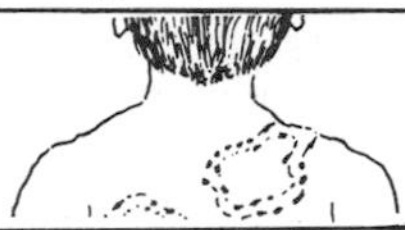	leprosy	191
	Small rings, sometimes with a small pit in the middle, found on the temple, nose, or neck. 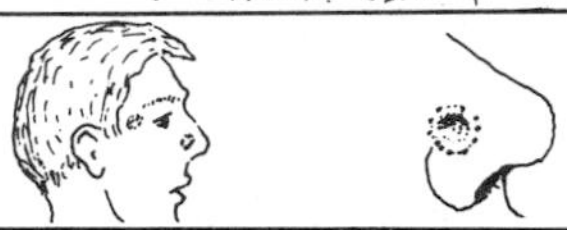	cancer of the skin	211
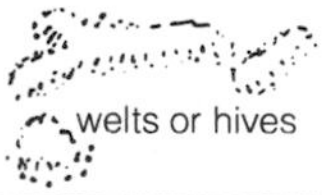 welts or hives	Very itchy rash, bumps, or patches. (They may appear and disappear rapidly.) 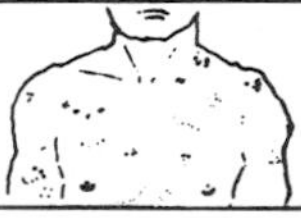	allergic reaction	203
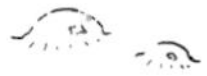 blisters 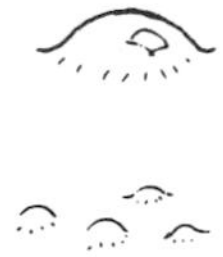	Blisters with bumps and much itching and weeping (oozing). 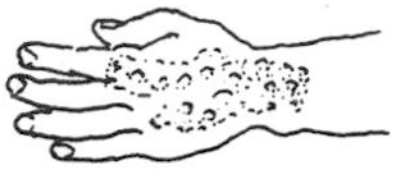	contact dermatitis (like poison ivy or sumac)	204
	Small blisters over the whole body, with some fever. 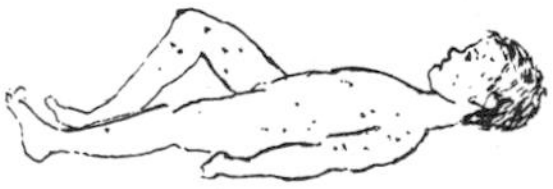	chickenpox	311
	A patch of painful blisters that appears only on one part of the body, often in a stripe or cluster. 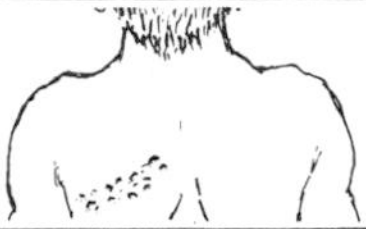	Herpes zoster (shingles)	204
	A gray or black bad smelling area with blisters and air pockets that spread. 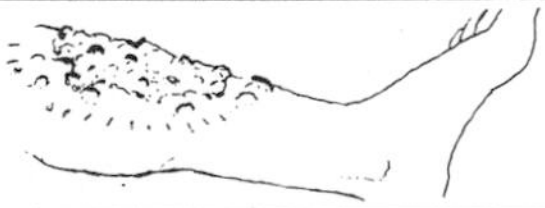	gas gangrene (very serious bacterial infection)	213
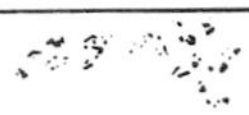 small reddish spots or a rash over the whole body; fever 	A rash that very sick children get over the whole body. 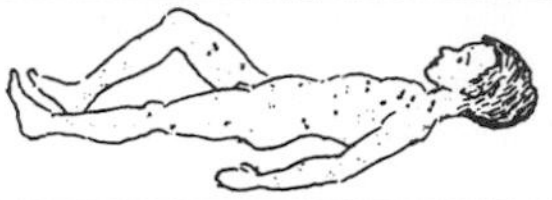	measles	311
	After a few days of fever a few small pinkish spots appear on the body; the person is very sick. 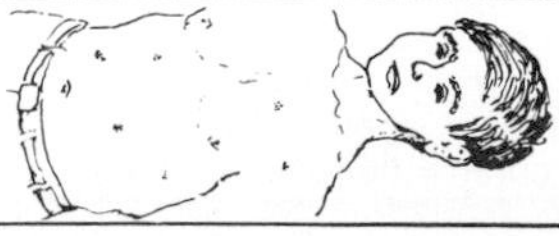	typhoid fever	188

SCABIES (SEVEN YEAR ITCH)

Scabies is especially common in children. It causes very itchy little bumps that can appear all over the body, but are most common:

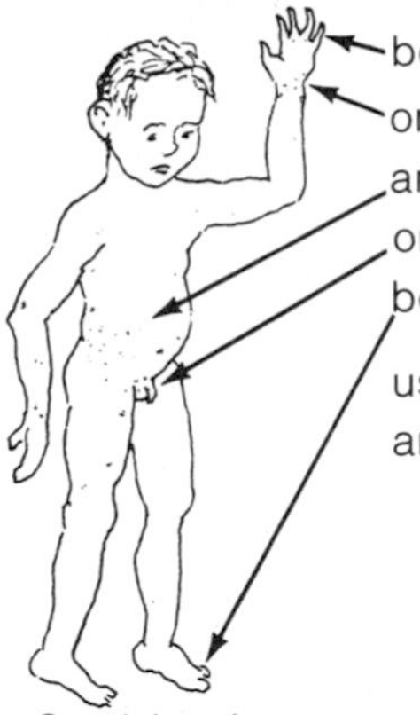

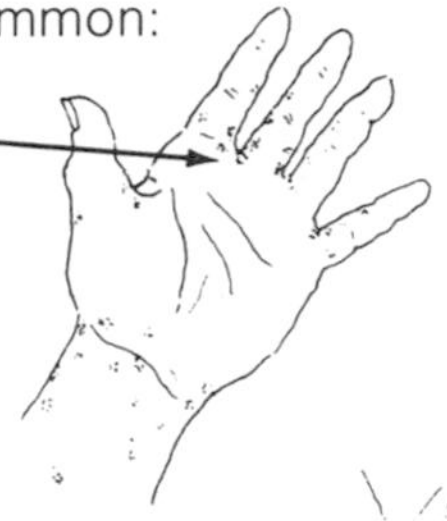

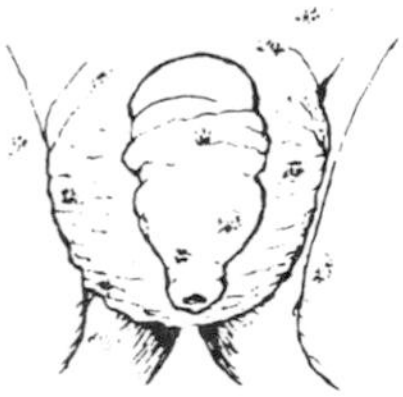

Small itchy sores on the penis and scrotum of young boys are almost always scabies.

Scabies is caused by little animals—similar to tiny ticks or chiggers—which make tunnels under the skin. It is spread by touching the affected skin or by clothes and bedding. Scratching can cause infection, producing sores with pus, and sometimes swollen lymph nodes or fever.

Treatment:

- If one person has scabies, everyone in his family should be treated.
- Personal cleanliness is of first importance. Bathe and change clothes daily.
- Cut fingernails very short to reduce spreading and infection.
- Wash all clothes and bedding or, better still, boil them and hang them in the sun.
- Make the following ointment from lindane (gamma benzene hexachloride, p. 373) and *Vaseline* (petroleum jelly, p. 371). In many countries lindane is sold as a sheep or cattle 'dip'.

  Wash the whole body vigorously with soap and hot water.

  Heat 15 parts *Vaseline* (or body oil) and mix well with 1 part lindane. Smear this ointment on the whole body (except the face—unless it is affected). Leave for 1 day and then bathe well.

  After treating, put on clean clothes and use clean bedding. Repeat treatment 1 week later.

- Instead of this ointment, you can put 4 drops of lindane on half a lemon. Leave it for 5 minutes and then rub the lemon over your whole body, except the face, starting with the areas most affected.

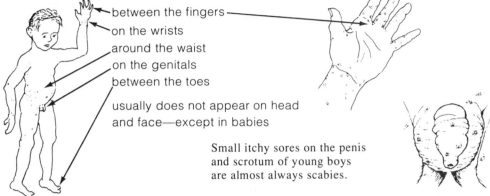

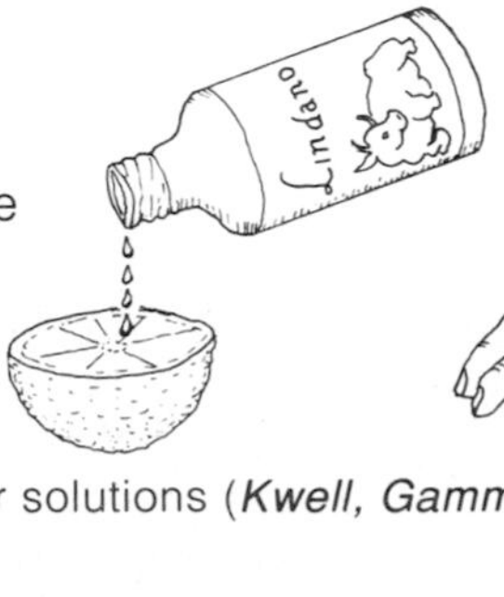

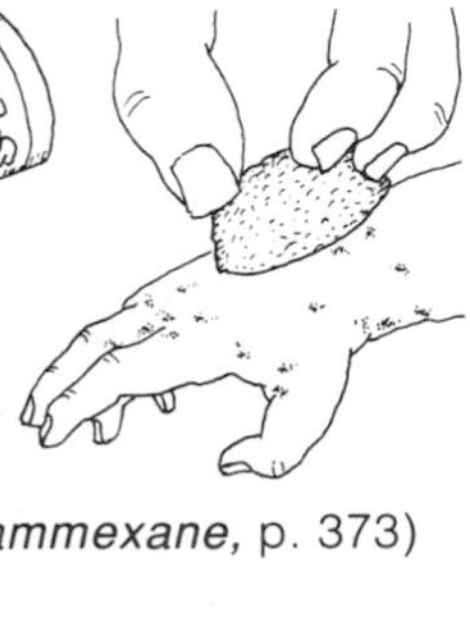

Note: Lindane comes in commercial ointments or solutions (***Kwell, Gammexane,*** p. 373) but these are more expensive.

CAUTION: Lindane can cause poisoning if used too often. Do not apply more than once a week and bathe well the day after treatment. Do not use lindane on babies under 1 year old. See the next page for some safer treatments.

- Sulfur powder mixed with lard or body oil—use 1 part sulfur to 10 parts lard or oil. Apply to whole body (except face) 3 times a day for 3 days.
- Benzyl benzoate lotion (see p. 373)
- Crotamiton (***Eurax,*** p. 373)

LICE

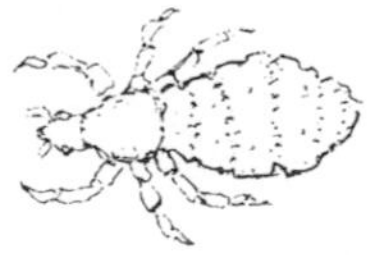

There are 3 kinds: head lice, body lice, and pubic lice (or 'crabs') that live in the hairy parts of the body. Lice cause itching, and sometimes skin infections and swollen lymph nodes. To avoid lice, take great care with personal cleanliness. Wash clothing and bedding often and hang them in the sun. Bathe and wash hair often. Check children's hair. If they have lice, treat them at once. Do not let a child with lice sleep with others.

Treatment:

For head and pubic lice: You can often get rid of lice without medicines by scrubbing the hair well with regular soap or shampoo for 10 minutes. Rinse well and comb thoroughly with a fine-tooth comb. Repeat every day for 10 days.

- If necessary, make a shampoo of lindane (p. 373), water, and soap (1 part lindane to 10 parts water). Wash hair, being careful not to get lindane in the eyes. Leave the shampoo for 10 minutes; then rinse well with clean water. Repeat a week later. Medications containing pyrethrins with piperonyl *(RID)* also work well for lice and are safer (see p. 373).
- To get rid of nits (lice eggs), soak hair with warm vinegar water (1 part vinegar to 1 part water) for half an hour, then comb it thoroughly with a fine-tooth comb.

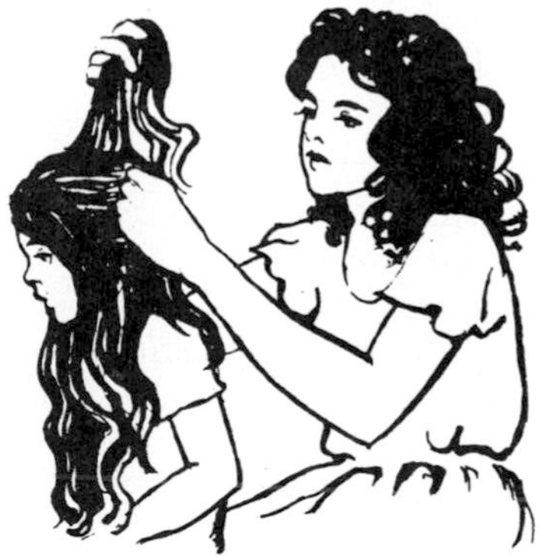

For body lice: Soak your whole body in a bath of hot water every day for 10 days. After each bath, wash your entire body thoroughly with soap and rinse well. Use a fine-tooth comb on any hairy places. If necessary, treat as for scabies. Keep clothing and bedding clean.

BEDBUGS

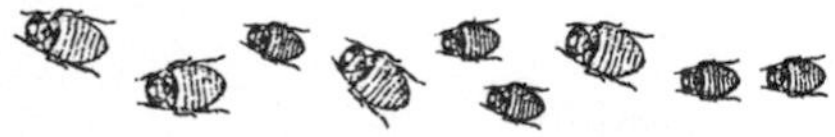

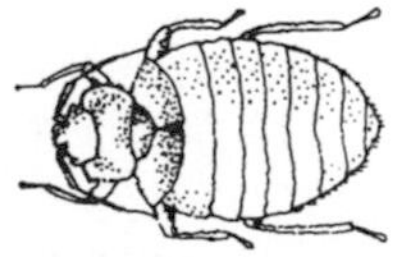

These are very small, flat, crawling insects that hide inside mattresses, bedding, furniture, and walls. They usually bite at night. The bites often appear in groups or lines.

To get rid of bedbugs, wash bedding and pour boiling water on cots and bed frames. Sprinkle sulfur on mattresses, cloth furniture, and rugs and do not use them for 3 weeks. Be sure to clean off the powder well before using again.

To prevent bedbugs, spread bedding, mats, and cots in the sun often.

TICKS AND CHIGGERS

Some dangerous infections or paralysis are spread by tick bites. But careful removal within a few hours usually prevents these problems. So check the whole body well after walking in areas where ticks are common.

When removing a tick that is firmly attached, take care that its head does not remain in the skin, since this can cause an infection. Never pull on the body of a tick. To remove a tick:

- With tweezers, grasp the tick as close as possible to its mouth—the part sticking into the skin. (Try not to squeeze its swollen belly.) Pull the tick out gently but firmly. Do not touch the removed tick. Burn it.
- Or, hold a lit cigarette near it. Or put some alcohol on it.

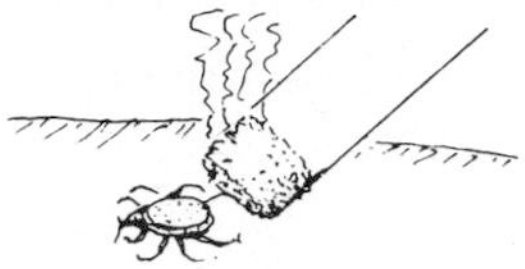

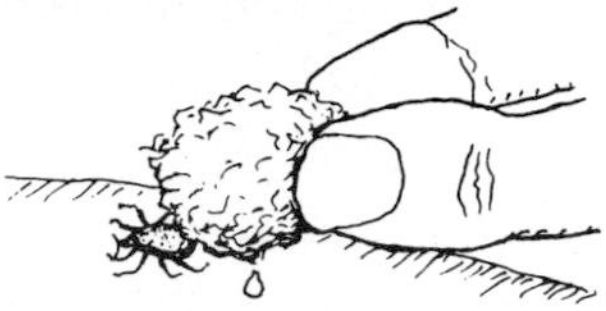

To remove very small ticks or chiggers, use one of the remedies recommended for scabies (see p. 199). To relieve itching or pain caused by tick or chigger bites, take aspirin and follow the instructions for treatment of itching on p. 203.

To help prevent chiggers and ticks from biting you, dust sulfur powder on your body before going into the fields or forests. Especially dust ankles, wrists, waist, and underarms.

SMALL SORES WITH PUS

Skin infections in the form of small sores with pus often result from scratching insect bites, scabies, or other irritations with dirty fingernails.

Treatment and Prevention:

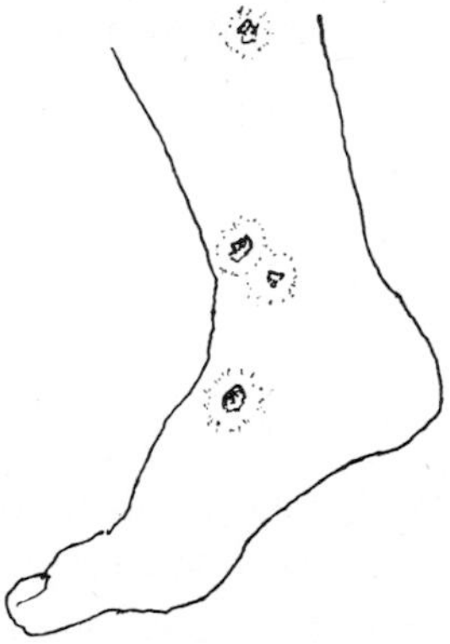

- Wash the sores well with soap and cooled, boiled water, gently soaking off the scabs. Do this daily as long as there is pus.
- Leave small sores open to the air. Bandage large sores and change the bandage frequently.
- If the skin around a sore is red and hot, or if the person has a fever, red lines coming from the sore, or swollen lymph nodes, use an antibiotic—such as penicillin tablets (p. 351) or sulfa tablets (p. 358).
- Do not scratch. This makes the sores worse and can spread infection to other parts of the body. Cut the fingernails of small children very short. Or put gloves or socks over their hands so they cannot scratch.
- Never let a child with sores or any skin infection play or sleep with other children. These infections are easily spread.

IMPETIGO

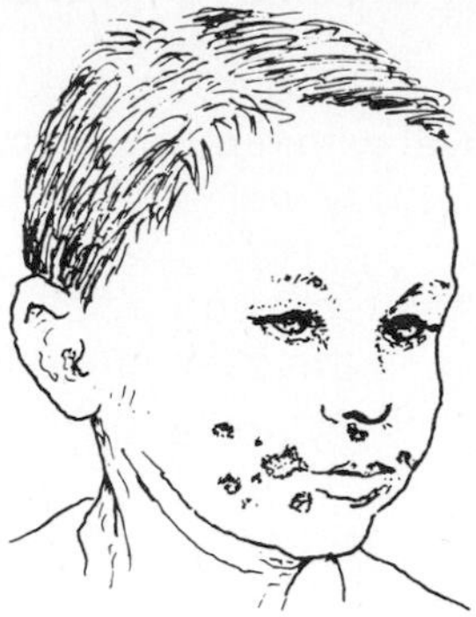

This is a bacterial infection that causes rapidly spreading sores with shiny, yellow crusts. It often occurs on children's faces especially around the mouth. Impetigo can spread easily to other people from the sores or contaminated fingers.

Treatment:

- Wash the affected part with soap and cooled, boiled water 3 to 4 times each day, gently soaking off the crusts.
- After each washing, paint the sores with gentian violet (p. 371) or spread on an antibiotic cream containing bacitracin such as ***Polysporin*** (p. 371).
- If the infection is spread over a large area or causes fever, give penicillin tablets (p. 351) or dicloxacillin (p. 351). If the person is allergic to penicillin, or if these medicines do not seem to be helping, give erythromycin (p. 355) or co-trimoxazole (p. 358).

Prevention:

- Follow the Guidelines of Personal Cleanliness (p. 133). Bathe children daily and protect them from bedbugs and biting flies. If a child gets scabies, treat him as soon as possible.
- Do not let a child with impetigo sleep or play with other children. Begin treatment at the first sign.

BOILS AND ABSCESSES

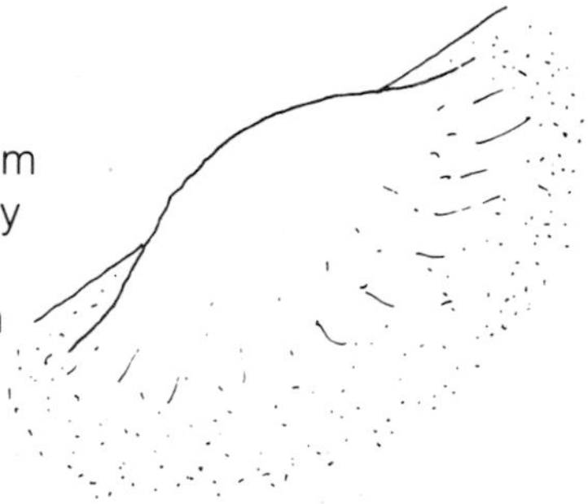

A boil, or abscess, is an infection that forms a sac of pus under the skin. This can happen when the root of a hair gets infected. Or it can result from a puncture wound or an injection given with a dirty needle. A boil is painful and the skin around it becomes red and hot. It can cause swollen lymph nodes and fever.

Treatment:

- Put hot compresses over the boil several times a day (see p. 195).
- Let the boil break open by itself. After it opens, keep using hot compresses. Allow the pus to drain, but never press or squeeze the boil, since this can cause the infection to spread to other parts of the body.
- If the abscess is very painful and does not open after 2 or 3 days of hot soaks, it may help to have it cut open so the pus can drain out. This will quickly reduce the pain. If possible, get medical help.
- If the boil causes swollen nodes or fever, take penicillin tablets (p. 351) or erythromycin (p. 355).

ITCHING RASH, WELTS, OR HIVES (ALLERGIC REACTIONS IN THE SKIN)

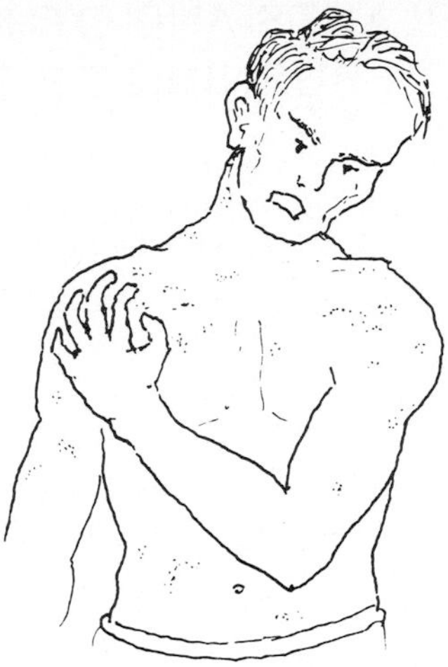

Touching, eating, injecting, or breathing certain things can cause an itching rash or ***hives*** in allergic persons. For more details, see Allergic Reactions, p. 166.

Hives are thick, raised spots or patches that look like bee stings and itch like mad. They may come and go rapidly or move from one spot to another.

Be on the watch for any reaction caused by certain medicines, especially injections of penicillin and the antivenoms or antitoxins made from horse serum. A rash or hives may appear from a few minutes up to 10 days after the medicine has been injected.

If you get an itching rash, hives, or any other allergic reaction after taking or being injected with any medicine, stop using it and never use that medicine again in your life!
This is very important to prevent the danger of ALLERGIC SHOCK (see p. 70).

Treatment of itching:

- Bathe in cool water or use cool compresses—cloths soaked in cold water or ice water.

- Compresses of cool oatmeal water also calm itching. Boil the oatmeal in water, strain it, and use the water when cool. (Starch can be used instead of oats.)

- If itching is severe, take an antihistamine like chlorpheniramine (p. 387).

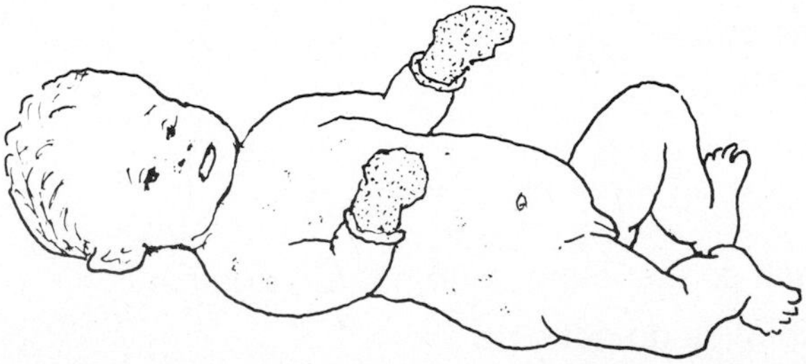

- To protect a baby from scratching himself, cut his fingernails very short, or put gloves or socks over his hands.

PLANTS AND OTHER THINGS THAT CAUSE ITCHING OR BURNING OF THE SKIN

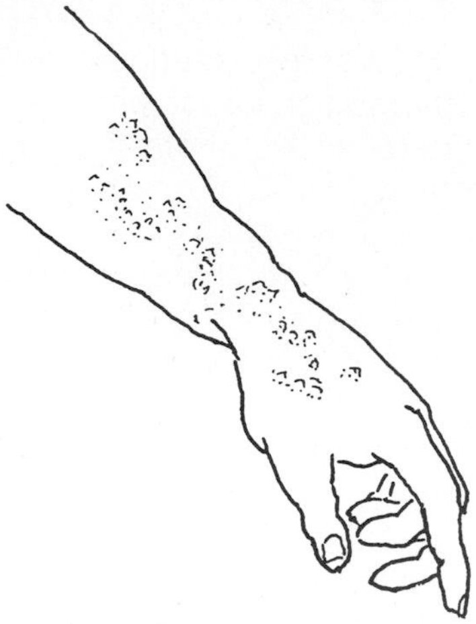

Nettles, 'stinging trees', sumac, 'poison ivy', and many other plants may cause blisters, burns, or hives with itching when they touch the skin. Juices or hairs of certain caterpillars and other insects produce similar reactions.

In allergic persons rashes or 'weeping' sore patches may be caused by certain things that touch or are put on the skin. Rubber shoes, watchbands, ear drops and other medicines, face creams, perfumes, or soaps may cause such problems.

Treatment:

All these irritations go away by themselves when the things that cause them no longer touch the skin. A paste of oatmeal and cool water helps calm the itching. Aspirin or antihistamines (p. 386) may also help. In severe cases, you can use a cream that contains cortisone or a cortico-steroid (see p. 371). To prevent infection, keep the irritated areas clean.

SHINGLES (HERPES ZOSTER)

Signs:

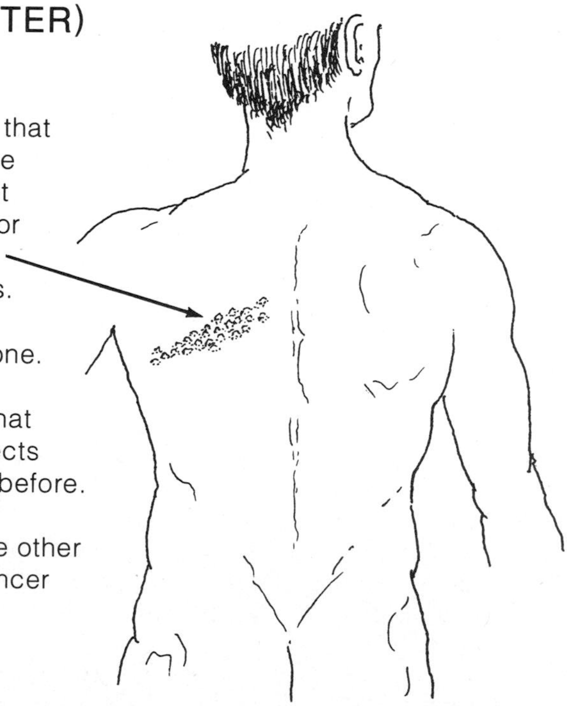

A line or patch of painful blisters that suddenly appears on one side of the body is probably shingles. It is most common on the back, chest, neck, or face. The blisters usually last 2 or 3 weeks, then go away by themselves. Sometimes the pain continues or returns long after the blisters are gone.

Shingles is caused by the virus that causes chickenpox and usually affects persons who have had chickenpox before. It is not dangerous. (However, it is occasionally a warning sign of some other more serious problem—perhaps cancer or AIDS, p. 399.)

Treatment:

- Put light bandages over the rash so that clothes do not rub against it.
- Take aspirin for the pain. (Antibiotics do not help.)

RINGWORM, TINEA (FUNGUS INFECTIONS)

Fungus infections may appear on any part of the body, but occur most frequently on:

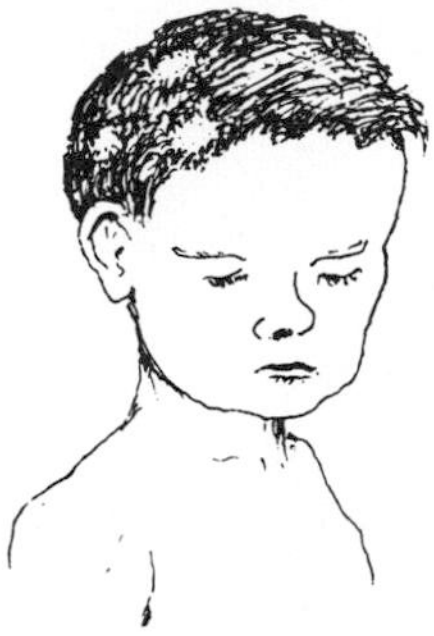
the scalp (tinea)

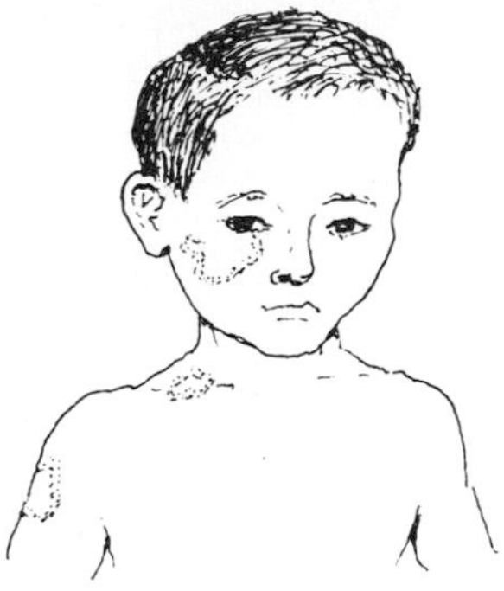
the parts without hair (ringworm)

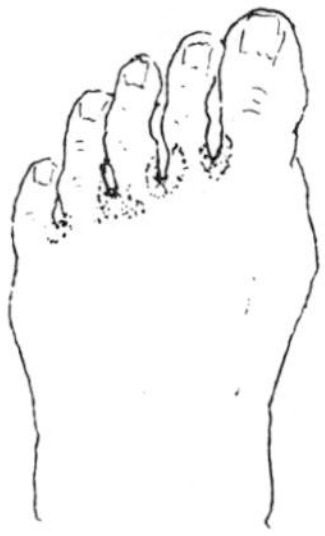
between the toes or fingers (athlete's foot)

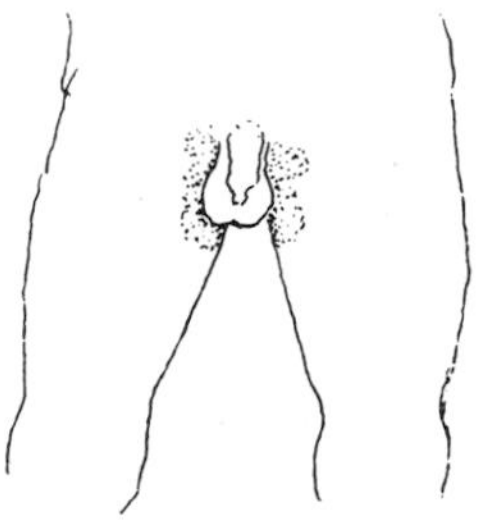
between the legs (jock itch)

Most fungus infections grow in the form of a ring. They often itch. Ringworm of the head can produce round patches with scales and loss of hair. Finger and toe nails infected with the fungus become rough and thick.

Treatment:

- Soap and water. Washing the infected part every day with soap and water may be all that is needed.
- Do your best to keep the affected areas dry and exposed to the air or sunlight. Change underwear or socks often, especially when sweaty.
- Use a cream of sulfur and lard (1 part sulfur to 10 parts lard).
- Creams and powders with salicylic or undecylenic acid, or tolnaftate (*Tinactin*, p. 372) help cure the fungus between the fingers, toes, and groin.
- For severe tinea of the scalp, or any fungus infection that is widespread or does not get better with the above treatments, take griseofulvin, 1 gram a day for adults and half a gram a day for children (p. 372). It may be necessary to keep taking it for weeks or even months to completely control the infection.
- Many tineas of the scalp clear up when a child reaches puberty (11 to 14 years old). Severe infections forming large swollen patches with pus should be treated with compresses of warm water (p. 195). It is important to pull out all of the hair from the infected part. Use griseofulvin, if possible.

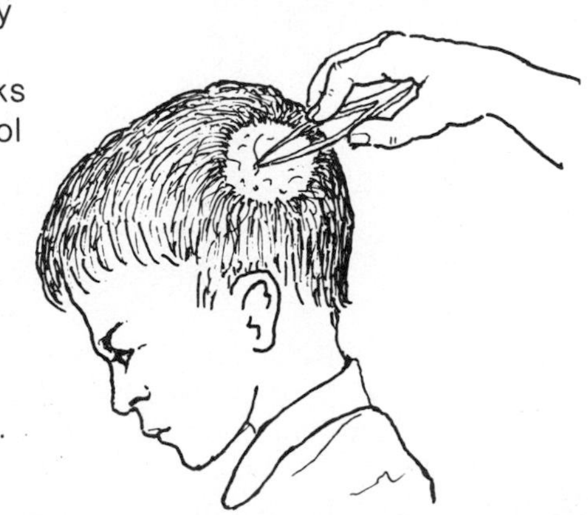

How to prevent fungal infections:

Ringworm and all other fungus infections are ***contagious*** (easily spread). To prevent spreading them from one child to others:

- Do not let a child with a fungal infection sleep with the others.
- Do not let different children use the same comb, or use each other's clothing or towel, unless these are washed or well cleaned first.
- Treat an infected child at once.

WHITE SPOTS ON THE FACE AND BODY

Tinea versicolor is a mild fungus infection that causes small dark or light spots with a distinct and irregular border that are often seen on the neck, chest, and back. The spots may be slightly scaly but usually do not itch. They are of little medical importance.

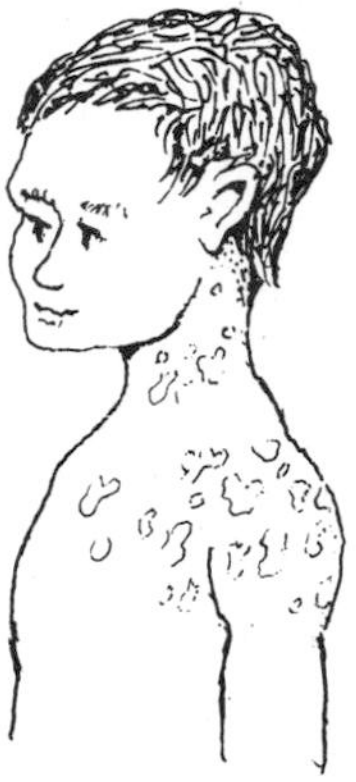

Treatment:

- Make a cream with sulfur and lard (1 part sulfur to 10 parts lard) and apply it to the whole body every day until they disappear. Or use an anti-fungal cream (p. 372).
- Sodium thiosulfate works better. This is the 'hypo' photographers use when developing film. Dissolve a tablespoon of sodium thiosulfate in a glass of water and apply it to the whole upper body. Then rub the skin with a piece of cotton dipped in vinegar.
- To prevent the spots from returning, it is often necessary to repeat this treatment every 2 weeks.
- Selenium sulfide (p. 372) or Whitfield's ointment may also help.

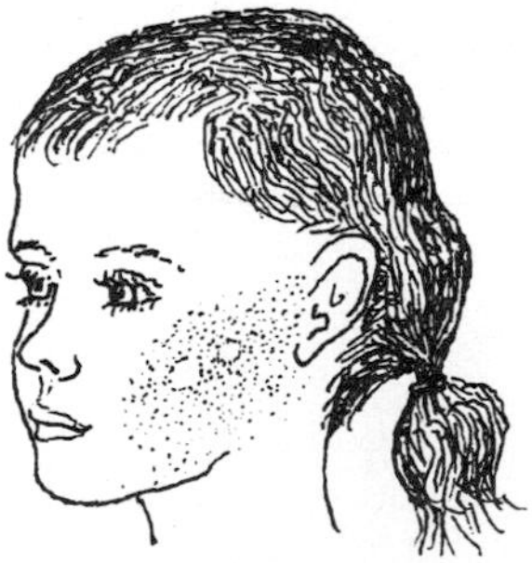

There is **another kind of small whitish spot** that is common on the cheeks of dark-skinned children who spend a lot of time in the sun. The border is less clear than in tinea versicolor. These spots are not an infection and are of no importance. Usually they go away as the child grows up. Avoid harsh soaps and apply oil. No other treatment is needed.

Contrary to popular opinion, none of these types of white spots is a sign of anemia. They will not go away with tonics or vitamins. The spots that are only on the cheeks do not need any treatment.

CAUTION: Sometimes pale spots are early signs of **leprosy** (see p. 191). Leprosy spots are never completely white and may have **reduced feeling** when pricked by a pin. If leprosy is common in your area, have the child checked.

Vitiligo (White Areas of the Skin)

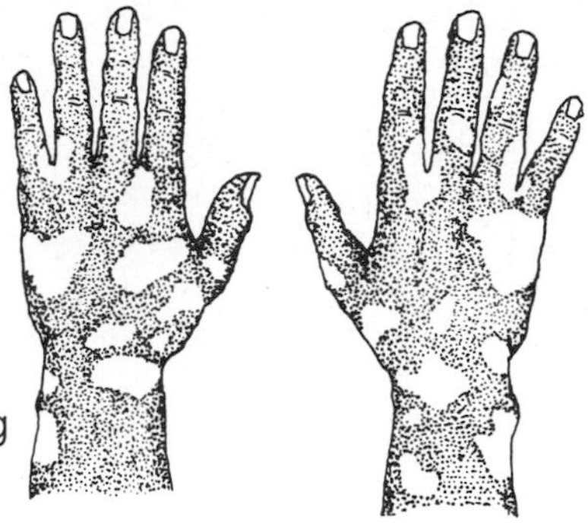

In some persons, certain areas of the skin lose their natural color (pigment). Then white patches appear. These are most common on the hands, feet, face, and upper body. This loss of normal skin color—called vitiligo—is not an illness. It can be compared to white hair in older people. No treatment helps or is needed, but the white skin should be protected from sunburn—with clothing or an ointment of zinc oxide. Also, special coloring creams can help make the spots less noticeable.

Other Causes of White Skin Patches

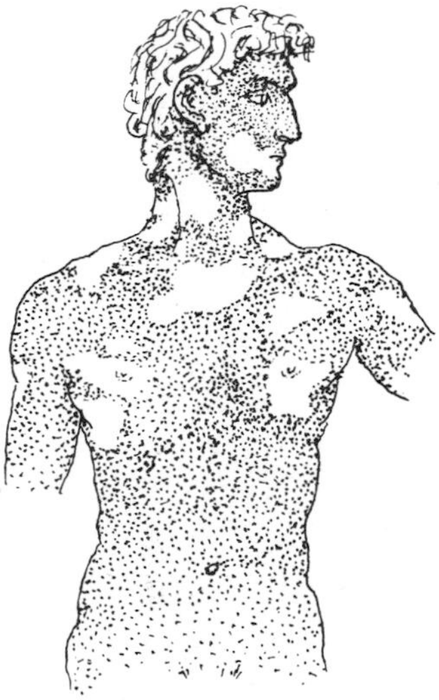

Certain diseases may cause white spots that look like vitiligo. In Latin America an infectious disease called **pinta** starts with bluish or red pimples and later leaves pale or white patches.

Treatment of pinta is 2.4 million units of benzathine penicillin injected into the buttocks (1.2 million units in each buttock). For a person allergic to penicillin give tetracycline or erythromycin, 500 mg. 4 times each day for 15 days.

Some fungus infections also cause whitish spots (see tinea versicolor, on the opposite page).

General or patchy, partial loss of skin and hair color in children may be caused by severe malnutrition (kwashiorkor, p.113; or pellagra, p. 208).

MASK OF PREGNANCY

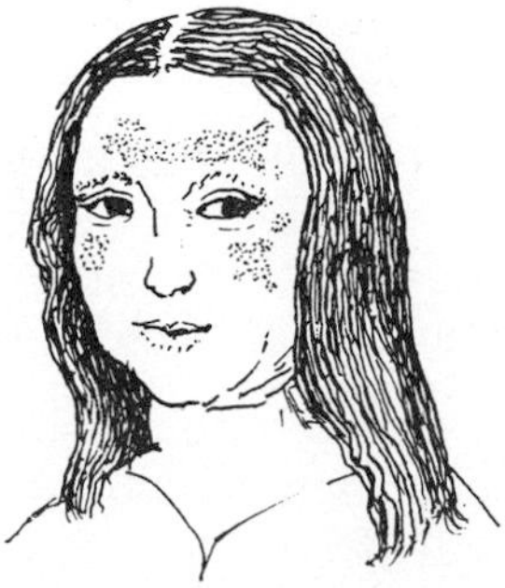

During pregnancy many women develop dark, olive-colored areas on the skin of the face, breasts, and down the middle of the belly. Sometimes these disappear after the birth and sometimes not. These marks also appear sometimes on women who are taking birth control pills.

They are completely normal and do not indicate weakness or sickness. No treatment is needed.

PELLAGRA
AND OTHER SKIN PROBLEMS DUE TO MALNUTRITION

Pellagra is a form of malnutrition that affects the skin and sometimes the digestive and nervous systems. It is very common in places where people eat a lot of maize (corn) or other starchy foods and not enough beans, meat, fish, eggs, vegetables, and other body-building and protective foods (see p. 110).

Skin signs in malnutrition (see the pictures on the following page):

In adults with pellagra the skin is dry and cracked; it peels like sunburn on the parts where the sun hits it, especially:

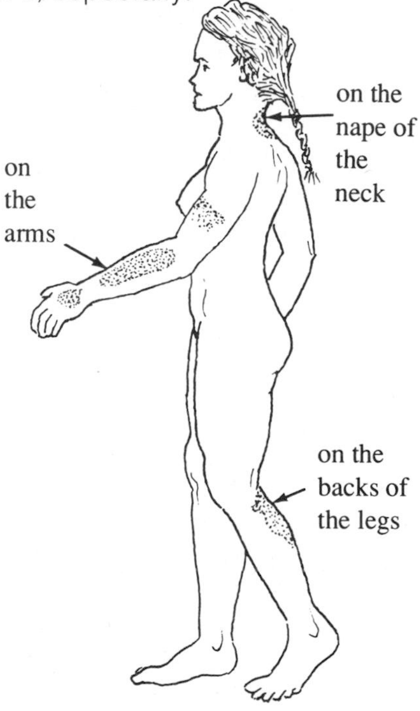

In malnourished children, the skin of the legs (and sometimes arms) may have dark marks, like bruises, or even peeling sores; the ankles and feet may be swollen (see p. 113).

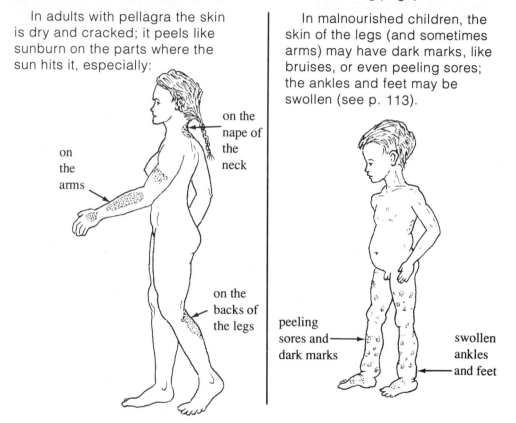

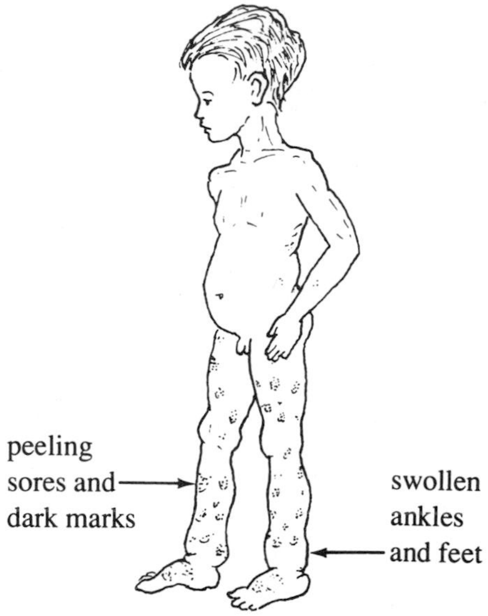

When these conditions exist, often there are also other signs of malnutrition: swollen belly; sores in the corners of the mouth; red, sore tongue; weakness; loss of appetite; failure to gain weight; etc. (see Chapter 11, p. 112 and 113).

Treatment:

- Eating nutritious foods cures pellagra. Every day a person should try to eat beans, lentils, groundnuts, or some chicken, fish, eggs, meat, or cheese. When you have a choice, it is also better to use wheat (preferably whole wheat) instead of maize (corn).

- For severe pellagra and some other forms of malnutrition, it may help to take vitamins, but **good food is more important.** Be sure the vitamin formula you use is high in the B vitamins, especially niacin. Brewer's yeast is a good source of B vitamins.

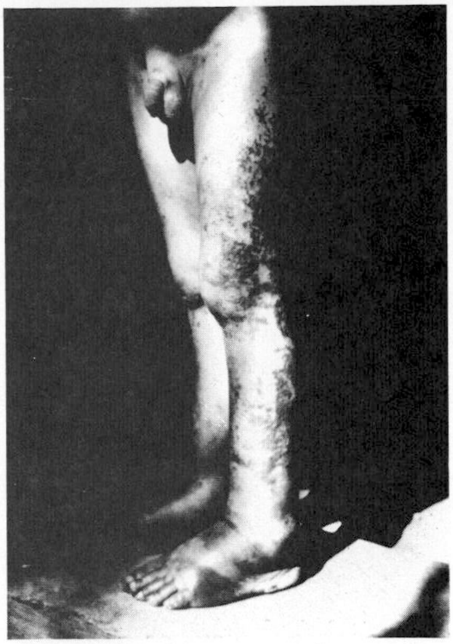

BEFORE
THIS BOY
BEGAN TO
EAT WELL

AND
AFTER

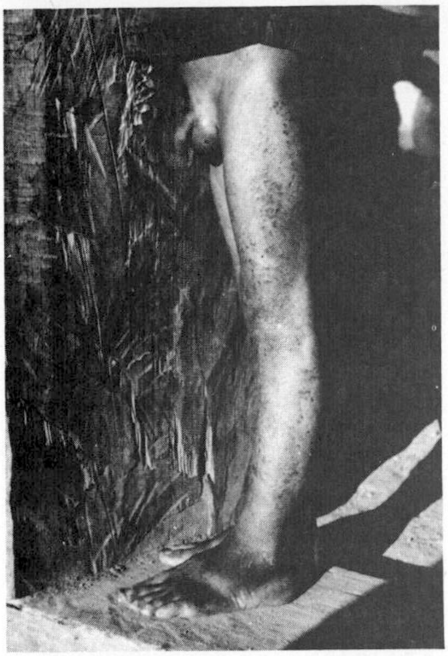

The swelling and dark spots on this boy's legs and feet are the result of poor nutrition. He was eating mostly maize (corn) without any foods rich in proteins and vitamins.

One week after he began to eat beans and eggs along with the maize, the swelling was gone and the spots had almost disappeared.

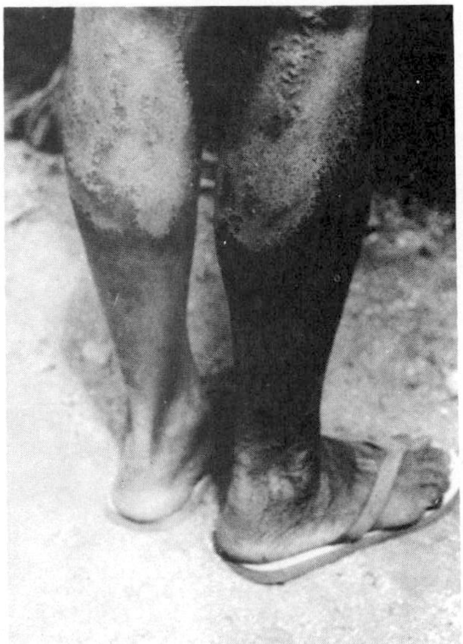

The 'burnt' skin on the legs of this woman is a sign of pellagra —which results from not eating well (see p. 208).

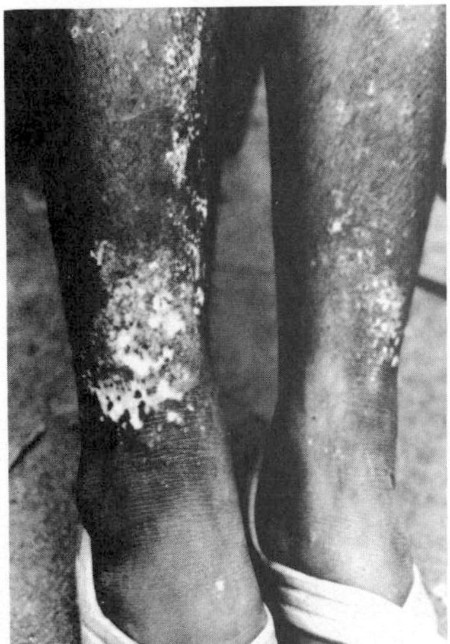

The white spots on the legs of this woman are due to an infectious disease called pinta (see p. 207).

WARTS (VERRUCAE)

Most warts, especially those in children, last 3 to 5 years and go away by themselves. Flat, painful wart-like spots on the sole of the foot are often 'plantar warts'. (Or they may be corns. See below.)

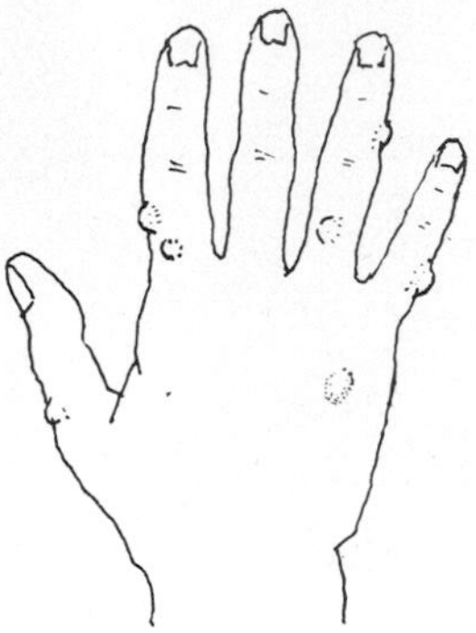

Treatment:

- Magical or household cures often get rid of warts. But it is safer not to use strong acids or poisonous plants, as these may cause burns or sores much worse than the warts.
- Painful plantar warts sometimes can be removed by a health worker.
- For warts on the penis or vagina, see p. 402.

CORNS

A corn is a hard, thick part of the skin. It forms where sandals or shoes push against the skin, or one toe presses against another. Corns can be very painful.

Treatment:

- Get sandals or shoes that do not press on the corns.
- To make corns hurt less, do this:

1. Soak the foot in warm water for 15 minutes.

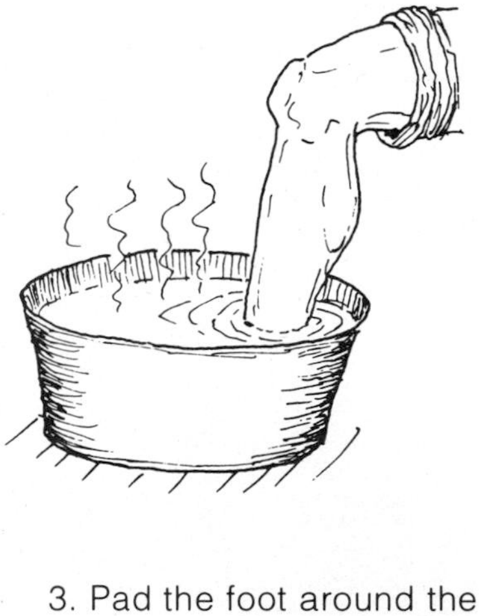

2. With a file or rasp, trim down the corn until it is thin.

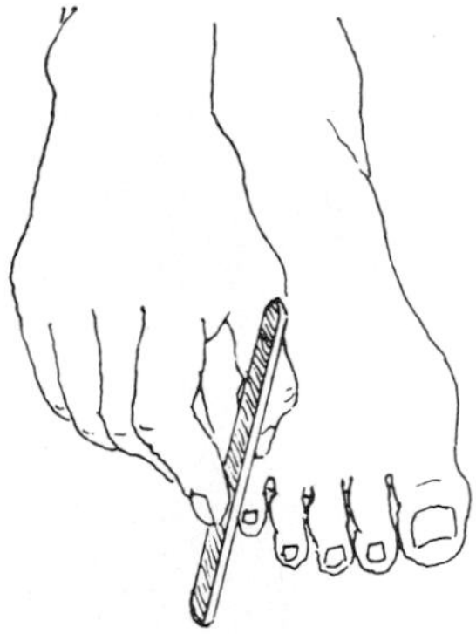

3. Pad the foot around the corn so that it will not press against the shoe or another toe. Wrap the foot or toe in a soft cloth to make a thick pad and cut a hole around the corn.

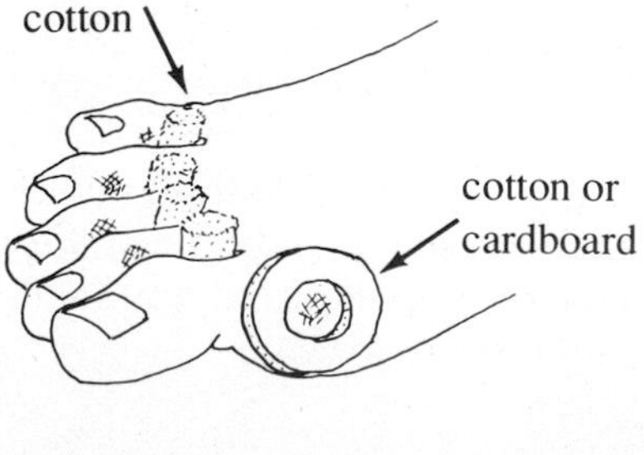

PIMPLES AND BLACKHEADS (ACNE)

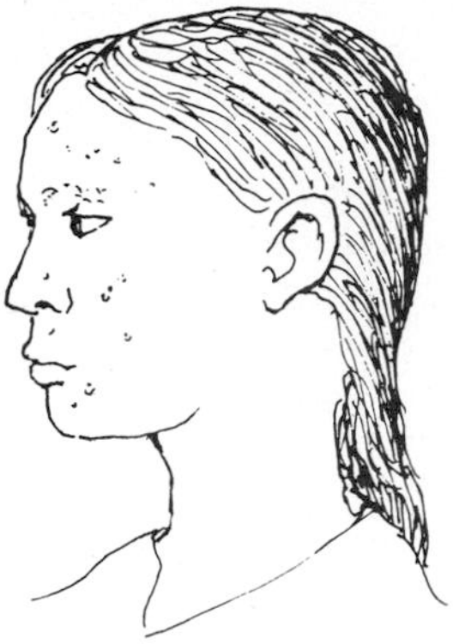

Young people sometimes get pimples on their face, chest, or back—especially if their skin has too much oil in it. ***Pimples*** are little lumps that form tiny white 'heads' of pus or ***blackheads*** of dirt. Sometimes they can become quite sore and large.

Treatment:

- Wash the face twice a day with soap and hot water.
- Wash the hair every 2 days, if possible.
- Sunshine helps clear pimples. Let the sunlight fall on the affected parts of the body.
- Eat as well as possible, drink a lot of water, and get enough sleep.
- Do not use skin or hair lotions that are waxy, oily, or greasy.
- Before you go to bed, put a mixture of alcohol with a little sulfur on the face (10 parts alcohol to 1 part sulfur).
- For serious cases forming lumps and pockets of pus, if these do not get better with the methods already described, tetracycline may help. Take 1 capsule 4 times a day for 3 days and then 2 capsules daily. It may be necessary to take 1 or 2 capsules daily for months.

CANCER OF THE SKIN

Skin cancer is most frequent in light-skinned persons who spend a lot of time in the sun. It usually appears in places where the sun hits with most force, especially:

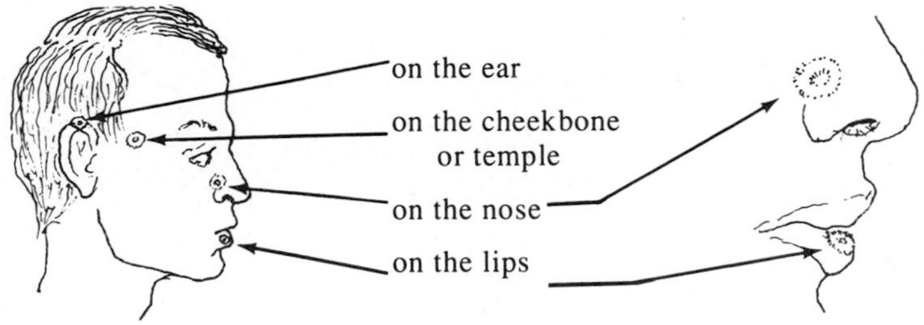

Skin cancer may take many forms. It usually begins as a little ring the color of pearl with a hole in the center. It grows little by little.

Most cancers of the skin are not dangerous if treated in time. Surgery is needed to remove them. If you have a chronic sore that might be skin cancer, see a health worker.

To prevent skin cancer, light-skinned persons should protect themselves from the sun and always wear a hat. Persons who have suffered from cancer of the skin and have to work in the sun can buy special creams that protect them. Zinc oxide ointment is cheap and works well.

TUBERCULOSIS OF THE SKIN OR LYMPH NODES

The same microbe that causes tuberculosis of the lungs also sometimes affects the skin, causing painless

tumors that disfigure,

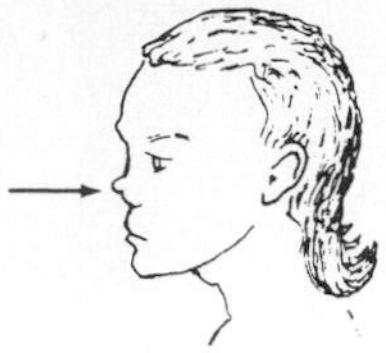

chronic patches of sores,

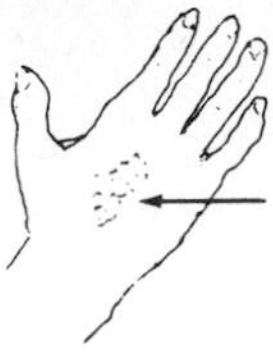

skin ulcers,

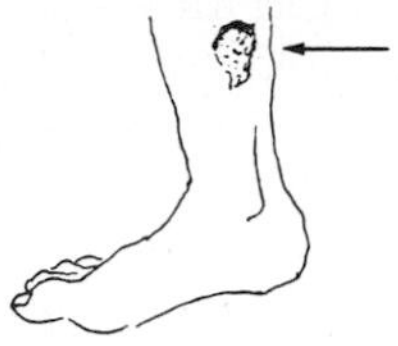

or

big warts.

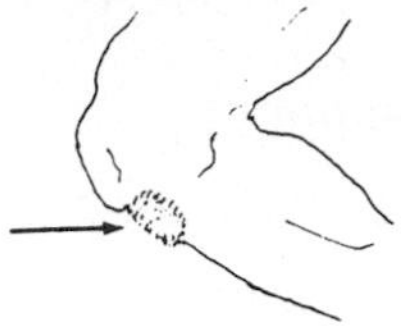

As a rule, TB of the skin develops slowly, lasts a long time, and keeps coming back over a period of months or years.

Also, tuberculosis sometimes infects the lymph nodes—most often those of the neck or in the area behind the collar bone, between the neck and the shoulder. The nodes become large, open, drain pus, seal closed for a time, and then open and drain again. Usually **they are not painful.**

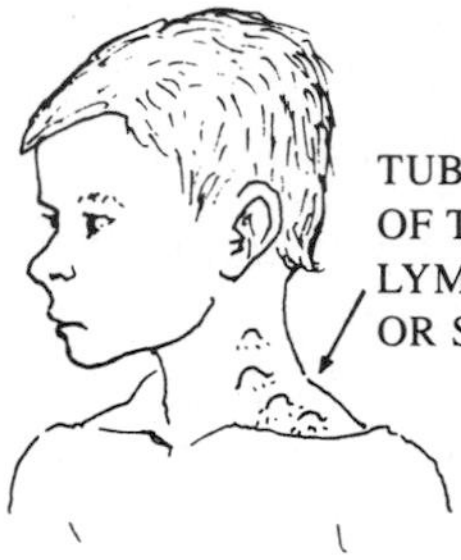

TUBERCULOSIS OF THE LYMPH NODES, OR SCROFULA

Treatment:

In the case of any chronic sore, ulcer, or swollen lymph nodes, it is best to seek medical advice. Tests may be needed to learn the cause. Tuberculosis of the skin is treated the same as tuberculosis of the lungs (see p. 180). To keep the infection from returning, the medicines must be taken for many months after the skin looks well.

ERYSIPELAS AND CELLULITIS

Erysipelas (or St. Anthony's fire) is a very painful acute (sudden) infection in the skin. It forms a hot, bright red, swollen patch with a sharp border. The patch spreads rapidly over the skin. It often begins on the face, at the edge of the nose. This usually causes swollen lymph nodes, fever, and chills.

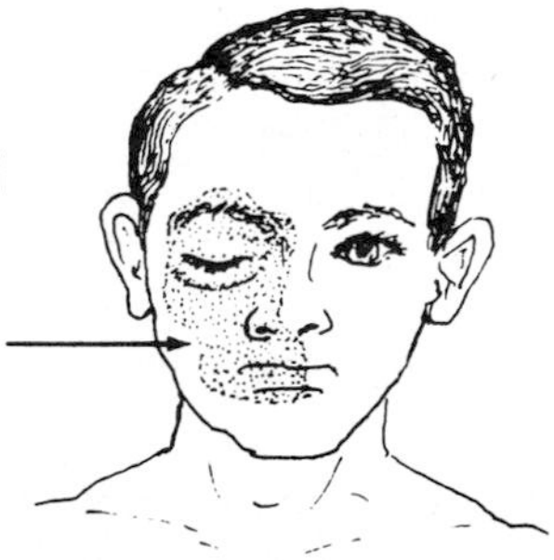

Cellulitis is also a very painful, acute infection of the skin that can appear anywhere on the body. It usually occurs after a break in the skin. The infection is deeper and the borders of the patch are less clear than with erysipelas.

Treatment:

For both erysipelas and cellulitis, begin treatment as soon as possible. Use an antibiotic: penicillin tablets, 400,000 units, 4 times a day; in serious cases, injectable procaine penicillin, 800,000 units daily (see p. 353). Continue using the antibiotic for 2 days after all signs of infection are gone. Also use hot compresses—and aspirin for pain.

GANGRENE (GAS GANGRENE)

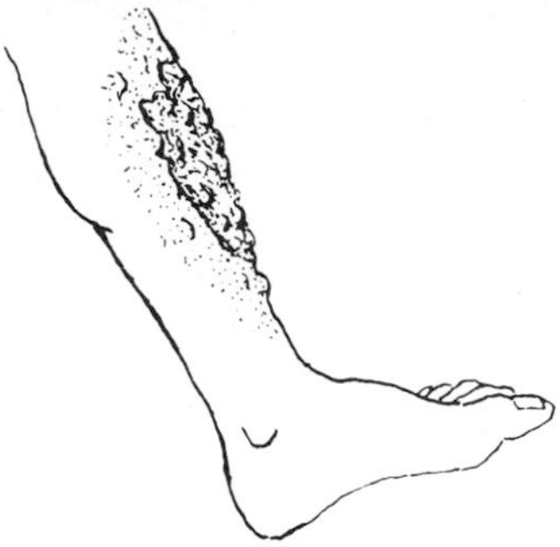

This is a very dangerous infection of a wound, in which a foul-smelling gray or brown liquid forms. The skin near the wound may have dark blisters and the flesh may have air bubbles in it. The infection begins between 6 hours and 3 days after the injury. It quickly gets worse and spreads fast. Without treatment it causes death in a few days.

Treatment:

- Open up the wound as wide as possible. Wash it out with cool, boiled water and soap. Clean out the dead and damaged flesh. If possible, flood the wound with hydrogen peroxide every 2 hours.
- Inject penicillin (crystalline if possible), 1,000,000 (a million) units every 3 hours.
- **Leave the wound uncovered so that air gets to it. Get medical help.**

ULCERS OF THE SKIN CAUSED BY POOR CIRCULATION

Skin ulcers, or large, open sores, have many causes (see p. 20). However, chronic ulcers on the ankles of older persons, especially in women with varicose veins, usually come from poor circulation. The blood is not moved fast enough through the legs. Such ulcers may become very large. The skin around the ulcer is dark blue, shiny, and very thin. Often the foot is swollen.

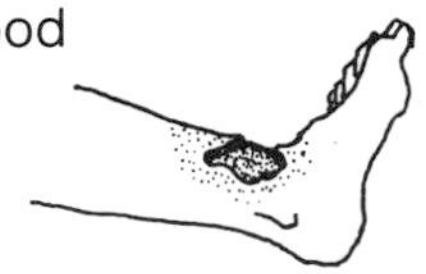

Treatment:

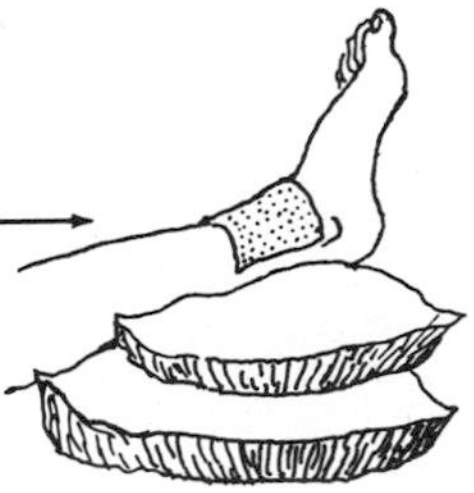

- These ulcers heal very slowly—and only if great care is taken. Most important: **keep the foot up** high as often as possible. Sleep with it on pillows. During the day, rest with the foot up high every 15 or 20 minutes. **Walking helps the circulation, but standing in one place and sitting with the feet down are harmful.**
- Put warm compresses of weak salt water on the ulcer—1 teaspoon salt to a liter of boiled water. Cover the ulcer loosely with sterile gauze or a clean cloth. **Keep it clean.**
- Support the varicose veins with elastic stockings or bandages. Continue to use these and to keep the feet up after the ulcer heals. Take great care not to scratch or injure the delicate scar.

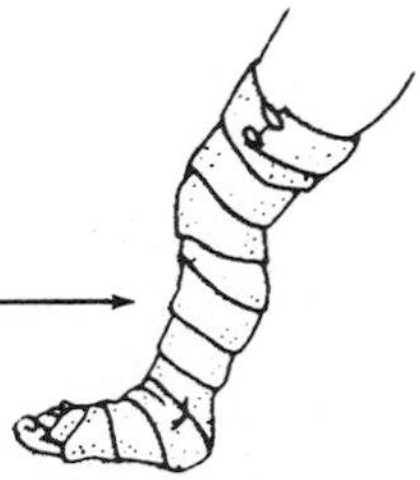

- Treating the ulcers with honey or sugar may help (see p. 214).

Prevent skin ulcers—care for varicose veins early (see p. 175).

BED SORES (PRESSURE SORES)

These chronic open sores appear in persons so ill they cannot roll over in bed, especially in sick old persons who are very thin and weak. The sores form over bony parts of the body where the skin is pressed against the bedding. They are most often seen on the buttocks, back, shoulders, elbows, or feet.

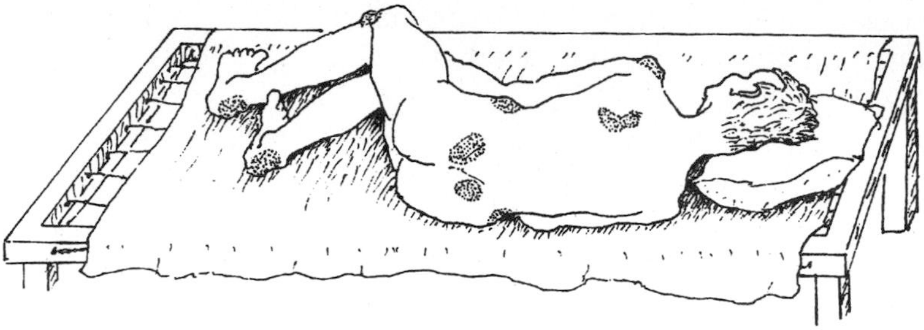

For a more complete discussion of pressure sores, see ***Disabled Village Children,*** Chapter 24.

How to prevent bed sores:

- Turn the sick person over every hour: face up, face down, side to side.
- Bathe him every day and rub his skin with baby oil.
- Use soft bed sheets and padding. Change them daily and each time the bedding gets dirty with urine, stools, vomit, etc.
- Put cushions under the person in such a way that the bony parts rub less.

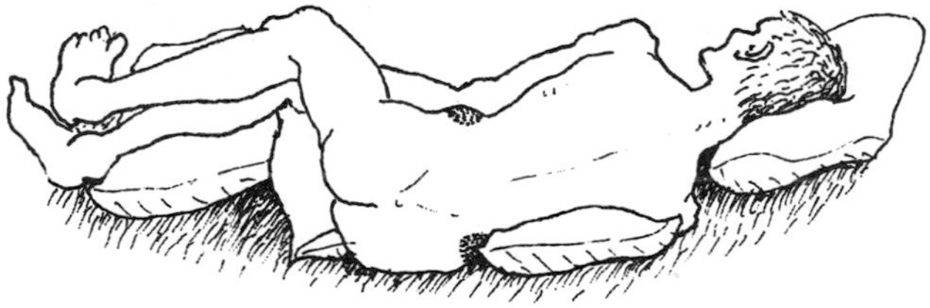

- Feed the sick person as well as possible. If he does not eat well, extra vitamins and iron may help (see p. 118).
- A child who has a severe chronic illness should be held often on his mother's lap.

Treatment:

- Do all the things mentioned above.
- 3 times a day, wash the sores with cool, boiled water mixed with mild soap. Gently remove any dead flesh. Rinse well with cool, boiled water.
- To fight infection and speed healing, fill the sore with honey, sugar, or molasses. (A paste made of honey and sugar is easiest to use.) It is important to clean and refill the sore at least 2 times a day. If the honey or sugar becomes too thin with liquid from the sore, it will feed germs rather than kill them.

SKIN PROBLEMS OF BABIES

Diaper Rash

Reddish patches of irritation between a baby's legs or buttocks may be caused by urine in his diapers (nappy) or bedding.

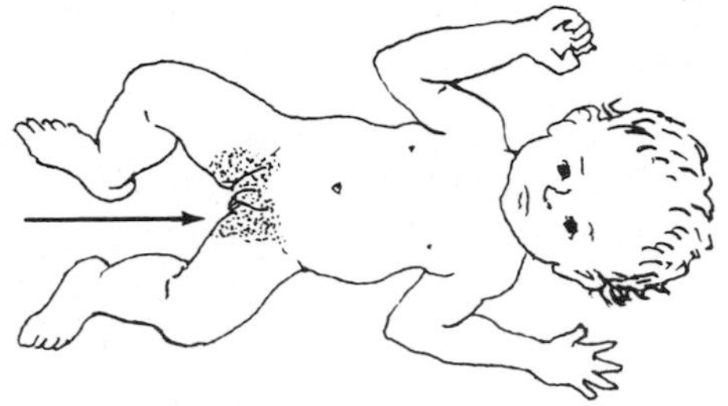

Treatment:

- Bathe the child daily with lukewarm water and mild soap. Dry her carefully.
- **To prevent or cure the rash, the child should be kept naked, without diapers, and he should be taken out into the sun.**

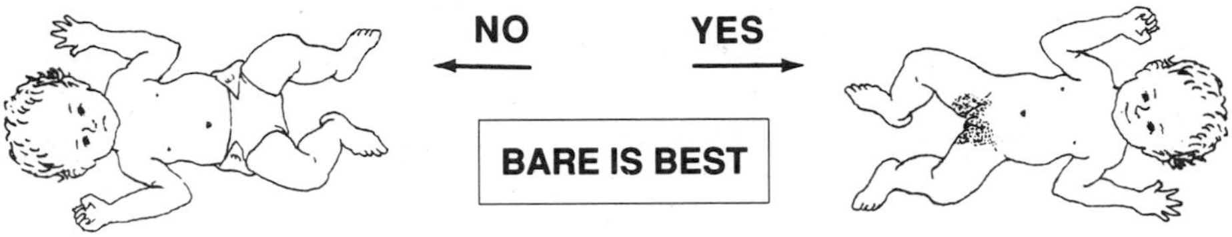

- If diapers are used, change them often. After washing the diapers, rinse them in water with a little vinegar.
- It is best not to use talc (talcum powder), but if you do, wait until the rash is gone.

Cradle Cap (Seborrhea, Dandruff)

Cradle cap is an oily, yellow crust that forms on a baby's scalp. The skin is often red and irritated. Cradle cap usually results from not washing the baby's head often enough, or from keeping the head covered.

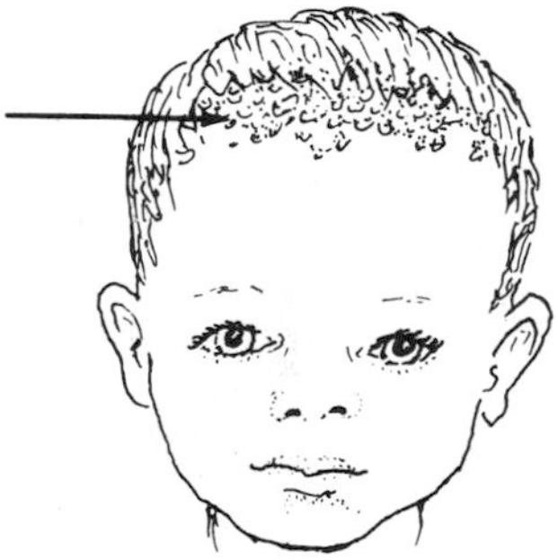

Treatment:

- Wash the head daily. If possible use a medicated soap (see p. 371).
- Gently clean off all the dandruff and crust. To loosen the scales and crust, first wrap the head with towels soaked in lukewarm water.
- Keep the baby's head **uncovered,** open to the air and sunlight.

DO NOT COVER A BABY'S HEAD WITH A CAP OR CLOTH. KEEP THE HEAD UNCOVERED.

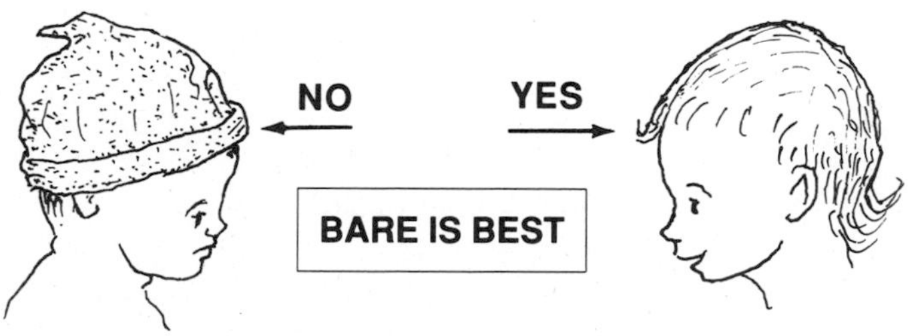

- If there are signs of infection, treat as for impetigo (see p. 202).

ECZEMA (RED PATCHES WITH LITTLE BLISTERS)

Signs:

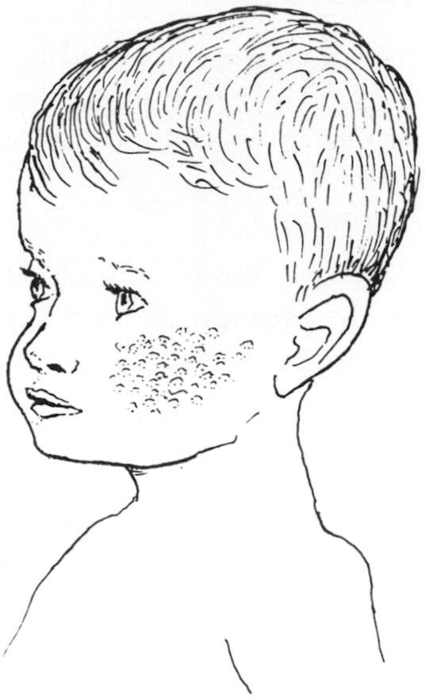

- In small children: a red patch or rash forms on the cheeks or sometimes on the arms and hands. The rash consists of small sores or blisters that ooze or weep (burst and leak fluid).
- In older children and grown-ups: eczema is usually drier and is most common behind the knees and on the inside of the elbows.
- It does not start as an infection but is more like an allergic reaction.

Treatment:

- ♦ Put cold compresses on the rash.
- ♦ If signs of infection develop (p. 88), treat as for impetigo (p. 202).
- ♦ Let the sunlight fall on the patches.
- ♦ In difficult cases, use a cortisone or cortico-steroid cream (see p. 371). Or coal tar may help. Seek medical advice.

PSORIASIS

Signs:

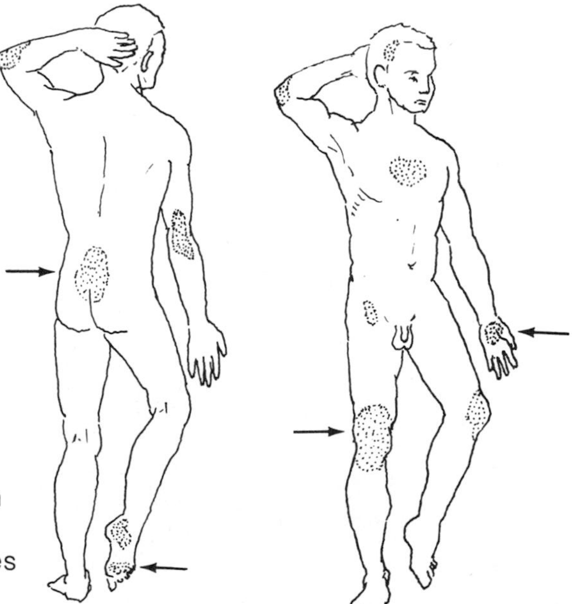

- Thick, rough patches of reddish or blue-gray skin covered with whitish or silver-colored scales. The patches appear most commonly in the parts shown in the drawings.
- The condition usually lasts a long time or keeps coming back. It is not an infection and is not dangerous.

Treatment:

- ♦ Leaving the affected skin open to the sunlight often helps.
- ♦ Bathing in the ocean sometimes helps.
- ♦ Seek medical advice. Treatment must be continued for a long time.

CHAPTER 16

THE EYES

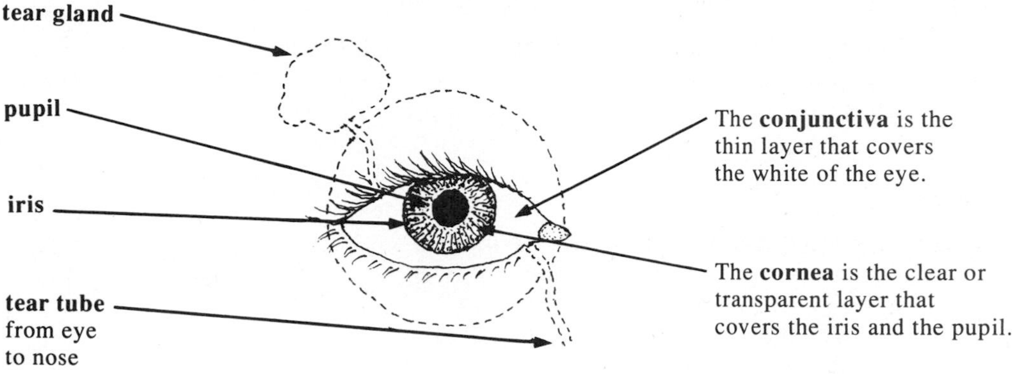

tear gland
pupil
iris
tear tube from eye to nose
The **conjunctiva** is the thin layer that covers the white of the eye.
The **cornea** is the clear or transparent layer that covers the iris and the pupil.

DANGER SIGNS

The eyes are delicate and need good care. Get medical help fast when any of the following danger signs occurs:

1. Any injury that cuts or ruptures (goes through) the eyeball.
2. Painful, grayish spot on the cornea, with redness around the cornea (corneal ulcer).
3. Great pain inside the eye (possibly iritis or glaucoma).
4. A big difference in the size of the pupils when there is pain in the eye or the head.

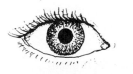

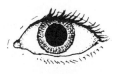

A big difference in the size of the pupils may come from brain damage, stroke, injury to the eye, glaucoma, or iritis. (A small difference is normal in some people.)

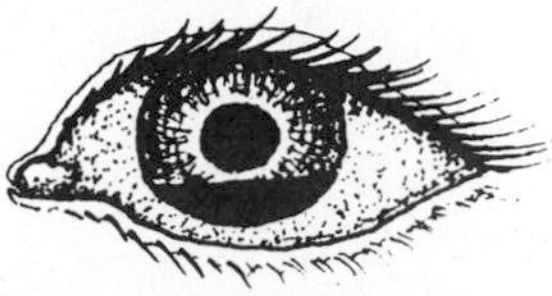

5. Blood behind the cornea inside the eyeball (see p. 225).
6. If vision begins to fail in one or both eyes.
7. Any eye infection or inflammation that does not get better after 5 or 6 days of treatment with an antibiotic eye ointment.

INJURIES TO THE EYE

All injuries to the eyeball must be considered dangerous, for they may cause blindness.

Even small cuts on the **cornea** (the transparent layer covering the pupil and iris) may get infected and harm the vision if not cared for correctly.

If a wound to the eyeball is so deep that it reaches the black layer beneath the outer white layer, this is especially dangerous.

If a blunt injury (as with a fist) causes the eyeball to fill with blood, the eye is in danger (see p. 225). Danger is especially great if pain suddenly gets much worse after a few days, for this is probably acute glaucoma (p. 222).

Treatment:

- If the person still sees well with the injured eye, put an antibiotic eye ointment (p. 378) in the eye and cover it with a soft, thick bandage. If the eye is not better in a day or two, get medical help.
- If the person cannot see well with the injured eye, if the wound is deep, or if there is blood inside the eye behind the cornea (p. 225), cover the eye with a clean bandage and go for medical help at once. **Do not press on the eye.**
- **Do not** try to remove thorns or splinters that are tightly stuck in the eyeball. Get medical help.

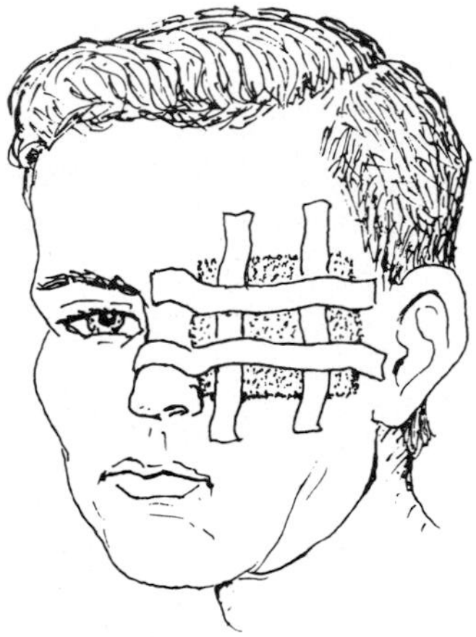

HOW TO REMOVE A SPECK OF DIRT FROM THE EYE

Have the person close her eyes and look to the left, the right, up and down. Then, while you hold her eye open, have her look up and then down. This will make the eye produce more tears and the dirt often comes out by itself.

Or you can try to remove the bit of dirt or sand by flooding the eye with clean water (p. 219) or by using the corner of a clean cloth or some moist cotton. If the particle of dirt is under the upper lid, look for it by turning the lid up over a thin stick. The person should look down while you do this:

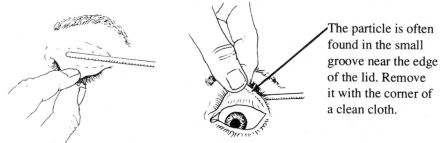

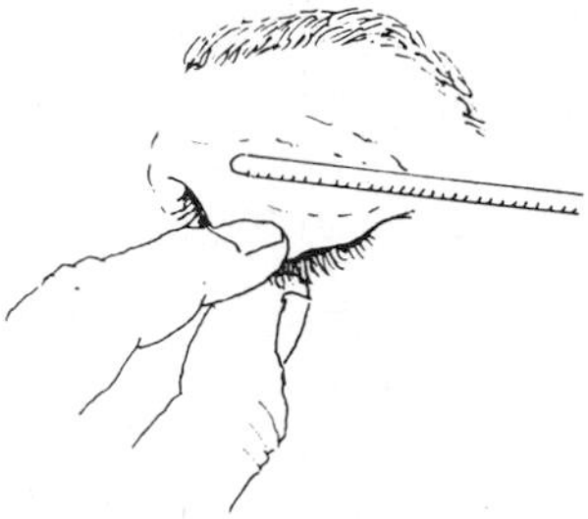

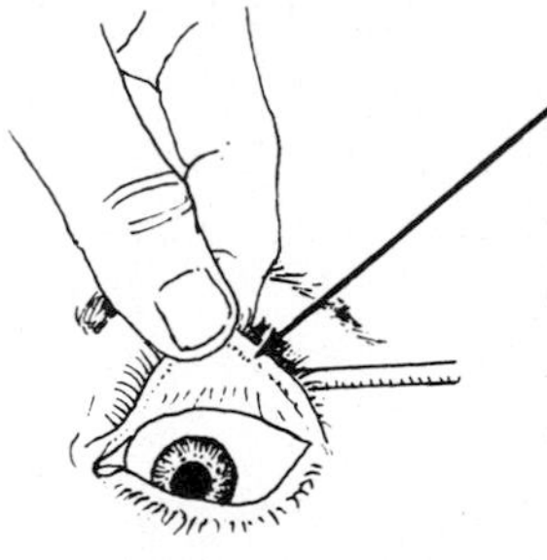

The particle is often found in the small groove near the edge of the lid. Remove it with the corner of a clean cloth.

If you cannot get the particle out easily, use an antibiotic eye ointment, cover the eye with a bandage, and go for medical help.

CHEMICAL BURNS OF THE EYE

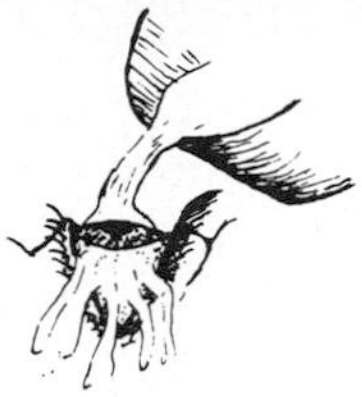

Battery acid, lye, gasoline, or a pesticide that gets into the eye can be dangerous. Hold open the eye. **Immediately flood the eye with clean, cool water. Keep flooding for 30 minutes,** or until it stops hurting. Do not let the water get into the other eye.

RED, PAINFUL EYES—DIFFERENT CAUSES

Many different problems cause red, painful eyes. Correct treatment often depends on finding the cause, so be sure to check carefully for signs of each possibility. This chart may help you find the cause:

foreign matter (bit of dirt, etc.) in the eye (p. 218)	usually affects **one eye only;** redness and pain variable
burns or harmful liquids (p. 219)	one or both eyes; redness and pain variable
'pink eye' (conjunctivitis, p. 219) hay fever (allergic conjunctivitis, p. 165) trachoma (p. 220) measles (p. 311)	usually **both eyes** (may start or be worse in one) usually reddest at outer edge 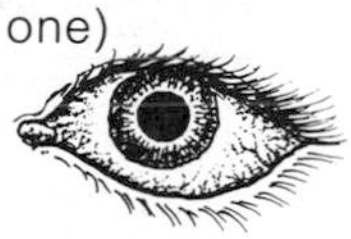 'burning' pain, usually mild
acute glaucoma (p. 222) iritis (p. 221) scratch or ulcer on the cornea (p. 224)	usually **one eye only;** reddest next to the cornea 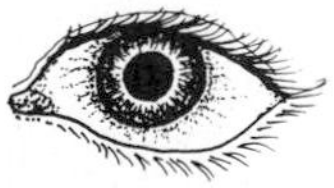 pain often great

'PINK EYE' (CONJUNCTIVITIS)

This infection causes redness, pus, and mild 'burning' in one or both eyes. Lids often stick together after sleep. It is especially common in children.

Treatment:

First clean pus from the eyes with a clean cloth moistened with boiled water. Then put in antibiotic eye ointment (p. 378). Pull down the lower lid and put a little bit of ointment **inside,** like this: Putting ointment outside the eye does no good.

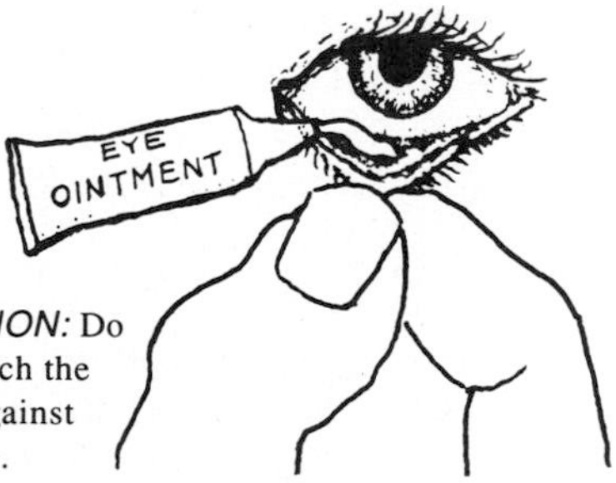

CAUTION: Do not touch the tube against the eye.

Prevention:

Most conjunctivitis is very contagious. The infection is easily spread from one person to another. Do not let a child with pink eye play or sleep with others, or use the same towel. Wash hands after touching eyes.

TRACHOMA

Trachoma is a chronic infection that slowly gets worse. It may last for months or many years. If not treated early, it sometimes causes blindness. It is spread by touch or by flies, and is most common where people live in poor, crowded conditions.

Signs:

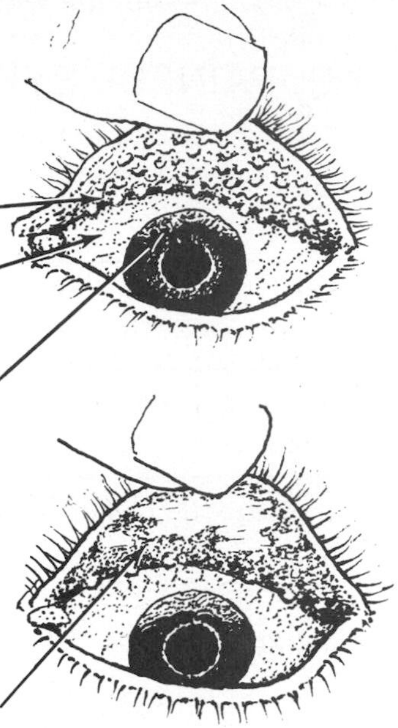

- Trachoma begins with red, watery eyes, like ordinary conjunctivitis.
- After a month or more, small, pinkish gray lumps, called follicles, form inside the upper eyelids. To see these, turn back the lid as shown on p. 218.
- The white of the eye is a little red.
- After a few months, if you look very carefully, or with a magnifying glass, you may see that the top edge of the cornea looks grayish, because it has many tiny new blood vessels in it *(pannus).*
- The combination of both follicles and pannus is almost certainly trachoma.
- After several years, the follicles begin to disappear, leaving whitish scars.

These scars make the eyelids thick and may keep them from opening or closing all the way.

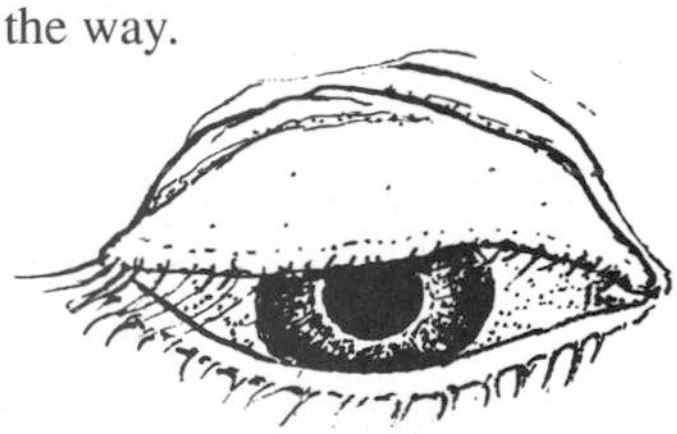

Or the scarring may pull the eyelashes down into the eye, scratching the cornea and causing blindness.

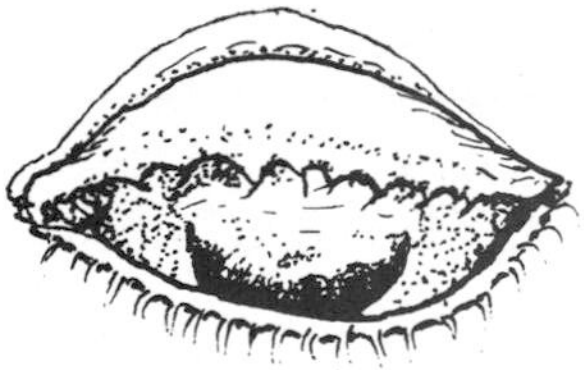

Treatment of trachoma:

Put 1% tetracycline or erythromycin eye ointment (p. 378) inside the eye 3 times each day, or 3% tetracycline or erythromycin eye ointment 1 time each day. Do this for 30 days. For a complete cure, also take tetracycline (p. 356), erythromycin (p. 355) or a sulfonamide (p. 358) by mouth for 2 to 3 weeks.

Prevention:

Early and complete treatment of trachoma helps prevent its spread to others. All persons living with someone who has trachoma, especially children, should have their eyes examined often and if signs appear, they should be treated early. Washing the face every day can help prevent trachoma. Also, it is very important to follow the Guidelines of Cleanliness, explained in Chapter 12.

Cleanliness helps prevent trachoma.

INFECTED EYES IN NEWBORN BABIES (NEONATAL CONJUNCTIVITIS)

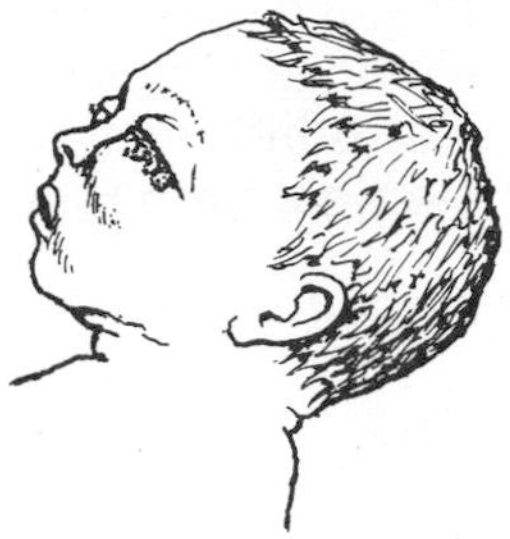

In the first 2 days of life, if a newborn baby's eyes get red, swell, and have a lot of pus in them, this is probably **gonorrhea** (p. 236). It must be treated **at once** to prevent the baby from going blind. If the eye infection begins between 1 and 3 weeks after birth, she may have **chlamydia.** The baby has picked up one or both of these diseases from the mother at birth.

Treatment for gonorrhea:

- Give one injection of 50 to 75 mg. of kanamycin (see p. 359). Or, penicillin sometimes works: inject 200,000 units of crystalline penicillin twice a day for 3 days. Or, try 1/2 teaspoon of co-trimoxazole syrup by mouth 2 times a day for a week (see p. 358). (If available, one injection of 125 mg. of ceftriaxone is the best treatment.)
- Also use tetracycline or erythromycin eye ointment: put a little in the baby's eyes every hour for the first day, and then 3 times a day for 2 weeks. (First clean out the pus as described on p. 219.)

Treatment for chlamydia: Treat with tetracycline or erythromycin ointment as described above. Also give erythromycin syrup by mouth, 30 mg. 4 times a day for 2 weeks. (This will treat pneumonia, which often affects babies with chlamydia.)

Prevention:

All babies' eyes should be protected against gonorrhea and chlamydia, especially the eyes of babies whose mothers may have these diseases or whose fathers have pain when passing urine. (Mothers may have gonorrhea or chlamydia without knowing it.)

Put a little 1 % tetracycline, erythromycin or chloramphenicol eye ointment in each eye at birth (see p. 379). Or, if you do not have eye ointment, put a drop of 1% silver nitrate solution **once only** in each eye at birth.

If a baby develops gonorrhea or chlamydia of the eyes, **both** parents should be treated for these infections (p. 236).

IRITIS (INFLAMMATION OF THE IRIS)

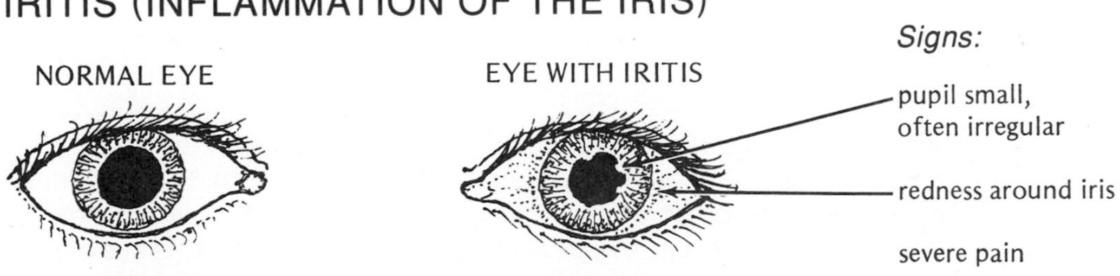

Iritis usually happens in one eye only. Pain may begin suddenly or gradually. The eye waters a lot. It hurts more in bright light. The eyeball hurts when you touch it. There is no pus as with conjunctivitis. Vision is usually blurred.

This is an emergency. Antibiotic ointments do not help. **Get medical help.**

GLAUCOMA

This dangerous disease is the result of too much pressure in the eye. It usually begins after the age of 40 and is a common cause of blindness. **To prevent blindness, it is important to recognize the signs of glaucoma and get medical help fast.**

There are 2 forms of glaucoma.

ACUTE GLAUCOMA:

This starts suddenly with a headache or severe pain in the eye. The eye becomes red, the vision blurred. The eyeball feels hard to the touch, like a marble. There may be vomiting. The pupil of the bad eye is bigger than that of the good eye.

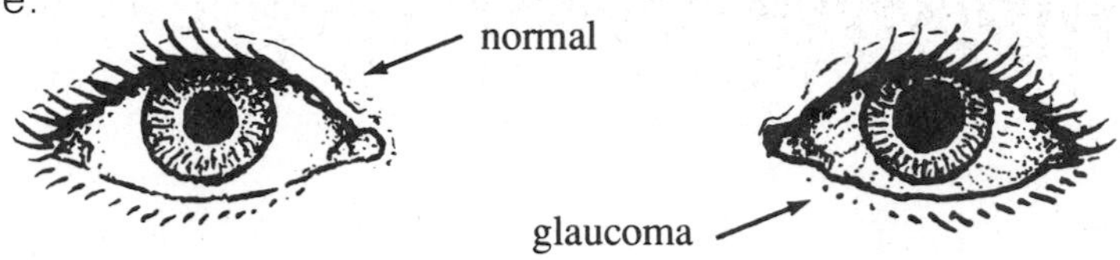

If not treated very soon, acute glaucoma will cause blindness within a few days. Surgery is often needed. **Get medical help fast.**

CHRONIC GLAUCOMA:

The pressure in the eye rises slowly. Usually there is no pain. Vision is lost slowly, starting from the side, and often the person does not notice the loss. Testing the side vision may help detect the disease.

TEST FOR GLAUCOMA

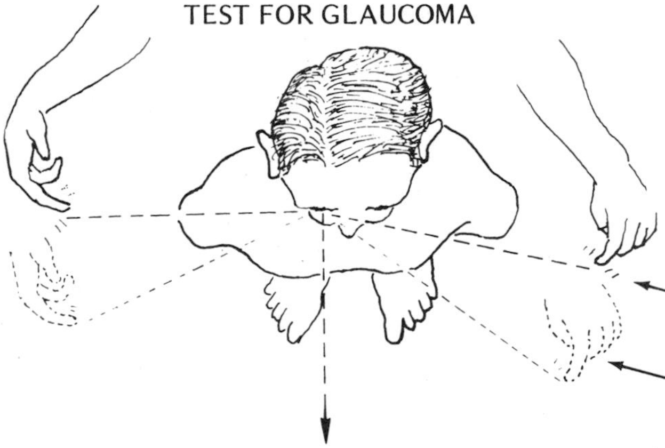

Have the person cover one eye, and with the other look at an object straight ahead of him. Note when he can first see moving fingers coming from behind on each side of the head.

Normally fingers are first seen here.

In glaucoma, finger movement is first seen more toward the front.

If discovered early, treatment with special eyedrops (pilocarpine) may prevent blindness. Dosage should be determined by a doctor or health worker who can measure the eye pressure periodically. Drops must be used for the rest of one's life. When possible, eye surgery is usually the surest form of treatment.

Prevention:

Persons who are over 40 years old or have relatives with glaucoma should try to have their eye pressure checked once a year.

INFECTION OF THE TEAR SAC (DACRYOCYSTITIS)

Signs:

Redness, pain, and swelling beneath the eye, next to the nose. The eye waters a lot. A drop of pus may appear in the corner of the eye when the swelling is gently pressed.

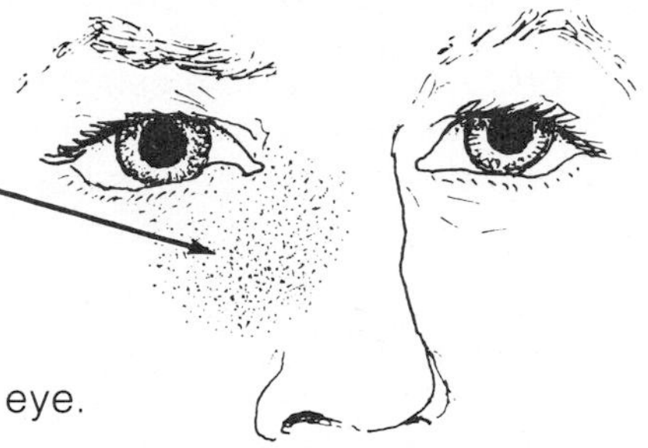

Treatment:

- Apply hot compresses.
- Put antibiotic eye drops or ointment in the eye.
- Take penicillin (p. 351).

TROUBLE SEEING CLEARLY

Children who have trouble seeing clearly or who get headaches or eye pain when they read may need glasses. Have their eyes examined.

In older persons, it is normal that, with passing years, it becomes more difficult to see close things clearly. Reading glasses often help. Pick glasses that let you see clearly about 40 cm. (15 inches) away from your eyes. If glasses do not help, see an eye doctor.

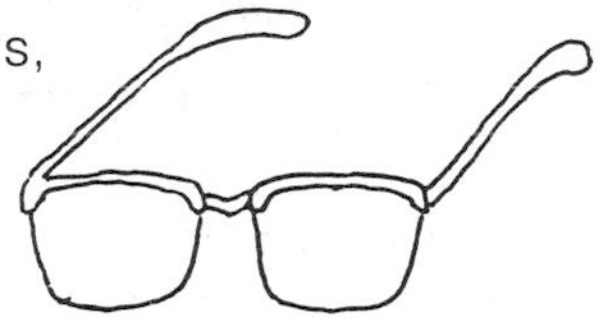

CROSS-EYES AND A WANDERING OR 'LAZY' EYE (STRABISMUS, 'SQUINT')

If the eye sometimes wanders like this, but at other times looks ahead normally, usually you need not worry. The eye will grow straighter in time. But if the eye is always turned the wrong way, and if the child is not treated at a very early age, she may never see well with that eye. See an eye doctor as soon as possible to find out if patching of the good eye, surgery, or special glasses might help.

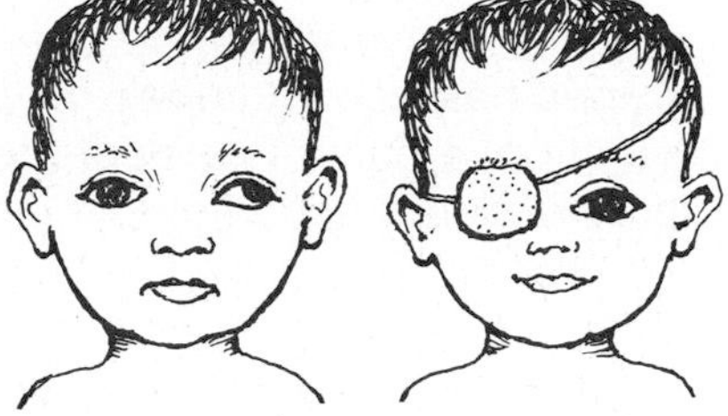

Surgery done at a later age can usually straighten the eye and improve the child's appearance, but it will not help the weak eye see better.

IMPORTANT: The eyesight of every child should be checked as early as possible (best around 4 years). You can use an 'E' chart (see *Helping Health Workers Learn,* p. 24-13). Test each eye separately to discover any problem that affects only one eye. If sight is poor in one or both eyes, see an eye doctor.

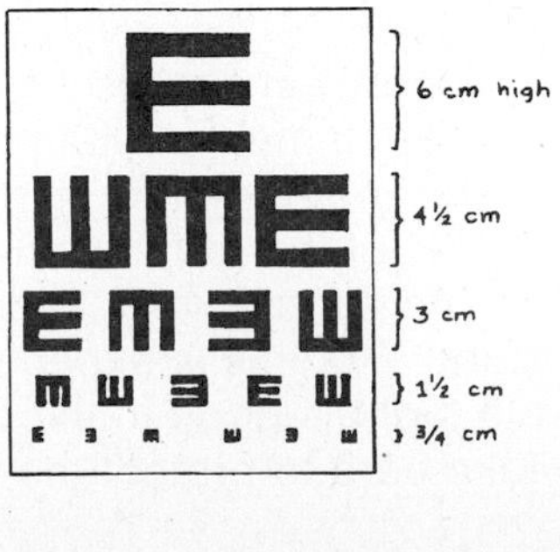

STY (HORDEOLUM)

A red, swollen lump on the eyelid, usually near its edge. To treat, apply warm, moist compresses with a little salt in the water. Use of an antibiotic eye ointment 3 times a day will help prevent more sties from occurring.

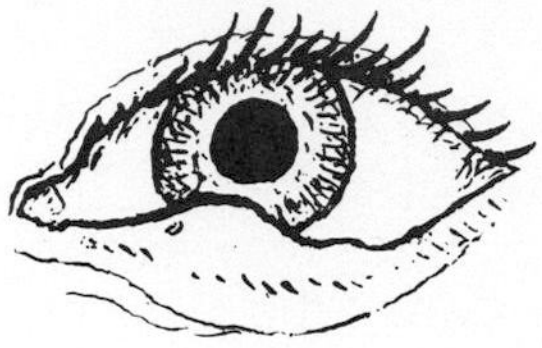

PTERYGIUM

A fleshy thickening on the eye surface that slowly grows out from the edge of the white part of the eye near the nose and onto the cornea; caused in part by sunlight, wind, and dust. Dark glasses may help calm irritation and slow the growth of a pterygium. It should be removed by surgery before it reaches the pupil. Unfortunately, after surgery a pterygium often grows back again.

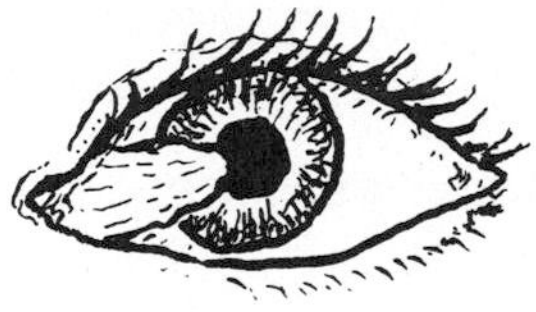

Folk treatments using powdered shells do more harm than good. To help calm itching and burning you can try using cold compresses. Or use eye drops of camomile (well boiled, then cooled, and without sugar).

A SCRAPE, ULCER, OR SCAR ON THE CORNEA

When the very thin, delicate surface of the cornea has been scraped, or damaged by infection, a painful **corneal ulcer** may result. If you look hard in a good light, you may see a grayish or less shiny patch on the surface of the cornea.

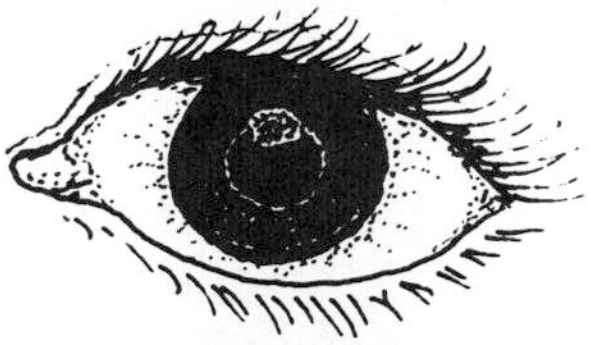

If not well cared for, a corneal ulcer can cause blindness. Apply antibiotic eye ointment, 4 times a day for 7 days, give penicillin (p. 351), and cover the eye with a patch. If the eye is not better in 2 days, get medical help.

A **corneal scar** is a painless, white patch on the cornea. It may result from a healed corneal ulcer, burn, or other injury to the eye. If both eyes are blind but the person still sees light, surgery (corneal transplant) to one eye may return its sight. But this is expensive. If one eye is scarred, but sight is good in the other, avoid surgery. Take care to protect the good eye from injury.

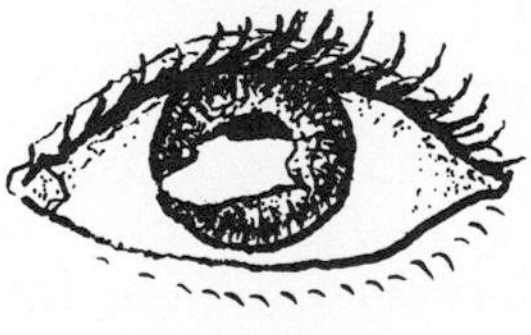

BLEEDING IN THE WHITE OF THE EYE

A painless, blood-red patch in the white part of the eye occasionally appears after lifting something heavy, coughing hard (as with whooping cough), or being hit on the eye. The condition results from the bursting of a small vessel. It is harmless, like a bruise, and will slowly disappear without treatment in about 2 weeks.

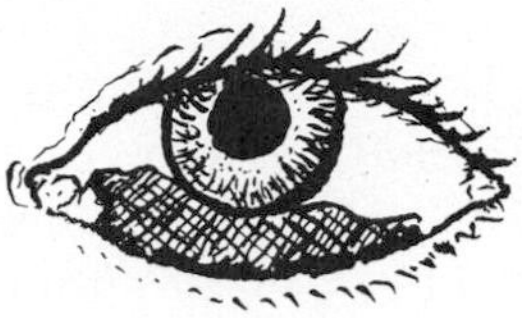

Small red patches are common on the eyes of newborn babies. No treatment is needed.

BLEEDING BEHIND THE CORNEA (HYPHEMA)

Blood behind the cornea is a danger sign. It usually results from an injury to the eye with a blunt object, like a fist. If there is pain and loss of sight, refer the person to an eye specialist immediately. If the pain is mild and there is not loss of sight, patch both eyes and keep the person at rest in bed for several days. If after a few days the pain becomes much worse, there is probably hardening of the eye (glaucoma, p. 222). Take the person to an eye doctor **at once.**

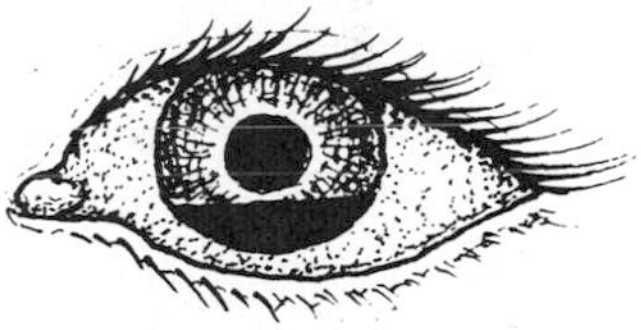

PUS BEHIND THE CORNEA (HYPOPYON)

Pus behind the cornea is a sign of severe *inflammation.* It is sometimes seen with corneal ulcers and is a sign that the eye is in danger. Give penicillin (p. 351) and get medical help at once. If the ulcer is treated correctly, the hypopyon will often clear up by itself.

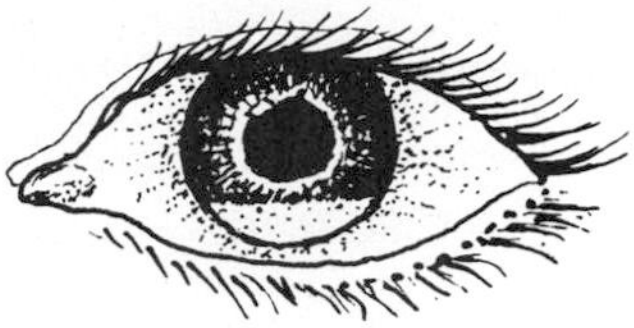

CATARACT

The lens of the eye, behind the pupil, becomes cloudy, making the pupil look gray or white when you shine a light into it. Cataract is common in older persons, but also occurs, rarely, in babies. If a blind person with cataracts can still tell light from dark and notice movement, surgery may let him see again. However, he will need strong glasses afterward, which take time to get used to. Medicines do not help cataracts. (Now sometimes during surgery an artificial lens is put inside the eye—so that strong eyeglasses are not needed.)

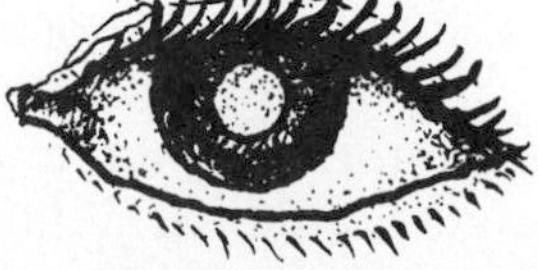

NIGHT BLINDNESS AND XEROPHTHALMIA (VITAMIN A DEFICIENCY)

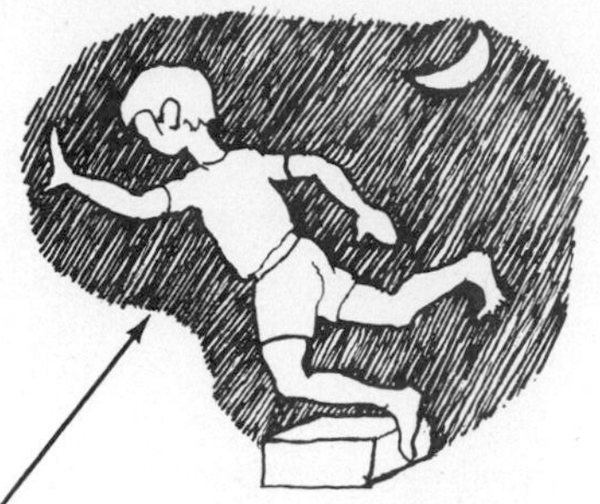

This eye disease is most common in children between 1 and 5 years of age. It comes from not eating enough foods with vitamin A. If not recognized and treated early, it can make the child blind.

Signs:

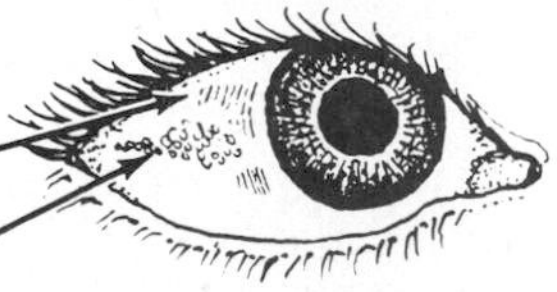

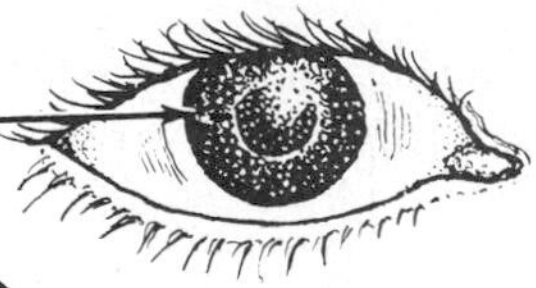

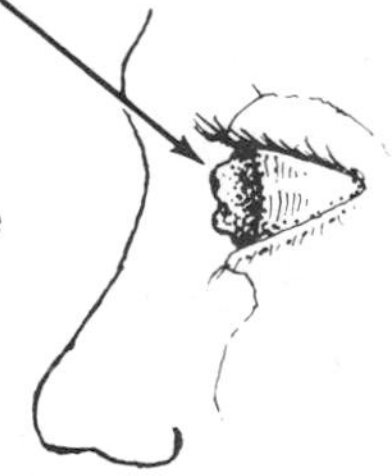

- At first, the child may have **night blindness.** He cannot see as well in the dark as other people can.
- Later, he develops **dry eyes** (xerophthalmia). The white of the eyes loses its shine and begins to wrinkle.
- Patches of little gray bubbles (Bitot's spots) may form in the eyes.
- As the disease gets worse, the cornea also becomes dry and dull, and may develop little pits.
- Then the cornea may quickly grow soft, bulge, or even burst. Usually there is no pain. Blindness may result from infection, scarring, or other damage.
- Xerophthalmia often begins, or gets worse, when a child is sick with another illness like diarrhea, whooping cough, tuberculosis, or measles. **Examine the eyes of all sick and underweight children.** Open the child's eyes and look for signs of vitamin A deficiency.

Prevention and treatment:

Xerophthalmia can easily be prevented by eating foods that have vitamin A. Do the following:

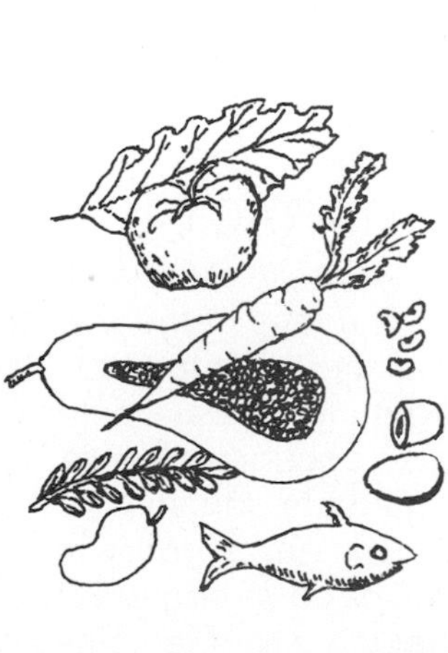

- ♦ Breast feed the baby—up to 2 years, if possible.
- ♦ After the first 6 months, begin giving the child foods rich in vitamin A, such as dark green leafy vegetables, and yellow or orange fruits and vegetables such as papaya (paw paw), mango, and squash. Whole milk, eggs, and liver are also rich in vitamin A.
- ♦ If the child is not likely to get these foods, or if he is developing signs of night blindness or xerophthalmia, give him vitamin A, 200,000 units (60 mg. retinol, in capsule or liquid) once every 6 months (p. 392). Babies under 1 year of age should get 100,000 units.

- If the condition is already fairly severe, give the child 200,000 units of vitamin A the first day, 200,000 units the second day, and 200,000 units 14 days later. Babies under 1 year old should get half that amount (100,000 units).
- In communities where xerophthalmia is common, give 200,000 units of vitamin A once every 6 months to women who are breast feeding, and also to pregnant women during the second half of their pregnancy.

WARNING: Too much vitamin A is poisonous. Do not give more than the amounts advised here.

If the condition of the child's eye is severe, with a dull, pitted, or bulging cornea, get medical help. The child's eye should be bandaged, and he should receive vitamin A at once, preferably an injection of 100,000 units.

Dark green leafy vegetables, and yellow or orange fruits and vegetables, help prevent blindness in children.

SPOTS OR 'FLIES' BEFORE THE EYES (MOUCHES VOLANTES)

Sometimes older persons complain of small moving spots when they look at a bright surface (wall, sky). The spots move when the eyes move and look like tiny flies. These spots are usually harmless and need no treatment. But if they appear suddenly in large numbers and vision begins to fail from one side, this could be a medical emergency (detached retina). **Seek medical help at once.**

DOUBLE VISION

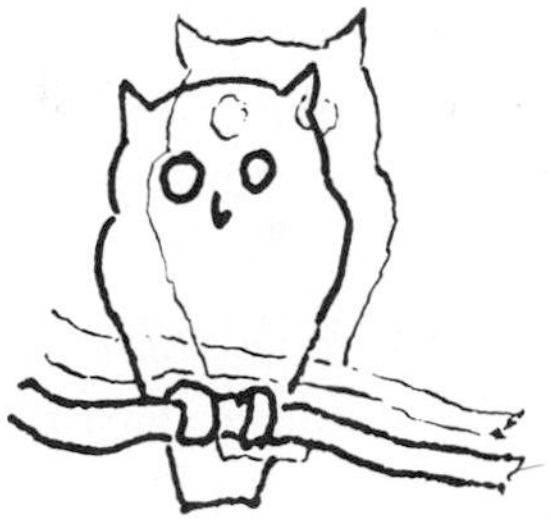

Seeing double can have many causes.

If double vision comes suddenly, is chronic, or gradually gets worse, it is probably a sign of a serious problem. Seek medical help.

If double vision occurs only from time to time, it may be a sign of weakness or exhaustion, perhaps from malnutrition. Read Chapter 11 on good nutrition and try to eat as well as possible. If sight does not improve, get medical help.

RIVER BLINDNESS (ONCHOCERCIASIS)

This disease is common in many parts of Africa and certain areas of southern Mexico, Central America, and northern South America. The infection is caused by tiny worms that are carried from person to person by small, hump-backed flies or gnats known as black flies (simulids).

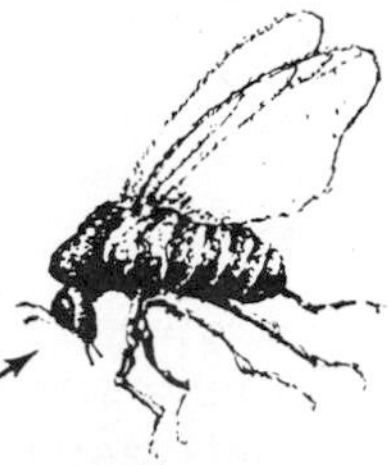

BLACK FLY

actual size →

The worms are 'injected' into a person when an infected black fly bites him.

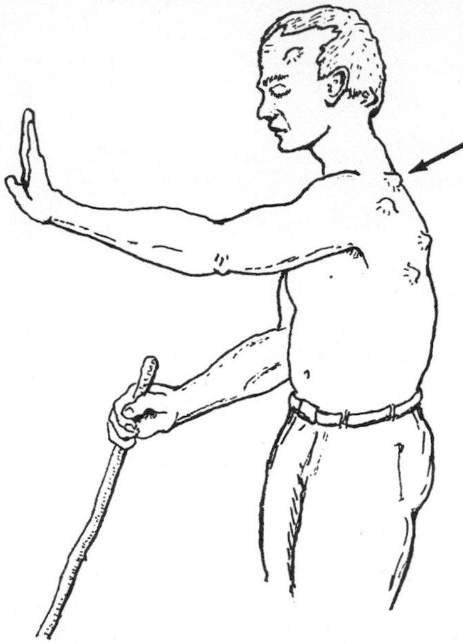

Signs of river blindness:

- Several months after a black fly bites and the worms enter the body, lumps begin to form under the skin. In the Americas the lumps are most common on the head and upper body; in Africa on the chest, the lower body, and thighs. Often there are no more than 3 to 6 lumps. They grow slowly to a size of 2 to 3 cm. across. They are usually painless.
- There may be itching when the baby worms are spreading.
- Pains in the back, shoulder or hip joints, or 'general pains all over'.
- Enlargement of the lymph nodes in the groin.
- Thickening of the skin on the back or belly, with big pores like the skin of an orange. To see this, look at the skin with light shining across it from one side.
- If the disease is not treated, the skin gradually becomes more wrinkled, like an old man's. White spots and patches may appear on the front of the lower legs. A dry rash may appear on the lower limbs and trunk.
- Eye problems often lead to blindness. First there may be redness and tears, then signs of iritis (p. 221). The cornea becomes dull and pitted as in xerophthalmia (p. 226). Finally, sight is lost because of corneal scarring, cataract, glaucoma, or other problems.

Treatment of river blindness:

Early treatment can prevent blindness. In areas where river blindness is known to occur, seek medical testing and treatment when the first signs appear.

- Ivermectin ***(Mectizan)*** is the best medicine for river blindness, and it may be available at no cost through your local health department. Diethylcarbamazine and suramin are other medicines used to treat river blindness, but these can sometimes do more harm than good, especially when eye damage has already begun. They should only be given by experienced health workers. For dosage and precautions on all these medicines, see p. 378.
- Antihistamines help reduce itching (p. 386).
- Early surgical removal of the lumps lowers the number of worms.

Prevention:

- Black flies breed in fast-running water. Clearing brush and vegetation back from the banks of fast-running streams may help reduce the number.
- Avoid sleeping out-of-doors—especially in the daytime, which is when the flies usually bite.
- Cooperate with programs for the control of black flies.
- **Early treatment prevents blindness and reduces spread of the disease.**

CHAPTER

THE TEETH, GUMS, AND MOUTH

17

CARE OF THE TEETH AND GUMS

Taking good care of teeth and gums is important because:

- Strong, healthy teeth are needed to chew and digest food well.
- Painful cavities (holes in the teeth caused by decay) and sore gums can be prevented by good tooth care.
- Decayed or rotten teeth caused by lack of cleanliness can lead to serious infections that may affect other parts of the body.

To keep the teeth and gums healthy:

1. **Avoid sweets.** Eating a lot of sweets (sugar cane, candy, pastry, tea or coffee with sugar, soft or fizzy drinks like colas) rots the teeth quickly.

Do not accustom children to sweets or soft drinks if you want them to have good teeth.

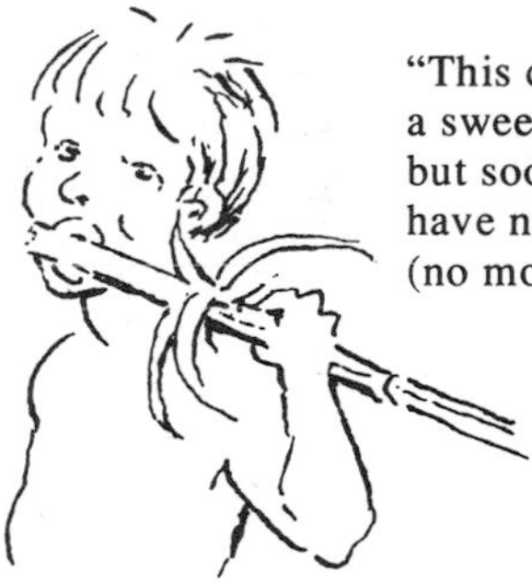

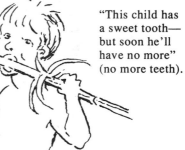

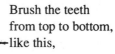

"This child has a sweet tooth—but soon he'll have no more" (no more teeth).

2. **Brush teeth well every day**—and always brush immediately after eating anything sweet. Start brushing your children's teeth as the teeth appear. Later, teach them to brush their teeth themselves, and watch to see that they do it right.

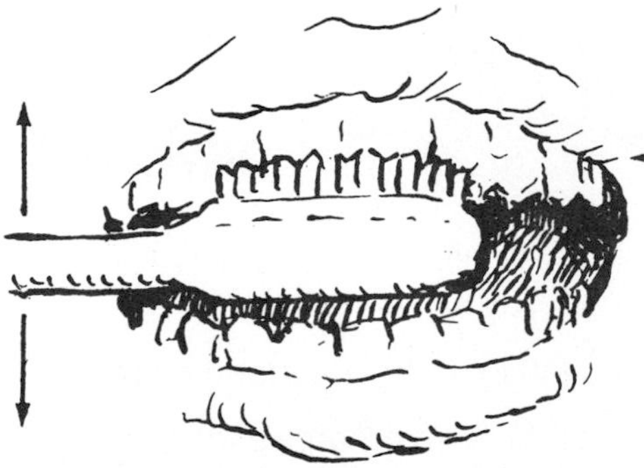

Brush the teeth from top to bottom, like this,

not just from side to side.

Brush the front, back, top, and bottom of all teeth.

3. In areas where there is not enough natural **fluoride** in water and foods, putting fluoride in the drinking water or directly on teeth helps prevent cavities. Some health programs put fluoride on children's teeth once or twice a year. Also, most foods from the sea contain a large amount of fluoride.

CAUTION: Fluoride is poisonous if more than a small amount is swallowed. Use with care and keep it out of the reach of children. Before adding fluoride to drinking water, try to get the water tested to see how much fluoride is needed.

4. **Do not bottle feed older babies.** Continual sucking on a bottle bathes the baby's teeth in sweet liquid and causes early decay. (It is best not to bottle feed at all. See p. 271.)

A TOOTHBRUSH IS NOT NECESSARY

You can use the twig of a tree, like this:

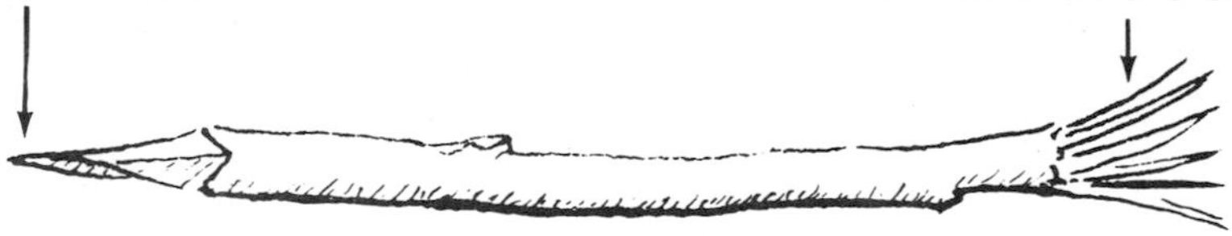

Sharpen this end to clean between the teeth.
Chew on this end and use the fibers as a brush.

Or tie a piece of rough towel around the end of a stick, or wrap it around your finger, and use it as a toothbrush.

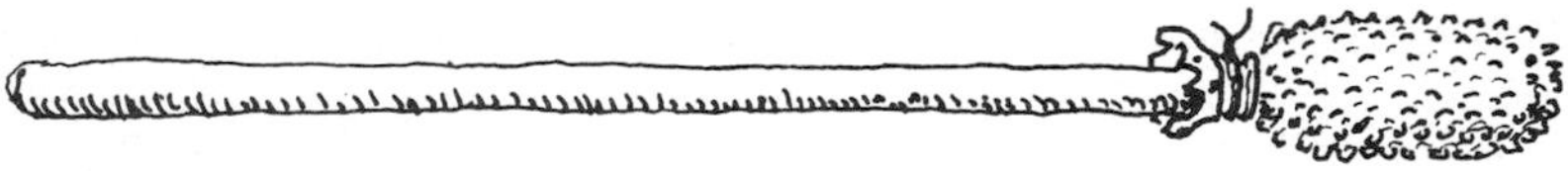

TOOTHPASTE IS NOT NECESSARY

Just water is enough, if you rub well. Rubbing the teeth and gums with something soft but a little rough is what cleans them. Some people rub their teeth with powdered charcoal or with salt. Or you can make a tooth powder by mixing salt and bicarbonate of soda (baking soda) in equal amounts. To make it stick, wet the brush before putting it in the powder.

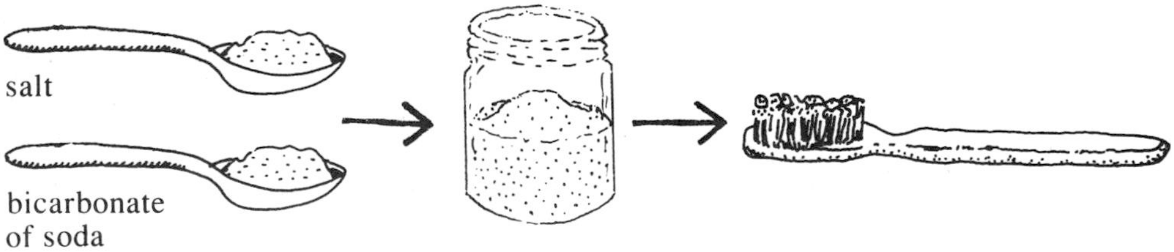

IF A TOOTH ALREADY HAS A CAVITY (a hole caused by rot)

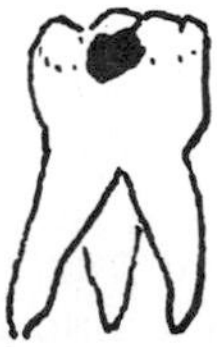

To keep it from hurting as much or forming an abscess, avoid sweet things and brush well after every meal.

If possible, see a dental worker right away. If you go soon enough, he can often clean and fill the tooth so it will last for many years.

When you have a tooth with a cavity, do not wait until it hurts a lot. Have it filled by a dental worker right away.

TOOTHACHES AND ABSCESSES

To calm the pain:

- ♦ Clean the hole in the tooth wall, removing all food particles. Then rinse the mouth with warm salt water.
- ♦ Take a pain medicine like aspirin.
- ♦ If the tooth infection is severe (swelling, pus, large tender lymph nodes), use an antibiotic: tablets of penicillin (p. 351) or sulfonamide (p. 358), or tetracycline capsules (for adults only. See p. 356).

If the pain and swelling do not go away or keep coming back, the tooth should probably be pulled.

Treat abscesses right away—before the infection spreads to other parts of the body.

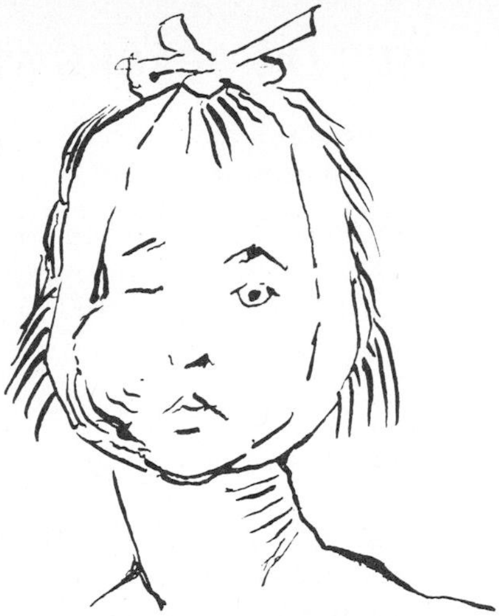

A toothache results when a cavity becomes infected.

An *abscess* results when the infection reaches the tip of a root and forms a pocket of pus.

AN INFECTION OF THE GUMS (PYORRHEA)

Inflamed (red and swollen), painful gums that bleed easily are caused by:

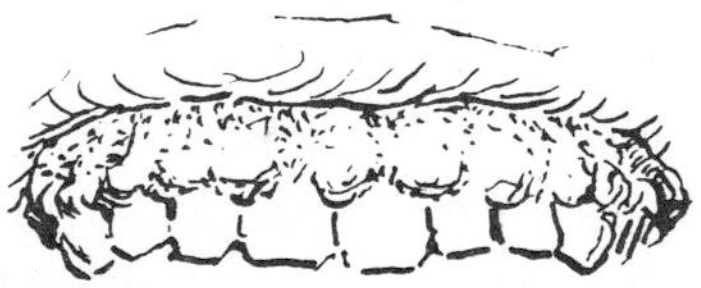

1. Not cleaning the teeth and gums well or often enough.
2. Not eating enough nutritious foods (malnutrition).

Prevention and treatment:

- ♦ Brush teeth well after each meal, removing food that sticks between the teeth. Also, if possible, scrape off the dark yellow crust (tartar) that forms where the teeth meet the gums. It helps to **clean under the gums** regularly by passing a strong thin thread (or dental floss) between the teeth. At first this will cause a lot of bleeding, but soon the gums will be healthier and bleed less.
- ♦ Eat protective foods rich in vitamins, especially eggs, meat, beans, dark green vegetables, and fruits like oranges, lemons, and tomatoes (see Chapter 11). Avoid sweet, sticky, and stringy foods that get stuck between the teeth.

Note: Sometimes medicines for fits (epilepsy), such as phenytoin *(Dilantin)*, cause swelling and unhealthy growth of the gums (see p. 390). If this happens, consult a health worker and consider using a different medicine.

SORES OR CRACKS AT THE CORNERS OF THE MOUTH

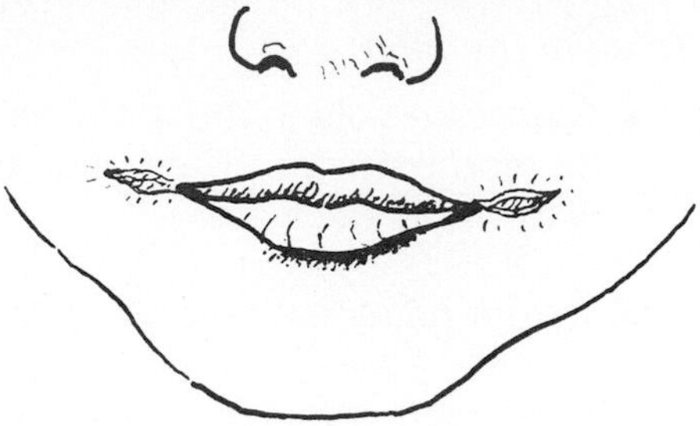

Narrow sores at the corners of children's mouths are often a sign of malnutrition.

Children with these sores should eat foods rich in vitamins and proteins: like milk, meat, fish, nuts, eggs, fruits, and green vegetables.

WHITE PATCHES OR SPOTS IN THE MOUTH

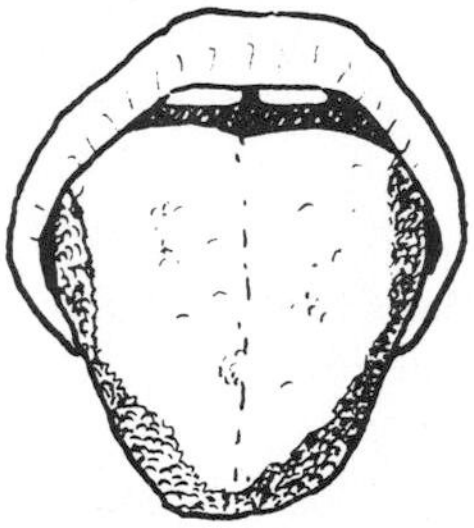

The tongue is coated with white 'fur'. Many illnesses cause a white or yellowish coating on the tongue and roof of the mouth. This is common when there is a fever. Although this coating is not serious, it helps to rinse the mouth with a solution of warm water with salt and bicarbonate of soda several times a day.

Tiny white spots, like salt grains, in the mouth of a child with fever may be an early sign of measles (p. 311).

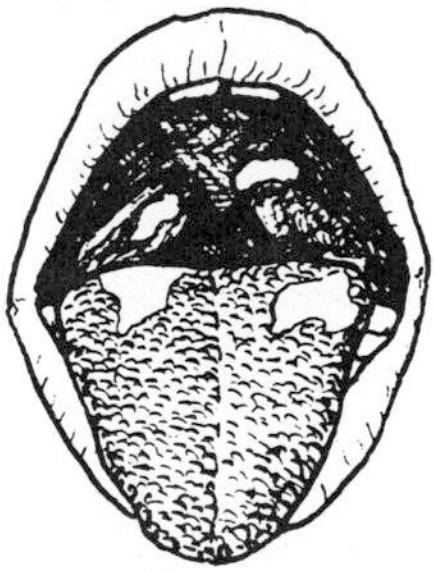

Thrush: small white patches on the inside of the mouth and tongue that look like milk curds stuck to raw meat. They are caused by a fungus or yeast infection called moniliasis (see p. 242). Thrush is common in newborn babies, in persons with the AIDS virus, and in persons using certain antibiotics, especially tetracycline or ampicillin.

Unless it is very important to keep taking the antibiotic, stop taking it. Paint the inside of the mouth with gentian violet. Chewing garlic or eating yogurt may also help. In severe cases, use nystatin (p. 373).

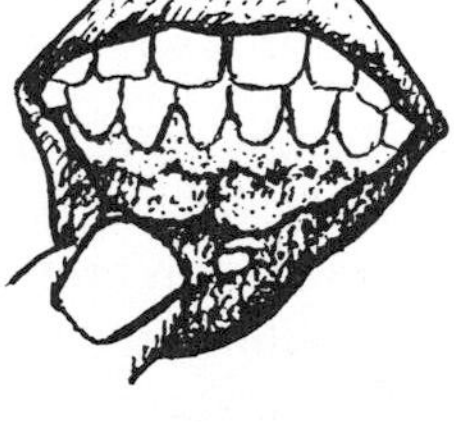

Canker sores: small, white, painful spots inside the lip or mouth. May appear after fever or stress (worry). In 1 to 3 weeks they go away. Rinse mouth with salt water, or put on a little hydrogen peroxide or cortico-steroid ointment (p. 371). Antibiotics do not help.

COLD SORES AND FEVER BLISTERS

Small painful blisters on lips (or genitals) that break and form scabs. May appear after fever or stress. Caused by a herpes virus. They heal after 1 or 2 weeks. Holding ice on the sores for several minutes, several times a day may help them to heal faster. Putting alum, camphor, or bitter plant juices (see Cardon, p. 13) on them may help. No medications do much good. For information about herpes on the genitals, see p. 402 .

For more information on caring for the teeth and gums, see ***Where There Is No Dentist,*** also available from the Hesperian Foundation.

CHAPTER 18

THE URINARY SYSTEM AND THE GENITALS

The urinary system or *tract* serves the body by removing waste material from the blood and getting rid of it in the form of *urine:*

The *kidneys* filter the blood and form the urine.

The *ureters* are tubes that carry urine to the bladder.

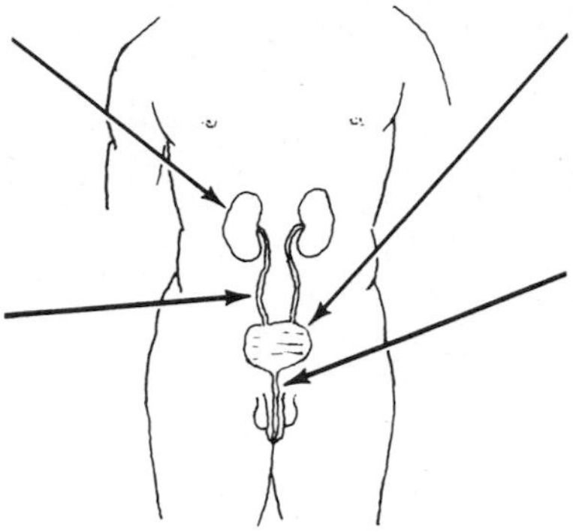

The *bladder* is a bag that stores the urine. As it fills, it stretches and gets bigger.

The urine tube or *urinary canal (urethra)* carries urine out through the penis in men or to a small opening between the lips of the vagina in women.

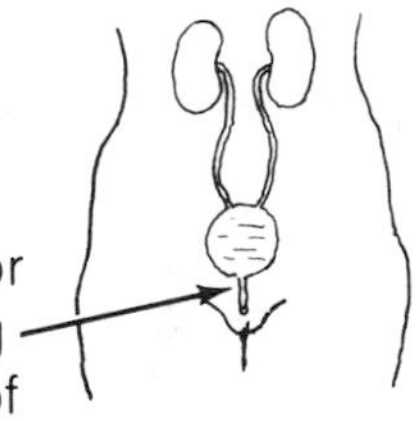

The genitals are the sex organs.

The man:

bladder

urine canal

penis or male sex organ

scrotum or sac that holds the testicles

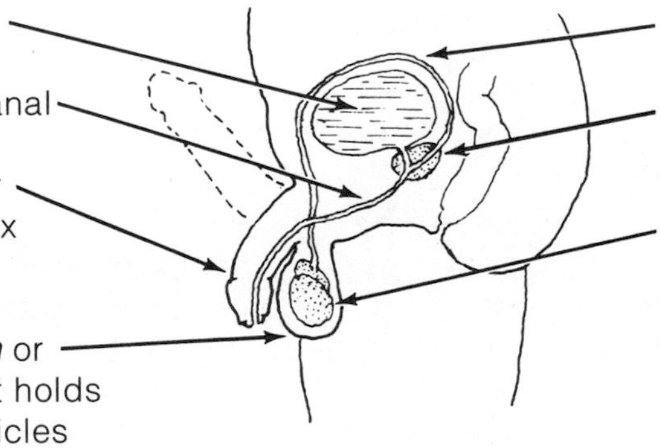

sperm tube

The *prostate gland* makes the liquid that carries the sperm.

The *testicles* make the *sperm,* or microscopic cells with tails that join with the egg of a woman and make her pregnant.

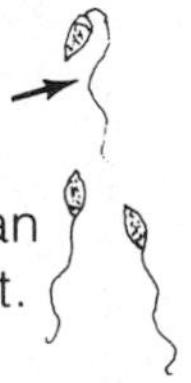

The woman:

outer lip of the vagina

inner lip

anus: end of the intestine

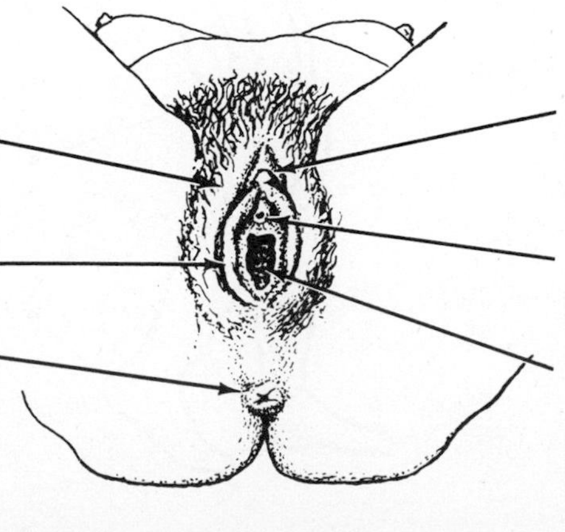

clitoris: a sensitive part somewhat like a small penis

urinary opening: hole where urine comes out

opening to the *vagina* or birth canal. (For inside view, see p. 280.)

PROBLEMS OF THE URINARY TRACT

There are many different disorders of the urinary tract. They are not always easy to tell apart. And the same illness can show itself differently in men and women. Some of these disorders are not serious, while others can be very dangerous. A dangerous illness may begin with only mild symptoms. It is often difficult to identify these disorders correctly by simply using a book like this one. Special knowledge and tests may be needed. When possible, seek advice from a health worker.

Common **problems with urinating** include:

1. Urinary tract infections. These are most common in women. (Sometimes they start after sexual contact, but may come at other times, especially during pregnancy.)
2. Kidney stones, or bladder stones.
3. Prostate trouble (difficulty passing urine caused by an enlarged prostate gland; most common in older men).
4. Gonorrhea or chlamydia (infectious diseases spread by sexual contact that often cause difficulty or pain in passing urine).
5. In some parts of the world schistosomiasis is the most common cause of blood in the urine. This is discussed with other worm infections. See page 146.

Urinary Tract Infections

Signs:

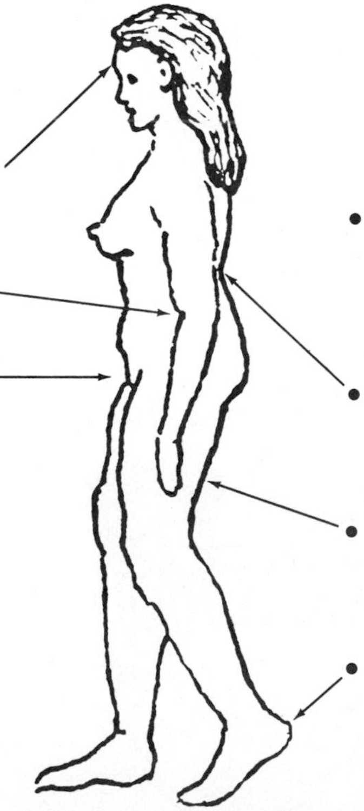

- Sometimes fever and chills or headache.
- Sometimes pain in the side.
- Painful urination and need to urinate very often.
- Unable to hold in urine (especially true for children).
- Urine may be cloudy or reddish (bloody).
- Sometimes it feels as though the bladder does not empty completely.
- Sometimes there is pain in the lower back (kidneys).
- Sometimes the pain seems to go down the legs.
- In serious cases (kidney disease) the feet and face may swell.

Many women suffer from urinary infections. In men they are much less common. Sometimes the only symptoms are **painful urination** and the **need to urinate often.** Other common signs are **blood in the urine** and **pain in the lower belly.** Pain in the mid or lower back, often spreading around the sides below the ribs, with fever, indicates a more serious problem.

Treatment:

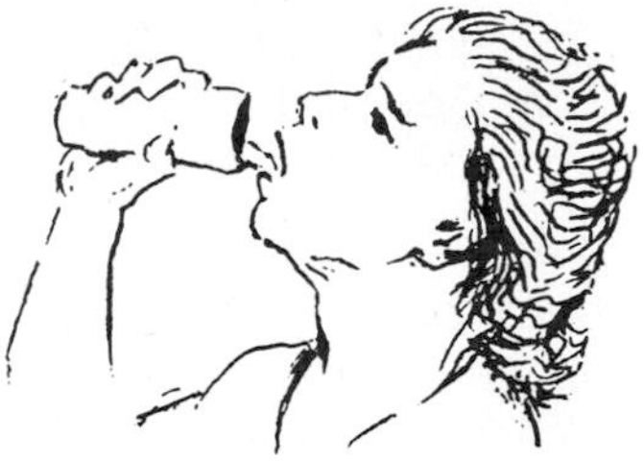

- **Drink a lot of water.** Many minor urinary infections can be cured by simply drinking a lot of water, without the need for medicine. Drink at least 1 glass every 30 minutes for 3 to 4 hours, and get into the habit of drinking lots of water. (But if the person cannot urinate or has swelling of the hands and face, she should not drink much water.)
- If the person does not get better by drinking a lot of water, or if she has a fever, she should take pills of co-trimoxazole or another sulfonamide (p. 358), ampicillin (p. 353), or tetracycline (p. 356). Pay careful attention to dosage and precautions. To completely control the infection it may be necessary to take the medicine for 10 days or more. It is important to drink a lot of water while taking these medicines, especially the sulfonamides.
- If the person does not get better quickly, seek medical advice.
- Some new medicines take away the pain **but do not cure** urinary tract infections. Do not use them for more than 2 days.

Kidney or Bladder Stones:

Signs:

- The first sign is often sharp or severe pain in the lower back, the side, or the lower belly, or in the base of the penis in men.
- Sometimes the urinary tube is blocked so the person has difficulty passing urine—or cannot pass any. Or drops of blood may come out when the person begins to urinate.
- There may be a urinary infection at the same time.

Treatment:

- The same as for the urinary infections described above.
- Also give aspirin or another painkiller and an antispasmodic (see p. 381).
- If you cannot pass urine, try to do it lying down. This sometimes allows a stone in the bladder to roll back and free the opening to the urinary tube.
- In severe cases, get medical help. Sometimes surgery is needed.

Enlarged Prostate Gland:

This condition is most common in men over 40 years old. It is caused by a swelling of the prostate gland, which is between the bladder and the urinary tube (urethra).

- The person has difficulty in passing urine and sometimes in having a bowel movement. The urine may only dribble or drip or become blocked completely. Sometimes the man is not able to urinate for days.
- If he has a fever, this is a sign that infection is also present.

Treatment for an enlarged prostate:

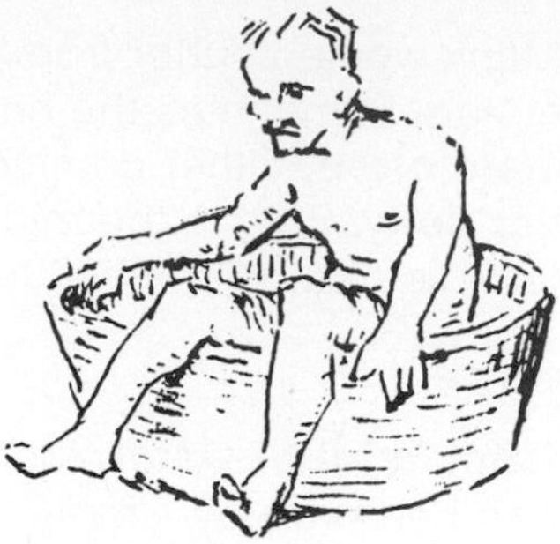

- If the person cannot urinate, he should try sitting in a tub of hot water, like this: If this does not work, a catheter may be needed (p. 239).
- If he has a fever, use an antibiotic such as ampicillin (p. 353) or tetracycline (p. 356).
- Get medical help. Serious or chronic cases may require surgery.

Note: Both prostate trouble and gonorrhea (or chlamydia) can also make it hard to pass urine. In older men it is more likely to be an enlarged prostate. However, a younger man—especially one who has recently had sex with an infected person—probably has gonorrhea or chlamydia.

DISEASES SPREAD BY SEXUAL CONTACT (SEXUALLY TRANSMITTED DISEASES)

On the following pages, we discuss some common diseases spread by sexual contact (STD): **gonorrhea, chlamydia, syphilis,** and **bubos. AIDS,** a new, dangerous illness, and some sexually transmitted diseases that cause sores on the genitals **(genital herpes, genital warts,** and **chancroid)** are discussed in the Blue Pages—see p. 399 to 403.

Gonorrhea (clap, VD, the drip) and Chlamydia:

These diseases are usually spread by sexual contact, and have the same early signs. Often a person has both gonorrhea and chlamydia at the same time, so usually both diseases should be treated.

Signs:

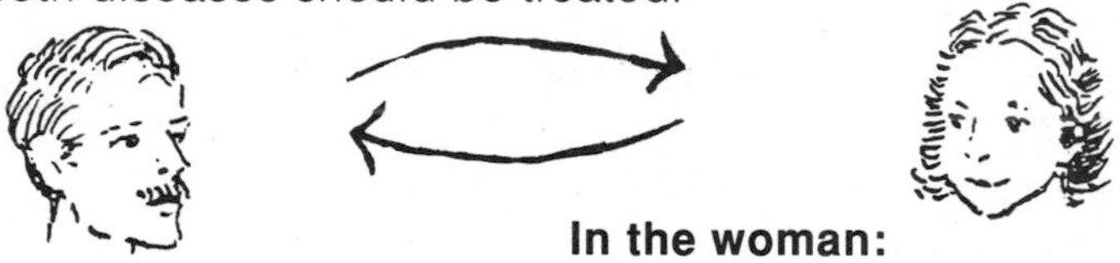

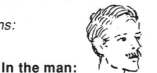

In the man:

- Pain or difficulty with urination.
- Drops of pus from the penis.
- Sometimes there is painful swelling of the testicles.

After weeks or months:

- Painful swelling in one or both knees, ankles or wrists, or many other problems.
- Rash or sores all over the body.
- He may become sterile (cannot make a woman pregnant).

In the woman:

- **At first, there are often no symptoms** (she may feel a little pain when urinating or have a slight vaginal discharge).
- If a pregnant woman with gonorrhea is not treated before giving birth, the infection may get in the baby's eyes and make him blind (see p. 221).

After weeks or months:

- Pain in the lower belly (pelvic inflammatory disease, p. 243).
- Menstrual problems.
- She may become *sterile.*
- Urinary problems (p. 234).

In a man, the first signs begin 2 to 5 days (or up to 3 weeks or more) after sexual contact with an infected person. In a woman, signs may not show up for weeks or months. But **a person who does not show any signs can give the disease to someone else,** starting a few days after becoming infected.

Treatment:

- In the past, gonorrhea was usually treated with penicillin. But now in many areas the disease has become *resistant* to penicillin, so other antibiotics must be used. It is best to seek local advice about which medicines are effective, available, and affordable in your area. Medicines used to treat gonorrhea and chlamydia are listed on p. 360. If the drip and pain have not gone away in 2 or 3 days after trying a treatment, the gonorrhea could be *resistant* to the medicine, or the person could have chlamydia.
- If a woman has gonorrhea or chlamydia and also has fever and pain in the lower belly, she may have pelvic inflammatory disease (see p. 243).
- Everyone who has had sex with a person known to have gonorrhea or chlamydia should also be treated, especially wives of men who are infected. Even if the wife shows no signs, she is probably infected. If she is not treated at the same time, she will give the disease back to her husband again.
- Protect the eyes of all newborn babies from chlamydia and especially gonorrhea, which can cause blindness (see p. 221). For treatment see p. 379.

CAUTION: A person with gonorrhea or chlamydia may also have syphilis without knowing it. Sometimes it is best to go ahead and give the full treatment for syphilis, because the gonorrhea or chlamydia treatment may prevent the first syphilis symptoms, **but may not cure the disease.**

For prevention of these and other sexually transmitted diseases, see p. 239.

Syphilis:

Syphilis is a common and dangerous disease that is spread from person to person through sexual contact.

Signs:

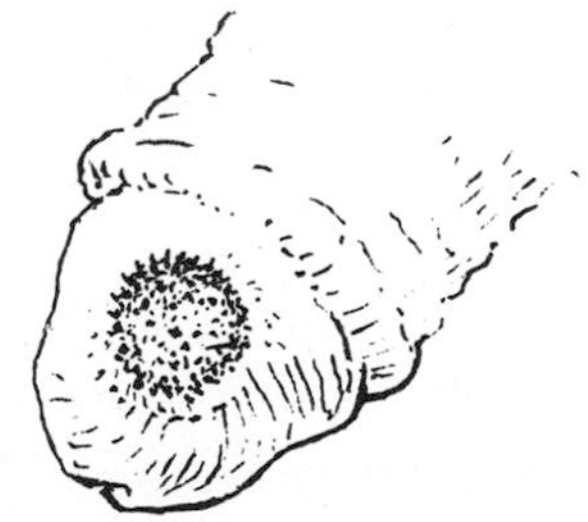

- The first sign is usually a sore, called a *chancre.* It appears 2 to 5 weeks after sexual contact with a person who has syphilis. The chancre may look like a pimple, a blister, or an open sore. It usually appears in the genital area of the man or woman (or less commonly on the lips, fingers, anus, or mouth). This sore is full of germs, which are easily passed on to another person. **The sore is usually painless, and if it is inside the vagina, a woman may not know she has it—but she can easily infect other persons.**
- The sore only lasts a few days and then goes away by itself without treatment. **But the disease continues spreading through the body.**

- Weeks or months later, there may be sore throat, mild fever, mouth sores, or swollen joints. Or any of these signs may appear on the skin:

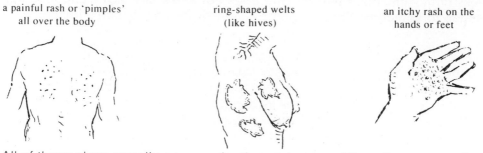

a painful rash or 'pimples' all over the body

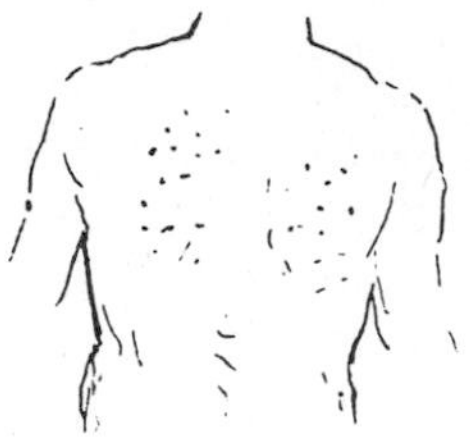

ring-shaped welts (like hives)

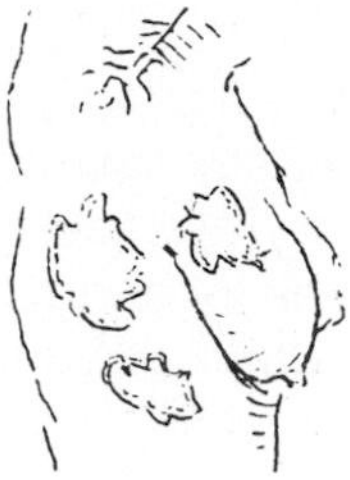

an itchy rash on the hands or feet

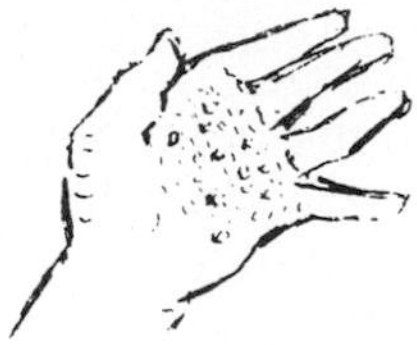

All of these signs usually go away by themselves, and then the person often thinks he is well—but the disease continues. **Without adequate treatment, syphilis can invade any part of the body, causing heart disease, paralysis, insanity, and many other problems.**

CAUTION: If any strange rash or skin condition shows up days or weeks after a pimple or sore appears on the genitals, it may be syphilis. Get medical advice.

Treatment for syphilis: **(For complete cure, the full treatment is essential.)**

- **If signs have been present less than 1 year,** inject 2.4 million units of benzathine penicillin all at once. Put half the dose in each buttock (see p. 353). Persons allergic to penicillin can take tetracycline, 500 mg., 4 times each day for 15 days.
- **If signs have been present more than 1 year,** inject 2.4 million units of benzathine penicillin—half in each buttock—once a week for 3 weeks, for a total of 7.2 million units. If allergic to penicillin, take tetracycline, 500 mg., 4 times each day for 30 days.
- If there is any chance that someone has syphilis, she should immediately see a health worker. Special blood tests may be needed. If tests cannot be made, the person should be treated for syphilis in any case.
- Everyone who has had sexual contact with a person known to have syphilis should also be treated, especially husbands or wives of those known to be infected.

Note: Pregnant or breast feeding women who are allergic to penicillin can take erythromycin in the same dosage as tetracycline (see p. 356).

To prevent syphilis, see the next page.

Bubos: Bursting Lymph Nodes in the Groin (Lymphogranuloma Venereum)

Signs:

- **In a man:** Large, dark lumps in the groin that open to drain pus, scar up, and open again.
- **In a woman:** Lymph nodes similar to those in the man. Or painful, oozing sores in the anus.

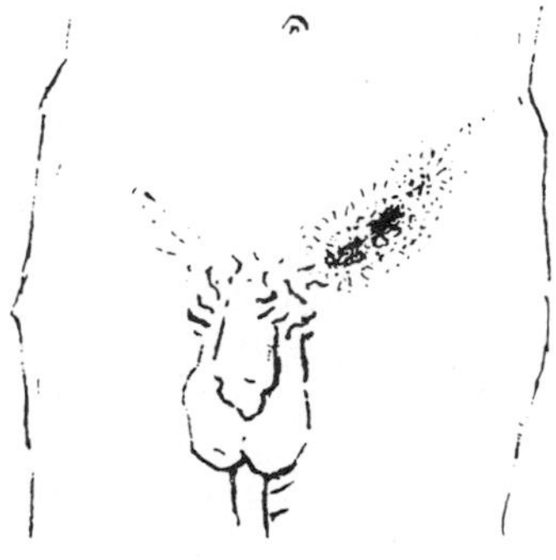

Treatment:

- See a health worker.
- Give adults 250 mg. capsules of tetracycline, 2 capsules, 4 times a day for 14 days.
- Avoid sex until the sores are completely healed.

Note: Bubos in the groin can also be a sign of chancroid (see p. 403).

HOW TO PREVENT SPREADING SEXUALLY TRANSMITTED DISEASES

1. **Be careful with whom you have sex:** Someone who has sex with many different persons is more likely to catch these diseases. Prostitutes are especially likely to be infected. To avoid infection, have sex only with one faithful partner. If you have sex with anyone else, **always use a condom.** (Use of condoms helps prevent sexually transmitted diseases, but does not assure complete protection.)

2. **Get treatment right away:** It is very important that all persons infected with a sexually transmitted disease get treatment at once so that they do not infect other people. Do not have sex with anyone until 3 days after treatment is finished. (Unfortunately there is still no effective treatment for AIDS.)

3. **Tell other people if they need treatment:** When a person finds out that he or she has a sexually transmitted disease, he should tell everyone with whom he has had sex, so that they can get treatment, too. It is especially important that a man tell a woman, because without knowing she has the disease she can pass it on to other people, her babies may become infected or blind, and in time she may become sterile or very ill herself.

4. **Help others:** Insist that friends who may have a sexually transmitted disease get treatment at once, and that they avoid all sexual contact until they are cured.

HOW AND WHEN TO USE A CATHETER (A RUBBER TUBE TO DRAIN URINE FROM THE BLADDER)

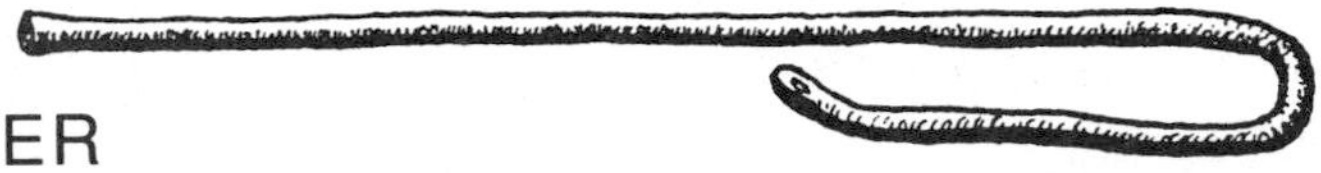

When to use and when not to use a catheter:

- **Never use a catheter unless it is absolutely necessary** and it is impossible to get medical help in time. Even careful use of a catheter sometimes causes dangerous infection or damages the urinary canal.
- If any urine is coming out at all, do not use the catheter.
- If the person cannot urinate, first have him try to urinate while sitting in a tub of warm water (p. 236). Begin the recommended medicine (for gonorrhea or prostate trouble) at once.
- If the person has a very full, painful bladder and cannot urinate, or if he or she begins to show signs of poisoning from urine, then and only then use a catheter.

Signs of urine poisoning (uremia):

- The breath smells like urine.
- The feet and face swell.
- Vomiting, distress, confusion.

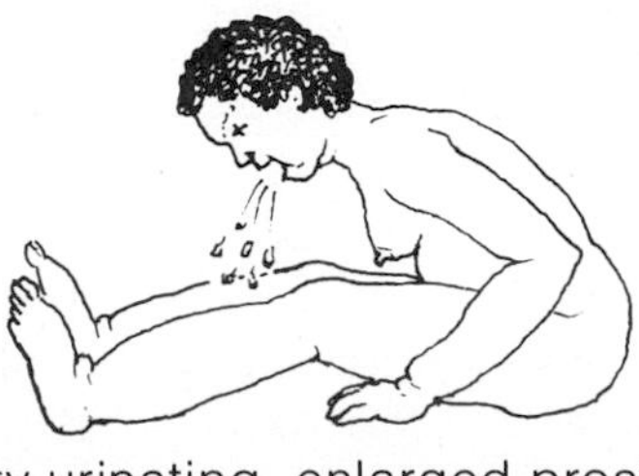

Note: People who have suffered from difficulty urinating, enlarged prostate, or kidney stones should buy a catheter and keep it handy in case of emergency.

HOW TO PUT IN A CATHETER

1. Boil the catheter (and any syringe or instrument you may be using) for 15 minutes.

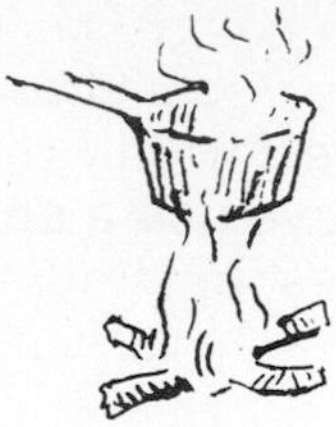

2. Wash well under foreskin or between vaginal lips and surrounding areas.

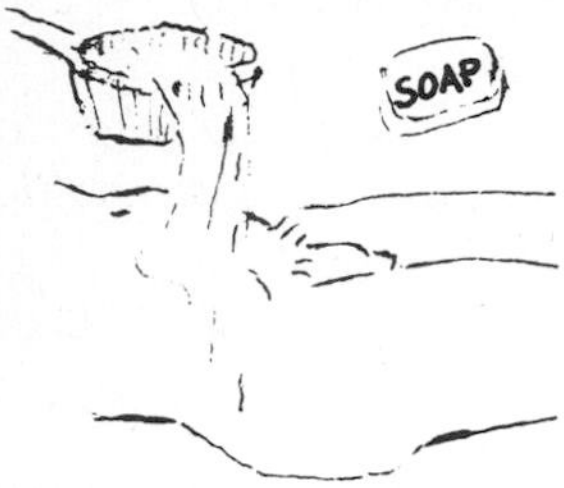

3. Wash hands—if possible with surgical soap (like *Betadine*). After washing, touch only things that are sterile or very clean.

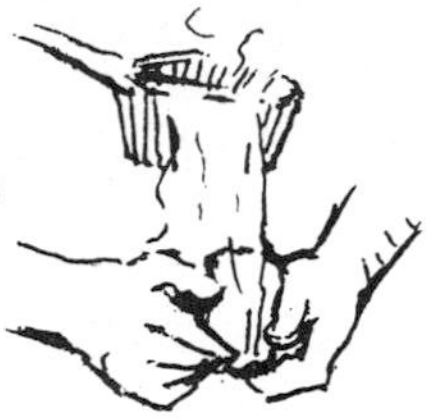

4. Put very clean cloths under and around the area.

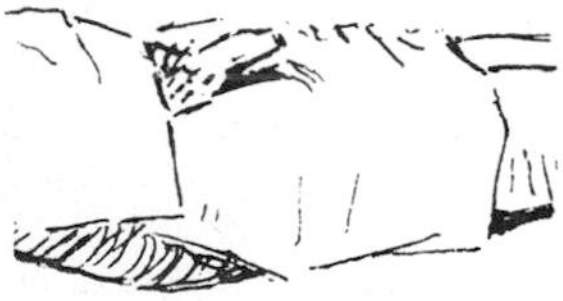

5. Put on sterile gloves—or rub hands well with alcohol or surgical soap.

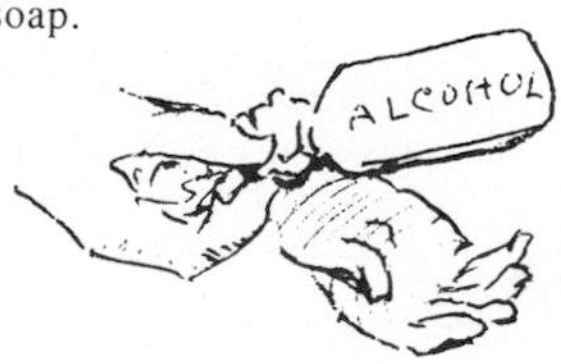

6. Cover the catheter with a sterile lubricant (slippery cream) like *K-Y Jelly* that dissolves in water (not oil or *Vaseline*).

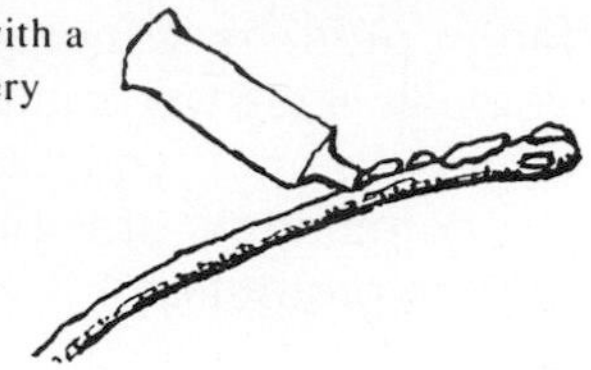

7. Pull back foreskin or open the vaginal lips,

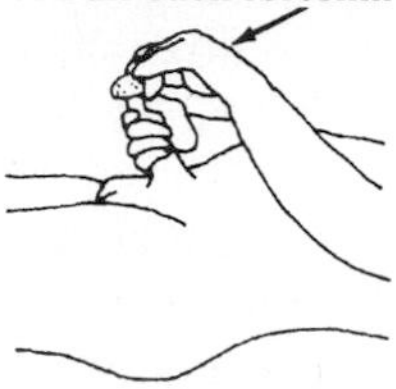

and wipe the urine opening with a sterile cotton wetted with soap.

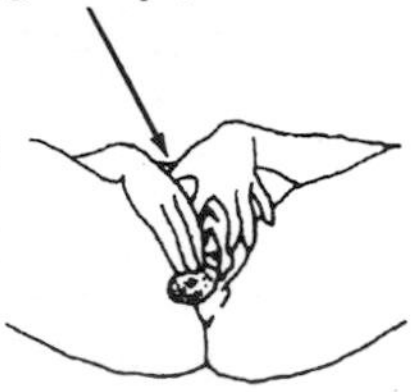

8. Holding the foreskin back or the lips open, gently put the catheter into the urine hole. Twist it as necessary but DO NOT FORCE IT.

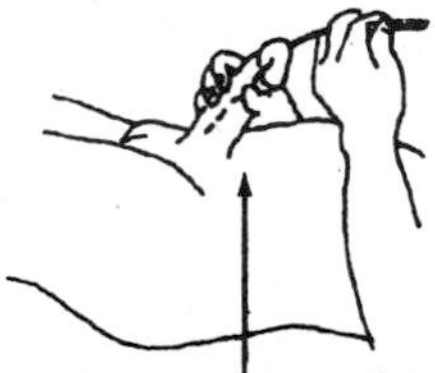

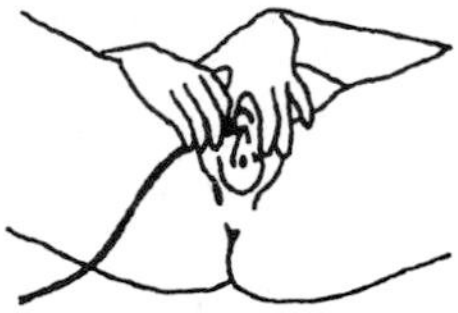

Hold the penis straight at this angle.

9. For a man, push the catheter in until urine starts coming out—then 3 cm. more

Note: A woman's urinary tube is much shorter than a man's.

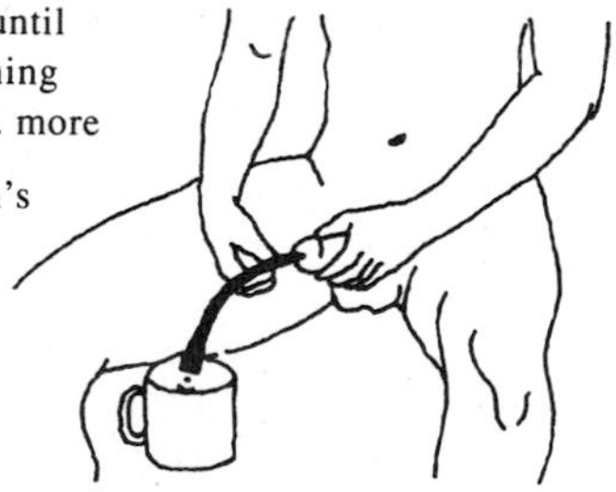

Important: If the person shows signs of urine poisoning, or if the bladder has been over-full and stretched, do not let the urine come out all at once: instead, let it out very slowly (by pinching or plugging the catheter), little by little over an hour or 2.

Sometimes a woman cannot urinate after giving birth. If more than 6 hours pass and her bladder seems full, she may need a catheter put in. If her bladder does not feel full, do not use a catheter but have her drink lots of water.

For more information on catheter use, see ***Disabled Village Children,*** Chapter 25.

PROBLEMS OF WOMEN

Vaginal Discharge
(a mucus or pus-like stuff that comes from the vagina)

All women normally have a small amount of vaginal discharge, which is clear, milky, or slightly yellow. If there is no itching or bad smell, there is probably no problem.

But many women, especially during pregnancy, suffer from a discharge often with itching in the vagina. This discharge may be caused by various infections. Most of them are bothersome, but not dangerous. However, an infection caused by gonorrhea or chlamydia can harm a baby at birth (see p. 221).

1. **A thin and foamy, greenish-yellow or whitish, foul-smelling discharge with itching.** This is probably an infection of **Trichomonas.** It may burn to urinate. Sometimes the genitals hurt or are swollen. The discharge may contain blood.

Treatment:

- It is very important to keep the genitals clean.
- A vaginal wash, or ***douche,*** with warm water and distilled vinegar will help. If there is no vinegar, use lemon juice in water.

IMPORTANT: Let water enter slowly during about 3 minutes. Do not put the tube more than 3 inches into the vagina.

For the douche, use 6 teaspoons of vinegar in 1 liter of boiled, cooled water.

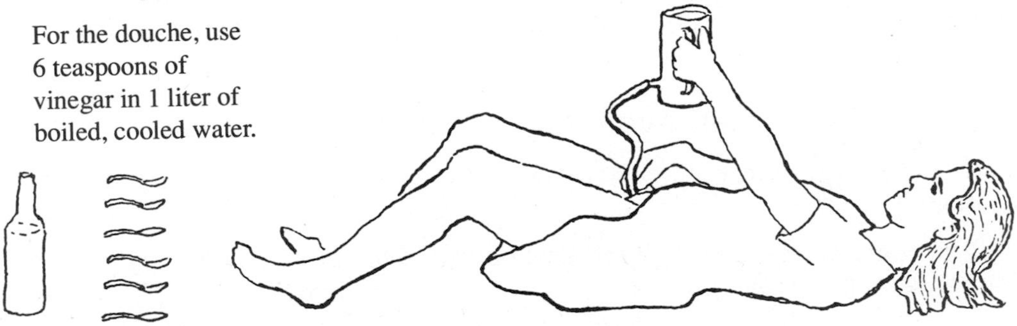

CAUTION: Do not douche in the last 4 weeks of pregnancy, or for 6 weeks after giving birth. If the discharge is troublesome, nystatin vaginal inserts may help (see #2 on the next page).

- You can also use a clove of garlic as a vaginal insert. (Peel the garlic, taking care not to puncture it. Wrap it in a piece of clean cloth or gauze, and put it into the vagina.)
- Use the douche 2 times during the day, and each night insert a new clove of garlic. Do this for 10 to 14 days.
- If this does not help, use vaginal inserts that contain metronidazole or other medication recommended for Trichomonas, or take metronidazole by mouth. For precautions and instructions, see page 370.

IMPORTANT: It is likely that the husband of a woman with Trichomonas has the infection, too, even though he does not feel anything. (Some men with Trichomonas have a burning feeling when urinating.) If a woman is treated with metronidazole, her husband should also take it by mouth at the same time.

2. **White discharge that looks like cottage cheese or buttermilk, and smells like mold, mildew, or baking bread.** This could be a yeast infection (moniliasis, Candida). Itching may be severe. The lips of the vagina often look bright red and hurt. It may burn to urinate. This infection is especially common in pregnant women or in those who are sick, diabetic (p. 127), or have been taking antibiotics, or birth control pills.

Treatment: Douche with vinegar-water (see p. 241) or dilute gentian violet, 2 parts gentian violet to 100 parts water (2 teaspoons to a half liter). Or use nystatin vaginal tablets or any other vaginal inserts for moniliasis or Candida. For dosage and instructions see page 370. Putting unsweetened yogurt in the vagina is said to be a useful home remedy to help control yeast infections. **Never use antibiotics for a yeast infection. They can make it worse.**

3. **Thick, milky discharge with a rancid smell.** This could be an infection caused by bacteria. Special tests may be needed to tell this from a Trichomonas infection. Douche with vinegar-water (p. 241), or with povidone-iodine (*Betadine:* 6 teaspoons in 1 liter of water). Also, you can try inserting a clove of garlic every night for 2 weeks (see p. 241). If none of these treatments works, try metronidazole (see p. 369).

4. **Watery, brown, or gray discharge, streaked with blood; bad smell; pain in the lower belly.** These are signs of more serious infections, or possibly cancer (p. 280). If there is fever, use antibiotics (if possible, ampicillin together with tetracycline—see p. 353 and 356). **Get medical help right away.**

Important: If any discharge lasts a long time, or does not get better with treatment, see a health worker.

How a Woman Can Avoid Many Infections:

1. Keep the genital area clean. When you bathe (daily if possible) wash well with mild soap.

2. Urinate after sexual contact. This helps prevent urinary infections (but will not prevent pregnancy).

3. Be sure to clean yourself carefully after each bowel movement. Always wipe from front to back:

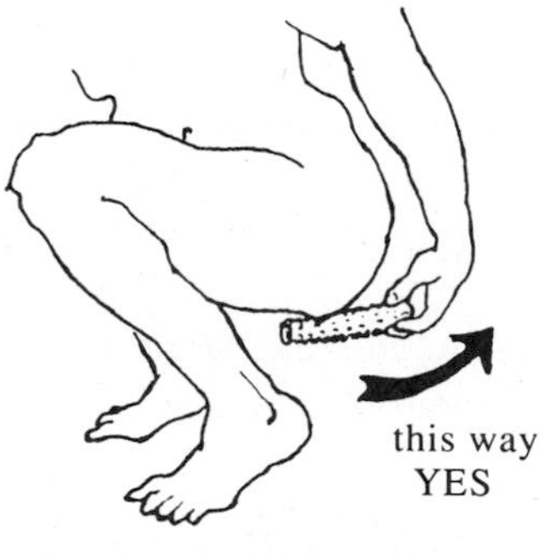

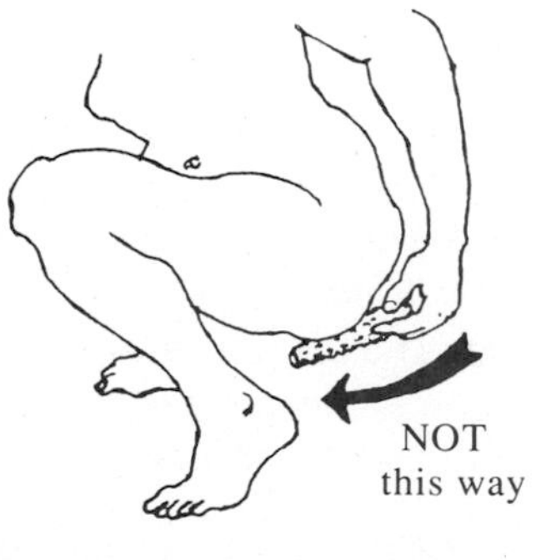

Wiping forward can spread germs, amebas, or worms into the urinary opening and vagina. Also take care to wipe little girls' bottoms from front to back and to teach them, as they grow up, to do it the same way.

Pain or Discomfort in the Lower Central Part of a Woman's Belly

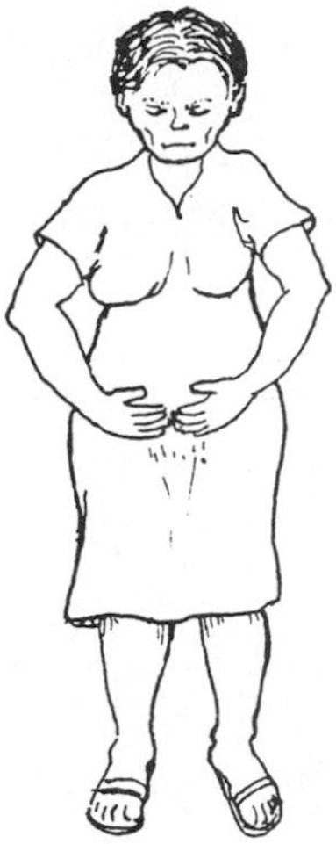

This can come from many different causes, which are discussed in different parts of this book. The following list, which includes a few key questions, will help you know where to look.

Possible causes of pain in the lower belly are:

1. **Menstrual discomfort** (p. 246). Is it worst shortly before or during the period?

2. **A bladder infection** (p. 234). One of the most common low mid-belly pains. Is urination very frequent or painful?

3. **Pelvic inflammatory disease.** This is almost always a late stage of gonorrhea or chlamydia (p. 236), with pain in the lower belly and fever. If these signs are mild, treat for gonorrhea (p. 360), and give tetracycline (p. 356) or erythromycin (p. 355) for 14 days. For more severe signs, also give 400 to 500 mg. of metronidazole 3 times a day for 10 days. If the woman is using an intrauterine device (IUD), it may need to be removed. See a health worker.

4. **Problems that are related to a lump or mass in the lower part of the belly.** These are discussed briefly on page 280 and include **ovarian cyst** and **cancer.** A special exam is needed, done by a trained health worker.

5. **Ectopic pregnancy** (when the baby begins to develop outside the womb—p. 280). Usually there is severe pain with irregular bleeding. The woman often has signs of early pregnancy (see p. 247), and feels dizzy and weak. **Get medical help immediately; her life is in danger.**

6. **Complications from an abortion** (p. 414). There may be fever, bleeding from the vagina with clots, belly pain, difficulty urinating, and shock. Start giving antibiotics as for childbirth fever (p. 276), and **get the woman to a hospital at once. Her life is in danger.**

7. **An infection or other problem of the gut or rectum** (p. 145). Is the pain related to eating or to bowel movements?

Some of the above problems are not serious. Others are dangerous. They are not always easy to tell apart. Special tests or examinations may be needed.

If you are unsure what is causing the pain, or if it does not get better soon, seek medical help.

MEN AND WOMEN WHO ARE NOT ABLE TO HAVE CHILDREN (INFERTILITY)

Sometimes a man and woman try to have children but the woman does not become pregnant. Either the man or woman may be infertile (unable to bring about pregnancy). Often nothing can be done to make a person fertile, but sometimes something can be done, depending on the cause.

COMMON CAUSES OF INFERTILITY:

1. **Sterility.** The person's body is such that he or she can never have children. Some men and women are born sterile.

2. **Weaknesses or a nutritional lack.** In some women severe anemia, poor nutrition, or lack of iodine may lower the chance of becoming pregnant. Or it may cause the unformed baby (embryo) to die, perhaps before the mother even knows she is pregnant (see Miscarriage, p. 281). A woman who is not able to become pregnant, or has had only miscarriages, should get enough nutritious food, use iodized salt, and if she is severely anemic, take iron pills (p. 247). These may increase her chance of becoming pregnant and having a healthy baby.

3. **Chronic infection,** especially pelvic inflammatory disease (see p. 243) due to gonorrhea or chlamydia, is a common cause of infertility in women. Treatment may help—if the disease has not gone too far. Prevention and early treatment of gonorrhea and chlamydia mean fewer sterile women.

4. **Men** are sometimes unable to make women pregnant because they have fewer sperms than is normal. It may help for the man to wait, without having sex, for several days before the woman enters her 'fertile days' each month, midway between her last menstrual period and the next (see Rhythm Method and Mucus Method, p. 291 and 292). This way he will give her his full amount of sperm when they have sex on days when she is able to become pregnant.

WARNING: Hormones and other medicines commonly given to men or women who cannot have babies almost never do any good, especially in men. Home remedies and magic cures are not likely to help either. Be careful not to waste your money for things that will not help.

If you are a woman and are not able to have a baby, there are still many possibilities for leading a happy and worthwhile life:

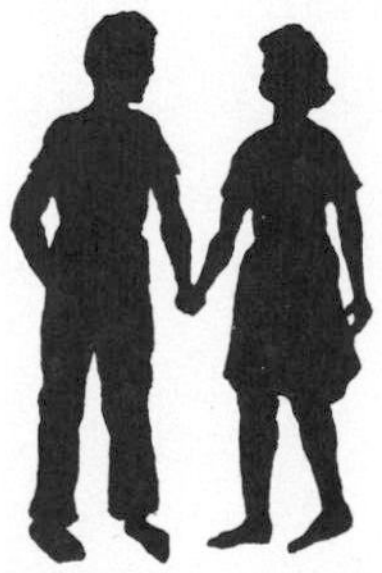

- Perhaps you can arrange to care for or adopt children who are orphans or need a home. Many couples come to love such children just as if they were their own.
- Perhaps you can become a health worker or help your community in other ways. The love you would give to your children, you can give to others, and all will benefit.
- You may live in a village where people look with shame on a woman who cannot have children. Perhaps you and others can form a group to help those who have special needs, and to show that having babies is not the only thing that makes a woman worthwhile.

CHAPTER 19

INFORMATION FOR MOTHERS AND MIDWIVES

THE MENSTRUAL PERIOD (MONTHLY BLEEDING IN WOMEN)

Most girls have their first 'period' or monthly bleeding between the ages of 11 and 16. This means that they are now old enough to become pregnant.

The normal period comes once every 28 days or so, and lasts 3 to 6 days. However, this varies a lot in different women.

Irregular or painful periods are common in adolescent (teenage) girls. This does not usually mean there is anything wrong.

If your menstrual period is painful:

There is no need for you to stay in bed. In fact, lying quietly can make the pain worse.

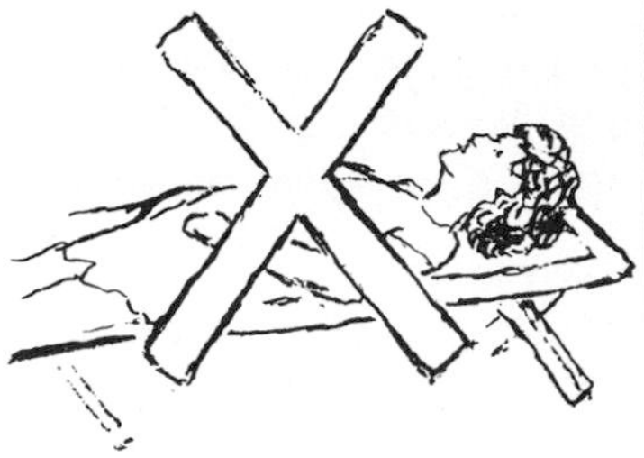

It often helps to walk around and do light work or exercises . . .

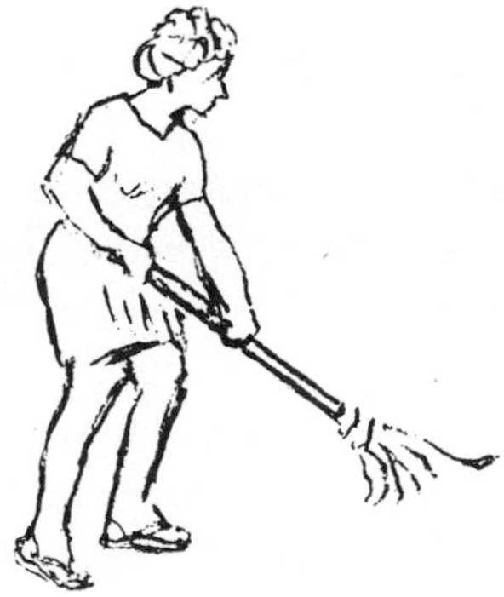

or to take hot drinks, or put your feet in hot water.

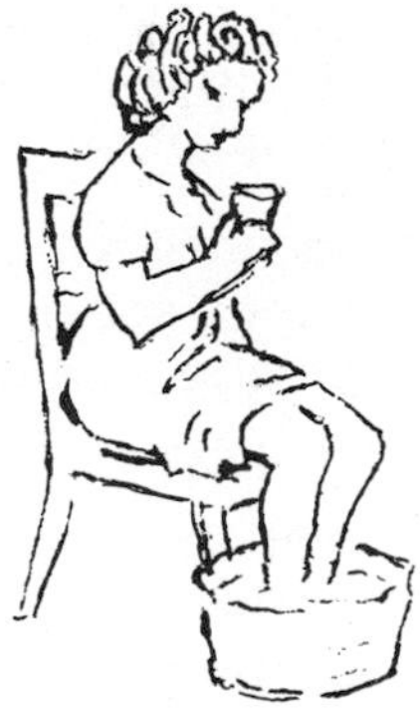

If it is very painful, it may help to take aspirin (p. 379) or ibuprofen (p. 380) and to lie down and put warm compresses on the belly.

During the period—as at all times—a woman should take care to keep clean, get enough sleep, and eat a well-balanced diet. She can eat everything she normally eats and can continue to do her usual work. It is not harmful to have sex during the menstrual period. (However, if one of the partners has the AIDS virus, the risk of infecting the other partner may be higher.)

Signs of menstrual problems:

- Some irregularity in the length of time between periods is normal for certain women, but for others it may be a sign of chronic illness, anemia, malnutrition, or possibly an infection or tumor in the womb.
- If a period does not come when it should, this may be a sign of pregnancy. But for many girls who have recently begun to menstruate, and for women over 40, it is often normal to miss or have irregular periods. Worry or emotional upset may also cause a woman to miss her period.
- If the bleeding comes later than expected, is more severe, and lasts longer, it may be a miscarriage (see p. 281).
- **If the menstrual period lasts more than 6 days, results in unusually heavy bleeding, or comes more than once a month, seek medical advice.**

THE MENOPAUSE (WHEN WOMEN STOP HAVING PERIODS)

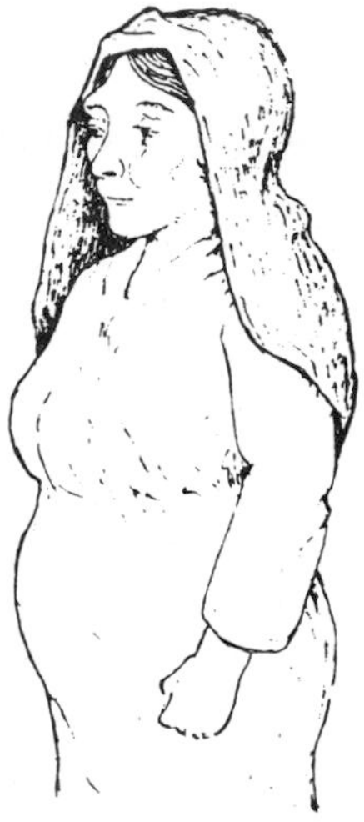

The *menopause* or *climacteric* is the time in a woman's life when the menstrual periods stop coming. After menopause, she can no longer bear children. In general, this 'change of life' happens between the ages of 40 and 50. The periods often become irregular for several months before they stop completely.

There is no reason to stop having sex during or after the menopause. But a woman can still become pregnant during this time. If she does not want to have more children, she should continue to use birth control for 12 months after her periods stop.

When menopause begins, a woman may think she is pregnant. And when she bleeds again after 3 or 4 months, she may think she is having a miscarriage. If a woman of 40 or 50 starts bleeding again after some months without, explain to her that it may be menopause.

During menopause, it is normal to feel many discomforts—anxiety, distress, 'hot flashes' (suddenly feeling uncomfortably hot), pains that travel all over the body, sadness, etc. After menopause is over, most women feel better again.

Women who have severe bleeding or a lot of pain in the belly during menopause, or who begin to bleed again after the bleeding has stopped for months or years, should seek medical help. An examination is needed to make sure they do not have cancer or another serious problem (see p. 280).

After menopause, a woman's bones may become weaker and break more easily. To prevent this, it helps to eat foods with calcium (see p. 116).

Because she will not have any more children, a woman may be more free now to spend time with her grandchildren or to become more active in the community. Some become midwives or health workers at this time in their lives.

PREGNANCY

Signs of pregnancy:

All these signs are normal:

- The woman misses her period (often the first sign).
- 'Morning sickness' (nausea or feeling you are going to vomit, especially in the morning). This is worse during the second and third months of pregnancy.
- She may have to urinate more often.
- The belly gets bigger.
- The breasts get bigger or feel tender.
- 'Mask of pregnancy' (dark areas on the face, breasts, and belly).
- Finally, during the fifth month or so, the child begins to move in the womb.

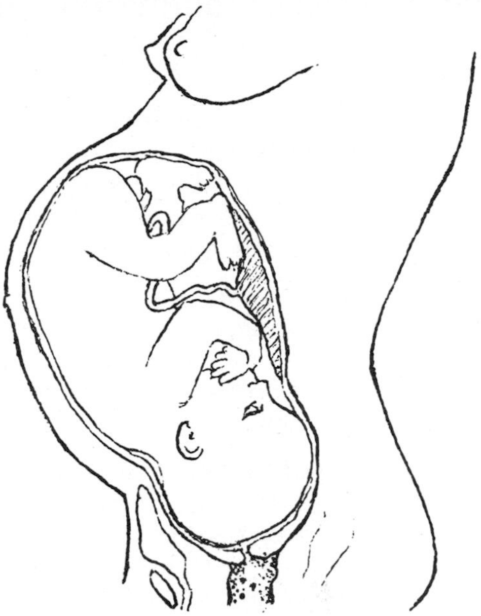

This is the normal position of the baby in the mother at 9 months.

How to Stay Healthy during Pregnancy

- Most important is to **eat enough** to gain weight regularly—especially if you are thin. It is also important to **eat well.** The body needs food rich in proteins, vitamins, and minerals, especially **iron.** (Read Chapter 11 in this book.)
- **Use iodized salt** to increase the chances that the child will be born alive and will not be retarded. (But to avoid swelling of the feet and other problems, do not use very much salt.)
- **Keep clean.** Bathe or wash regularly and brush your teeth every day.
- In the last month of pregnancy, it is best not to use a vaginal *douche* and to **avoid sexual contact** to keep from breaking the bag of water and causing an infection.
- **Avoid taking medicines** if at all possible. Some medicines can harm the developing baby. As a rule, only take medicines recommended by a health worker or doctor. (If a health worker is going to prescribe a medicine, and you think that you might be pregnant, tell her so.) You can take acetaminophen, or antacids once in a while if you need them. Vitamin and iron pills are often helpful and do no harm when taken in the right dosage.
- **Do not smoke or drink** during pregnancy. Smoking and drinking are bad for the mother and harm the developing baby.
- Stay far away from children with measles, especially **German measles** (see Rubella, p. 312).
- Continue to work and **get exercise,** but try not to get too tired.
- **Avoid poisons and chemicals.** They can harm the developing baby. Do not work near pesticides, herbicides, or factory chemicals—and do not store food in their containers. Try not to breathe fumes or powders from chemicals.

Minor Problems during Pregnancy

1. **Nausea or vomiting:** Normally, this is worse in the morning, during the second or third month of pregnancy. It helps to eat something dry, like crackers or dry bread, before you go to bed at night and before you get out of bed in the morning. Do not eat large meals but rather smaller amounts of food several times a day. Avoid greasy foods. Tea made from mint leaves also helps. In severe cases, take an antihistamine (see p. 386) when you go to bed and when you get up in the morning.

2. **Burning or pain** in the pit of the stomach or chest (acid indigestion and heartburn, see p. 128): Eat only small amounts of food at one time and drink water often. Antacids can help, especially those with calcium carbonate (see p. 382). It may also help to suck hard candy. Try to sleep with the chest and head lifted up some with pillows or blankets.

3. **Swelling of the feet:** Rest at different times during the day with your feet up (see p. 176). Eat less salt and avoid salty foods. Tea made from maize silk (corn silk) may help (see p. 12). If the feet are very swollen, and the hands and face also swell, seek medical advice. Swelling of the feet usually comes from the pressure of the child in the womb during the last months. It is worse in women who are anemic or malnourished. So **eat plenty of nutritious food.**

4. **Low back pain:** This is common in pregnancy. It can be helped by exercise and taking care to stand and sit with the back straight (p. 174).

5. **Anemia and malnutrition:** Many women in rural areas are anemic even before they are pregnant, and become more anemic during pregnancy. To make a healthy baby, a woman needs to **eat well.** If she is very pale and weak or has other signs of anemia and malnutrition (see p. 107 and 124), she needs to eat more protein and food with iron—foods like beans, groundnuts, chicken, milk, cheese, eggs, meat, fish, and dark green leafy vegetables. She should also take **iron pills** (p. 393), especially if it is hard to get enough nutritious foods. This way she will strengthen her blood to resist dangerous bleeding after childbirth. If possible, iron pills should also contain some **folic acid** and **vitamin C.** (Vitamin C helps the body make better use of the iron.)

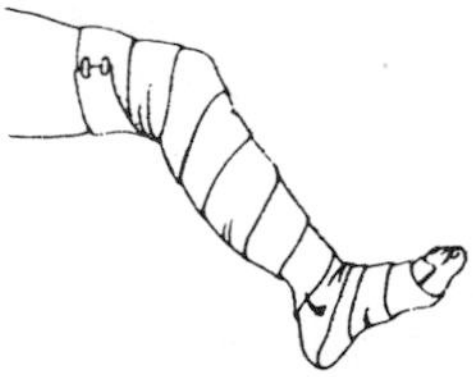

6. **Swollen veins (varicose veins):** These are common in pregnancy, due to the weight of the baby pressing on the veins that come from the legs. Put your feet up often, as high as you can (see p. 175). If the veins get very big or hurt, wrap them like this with an elastic bandage, or use elastic stockings. Take off the bandage or stockings at night.

7. **Piles (hemorrhoids):** These are varicose veins in the *anus.* They result from the weight of the baby in the womb.

To relieve the pain, kneel with the buttocks in the air like this: ⟶

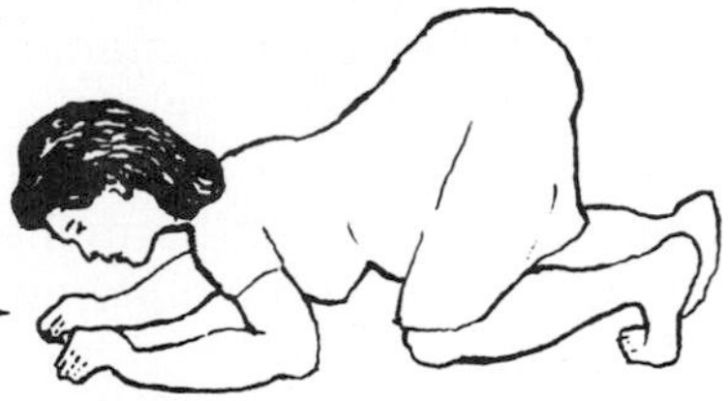

Or sit in a warm bath. Also see p. 175.

8. **Constipation:** Drink plenty of water. Eat fruits and food with a lot of natural fiber, like cassava or bran. Get plenty of exercise. **Do not take strong laxatives.**

Danger Signs in Pregnancy

1. **Bleeding:** If a woman begins to bleed during pregnancy, even a little, this is a danger sign. She could be having a miscarriage (losing the baby, p. 281) or the baby could be developing outside the womb (ectopic pregnancy, see p. 280). The woman should lie quietly and send for a health worker.

Bleeding late in pregnancy (after 6 months) may mean the ***placenta*** (afterbirth) is blocking the birth opening ***(placenta previa).*** Without expert help, the woman could quickly bleed to death. Do not do a vaginal exam or put anything inside her vagina. Try to get her to a hospital at once.

2. **Severe anemia:** The woman is weak, tired, and has pale or transparent skin (see The Signs of Anemia, p. 124). If not treated, she might die from blood loss at childbirth. If anemia is severe, a good diet is not enough to correct the condition in time. See a health worker and get pills of iron salts (see p. 393). If possible, she should have her baby in a hospital, in case extra blood is needed.

3. **Swelling** of the feet, hands, and face, with headache, dizziness, and sometimes blurred vision, are signs of **toxemia or poisoning of pregnancy.** Sudden weight gain, high blood pressure, and a lot of protein in the urine are other important signs. So if you can do so, go to a midwife or health worker who can measure these things.

To treat TOXEMIA OF PREGNANCY a woman should:

- Stay quiet and in bed.
- Eat foods rich in protein, but with only a little salt. Do not eat salty foods.
- If she does not get better quickly, has trouble seeing, swells more in the face or has fits (convulsions), get medical help fast! Her life is in danger!

To help prevent TOXEMIA OF PREGNANCY: eat nutritious food, make sure to get enough protein (p. 110) and use little salt (but do use a little).

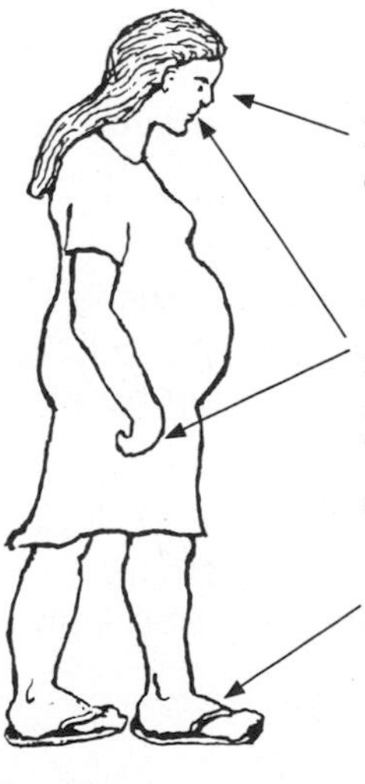
DURING THE LAST 3 MONTHS OF PREGNANCY:
If you have a headache or trouble seeing,
and
if your face and hands begin to swell, you may be suffering from TOXEMIA OF PREGNANCY.
GET MEDICAL HELP!
If only your feet swell, it probably is not serious. But watch for other signs of toxemia. Use little salt.

HIV/AIDS and Pregnancy

If woman has the AIDS virus, she can pass HIV to her baby while it is still in the womb or during birth. A medicine called nevirapine can help prevent the baby from getting HIV. Nevirapine is not expensive, and in some countries it is free.

A pregnant woman should take 200 mg. of nevirapine by mouth when her labor starts. Then, and even if the mother did not take nevirapine, give the baby about 6 mg. of liquid nevirapine (2mg./kg.) as soon as possible during the first 7 days after birth.

CHECK-UPS DURING PREGNANCY (PRENATAL CARE)

Many health centers and midwives encourage pregnant women to come for regular *prenatal* (before birth) check-ups and to talk about their health needs. If you are pregnant and have the chance to go for these check-ups, you will learn many things to help you prevent problems and have a healthier baby.

If you are a midwife, you can provide an important service to mothers-to-be (and babies-to-be) by inviting them to come for prenatal check-ups—or by going to see them. It is a good idea to see them **once a month for the first 6 months of pregnancy, twice a month during months 7 and 8,** and **once a week during the last month.**

Here are some important things prenatal care should cover:

1. **Sharing information**

Ask the mother about her problems and needs. Find out how many pregnancies she has had, when she had her last baby, and any problems she may have had during pregnancy or childbirth. Talk with her about ways she can help herself and her baby be healthy, including:

- **Eating right.** Encourage her to eat enough energy foods, and also foods rich in protein, vitamins, iron, and calcium (see Chapter 11).
- **Good hygiene** (Chapter 12 and p. 242).
- The importance of taking **few or no medicines** (p. 54).
- The importance of **not smoking** (p. 149), **not drinking alcoholic drinks** (p. 148), and **not using drugs** (p. 416 and 417).
- Getting enough **exercise and rest.**
- **Tetanus vaccination** to prevent tetanus in the newborn. (Give at the 6th, 7th, and 8th month if first time. If she has been vaccinated against tetanus before, give one booster during the 7th month.)

2. **Nutrition**

Does the mother look well nourished? Is she anemic? If so, discuss ways of eating better. If possible, see that she gets iron pills—preferably with folic acid and vitamin C. Advise her about how to handle morning sickness (p. 248) and heartburn (p. 128).

Is she gaining weight normally? If possible, weigh her each visit. Normally she should gain 8 to 10 kilograms during the nine months of pregnancy. If she stops gaining weight, this is a bad sign. Sudden weight gain in the last months is a danger sign. If you do not have scales, try to judge if she is gaining weight by how she looks.

Or make a simple scale:

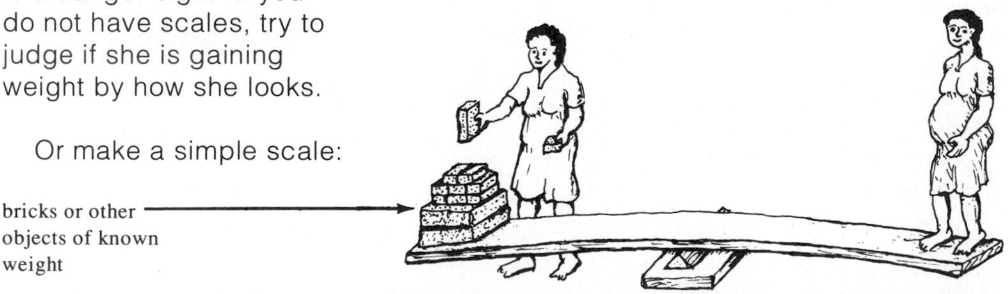
bricks or other objects of known weight

3. **Minor problems**

Ask the mother if she has any of the common problems of pregnancy. Explain that they are not serious, and give what advice you can (see p. 248).

4. **Signs of danger and special risk**

Check for each of the danger signs on p. 249. Take the mother's **pulse** each visit. This will let you know what is normal for her in case she has problems later (for example, shock from toxemia or severe bleeding). If you have a blood pressure cuff, take her **blood pressure** (see p. 410). And **weigh her.** Watch out especially for the following danger signs:

- sudden weight gain
- swelling of hands and face
- marked increase in blood pressure
- severe anemia (p. 124)
- any bleeding (p. 249)

} signs of toxemia of pregnancy (p. 249)

Some midwives may have paper 'dip sticks' or other methods for measuring the protein and sugar in the urine. High protein may be a sign of toxemia. High sugar could be a sign of diabetes (p. 127).

If any of the danger signs appear, see that the woman gets medical help as soon as possible. Also, check for **signs of special risk,** page 256. If any are present, it is safer if the mother gives birth in a hospital.

5. **Growth and position of the baby in the womb**

Feel the mother's womb each time she visits; or show her how to do it herself.

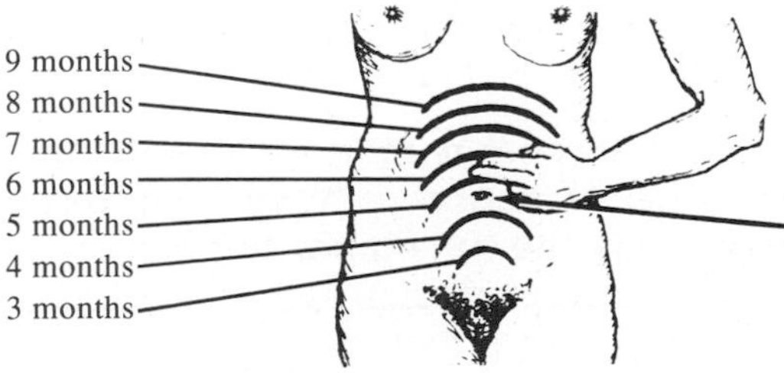

Normally the womb will be 2 fingers higher each month.

At 4 1/2 months it is usually at the level of the navel.

Each month write down how many finger widths the womb is above or below the navel. **If the womb seems too big or grows too fast,** it may mean the woman is having twins. Or the womb may have more water in it than normal. If so, you may find it more difficult to feel the baby inside. Too much water in the womb means greater risk of severe bleeding during childbirth and may mean the baby is deformed.

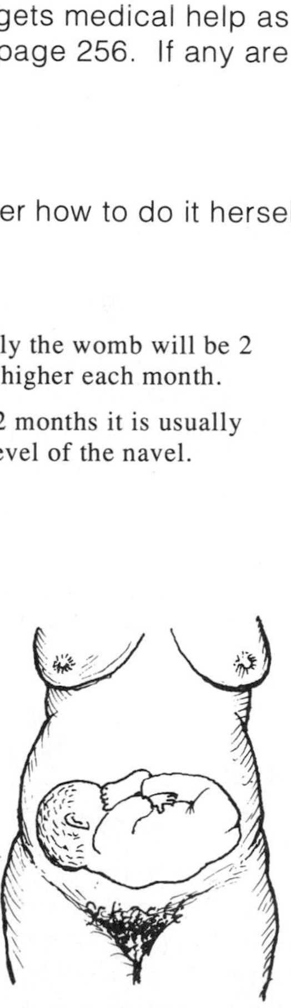

Try to feel the baby's position in the womb. If it appears to be lying sideways, the mother should go to a doctor **before** labor begins, because an operation may be needed. For checking the baby's position near the time of birth, see page 257.

6. **Baby's heartbeat (fetal heartbeat) and movement**

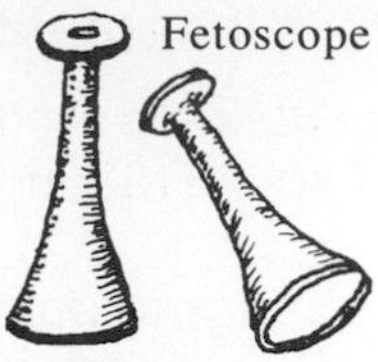
Fetoscope

After 5 months, listen for the baby's heartbeat and check for movement. You can try putting your ear against the belly, but it may be hard to hear. It will be easier if you get a *fetoscope*. (Or make one. Fired clay or hard wood works well.)

If the baby's heartbeat is heard loudest below the navel in the last month, the baby is head down and will probably be born head first.

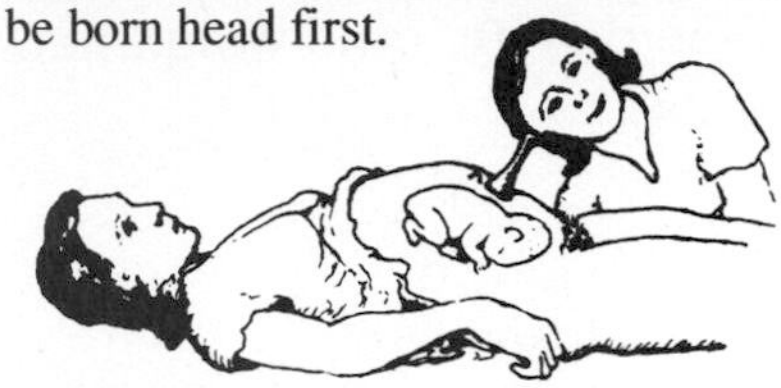

If the heartbeat is heard loudest above the navel, his head is probably up. It may be a breech birth.

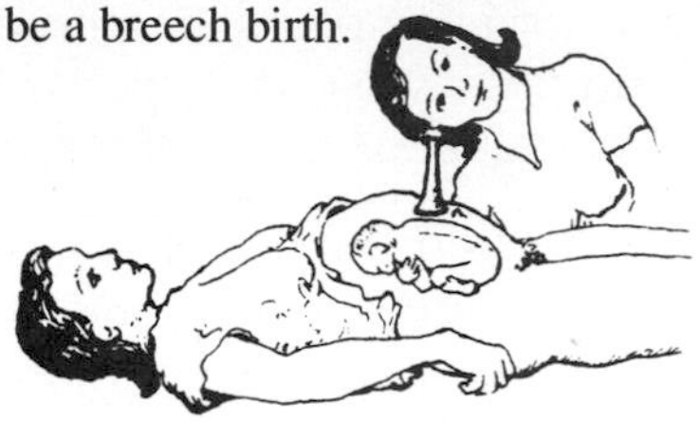

A baby's heart beats about twice as fast as an adult's. If you have a watch with a second hand, count the baby's heartbeats. From 120 to 160 per minute is normal. If less than 120, something is wrong. (Or perhaps you counted wrong or heard the mother's heartbeat. Check her pulse. The baby's heartbeat is often hard to hear. It takes practice.)

7. **Preparing the mother for labor**

As the birth approaches, see the mother more often. If she has other children, ask her how long labor lasted and if she had any problems. Perhaps suggest that she lie down to rest after eating, twice a day for an hour each time. Talk with her about ways to make the birth easier and less painful (see the next pages). You may want to have her practice deep, slow breathing, so that she can do this during the contractions of labor. Explain to her that relaxing during contractions, and resting between them, will help her save strength, reduce pain, and speed labor.

If there is any reason to suspect the labor may result in problems you cannot handle, send the mother to a health center or hospital to have her baby. Be sure she is near the hospital by the time labor begins.

HOW A MOTHER CAN TELL THE DATE WHEN SHE IS LIKELY TO GIVE BIRTH:

Start with the date the last menstrual period began, subtract 3 months, and add 7 days. For example, suppose your last period began May 10.

May 10 minus 3 months is February 10,
Plus 7 days is February 17.
The baby is likely to be born around February 17.

8. **Keeping records**

To compare your findings from month to month and see how the mother is progressing, it helps to keep simple records. On the next page is a sample record sheet. Change it as you see fit. A larger sheet of paper would be better. Each mother can keep her own record sheet and bring it when she comes for her check-up.

RECORD OF PRENATAL CARE

NAME ______________________ AGE ______ NUMBER OF CHILDREN _______ AGES ___________ DATE OF LAST CHILDBIRTH ______________

DATE OF LAST MENSTRUAL PERIOD ____________ PROBABLE DATE FOR BIRTH ___________ PROBLEMS WITH OTHER BIRTHS ____________________

MONTH	DATE OF VISIT	WHAT OFTEN HAPPENS	GENERAL HEALTH AND MINOR PROBLEMS	ANEMIA (how severe)?	DANGER SIGNS (see p. 249)	SWELLING (where? how much?)	PULSE	TEMP.	WEIGHT (estimate or measure)	BLOOD PRESSURE *	PROTEIN IN URINE *	SUGAR IN URINE *	POSITION OF BABY IN WOMB	SIZE OF WOMB (how many fingers above (+) or below (-) the navel?)	
1														-	
2		tiredness, nausea, and morning sickness												-	
3														-	
4		← womb at level of the navel												0	
5		← baby's heartbeat & 1st movements												+	TETANUS VACCINE
6														+	1st
7 (1st week)		some swelling of feet												+	2nd or booster
(3rd week)														+	
8 (1st week)		constipation												+	3rd
(3rd week)		heartburn												+	
9 (1st week)		varicose veins; shortness of breath												+	
(2nd week)		frequent urination												+	
(3rd week)														+	
(4th week)		← baby moves lower in belly												+	
														+	
BIRTH															

* These are included for midwives who have means of measuring or testing for this information.

THINGS A MOTHER SHOULD HAVE READY BEFORE GIVING BIRTH

Every pregnant woman should have the following things ready by the seventh month of pregnancy:

A lot of very clean cloths or rags.

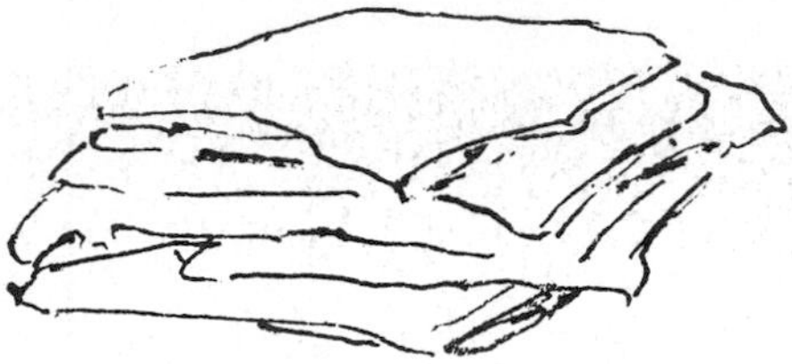

An antiseptic soap (or any soap).

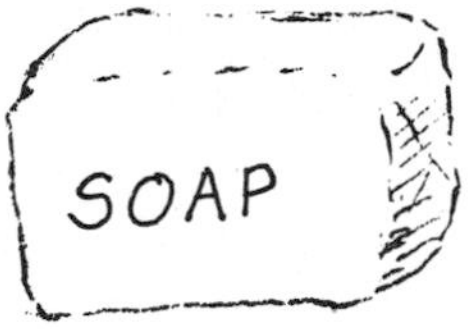

A clean scrub brush for cleaning the hands and fingernails.

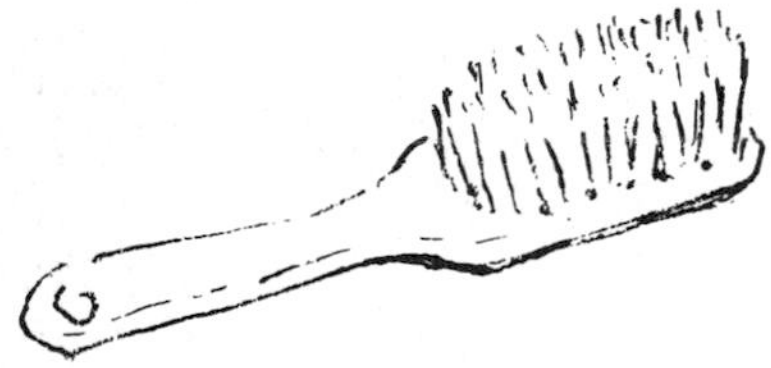

Alcohol for rubbing hands after washing them.

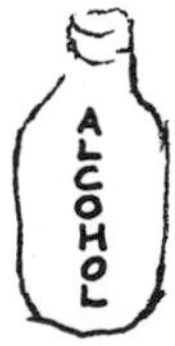

Clean cotton.

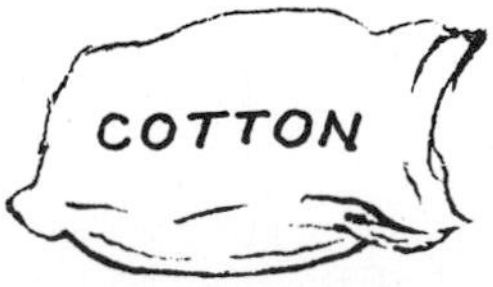

A new razor blade. (Do not unwrap until you are ready to cut the umbilical cord.)

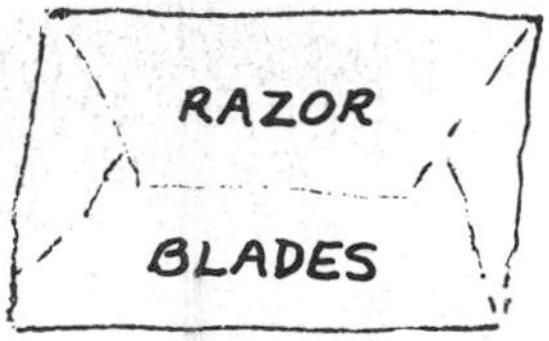

(If you do not have a new razor blade, have clean, rust-free scissors ready. Boil them just before cutting the cord.)

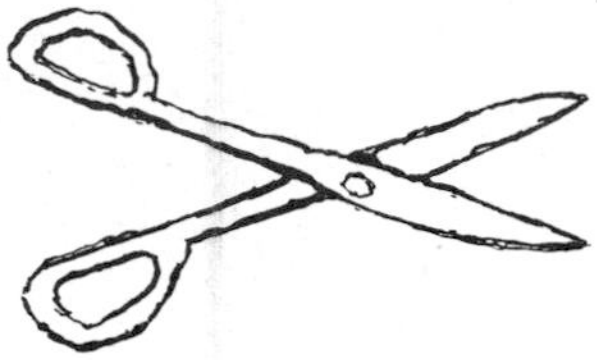

Sterile gauze or patches of thoroughly cleaned cloth for covering the navel.

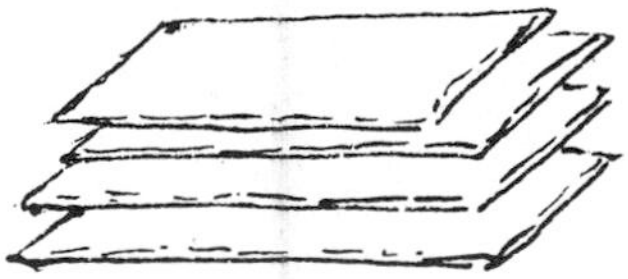

Two ribbons or strips of clean cloth for tying the cord.

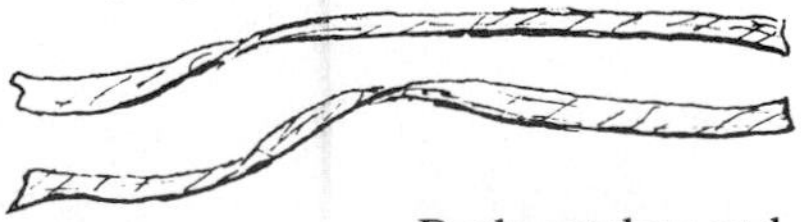

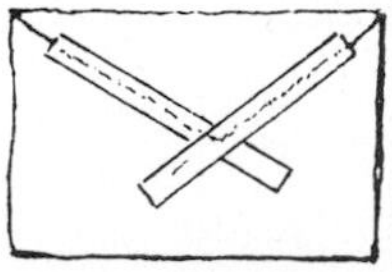

Both patches and ribbons should be wrapped and sealed in paper packets and then baked in an oven or ironed.

Additional Supplies
for the Well-Prepared Midwife or Birth Attendant

Flashlight (torch).

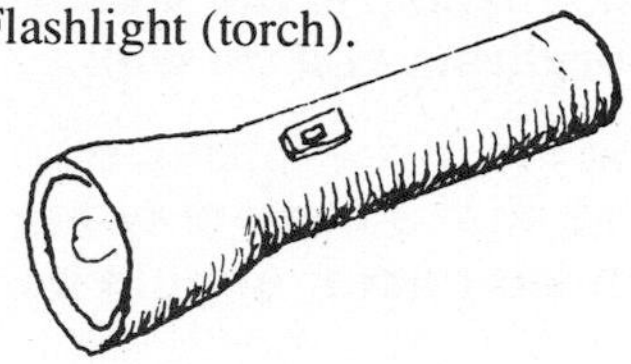

Fetoscope—or fetal stethoscope—for listening to the baby's heartbeat through the mother's belly.

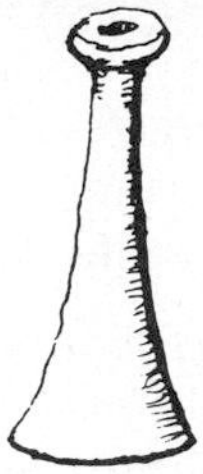

Suction bulb for sucking mucus out of the baby's nose and mouth.

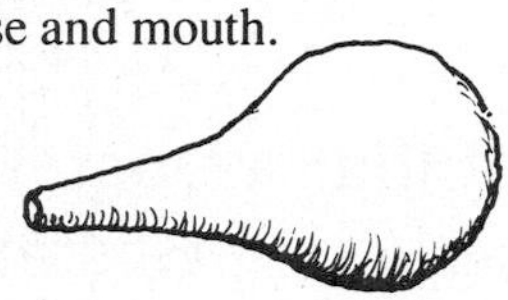

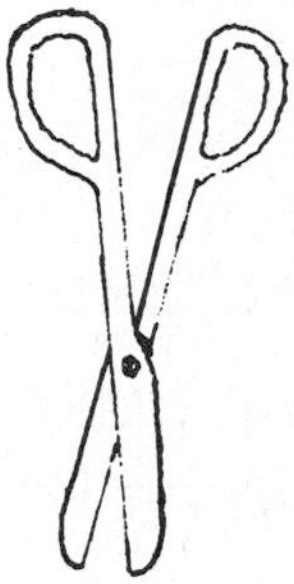

Blunt-tipped scissors for cutting the cord before the baby is all the way born (extreme emergency only).

Sterile syringe and needles.

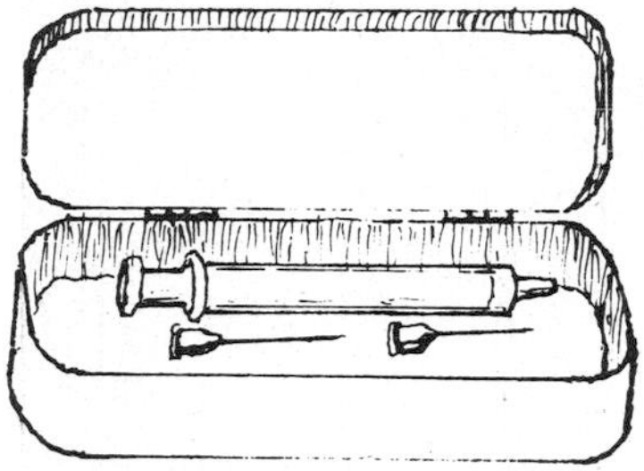

Two clamps (hemostats) for clamping the umbilical cord or clamping bleeding veins from tears of the birth opening.

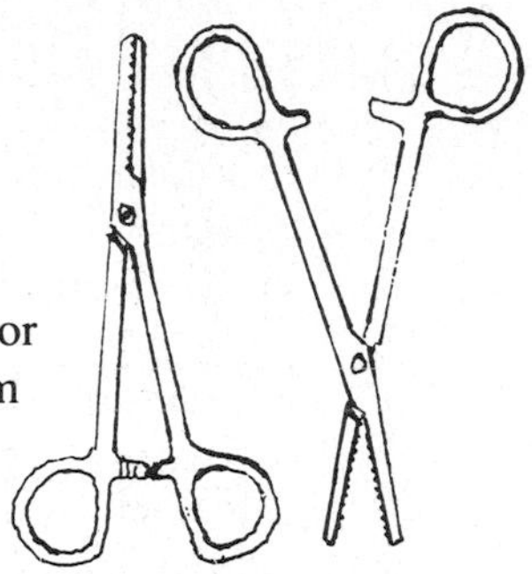

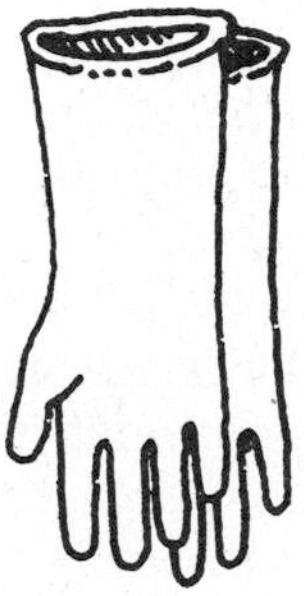

Rubber or plastic gloves (that can be sterilized by boiling, see p. 74) to wear while examining the woman, while the baby is coming out, when sewing tears in the birth opening, and for catching and examining afterbirth.

Several injections of ergonovine or ergometrine (see p. 391).

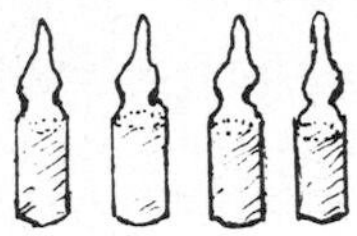

Sterile needle and gut thread for sewing tears in the birth opening

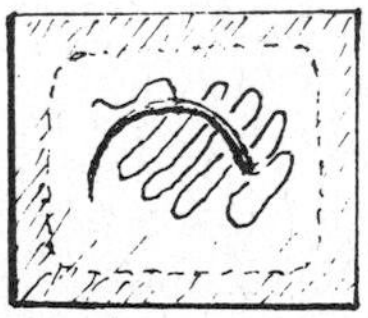

Two bowls—1 for washing hands and 1 for catching and examining the afterbirth.

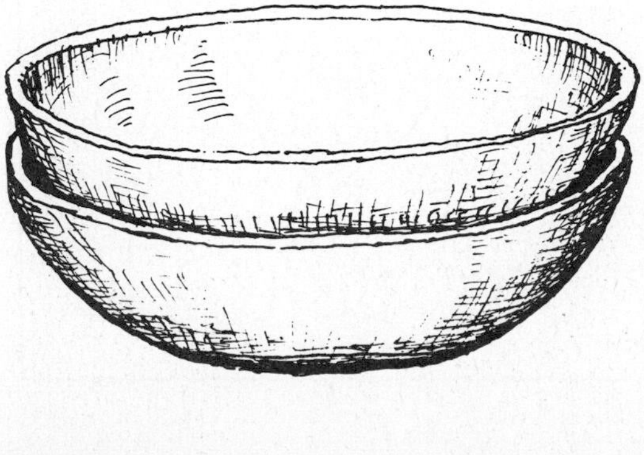

1% silver nitrate drops, tetracycline eye ointment, or erythromycin eye ointment for the baby's eyes to prevent dangerous infection (see p. 221).

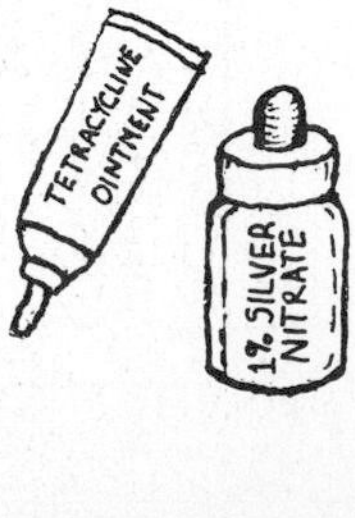

PREPARING FOR BIRTH

Birth is a natural event. When the mother is healthy and everything goes well, the baby can be born without help from anyone. In a normal birth, **the less the midwife or birth attendant does, the more likely everything will go well.**

Difficulties in childbirth do occur, and sometimes the life of the mother or child may be in danger. **If there is any reason to think that a birth may be difficult or dangerous, a skilled midwife or experienced doctor should be present.**

CAUTION: If you have a fever, cough, sore throat, or sores or infections on your skin at the time of the birth, it would be better for someone else to deliver the baby.

Signs of Special Risk that Make It Important that a Doctor or Skilled Midwife Attend the Birth—if Possible in a Hospital:

- If regular labor pains begin more than 3 weeks before the baby is expected.
- If the woman begins to bleed before labor.
- If there are signs of toxemia of pregnancy (see p. 249).
- If the woman is suffering from a chronic or acute illness.
- If the woman is very anemic, or if her blood does not clot normally (when she cuts herself).
- If she is under 15, over 40, or over 35 at her first pregnancy.
- If she has had more than 5 or 6 babies.
- If she is especially short or has narrow hips (p. 267).
- If she has had serious trouble or severe bleeding with other births.
- If she has diabetes or heart trouble.
- If she has a hernia.
- If it looks like she will have twins (see p. 269).
- If it seems the baby is not in a normal position in the womb.
- If the bag of waters breaks and labor does not begin within a few hours. (The danger is even greater if there is fever.)
- If the baby is still not born 2 weeks after 9 months of pregnancy.

THE BIRTHS WITH THE GREATEST CHANCE OF PROBLEMS ARE:

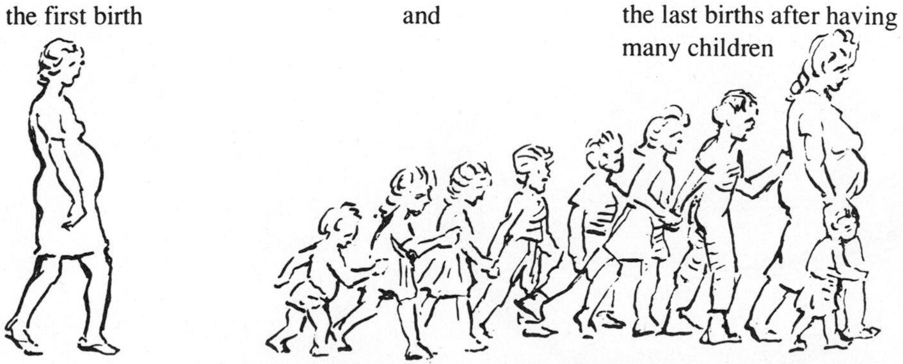
the first birth
and
the last births after having many children

Checking if the Baby Is in a Good Position

To make sure the baby is head down, in the normal position for birth, feel for his head, like this:

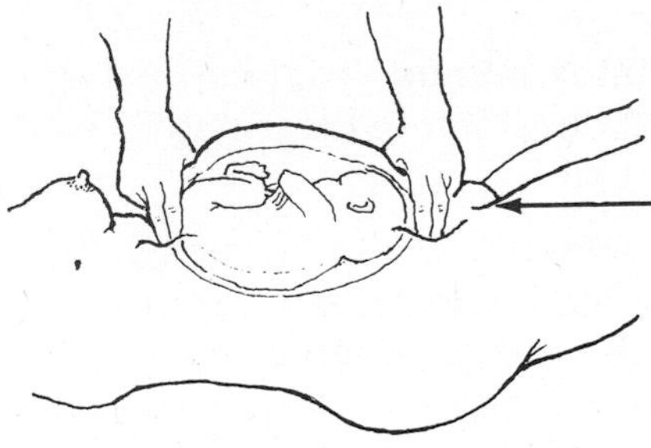

1. Have the mother breathe out all the way.

With the thumb and 2 fingers, push in here, just above the *pelvic* bone.

With the other hand, feel the top of the womb.

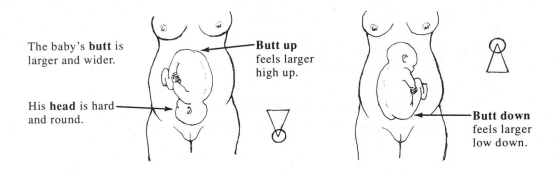

The baby's **butt** is larger and wider.

His **head** is hard and round.

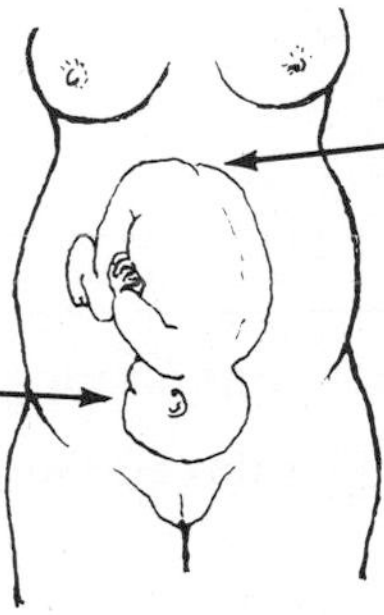

Butt up feels larger high up.

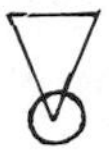

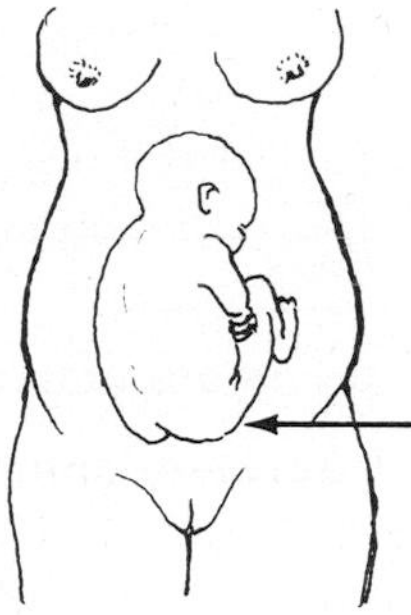

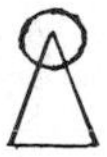

Butt down feels larger low down.

2. Push gently from side to side, first with one hand, then the other.

If the baby's butt is pushed gently sideways, the baby's whole body will move too.

But if the head is pushed gently sideways, it will bend at the neck and the back will not move.

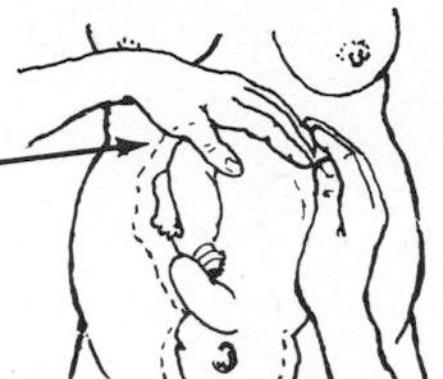

If the baby still is high in the womb, you can move the head a little. But if it has already engaged (dropped lower) getting ready for birth, you cannot move it.

A woman's first baby sometimes engages 2 weeks before labor begins. Later babies may not engage until labor starts.

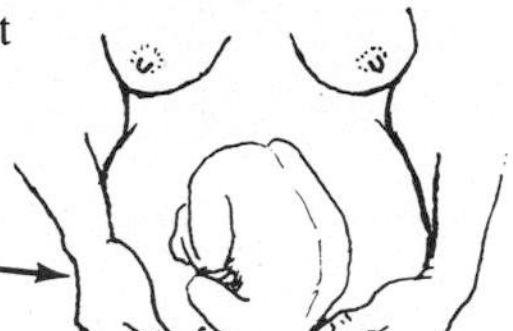

If the baby's head is *down,* his birth is likely to go well.
If the head is *up,* the birth may be more difficult (a breech birth), and it is safer for the mother to give birth in or near a hospital.
If the baby is *sideways,* the mother should have her baby in a hospital. She and the baby are in danger (see p. 267).

SIGNS THAT SHOW LABOR IS NEAR

- A few days before labor begins, usually **the baby moves lower** in the womb. This lets the mother breathe more easily, but she may need to urinate more often because of pressure on the bladder. (In the first birth these signs can appear up to 4 weeks before delivery.)
- A short time before the labor begins, **some thick mucus** (jelly) may come out. Or some mucus may come out for 2 or 3 days before labor begins. Sometimes it is tinted with blood. This is normal.
- The **contractions** (sudden tightening of the womb) or labor pains may start up to several days before childbirth; at first a long time usually passes between contractions—several minutes or even hours. When the contractions become stronger, regular, and more frequent, labor is beginning.
- Some women have a few **practice contractions** weeks before labor. This is normal. On rare occasions, a woman may have **false labor.** This happens when the contractions are coming strong and close together, but then stop for hours or days before childbirth actually begins. Sometimes walking, a warm bath, or resting will help calm the contractions if they are false, or bring on childbirth if they are real. Even if it is false labor, the contractions help to prepare the womb for labor.

Labor pains are caused by contractions or tightening of the womb.

Between contractions the womb is relaxed like this:

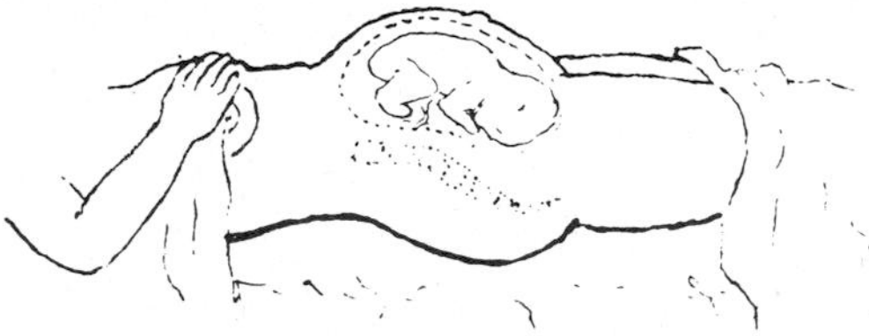

During contractions, the womb tightens and lifts up like this:

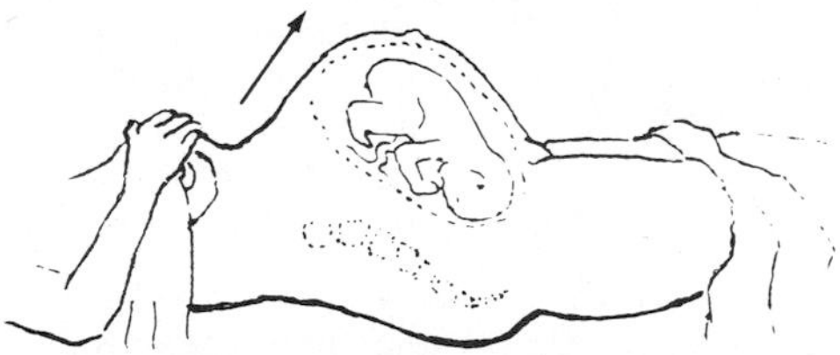

The contractions push the baby down farther. This causes the *cervix* or 'door of the womb' to open—a little more each time.

- The **bag of water** that holds the baby in the womb usually breaks with a flood of liquid sometime after labor has begun. If the waters break before the contractions start, this usually means the beginning of labor. After the waters break, the mother should keep very clean. Walking back and forth may help bring on labor more quickly. To prevent infection, avoid sexual contact, do not sit in a bath of water, and do not ***douche.*** If labor does not start within 12 hours, seek medical help.

THE STAGES OF LABOR

Labor has 3 parts or stages:

- The first stage lasts from the beginning of the strong contractions until the baby drops into the birth canal.
- The second stage lasts from the dropping of the baby into the birth canal until it is born.
- The third stage lasts from the birth of the baby until the placenta (afterbirth) comes out.

THE FIRST STAGE OF LABOR usually lasts 10 to 20 hours or more when it is the mother's first birth, and from 7 to 10 hours in later births. This varies a lot.

During the first stage of labor, the mother should not try to hurry the birth. It is natural for this stage to go slowly. The mother may not feel the progress and begin to worry. Try to reassure her. Tell her that most women have the same concern.

The mother should not try to push or bear down until the child is beginning to move down into the birth canal, and she feels she has to push.

The mother should keep her bowels and bladder empty.

If the bladder and the bowels are full, they get in the way when the baby is being born.

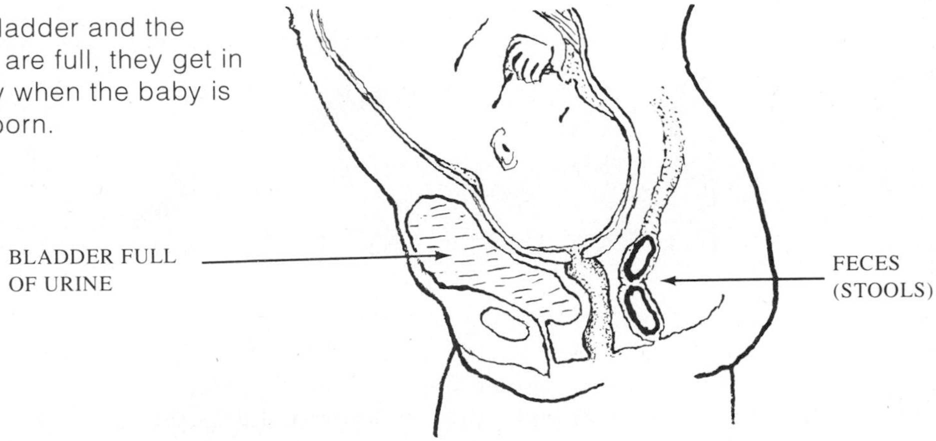

During labor, the mother should urinate often. If she has not moved her bowels in several hours, an enema may make labor easier. During labor the mother should drink water or other liquids often. Too little liquid in the body can slow down or stop labor. If labor is long, she should eat lightly, as well. If she is vomiting, she should sip a little Rehydration Drink, herbal tea, or fruit juices between each contraction.

During labor the mother should change positions often or get up and walk about from time to time. She should not lie flat on her back for a long time.

During the first stage of labor, the midwife or birth attendant should:

- Wash the mother's belly, genitals, buttocks, and legs well with soap and warm water. The bed should be in a clean place with enough light to see clearly.
- Spread clean sheets, towels, or newspapers on the bed and change them whenever they get wet or dirty.
- Have a new, unopened razor blade ready for cutting the cord, or boil a pair of scissors for 15 minutes. Keep the scissors in the boiled water in a covered pan until they are needed.

The midwife should **not** massage or push on the belly. She should **not** ask the mother to push or bear down at this time.

If the mother is frightened or in great pain, have her take deep, **slow,** regular breaths during each contraction, and breathe normally between them. This will help control the pain and calm her. Reassure the mother that the strong pains are normal and that they help to push her baby out.

THE SECOND STAGE OF LABOR, in which the child is born: Sometimes this begins when the bag of water breaks. It is often easier than the first stage and usually does not take longer than 2 hours. During the contractions the mother bears down (pushes) with all her strength. Between contractions, she may seem very tired and half asleep. This is normal.

To bear down, the mother should take a deep breath and push hard with her stomach muscles, as if she were having a bowel movement. If the child comes slowly after the bag of waters breaks, the mother can double her knees like this, while

squatting,

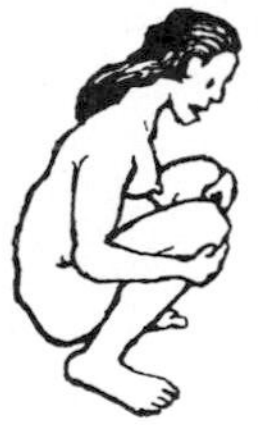

sitting propped up,

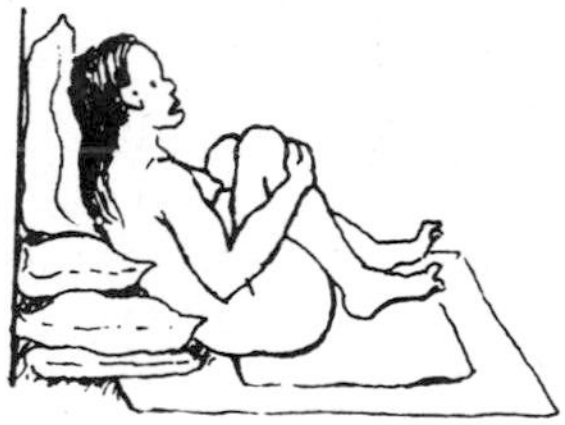

kneeling,

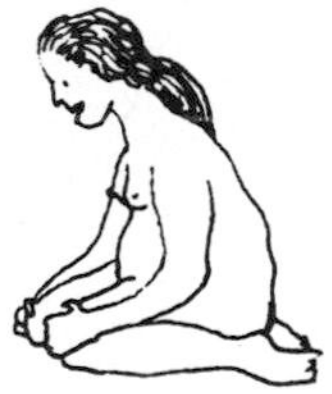

or lying down.

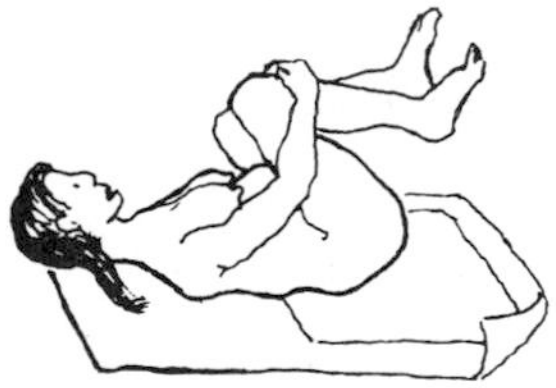

When the birth opening of the mother stretches, and the baby's head begins to show, the midwife or helper should have everything ready for the birth of the baby. At this time the mother should try **not** to push hard, so that the head comes out more slowly. This helps prevent tearing of the opening (see p. 269 for more details).

In a normal birth, the midwife NEVER needs to put her hand or finger inside the mother. This is the most common cause of dangerous infections of the mother after the birth.

When the head comes out, the midwife may support it, but must *never* pull on it.

If possible, **wear gloves to attend the birth**—to protect the health of the mother, baby, and midwife. Today this is more important than ever.

Normally the baby is born head first like this:

1.

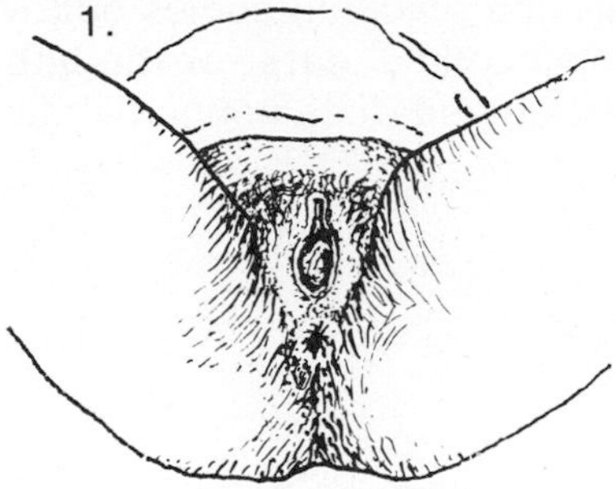

Now push hard.

2.

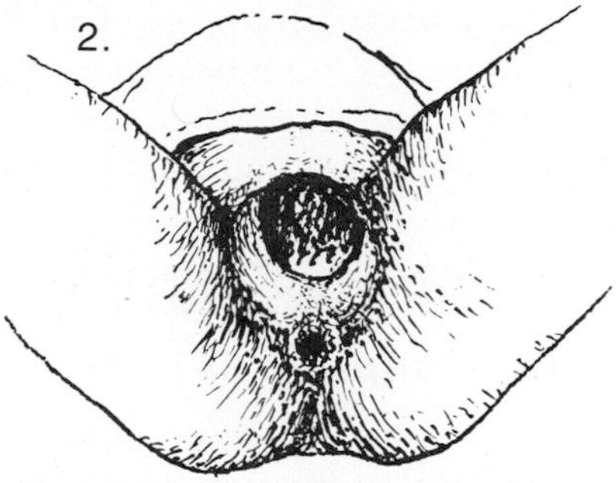

Now try not to push hard. Take many short, fast breaths. This helps prevent tearing the opening (see p. 269).

3.

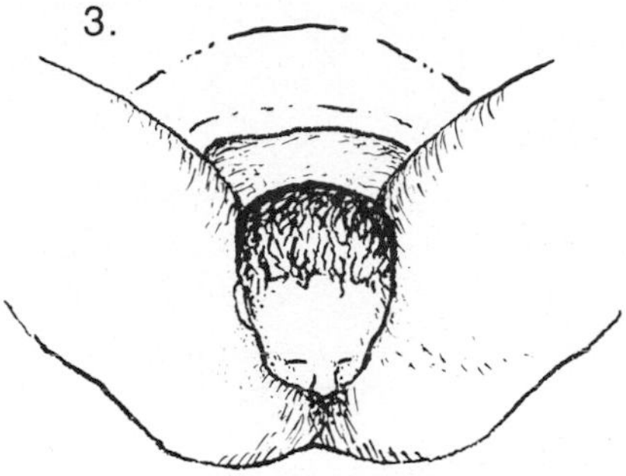

The head usually comes out face down. If the baby has feces (shit) in her mouth and nose, clean it out immediately (see p. 262).

4.

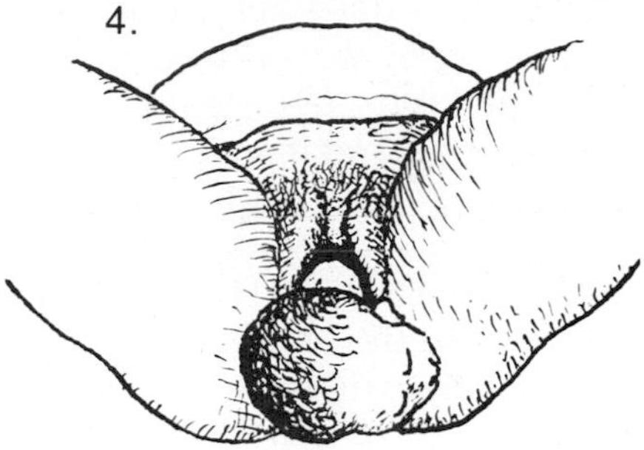

Then the baby's body turns to one side so the shoulders can come out.

If the shoulders get stuck after the head comes out:

1.

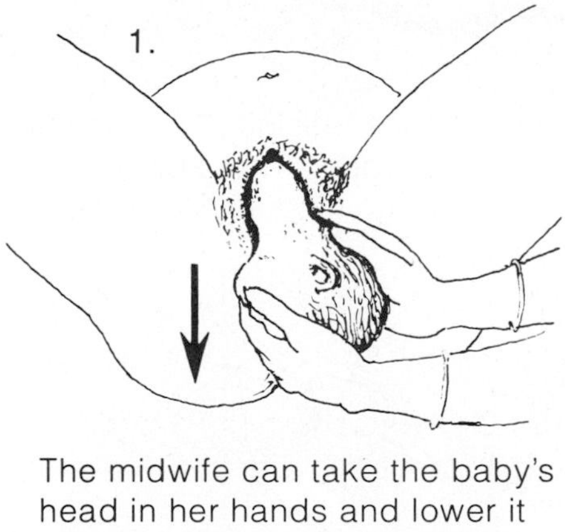

The midwife can take the baby's head in her hands and lower it very carefully, so the shoulder can come out.

2.

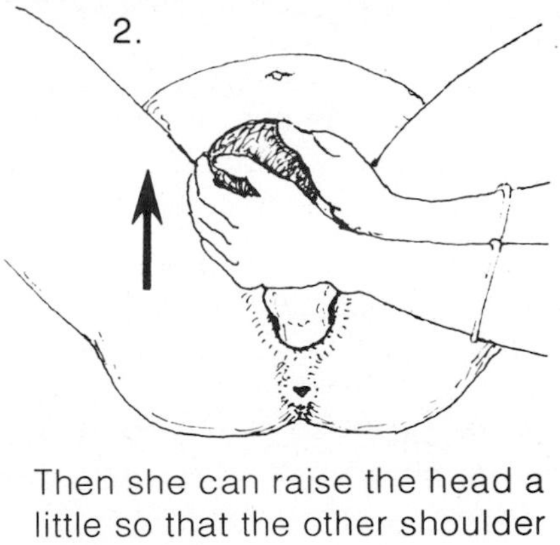

Then she can raise the head a little so that the other shoulder comes out.

All the force must come from the mother. The midwife should **never pull on the head, or twist or bend the baby's neck**, because this can harm the baby.

THE THIRD STAGE OF LABOR begins when the baby has been born and lasts until the placenta (afterbirth) comes out. Usually, the placenta comes out by itself 5 minutes to an hour after the baby. In the meantime, **care for the baby**. If there is a lot of bleeding (see p. 265) or if the placenta does not come out within 1 hour, seek medical help.

CARE OF THE BABY AT BIRTH

Immediately after the baby comes out:

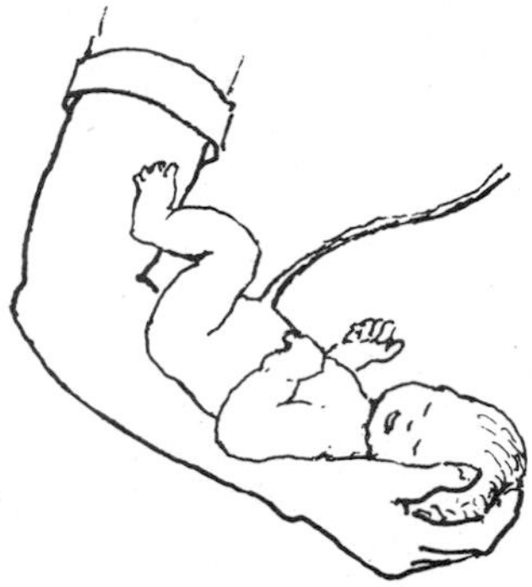

- Put the baby's head down so that the mucus comes out of his mouth and throat. Keep it this way until he begins to breathe.
- Keep the baby ***below*** the level of the mother until the cord is tied. (This way, the baby gets more blood and will be stronger.)
- If the baby does not begin to breathe right away, rub his back with a towel or a cloth.
- If he still does not breathe, clean the mucus out of his nose and mouth with a suction bulb or a clean cloth wrapped around your finger.
- If the baby has not begun to breathe within one minute after birth, start MOUTH-TO-MOUTH BREATHING **at once** (see p. 80).
- Wrap the baby in a clean cloth. It is very important not to let him get cold, especially if he is premature (born too early).

How to Cut the Cord

When the child is born, the cord pulses and is fat and blue. **WAIT.**

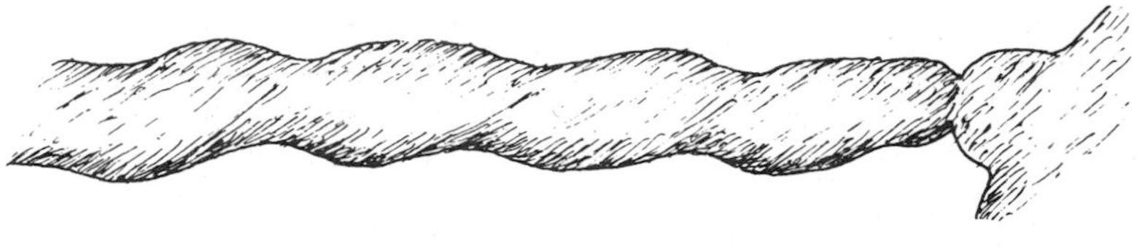

After a while, the cord becomes thin and white. It stops pulsing. Now tie it in 2 places with very clean, dry strips of cloth, string, or ribbon. These should have been recently ironed or heated in an oven. Cut between the ties, like this:

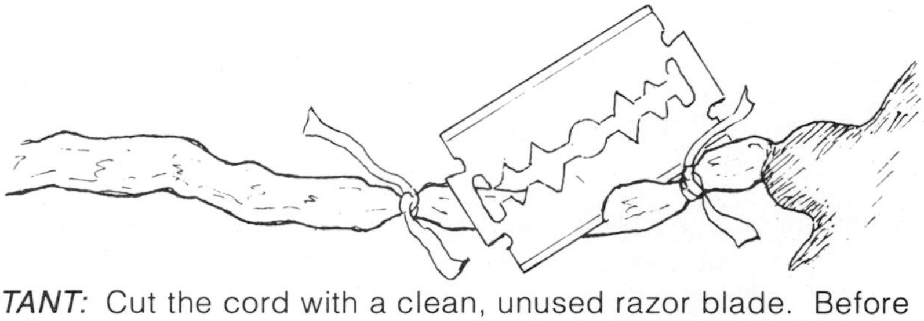

IMPORTANT: Cut the cord with a clean, unused razor blade. Before unwrapping it, wash your hands very well. Or wear clean rubber or plastic gloves. If you do not have a new razor blade, use freshly boiled scissors. **Always cut the cord close to the body of the newborn baby.** Leave only about 2 centimeters attached to the baby. These precautions help prevent tetanus (see p. 182).

Care of the Cut Cord

The most important way to protect the freshly cut cord from infection is to **keep it dry.** To help it dry out, **the air must get to it.** If the home is very clean and there are no flies, leave the cut cord uncovered and open to the air. If there are dust and flies, cover the cord lightly. It is best to use sterile gauze. Cut it with boiled scissors. Put it on like this:

1.

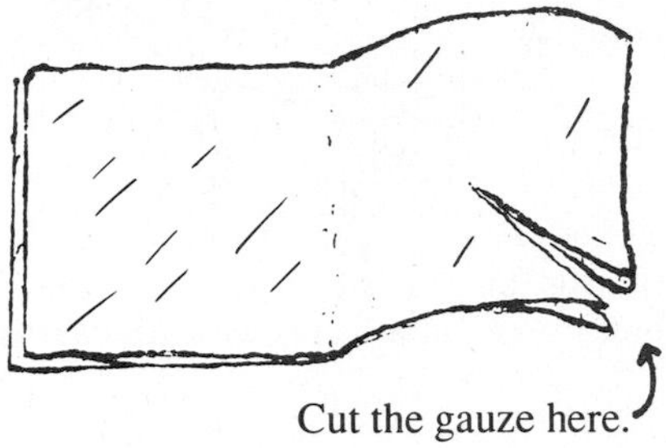

2.

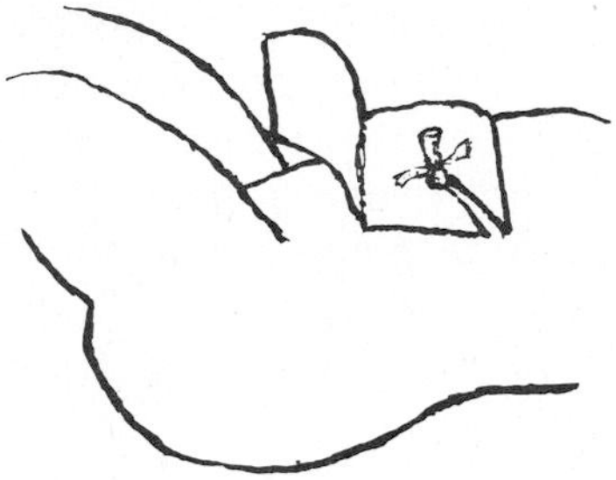

3.

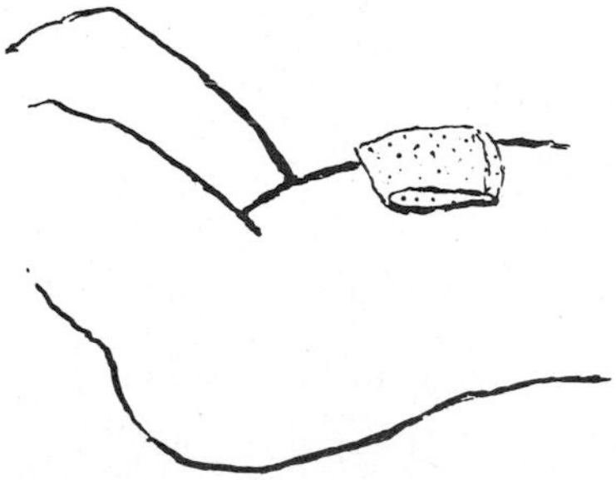

4.

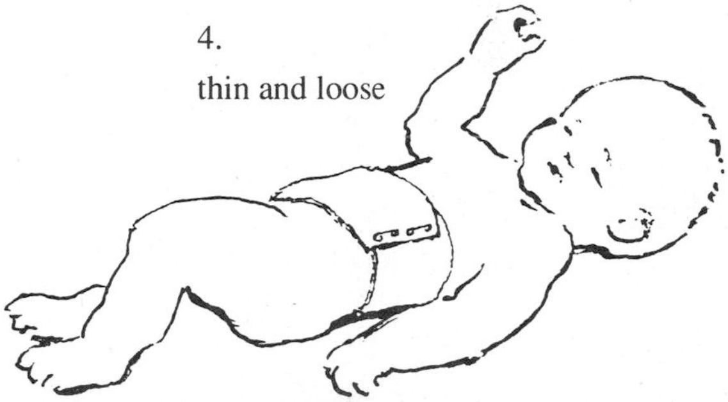

If you do not have sterile gauze, you can cover the navel with a very clean and freshly ironed cloth. It is better not to use a belly band, but if you want to use one, use a thin, light cloth, like cheesecloth, and be sure it is loose enough to let air under it, to keep the navel dry. Do not make it tight.

Be sure the baby's nappy (diapers) does not cover the navel, so that the cord does not get wet with urine.

Cleaning the Newborn Baby

With a warm, soft, damp cloth, gently clean away any blood or fluid.

It is better **not** to bathe the baby until after the cord drops off (usually 5 to 8 days). Then bathe him daily in warm water, using a mild soap.

Put the Newborn Baby to the Breast at Once

Place the baby at its mother's breast as soon as the baby is born. If the baby nurses, this will help to make the afterbirth come out sooner and to prevent or control heavy bleeding.

THE DELIVERY OF THE PLACENTA (AFTERBIRTH)

Normally, the placenta comes out 5 minutes to an hour after the baby is born, but sometimes it is delayed for many hours (see below).

Checking the afterbirth:

When the afterbirth comes out, pick it up and examine it to see if it is complete. If it is torn and there seem to be pieces missing, get medical help. A piece of placenta left inside the womb can cause continued bleeding or infection.

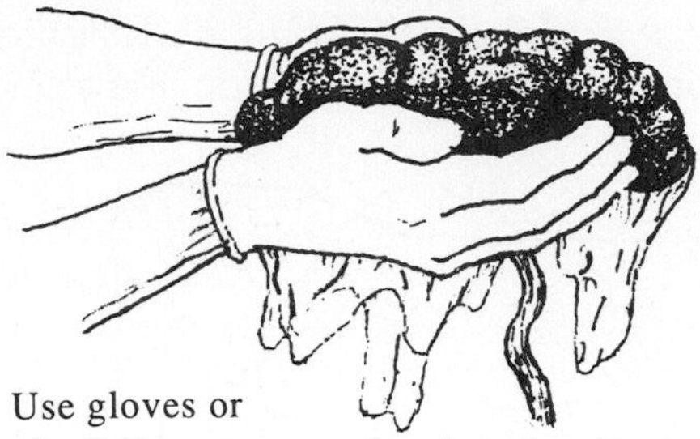

Use gloves or plastic bags on your hands to handle the placenta. Wash your hands well afterwards.

When the placenta is delayed in coming:

If the mother is not losing much blood, do nothing. **Do not pull on the cord.** This could cause dangerous hemorrhage (heavy bleeding). Sometimes the placenta will come out if the woman squats and pushes a little.

If the mother is losing blood, feel the womb (uterus) through the belly. If it is soft, do the following:

Massage the womb carefully, until it gets hard. This should make it contract and push out the placenta.

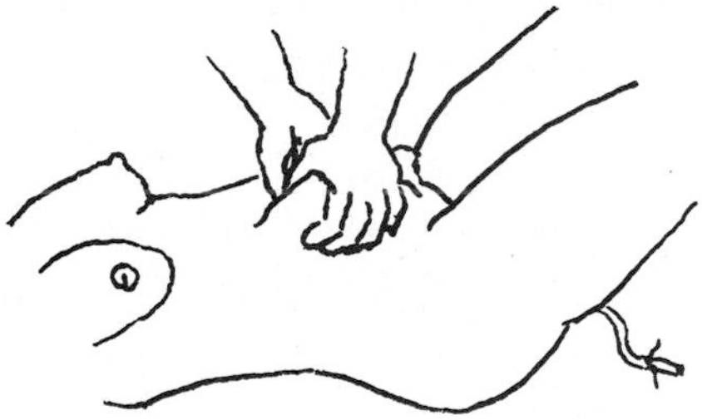

If the placenta does not come out soon, and bleeding continues, push downward on the top of the womb very carefully, while supporting the bottom of the womb like this.

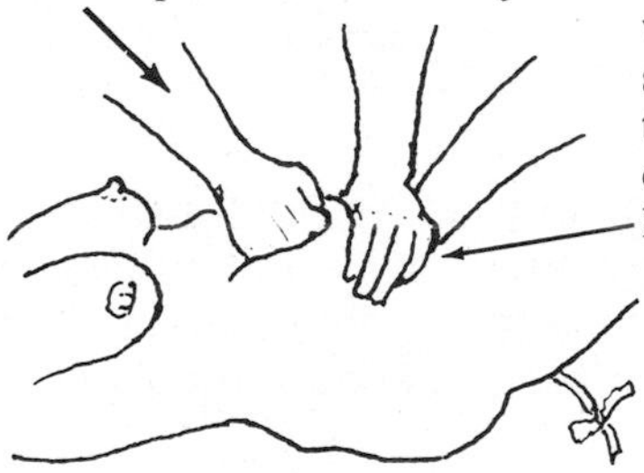

If the placenta still does not come out, and the heavy bleeding continues, try to control the bleeding (see next page) and seek medical help fast.

HEMORRHAGING (HEAVY BLEEDING)

When the placenta comes out, there is always a brief flow of blood. It normally lasts only a few minutes and not more than a quarter of a liter (1 cup) of blood is lost. (A little bleeding may continue for several days and is usually not serious.)

WARNING: Sometimes a woman may be bleeding severely inside without much blood coming out. Feel her belly from time to time. If it seems to be getting bigger, it may be filling with blood. Check her pulse often and watch for signs of shock (p. 77).

To help prevent or control heavy bleeding, **let the baby suck the mother's breast.** If the baby will not suck, have the husband (if possible) gently pull and massage the mother's nipples. This will cause her to produce a hormone (pituitrin) that helps control bleeding.

If heavy bleeding continues, or if the mother is losing a great deal of blood through a slow trickle, do the following:

- Get medical help fast. If the bleeding does not stop quickly, the mother may need to be given serum blood in a vein (a transfusion).
- If you have **ergonovine** or **oxytocin,** use it, following the instructions on the next page. (Use oxytocin instead of ergonovine if the placenta is still inside.)
- The mother should drink a lot of liquid (water, fruit juices, tea, soup, or Rehydration Drink—p. 152). If she grows faint or has a fast, weak pulse or shows other signs of **shock,** put her legs up and her head down (see p. 77).
- If the mother is losing a lot of blood, and is in danger of bleeding to death, try to stop the bleeding like this:

Massage the belly until you can feel the womb get hard.

If the bleeding stops, check every 5 minutes to make sure the womb stays hard. If it does not, massage it again.

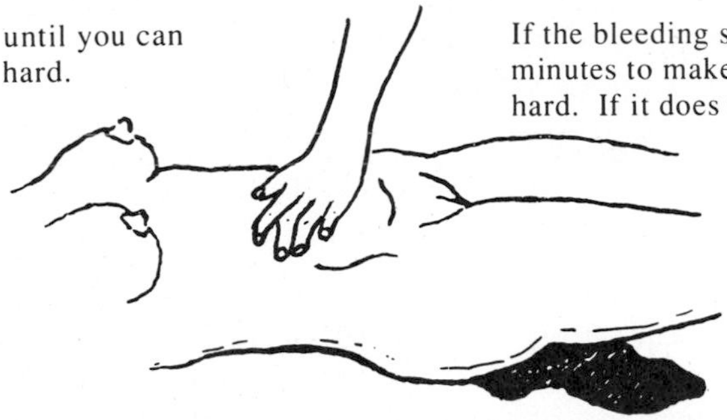

As soon as the womb gets hard and bleeding stops, stop massaging. Check it every minute or so. If it gets soft, massage it again.

- **If the bleeding continues** in spite of massaging the womb, do the following:

Using all of your weight, press down with both hands, one over the other, on the belly just below the navel. You should continue pressing down a long time after the bleeding stops.

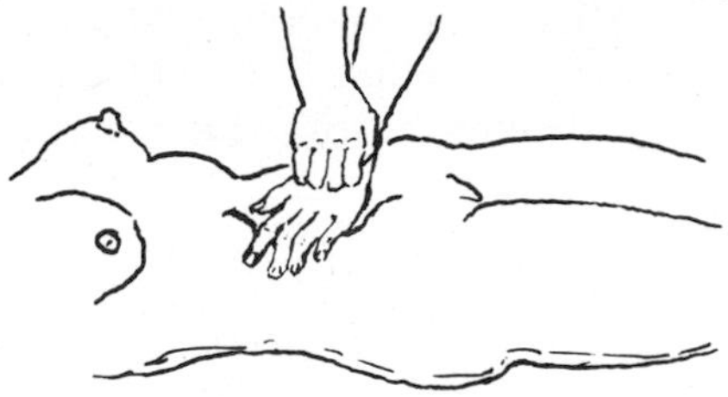

- If the bleeding is still not under control:

Press both hands into the belly above the womb. Scoop it up and fold it forward so the womb is pressed hard against the pubic bone. **Press as hard as you can,** using your weight if your muscles are not strong enough. Keep pressing for several minutes after the bleeding has stopped, or until you can get medical help.

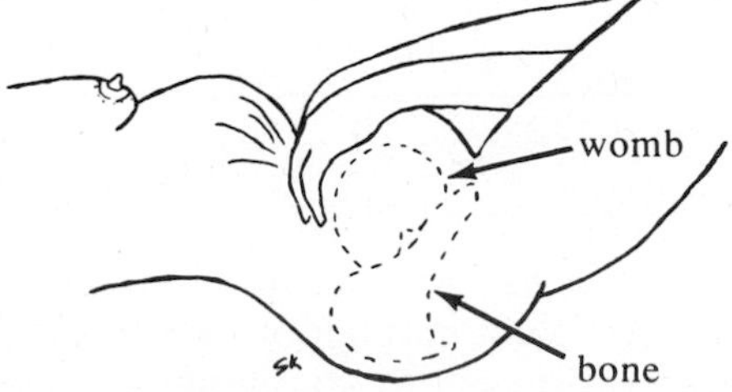

Note: Although some doctors use it, vitamin K does not help stop bleeding related to childbirth, miscarriage, or abortion. Do not use it.

THE CORRECT USE OF OXYTOCICS: ERGONOVINE, OXYTOCIN, *PITOCIN,* ETC.

Oxytocics are medicines that contain ergonovine, ergometrine, or oxytocin. They cause contractions of the uterus and its blood vessels. They are important but dangerous drugs. Used the wrong way, they can cause the death of the mother or the child in her womb. Used correctly, sometimes they can save lives. These are their correct uses:

1. **To control bleeding after childbirth.** This is the most important use of these medicines. In a case of heavy bleeding after the placenta has come out, inject one 0.2 mg. ampule (or give two 0.2 mg. tablets) of ergonovine or ergometrine maleate (*Ergotrate,* etc., p. 391) once every hour for 3 hours or until the bleeding is under control. After the bleeding is controlled, continue giving 1 ampule (or 1 pill) every 4 hours for 24 hours. If there is no ergonovine or if heavy bleeding starts before the placenta comes out, inject oxytocin (*Pitocin,* p. 391) instead.

IMPORTANT: Each expectant mother, and the midwife, should have ready enough ampules of oxytocin and ergonovine to combat heavy bleeding if it occurs. But these medicines should be used only in serious cases.

2. **To help prevent heavy bleeding after birth.** A woman who has suffered from heavy bleeding after previous births can be given 1 ampule (or 2 pills) of ergonovine immediately after the placenta comes out, and every 4 hours for the next 24 hours.

3. **To control the bleeding of a miscarriage** (p. 281). The use of oxytocics can be dangerous, and only a skilled health worker should use them. But, if the woman is rapidly losing blood and medical help is far away, use an oxytocic as suggested above. Oxytocin *(Pitocin)* is probably best.

WARNING: The use of *Ergotrate, Pitocin,* or *Pituitrin* to hasten childbirth or 'give strength' to the mother in labor is very dangerous for both her and the child. The times when oxytocics are needed before the baby is born are very rare, and it is better that only a trained birth attendant use them then. **Never use oxytocics before the child is born!**

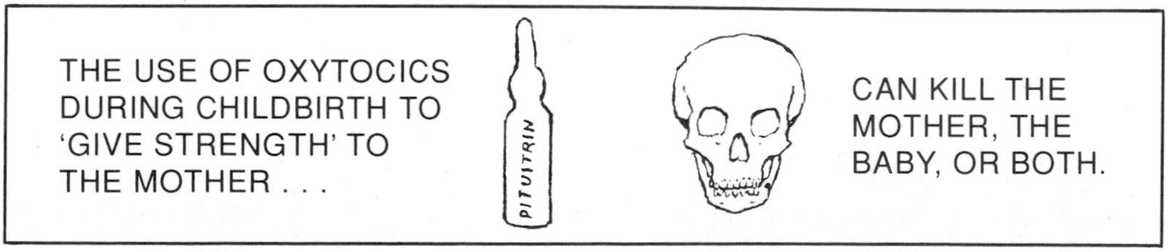
THE USE OF OXYTOCICS DURING CHILDBIRTH TO 'GIVE STRENGTH' TO THE MOTHER . . .
PITUITRIN
CAN KILL THE MOTHER, THE BABY, OR BOTH.

There is **no** safe medicine for giving strength to the mother or for making the birth quicker or easier.

If you want the woman to have enough strength for childbirth, have her eat plenty of nutritious foods during the 9 months of pregnancy (see p. 107). Also encourage her to space her children. Suggest that she not get pregnant again until enough time has passed for her to regain her full strength (see Family Planning, p. 283).

DIFFICULT BIRTHS

It is important to get medical help as quickly as possible when there is any serious problem during labor. Many problems or complications may come up, some more serious than others. Here are a few of the more common ones:

1. LABOR STOPS OR SLOWS DOWN, or lasts a very long time after being strong or after the waters break. This has several possible causes:

- **The woman may be frightened or upset.** This can slow down or even stop contractions. Talk to her. Help her to relax. Try to reassure her. Explain that the birth is slow, but there are no serious problems. Encourage her to change her position often and to drink, eat, and urinate. Stimulation (massage or milking motion) of the nipples can help speed labor.

- **The baby may be in an unusual position.** Feel the belly between contractions to see if the baby is **sideways.** Sometimes the midwife can turn the baby through **gentle** handling of the woman's belly. Try to work the baby around little by little between contractions, until the head is down. But **do not use force** as this could tear the womb or placenta, or pinch the cord. If the baby cannot be turned, try to get the mother to the hospital.

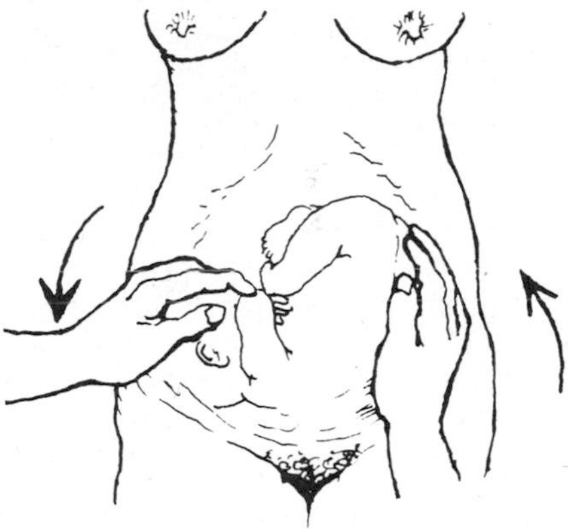

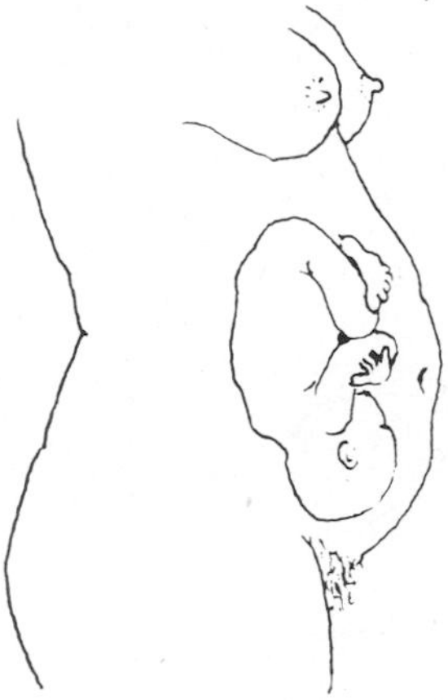

- **If the baby is facing forward** rather than backward, you may feel the lumpy arms and legs rather than the rounded back. This is usually no big problem, but labor may be longer and cause the woman more back pain. She should change positions often, as this may help turn the baby. Have her try on her hands and knees.

- **The baby's head may be too large to fit through the woman's hip bones** (pelvis). This is more likely in a woman with very narrow hips or a woman who is very much shorter than her husband. (It is very unlikely in a woman who has given normal birth before.) You may feel that the baby does not move down. If you suspect this problem, try to get the mother to a hospital as she may need an operation (Cesarean). **Women who have very narrow hips or are especially short should have at least their first child in or near a hospital.**

- **If the mother has been vomiting or has not been drinking liquids,** she may be dehydrated. This can slow down or stop contractions. Have her sip Rehydration Drink or other liquids after each contraction.

2. BREECH DELIVERY (the buttocks come out first). Sometimes the midwife can tell if the baby is in the breech position by feeling the mother's belly (p. 257) and listening to the baby's heartbeat (p. 252).

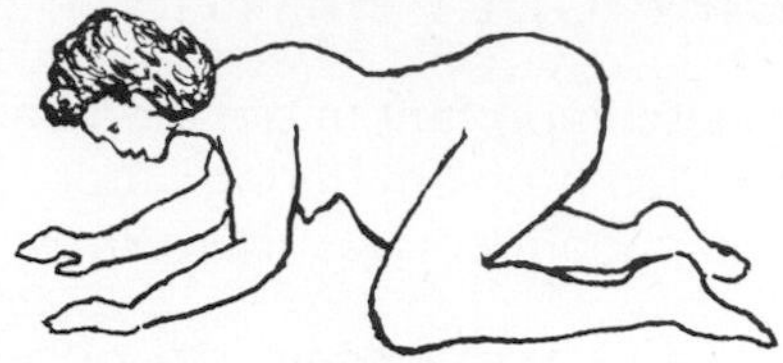

A breech birth may be easier in this position:

If the baby's legs come out, but not the arms, wash your hands very well, rub them with alcohol (or wear sterile gloves), and then . . .

slip your fingers inside and push the baby's shoulders toward the back, like this:

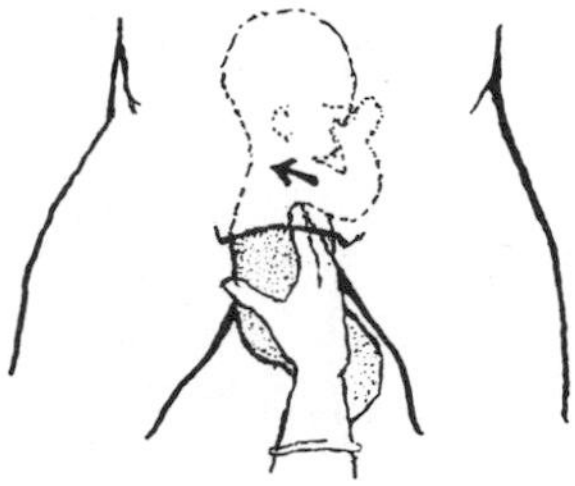

or press his arms against his body, like this:

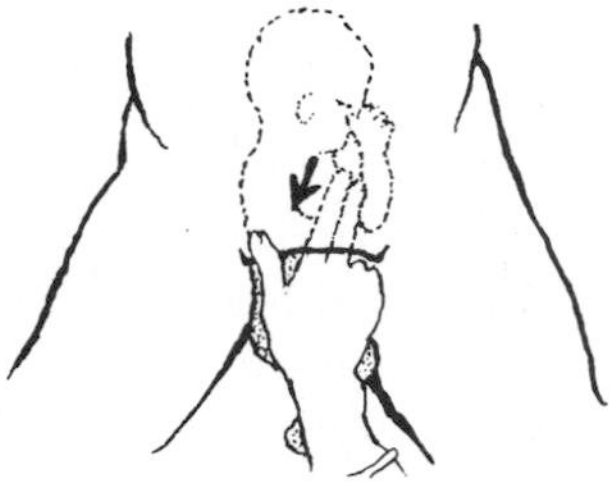

If the baby gets stuck, have the mother lie face up. Put your finger in the baby's mouth and push his head towards his chest. At the same time have someone push the baby's head down by pressing on the mother's belly like this→

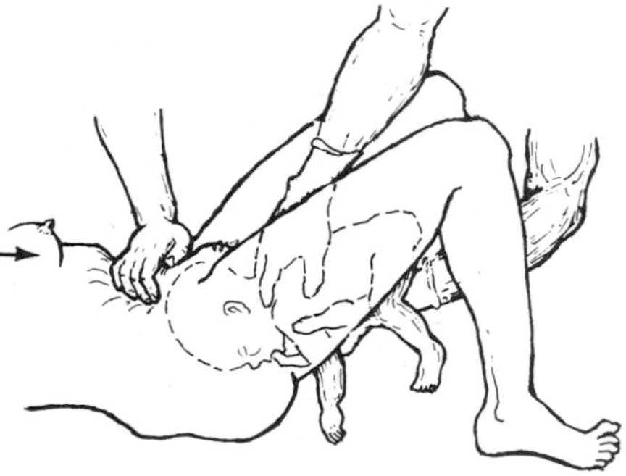

Have the mother push hard. But **never pull on the body of the baby.**

3. PRESENTATION OF AN ARM (hand first). If the baby's hand comes out first, get medical help right away. An operation may be needed to get the baby out.

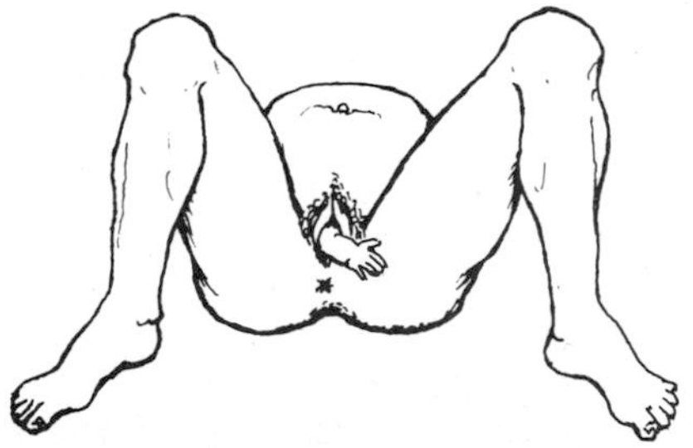

4. Sometimes the CORD IS WRAPPED AROUND THE BABY'S NECK so tightly he cannot come out all the way. Try to slip the loop of cord from around the baby's neck. If you cannot do this, you may have to clamp or tie and cut the cord. Use boiled blunt-tipped scissors.

5. FECES IN THE BABY'S MOUTH AND NOSE. When the waters break, if you see they contain a dark green (almost black) liquid, this is probably the baby's first stools (meconium). The baby may be in danger. If he breathes any of the feces into his lungs, he may die. As soon as his head is out, tell the mother not to push, but to take short, rapid breaths. Before the baby starts breathing, take time to suck the feces out of his nose and mouth with a suction bulb. Even if he starts breathing right away, keep sucking until you get all the feces out.

6. **TWINS.** Giving birth to twins is often more difficult and dangerous—both for the mother and babies—than giving birth to a single baby.

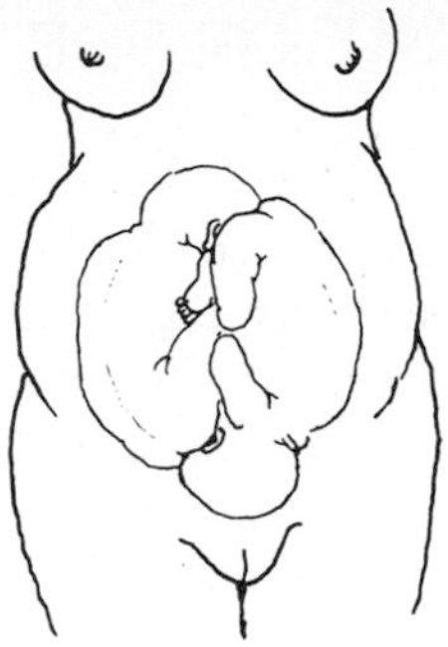

To be safe, the mother should give birth to twins in a hospital.

Because with twins labor often begins early, **the mother should be within easy reach of a hospital after the seventh month of pregnancy.**

Signs that a woman is likely to have twins:

- The belly grows faster and the womb is larger than usual, especially in the last months (see p. 251).
- If the woman gains weight faster than normal, or the common problems of pregnancy (morning sickness, backache, varicose veins, piles, swelling, and difficult breathing) are worse than usual, be sure to check for twins.
- If you can feel 3 or more large objects (heads and buttocks) in a womb that seems extra large, twins are likely.
- Sometimes you can hear 2 different heartbeats (other than the mother's)—but this is difficult.

During the last months, if the woman rests a lot and is careful to avoid hard work, twins are less likely to be born too early.

Twins are often born small and need special care. However, there is no truth in beliefs that twins have strange or magic powers.

TEARING OF THE BIRTH OPENING

The birth opening must stretch a lot for the baby to come out. Sometimes it tears. Tearing is more likely if it is the mother's first baby.

Tearing can usually be prevented if care is taken:

The mother should try to stop pushing when the baby's head is coming out. This gives her birth opening time to stretch. In order not to push, she should pant (take many short rapid breaths).

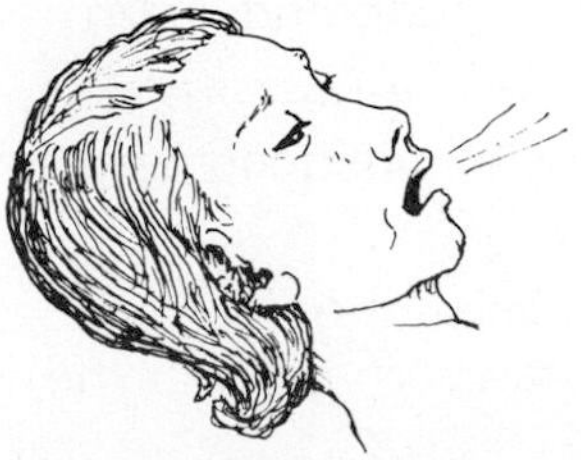

When the birth opening is stretching, the midwife can support it with one hand and with the other hand gently keep the head from coming too fast, like this:

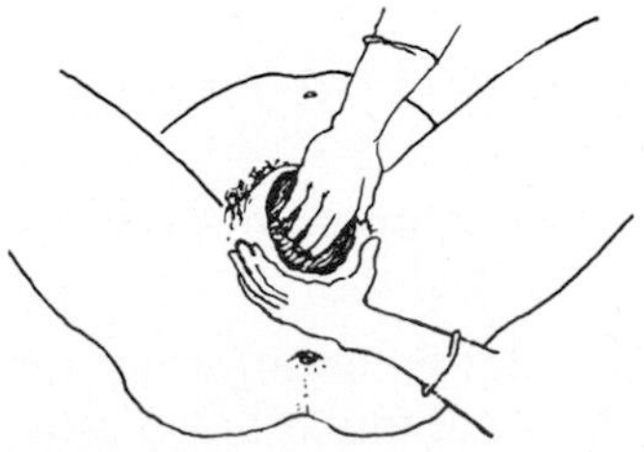

It may also help to put warm compresses against the skin below the birth opening. Start when it begins to stretch. You can also massage the stretched skin with oil.

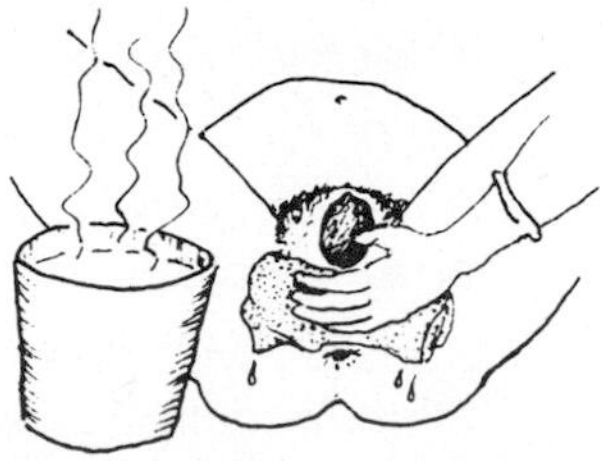

If a tear does happen, someone who knows how should carefully sew it shut after the placenta comes out (see p. 86 and 381).

CARE OF THE NEWBORN BABY

The Cord

To prevent the freshly cut cord from becoming infected, it should be kept **clean** and **dry.** The drier it is, the sooner it will fall off and the navel will heal. For this reason, it is better **not** to use a belly band, or if one is used, to keep it very loose (see p. 184 and 263).

The Eyes

To protect a newborn baby's eyes from dangerous conjunctivitis, put a drop of 1% silver nitrate, or a little tetracycline or erythromycin eye ointment, in each eye as soon as he is born (p. 221 and 365). This is especially important if either parent has ever had signs of gonorrhea or chlamydia (p. 236).

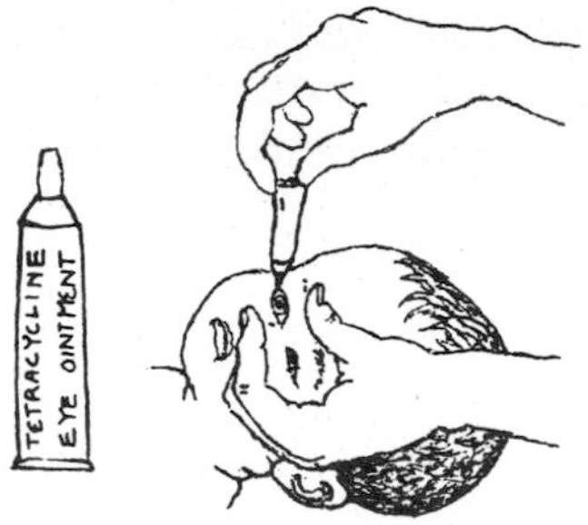

Keeping the Baby Warm—But Not Too Warm

Protect the baby from cold, but also from too much heat. Dress him as warmly as you feel like dressing yourself.

IN COLD WEATHER

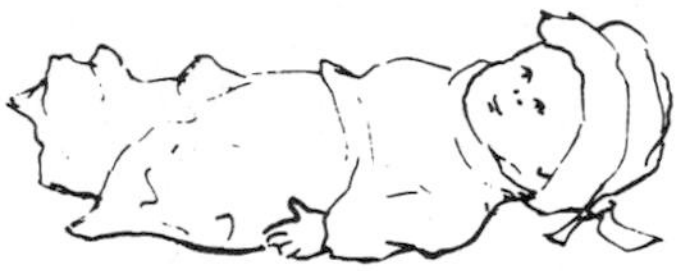

WRAP THE BABY WELL.

BUT IN HOT WEATHER (OR WHEN THE BABY HAS A FEVER)

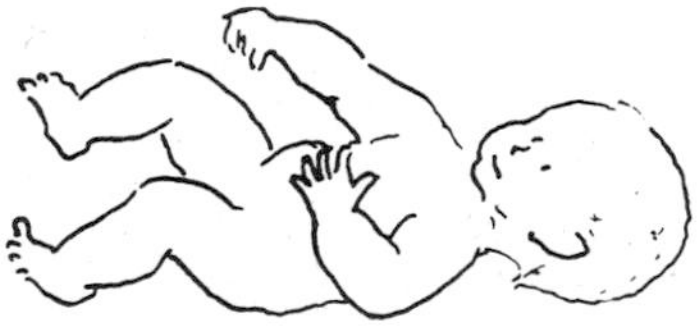

LEAVE HIM NAKED.

To keep a baby just warm enough, keep him close to his mother's body. This is especially important for a baby that is born early or very small. See 'Special Care for Small, Early, and Underweight Babies', p. 405.

Cleanliness

It is important to follow the Guidelines of Cleanliness as discussed in Chapter 12. Take special care with the following:

- Change the baby's diapers (nappy) or bedding each time he wets or dirties them. If the skin gets red, change the diaper more often—or better, leave it off! (See p. 215.)
- After the cord drops off, bathe the baby daily with mild soap and warm water.
- If there are flies or mosquitos, cover the baby's crib with mosquito netting or a thin cloth.
- Persons with open sores, colds, sore throat, tuberculosis, or other infectious illnesses should not touch or go near the newborn baby or the woman while she is giving birth.
- Keep the baby in a clean place away from smoke and dust.

Feeding

(Also see "The Best Diet for Small Children," p. 120.)

Breast milk is by far the best food for a baby. Babies who nurse on breast milk are healthier, grow stronger, and are less likely to die. This is why:

- Breast milk has a better balance of what the baby needs than does any other milk, whether fresh, canned, or powdered.
- Breast milk is clean. When other foods are given, especially by bottle feeding, it is very hard to keep things clean enough to prevent the baby from getting diarrhea and other sicknesses.
- The temperature of breast milk is always right.
- Breast milk has things in it (antibodies) that help protect the baby against certain illnesses, such as diarrhea, measles, and polio.

The mother should give her breast to the baby as soon as he is born. For the first few days the mother's breasts usually produce very little milk. This is normal. She should continue to **nurse her baby often**—at least every two hours. The baby's sucking will help her produce more milk.

If the baby seems healthy, gains weight, and wets her diaper (nappy) regularly, the mother is producing enough milk.

It is best for the baby if the mother gives him **only breast milk** for the first 4 to 6 months. After that, she should continue to breast feed her baby, but should begin to give him other nourishing foods also (see p. 122).

HOW A MOTHER CAN PRODUCE MORE BREAST MILK:

She should . . .

- drink plenty of liquids,
- eat as well as possible, especially milk, milk products, and body-building foods (see p. 110),
- get plenty of sleep and avoid getting very tired or upset,
- nurse her baby more often—at least every 2 hours.

BOTTLE-FED BABIES ARE MORE LIKELY TO GET SICK AND DIE.

BREAST-FED BABIES ARE HEALTHIER.

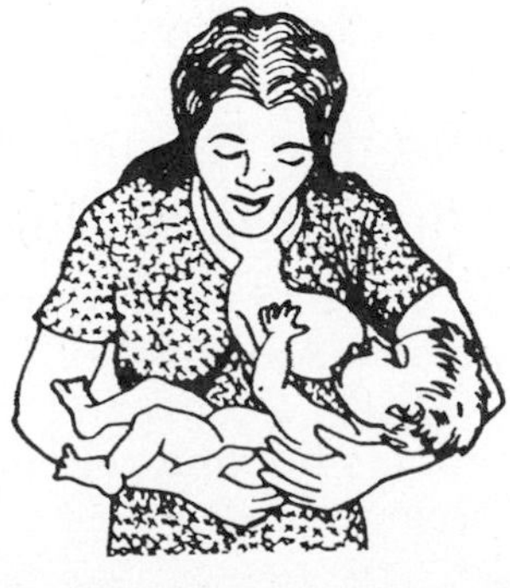

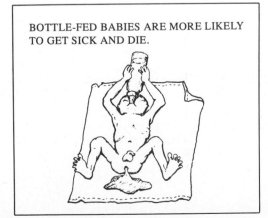

Care in Giving Medicines to the Newborn

Many medicines are dangerous for the newborn. Use only medicines you are sure are recommended for the newborn and use them only when they are absolutely necessary. Be sure you know the right dose and do not give too much. Chloramphenicol is especially dangerous to the newborn . . . and even more dangerous if the baby is premature or underweight (less than 2 kilograms).

ILLNESSES OF THE NEWBORN

It is very important to notice any problem or illness a baby may have—and to act quickly.

Diseases that take days or weeks to kill adults can kill a baby in a matter of hours.

Problems the Baby is Born with (Also see p. 316)

These may result from something that went wrong with the development of the baby in the womb or from damage to the baby while he was being born. Examine the baby carefully immediately after birth. If he shows any of the following signs, something is probably seriously wrong with him:

- If he does not breathe as soon as he is born.
- If his pulse cannot be felt or heard, or is less than 100 per minute.
- If his face and body are white, blue, or yellow after he has begun breathing.
- If his arms and legs are floppy—he does not move them by himself or when you pinch them.
- If he grunts or has difficulty breathing after the first 15 minutes.

Some of these problems may be caused by brain damage at birth. They are almost never caused by infection (unless the water broke more than 24 hours before birth). Common medicines probably will not help. Keep the baby warm, but not too warm (see p. 270). Try to get medical help.

If the newborn baby vomits or shits blood, or develops many bruises, she may need vitamin K (see p. 394).

If the baby does not urinate or have a bowel movement in the first 2 days, also seek medical help.

Problems that Result after the Baby is Born (in the first days or weeks)

1. **Pus or a bad smell from the navel (cord)** is a dangerous sign. Watch for early signs of tetanus (p. 182) or bacterial infection of the blood (p. 275). Soak the cord in alcohol and leave it open to the air. **If the skin around the cord becomes hot and red,** treat with ampicillin (p. 353) or with penicillin and streptomycin (p. 354).

2. Either **low temperature** (below 35°) or **high fever** can be a sign of infection. *High fever (above 39°) is dangerous for the newborn.* Take off all clothing and sponge the baby with cool (not cold) water as shown on page 76. Also look for signs of dehydration (see p. 151). If you find these signs, give the baby breast milk and also Rehydration Drink (p. 152).

3. **Fits (convulsions,** see p. 178). If the baby also has fever, treat it as just described. Be sure to check for dehydration. Fits that begin the day of birth could be caused by brain damage at birth. If fits begin several days later, look carefully for signs of tetanus (p. 182) or meningitis (p. 185).

4. **The baby does not gain weight.** During the first days of life, most babies lose a little weight. This is normal. After the first week, a healthy baby should gain about 200 gm. a week. By two weeks the healthy baby should weigh as much as he did at birth. If he does not gain weight, or loses weight, something is wrong. Did the baby seem healthy at birth? Does he feed well? Examine the baby carefully for signs of infection or other problems. If you cannot find out the cause of the problem and correct it, get medical help.

5. **Vomiting.** When healthy babies burp (or bring up air they have swallowed while feeding), sometimes a little milk comes up too. This is normal. Help the baby bring up air after feeding by holding him against your shoulder and patting his back gently, like this.

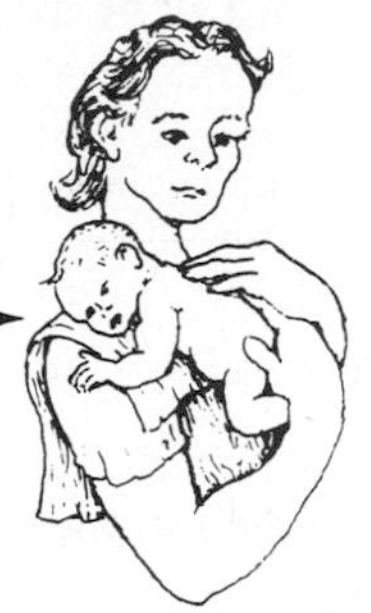

BURP YOUR BABY AFTER FEEDING.

If a baby vomits when you lay him down after nursing, try sitting him upright for a while after each feeding.

A baby who vomits violently, or so much and so often that he begins to lose weight or become dehydrated, is ill. If the baby also has diarrhea, he probably has a gut infection (p. 157). Bacterial infection of the blood (see the next pages), meningitis (p. 185), and other infections may also cause vomiting.

If the vomit is yellow or green, there may be a gut obstruction (p. 94), especially if the belly is very swollen or the baby has not been having bowel movements. Take the baby to a health center **at once.**

6. **The baby stops sucking well.** If more than 4 hours pass and the baby still will not nurse, this is a danger sign—especially if the baby seems very sleepy or ill, or if he cries or moves differently from normal. Many illnesses can cause these signs, but the most common and dangerous causes in the first 2 weeks of life are a **bacterial infection of the blood** (see next 2 pages) and **tetanus** (p. 182).

A baby who stops nursing during the second to fifth day of life may have a bacterial infection of the blood.

A baby who stops nursing during the fifth to fifteenth day may have tetanus.

If a Baby Stops Sucking Well or Seems Ill

Examine him carefully and completely as described in Chapter 3. Be sure to check the following:

- Notice if the baby has **difficulty breathing.** If the nose is stuffed up, suck it out as shown on page 164. Fast breathing (50 or more breaths a minute), blue color, grunting, and sucking in of the skin between the ribs with each breath are signs of pneumonia (p. 171). Small babies with pneumonia often do not cough; sometimes none of the common signs are present. If you suspect pneumonia, treat as for a bacterial infection of the blood (see the next page).

- Look at the baby's **skin color.**

  If the lips and face are blue, consider pneumonia (or a heart defect or other problem the baby was born with).

  If the face and whites of the eyes begin to get yellow (jaundiced) in the first day of life or after the fifth day, this is serious. Get medical help. Some yellow color between the second and fifth day of life is usually not serious. Give plenty of breast milk—by spoon if necessary. Take off all the baby's clothes and put him in bright light near a window (but not direct sunlight).

- Feel the **soft spot on top of the head** (fontanel). See p. 9.

If the soft spot is SUNKEN, the baby may be DEHYDRATED.

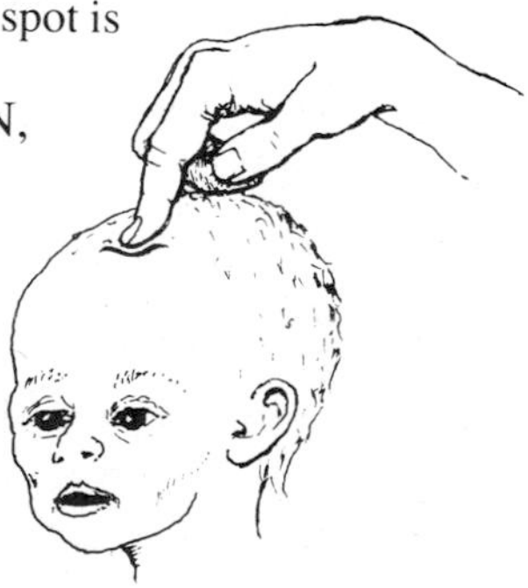

If the soft spot is SWOLLEN, the baby may have MENINGITIS.

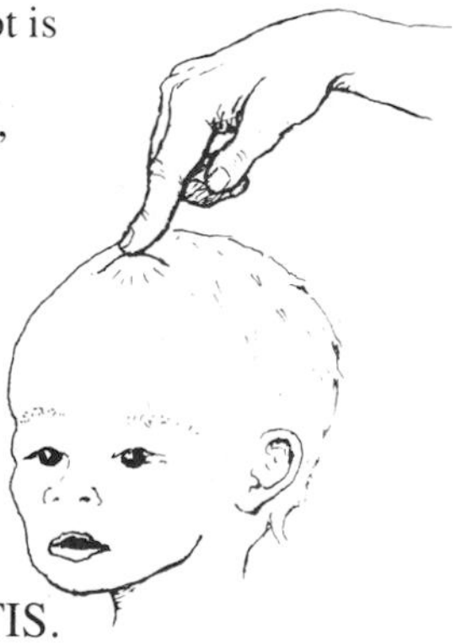

IMPORTANT: If a baby has meningitis and dehydration at the same time, the soft spot may feel normal. **Be sure to check for other signs** of both dehydration (see p. 151) and meningitis (see p. 185).

- **Watch the baby's movements and expression on his face.**

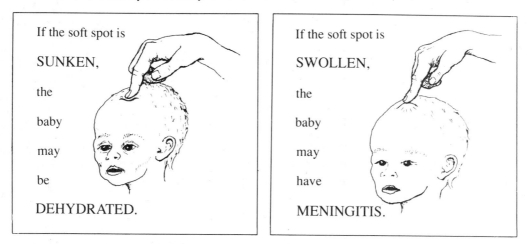

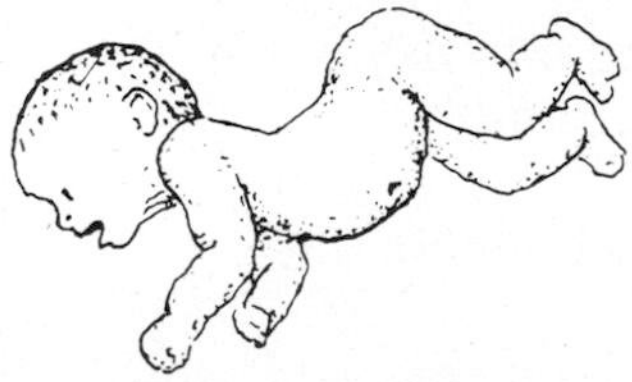

Stiffness of the body and/or strange movements may be signs of tetanus, meningitis, or brain damage from birth or fever. If, when the baby is touched or moved, the muscles of his face and body suddenly tighten, this could be tetanus. See if his jaw will open and check his knee reflexes (p. 183).

If the baby's eyes roll back or flutter when he makes sudden or violent movements, he probably does **not** have tetanus. Such fits **may** be caused by meningitis, but dehydration and high fever are more common causes. Can you put the baby's head between his knees? If the baby is too stiff for this or cries out in pain, it is probably meningitis (see p. 185).

- Look for signs of a bacterial infection in the blood.

Bacterial Infection in the Blood (Septicemia)

Newborn babies cannot fight infections well. Therefore, bacteria that enter the baby's skin or cord at the time of birth often get into the blood and spread through his whole body. Since this takes a day or two, septicemia is most common after the second day of life.

Signs:

Signs of infection in newborn babies are different from those in older children. In the baby, almost any sign could be caused by a serious infection in the blood. Possible signs are:

- does not suck well
- seems very sleepy
- very pale (anemic)
- vomiting or diarrhea
- fever or low temperature (below 35°)
- swollen belly
- yellow skin (jaundice)
- fits (convulsions)
- times when the baby turns blue

Each of these signs may be caused by something other than septicemia, **but if the baby has several of these signs at once, septicemia is likely.**

Newborn babies do not always have a fever when they have a serious infection. The temperature may be high, low, or normal.

Treatment when you suspect septicemia in the newborn:

- ♦ Inject 125 mg. of ampicillin (p. 353) 3 times a day. Or inject 150 mg. (250,000 units) of crystalline penicillin (p. 353) 3 times a day.
- ♦ If possible, also inject kanamycin (p. 359) or streptomycin (p. 354): Give 25 mg. of kanamycin **2 times a day;** or give 20 mg. of streptomycin for each kilogram the baby weighs (60 mg. for a 3 kilogram baby) **once a day.** Be careful not to give too much of either of these medicines!
- ♦ Be sure the baby has enough liquids. Spoon feed breast milk and Rehydration Drink, if necessary (see p. 152).
- ♦ Try to get medical help.

Infections in newborn babies are sometimes hard to recognize. Often there is no fever. If possible, get medical help. If not, treat with ampicillin as described above. Ampicillin is one of the safest and most useful antibiotics for babies.

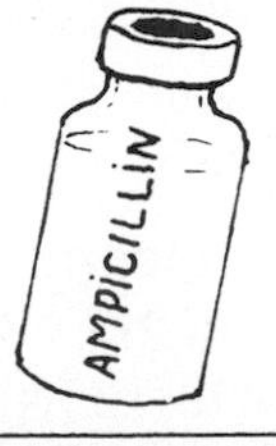

THE MOTHER'S HEALTH AFTER CHILDBIRTH

Diet and Cleanliness

As was explained in Chapter 11, after she gives birth to a baby, **the mother can and should eat every kind of nutritious food she can get.** She does not need to avoid any kind of food. Foods that are especially good for her are milk, cheese, chicken, eggs, meat, fish, fruits, vegetables, grains, beans, groundnuts, etc. If all she has is corn and beans, she should eat them both together at each meal. Milk and other dairy products help the mother make plenty of milk for her baby.

The mother can and should bathe in the first few days after giving birth. In the first week, it is better if she bathes with a wet towel and does not go into the water. **Bathing is not harmful following childbirth.** In fact, women who let many days go by without bathing may get infections that will make their skin unhealthy and their babies sick.

During the days and weeks following childbirth, the mother should:

eat nutritious foods and **bathe regularly.**

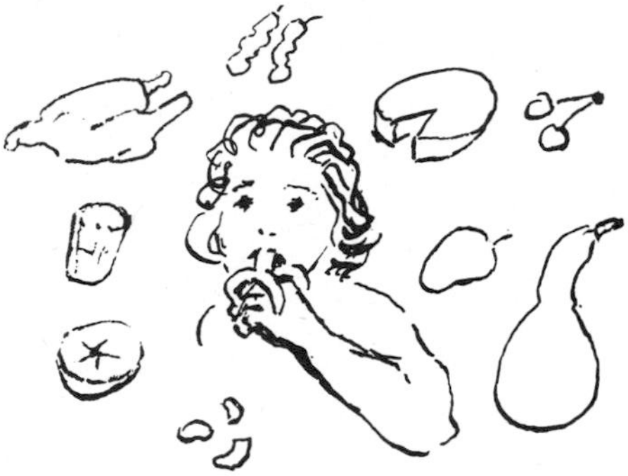

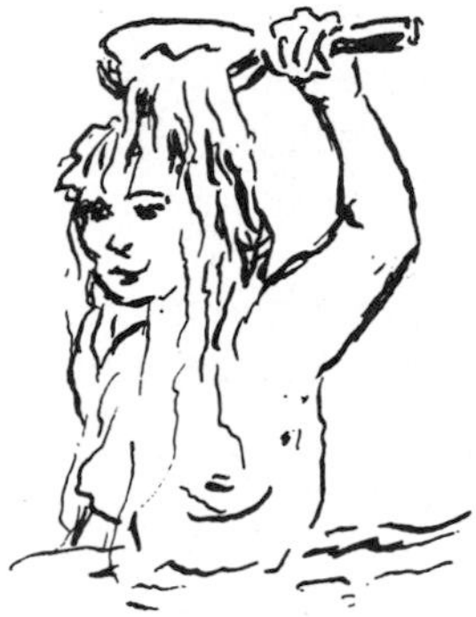

Childbirth Fever (Infection after Giving Birth)

Sometimes a mother develops fever and infection after childbirth, often because the midwife was not careful enough to keep everything very clean or because she put her hand inside the mother.

The signs of childbirth fever are: Chills or fever, headache or low back pain, sometimes pain in the belly, and a foul-smelling or bloody discharge from the vagina.

Treatment:

Give penicillin: injections of 500,000 units of procaine penicillin twice a day, or 2 pills of 400,000 units 4 times a day for a week (see p. 351). Ampicillin, co-trimoxazole, or tetracycline may be used instead.

Childbirth fever can be very dangerous. If the mother does not get well soon, get medical help. Very severe infections may need treatment with a stronger antibiotic (chloramphenicol, gentamicin, kanamycin, or a cephalosporin) in addition to high doses of penicillin or ampicillin.

BREAST FEEDING—AND CARE OF THE BREASTS

Taking good care of the breasts is important for the health of both the mother and her baby. The baby should begin to breast feed soon after it is born. A baby may want to breast feed right away or just lick the breast and be held. Encourage the baby to suck because it will help the milk to start flowing. This will also help the mother's womb to contract and the afterbirth to come out sooner. The mother's first milk is a thick yellow liquid (called colostrum). The first milk has everything a new baby needs to prevent infection and is rich in protein. **The first milk is very good for the baby, so...**

> **BEGIN BREAST FEEDING EARLY**
> **Put the baby to the mother's breast as soon as possible.**

Normally, the breasts make as much milk as the baby needs. If the baby empties them, they begin to make more. If the baby does not empty them, soon they make less. When a baby gets sick and stops sucking, after a few days the mother's breasts stop making milk. So when the baby can suck again, and needs a full amount of milk, there may not be enough. For this reason,

> **When a baby is sick and unable to take much milk,**
> **it is important that the mother keep producing lots of milk**
> **by milking her breasts with her hands.**

TO MILK THE BREASTS BY HAND

Take hold of the breast way back, like this,

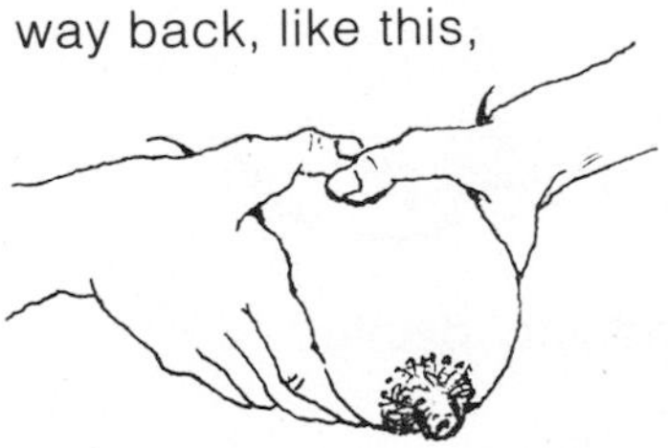

then move your hands forward, squeezing.

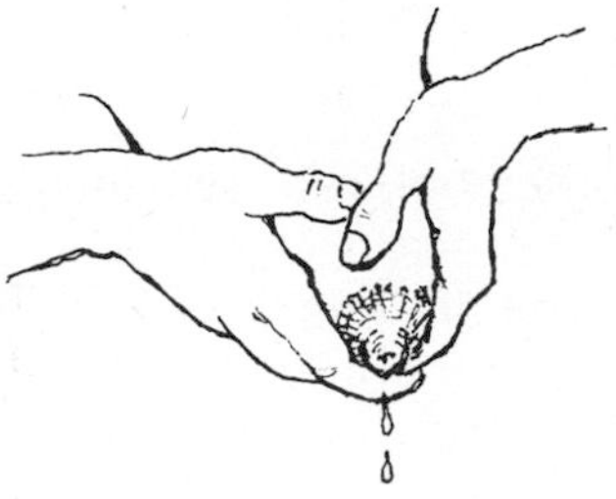

To squeeze the milk out, press behind the nipple .

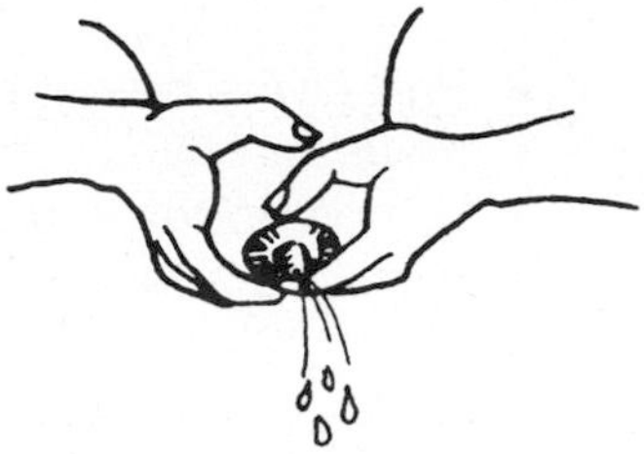

Another reason it is important to milk the breasts if the baby stops sucking is that this keeps the breasts from getting too full. When they are too full, they are painful. A breast that is painfully full is more likely to develop an abscess. Also, the baby may have trouble sucking when the breast is very full.

If your baby is too weak to suck, squeeze milk out of your breast by hand and give it to the baby by spoon or dropper.

Regular bathing will help to keep your breasts clean. It is not necessary to clean your breasts and nipples each time you breast feed your baby. Do **not** use soap to clean your breasts, as this may cause cracking of the skin, sore nipples, and infection.

Sore or Cracked Nipples

Sore or cracked nipples develop when the baby sucks only the nipple instead of taking the nipple and part of the breast when she is breast feeding.

Treatment:

It is important to keep breast feeding the baby even if it hurts. To avoid sore nipples, breast feed often, for as long as the baby wants to suck, and be sure the baby is taking as much of the breast into her mouth as she can. It also helps to change the baby's position each time she nurses.

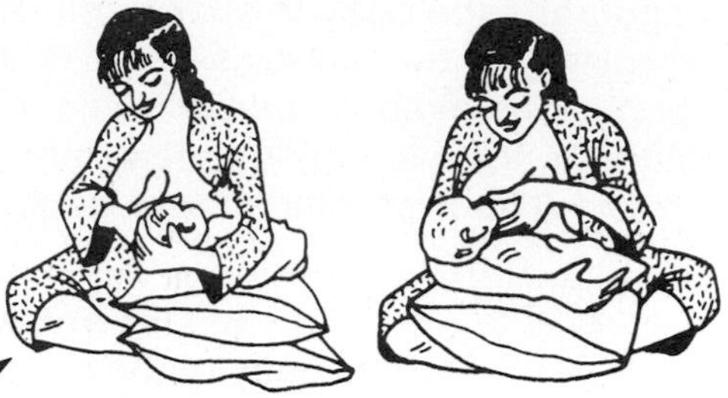

If only one nipple is sore, let the baby suck on the other side first, then let the baby suck from the sore nipple. After the baby is finished, squeeze out a little milk and rub the milk over the sore nipple. Let the milk dry before covering the nipple. The milk will help the nipple heal. If the nipple oozes a lot of blood or pus, milk the breast by hand until the nipple is healed.

Painful Breasts

Pain in the breast can be caused by a sore nipple or breasts that get very full and hard. The pain will often go away in a day or two if the baby breast feeds frequently and the mother rests in bed and drinks lots of liquids. Usually, antibiotics are not needed, but see the next section.

Breast Infection (Mastitis) and Abscess

Painful breasts and sore or cracked nipples can lead to an infection or abscess (pocket of pus).

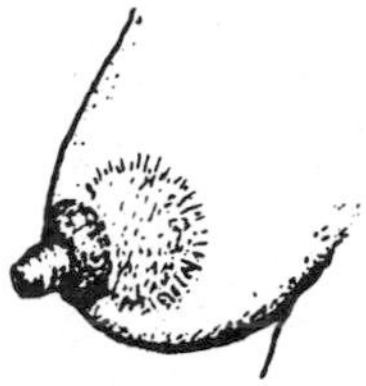

Signs

- Part of the breast becomes hot, red, swollen, and very painful.
- Fever or chills.
- Lymph nodes in the armpit are often sore and swollen.
- A severe abscess sometimes bursts and drains pus.

Treatment

- Keep breast feeding frequently, giving the baby the infected breast first, or milk the breast by hand, whichever is less painful.
- Rest and drink lots of liquids.
- Use hot compresses on the sore breast for 15 minutes before each feeding. Use cold compresses on the sore breast between feedings to reduce pain.
- Gently massage the sore breast while the baby is nursing.
- Take acetaminophen (p. 380) for pain.
- Use an antibiotic. Dicloxacillin is the best antibiotic to use (p. 351). Take 500 mg. by mouth, 4 times each day, for a full 10 days. Penicillin (p. 351), ampicillin (p.353) or erythromycin (p. 355) can also be used.

Prevention

- Keep the nipples from cracking (see above) and don't let the breasts get overfull.

Different kinds of breast lumps:

A painful, hot lump in the breast of a nursing mother is probably a breast abscess (infection). A painless breast lump may be cancer, or a *cyst*.

Breast Cancer

Cancer of the breast is fairly common in women, and is always dangerous. Successful treatment depends on spotting the first sign of possible cancer and getting medical care soon. Surgery is usually necessary.

Signs of breast cancer:

- The woman may notice a lump, often in this part of the breast.
- Or the breast may have an abnormal dent or dimple—or many tiny pits like the skin of an orange.
- Often there are large but painless lymph nodes in the armpit.
- The lump grows slowly.
- At first it usually does not hurt or get hot. Later it may hurt.

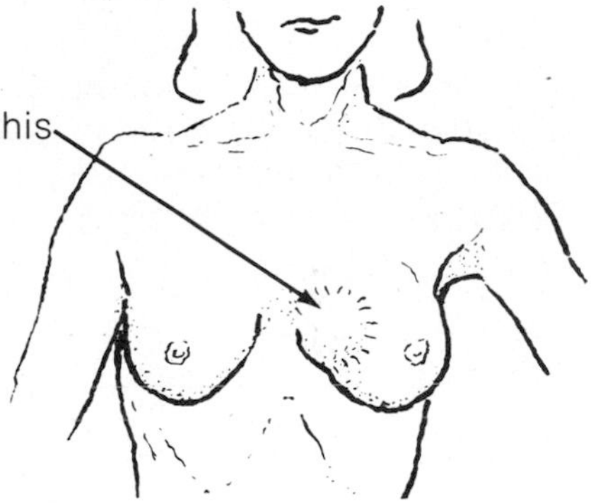

SELF-EXAMINATION OF THE BREASTS

Every woman should learn how to examine her own breasts for possible signs of cancer. She should do it once a month, preferably on the 10th day after her menstrual period started.

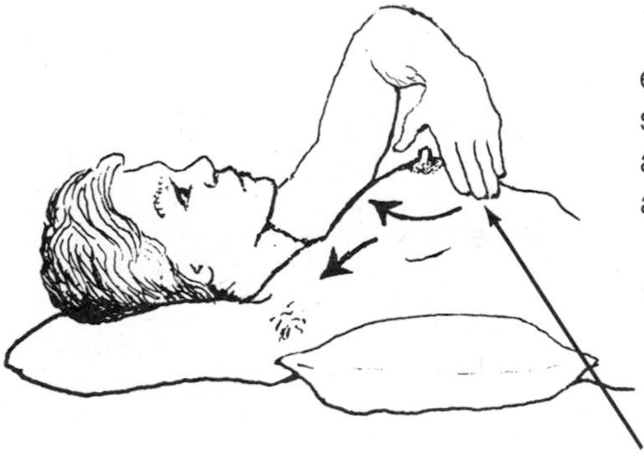

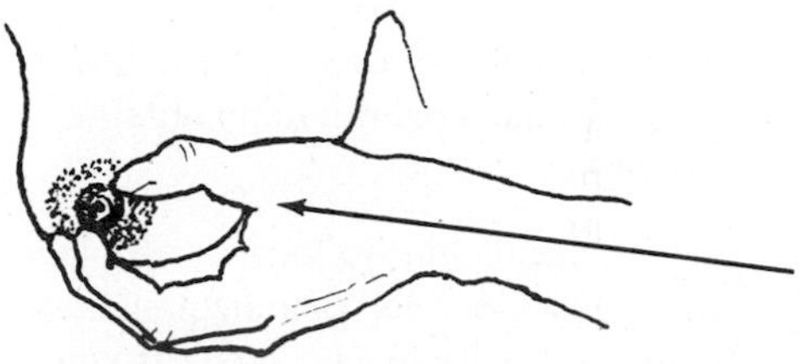

- Look at your breasts carefully for any new difference between the two in size or shape. Try to notice any of the above signs.
- While lying with a pillow or folded blanket under your back, feel your breasts with the flat of your fingers. Press your breast and roll it beneath your finger tips. Start near the nipple and go around the breast and up into the armpit.
- Then squeeze your nipples and check whether blood or a *discharge* comes out.

If you find a lump or any other abnormal sign, get medical advice. Many lumps are not cancer, but it is important to find out early.

LUMPS OR GROWTHS IN THE LOWER PART OF THE BELLY

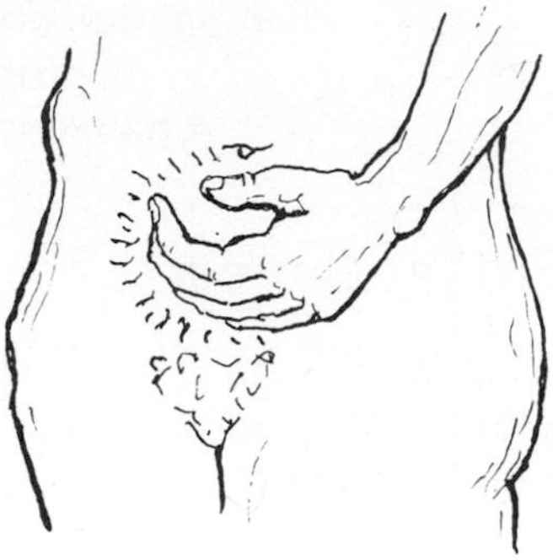

The most common lump is, of course, caused by the normal development of a baby. Abnormal lumps or masses may be caused by:

- a *cyst* or watery swelling in one of the ovaries
- by a baby that has accidentally begun to develop outside of the womb (ectopic pregnancy), or
- cancer

All 3 of these conditions are usually painless or mildly uncomfortable at first, and become very painful later. All require medical attention—usually surgery. If you find any unusual, gradually growing lump, seek medical advice.

Cancer of the Womb

Cancer of the uterus (womb), cervix (neck of the womb), or ovaries is most common in women over 40. The first sign may be *anemia* or unexplained bleeding. Later, an uncomfortable or painful lump in the belly may be noticed.

There is a special test called a Pap smear (Papanicolaou) to find cancer of the cervix when it is just beginning. Where it is available, all women over 20 should try to get one of these tests once a year.

At the first suspicion of cancer, seek medical help.

Home remedies are not likely to help.

Out-of-place or *Ectopic* Pregnancy

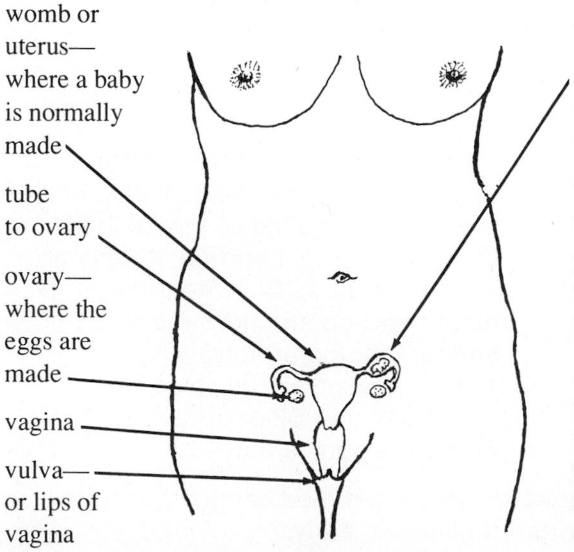

Sometimes a baby begins to form outside the womb, in one of the tubes that comes from the ovaries.

There may be abnormal menstrual bleeding together with signs of pregnancy—also severe cramps low in the belly and a painful lump **outside** the womb.

A baby that begins to form out of place usually cannot live. Ectopic pregnancy requires surgery in a hospital. **If you suspect this problem, seek medical advice soon, as dangerous bleeding could start any time.**

MISCARRIAGE (SPONTANEOUS ABORTION)

A miscarriage is the loss of the unborn baby. Miscarriages are most frequent in the first 3 months of pregnancy. Usually the baby is imperfectly formed, and this is nature's way of taking care of the problem.

Most women have one or more miscarriages in their lifetime. Many times they do not realize that they are having a miscarriage. They may think their period was missed or delayed, and then came back in a strange way, with big blood clots. A woman should learn to know when she is having a miscarriage, because it could be dangerous.

The embryo of a miscarriage may be no longer than 1 or 2 centimeters.

30 days

60 days

A woman who has heavy bleeding after she has missed one or more periods probably is having a miscarriage.

A miscarriage is like a birth in that the embryo (the beginning of the baby) and the placenta (afterbirth) must both come out. Heavy bleeding with big blood clots and painful cramps often continues until both are completely out.

Treatment:

The woman should rest and take aspirin (p. 379), ibuprofen (p. 380), or codeine (p. 384) for pain.

If heavy bleeding continues for many days:

- Get medical help. A simple operation may be needed to clean out the womb (dilatation and curettage, or D and C, or suction).
- Stay in bed until the heavy bleeding stops.
- If the bleeding is extreme, follow the instructions on page 266.
- If fever or other signs of infection develop, treat as for **Childbirth Fever** (see p. 276).
- A woman may continue to bleed a little for several days after the miscarriage. It will be similar to her menstrual flow (period).
- She should not *douche* or have sex for at least 2 weeks after the miscarriage, or until the bleeding stops.
- If she is using an IUD and has a miscarriage, serious infection may occur. **Seek medical help fast,** have the IUD removed, and give antibiotics.

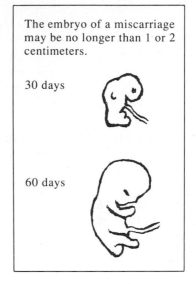

HIGH RISK MOTHERS AND BABIES

A note to midwives or health workers or anyone who cares:

Some women are more likely to have difficult births and problems following birth, and their babies are more likely to be underweight and sick. Often these are mothers who are single, homeless, poorly nourished, very young, mentally slow, or who already have malnourished or sickly children.

Often if a midwife, health worker, or someone else takes special interest in these mothers, and helps them find ways to get the food, care, and companionship they need, it can make a great difference in the well-being of both the mothers and their babies.

Do not wait for those in need to come to you. Go to them.

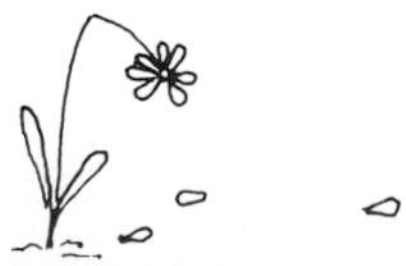

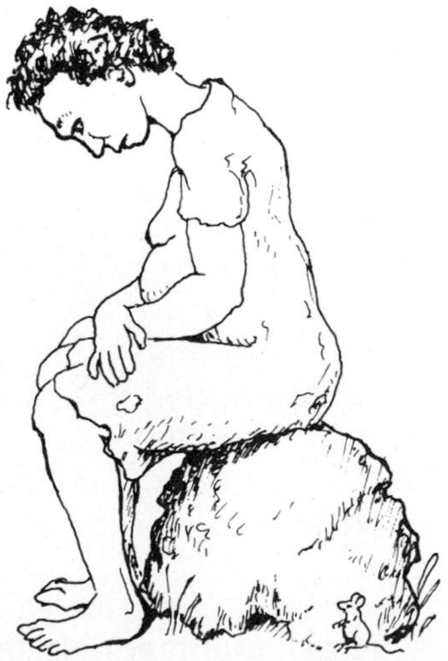

CHAPTER

20

Family Planning— Having the Number of Children You Want

BOTH THESE FAMILIES LIVE IN POOR COMMUNITIES:

This family lives where wealth is distributed unfairly.

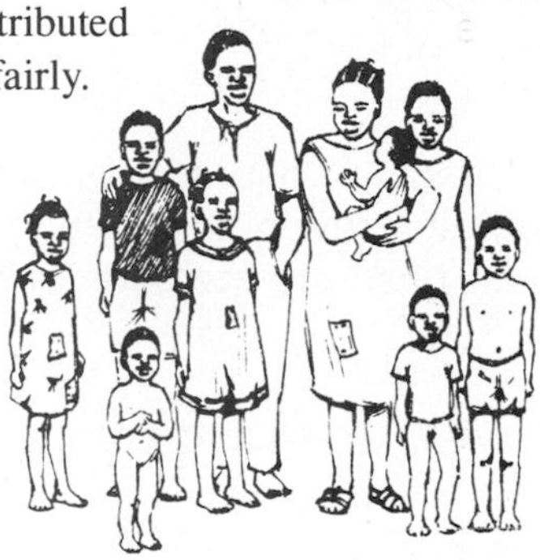

This family lives where resources are distributed fairly.

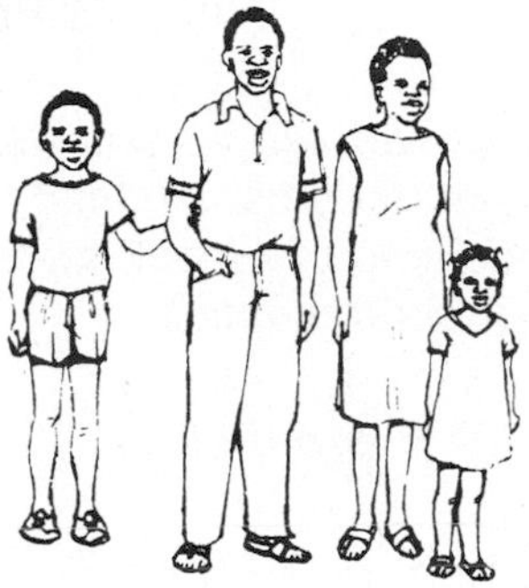

Some mothers and fathers want a lot of children—especially in countries where poor people are denied a fair share of land, resources, and social benefits. This is because children help with work and provide care for their parents in old age. In such areas, having just a few children may be a privilege only wealthier people can afford.

The situation is different in poor countries where resources and benefits are fairly distributed. Where employment, housing, and health care are guaranteed and where women have equal opportunities for education and jobs, people usually choose to have smaller families. This is in part because they do not need to depend on their children for economic security.

But in any society, it helps if a family has control over how many children they have, and when they have them.

When a mother has child after child, without much space between, she often becomes weak. Her babies are more likely to die (see p. 271). Also, after many pregnancies the danger is greater that she will die in childbirth, leaving many motherless children. Therefore many couples now choose to allow two or more years to pass between pregnancies, and avoid having a very large number of children.

If a man and woman have a lot of children, when the children grow up there may not be enough land for all of them to grow the food their families need. Children may begin to die of hunger. This is already happening in many areas.

Although most, if not all, hunger in the world today could be prevented if land and wealth were distributed fairly, the growing number of people is part of the problem. But the solution is not to force the poor to limit the number of children they have. Instead, the challenge is for societies to provide enough security so that the poor can afford to have few children.

FAMILY PLANNING

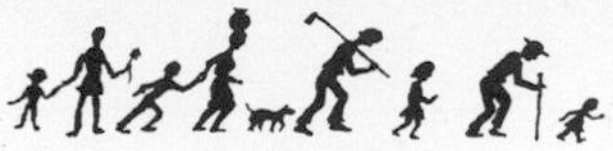

Different parents have different reasons for wanting to limit the size of their family. Some young parents may decide to delay having any children until they have worked and saved enough so that they can afford to care for them well. Some parents may decide that a small number of children is enough, and they never want more. Others may want to space their children several years apart, so that both the children and their mother will be healthier. Some parents may feel they are too old to have more children.

Family planning is having the number of children you want, when you want them.

When a man and woman decide when they want to have children, and when they do not, they can choose one of several methods to prevent the woman from becoming pregnant, for as long as she wishes. These are methods of ***birth control*** or ***contraception.***

Couples who want children but are not able to have them should see page 244.

IS FAMILY PLANNING GOOD - AND IS IT SAFE?

1. Is it good?

In some parts of the world there has been a lot of discussion about whether different forms of family planning are good or are safe. Some religions have been against any form of family planning except trying not to have sex. But an increasing number of religious leaders are realizing how important it is to the health and well-being of families and communities that people be able to use easier and surer methods of family planning.

Also, in many places women who get pregnant when they do not want a child will go for an ***abortion,*** to have the pregnancy removed. Where these abortions are legal, they can be done in health centers under sanitary conditions, and they are not usually dangerous to the woman. But where abortions are not permitted, many women get abortions illegally and secretly, often in dirty conditions and performed by unskilled persons. Thousands of women die from such abortions. If women are given the chance to use birth control methods, and information to use them wisely, many abortions, legal and illegal, would not be necessary. Much needless suffering and death could be prevented. (See Complications from Abortion, pages 414 and 415.)

Some people feel that much of the push for family planning comes from rich countries or persons who want to keep their control over the poor by controlling their numbers. The rich and powerful find it hard to accept that the way they manage the earth's land and resources strongly contributes to world hunger. They see only the growing numbers of people. In some countries professionals sterilize poor women by force or experiment on them with new or unsafe methods. For all these reasons social reformers and spokespersons for the poor often protest against family planning.

This is unfortunate. The object of attack should not be family planning, but rather its misuse. The attack should be against social injustice and the unfair distribution of land and wealth, and for equal rights for women. If used well, family planning can in fact help poor families, men and women, to gain strength to work for their basic human rights. But the decisions and responsibility for family planning must be in the hands of the people themselves.

Decide for yourself how you want to plan your family. Do not let anyone else decide for you.

2. Is it safe?

Whether or not different forms of birth control are safe has been much discussed. Often those who are against birth control for religious or political reasons try to scare women by talking about the risks. Some methods do have certain risks. However, the important thing all women should realize is that **family planning is safer than pregnancy,** especially for women less than 20 or more than 35 years old, and for women who have had many children.

The risk of serious illness or death resulting from pregnancy is many times greater than the risks involved in using any of the common methods of family planning.

There is much talk about the risks of taking birth control pills. But the risks with pregnancy are many times greater. The pill works so well in preventing pregnancy that for most women it is safer—in terms of protecting their lives—than any of the other 'less risky' but less effective methods.

CHOOSING A METHOD OF FAMILY PLANNING

On the following pages, several methods of family planning are described. Some work better for some people than others. Study these pages, and talk with your midwife, health worker, or doctor about what methods are available and are likely to work best for you. Differences in **effectiveness, safety, convenience, availability,** and **cost** should be considered. Husbands and wives should decide together, and share the responsibility.

AVERAGE EFFECTIVENESS OF DIFFERENT FORMS OF FAMILY PLANNING

Of each 20 women using this method . . .	on the average this many are likely to get pregnant in spite of the method . . .		and this many must (or should) stop the method because of problems.
PILL	1		1
CONDOM	2		
DIAPHRAGM	3		1
FOAM	4		
I. U. D.	1		5 + part
PULLING OUT	5		
STERILIZATION			*
INJECTIONS			2
IMPLANTS	part		1
SPONGE (HOME METHOD)	8		3
RHYTHM	7	COMBINED 5	
MUCUS	6		

* With sterilization, problems occasionally result from surgery but the method is permanent.

BIRTH CONTROL PILLS (ORAL CONTRACEPTIVES)

Birth control pills are made of chemicals (hormones) that normally occur in a woman's body. When taken correctly, the 'pill' is one of the most effective methods for avoiding pregnancy. However, certain women should not take birth control pills if they can use another method (see p. 288). Birth control pills do not prevent AIDS or any other sexually transmitted diseases. To prevent these diseases, use a condom (p. 290). If possible, birth control pills should be given by health workers, midwives, or other persons trained in their use.

The pills usually come in packets of 21 or 28 tablets. The packets of 21 are often less expensive, and of these, some brands are cheaper than others. The amount of medicine differs in different brands. To pick the kind that is right for you, see the GREEN PAGES, pages 394 and 395.

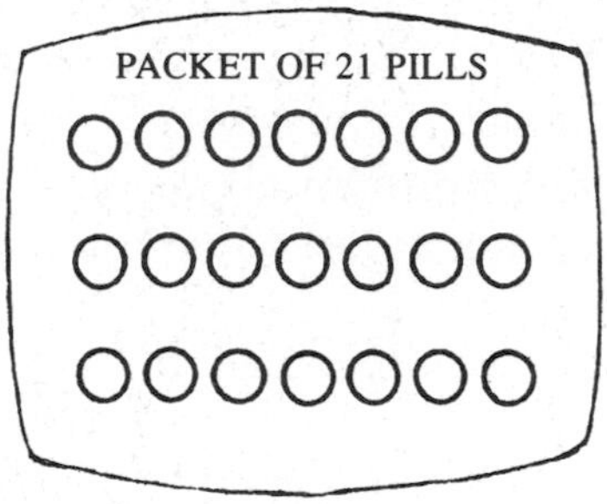

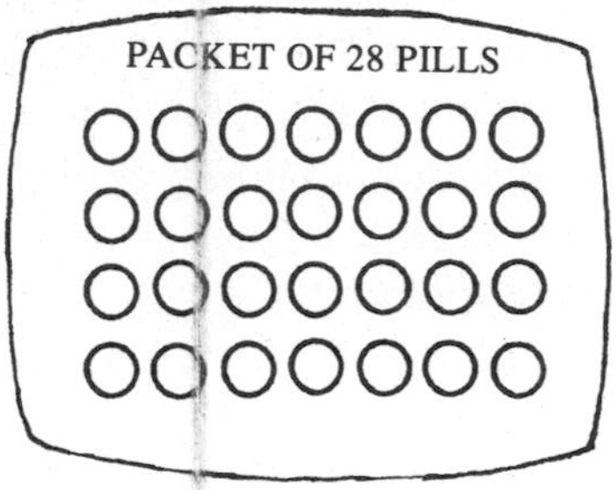

How to take the pills—packet of 21:

Take the first pill on the fifth day from the beginning of your period, counting the first day of the period as day 1. Then take 1 pill every day until the packet is finished (21 days). **Take your pills at the same time each day.**

After finishing the packet, wait 7 days before taking any more pills. Then begin another packet, 1 pill each day.

This way, you will take the pills for 3 weeks out of each month, then go 1 week without taking any. Normally, the menstrual period will come during the week when the pill is not taken. Even if the period does not come, start the new packet 7 days after finishing the last one.

If you do not want to get pregnant, it is important to take the pills as directed—1 every day. If you forget to take the pill one day, take it as soon as you realize this, or take 2 the next day.

Packet of 28 pills:

Take the first pill on the fifth day of the period, just as with the packets of 21. Take 1 a day. Seven of the pills will probably be a different size and color. Take these pills last (one a day) after the others have all been taken. The day after you finish the packet of 28, start another packet. Take 1 a day without ever missing a day, packet after packet, for as long as you want not to get pregnant.

No special diet must be followed when taking the pill. Even if you happen to get sick with a cold or another common illness while taking birth control pills, go right on taking them. If you stop taking the pills before the packet is used up, you may become pregnant.

Side effects:

Some women get a little morning sickness, swelling of the breasts, or other signs of pregnancy when they first start taking the pill. This is because the pill contains the same chemicals (hormones) that a woman's body puts into her blood when she is pregnant. These signs do not mean she is unhealthy or should stop taking the pill. They usually go away after the first 2 or 3 months. If the signs do not go away, she may need to change to a kind with a different amount of hormone. This is discussed in the GREEN PAGES (p. 394 and 395).

Most women bleed less than usual in their monthly period when they are taking the pill. This change is usually not important.

"Is it dangerous to take oral contraceptives?"

Like all medicines, birth control pills may cause serious problems in certain persons (see next pages), The most serious problems related to the pill are blood clots in the heart, lungs, or brain (see stroke, p. 327). This occurs most often in women over 35 who smoke tobacco. However, the chance of getting dangerous clots is higher when women get pregnant than when they take the pill. But for some women, both pregnancy and taking birth control pills have a higher risk. These women should use other methods of family planning.

A woman rarely becomes pregnant while taking the pill. But if this happens, **immediately stop taking the pill.** It can harm the developing baby.

Death related to taking the pill is rare. On the average, pregnancy and childbirth are 50 times more dangerous than taking the pill.

Of 15,000 women who become pregnant, this many are likely to die from problems of pregnancy or childbirth.

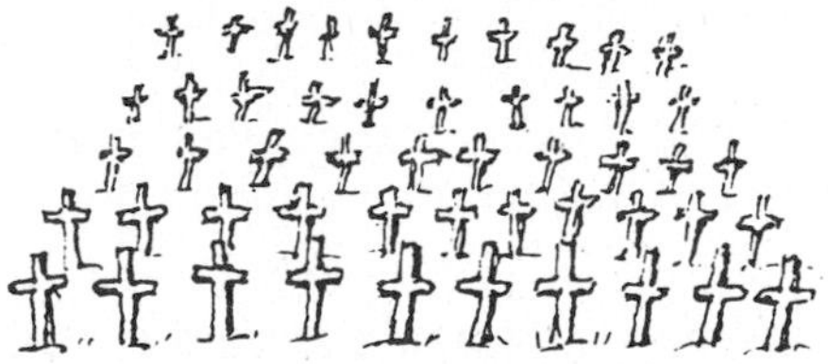

Of 15,000 women who take birth control pills, only 1 is likely to die from problems related to having taken the pills.

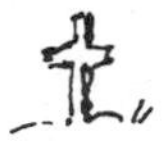

Conclusion:

IT IS MUCH SAFER TO TAKE THE PILL THAN TO BECOME PREGNANT.

EMERGENCY PILLS

If for whatever reason your family planning method was not used properly before sex, you can still avoid becoming pregnant by taking a larger-than-usual amount of some kinds of birth control pills, or special pills made for this purpose. But it only works if the pills are taken no later than 72 hours after having sex (see p. 396).

Who Should Not Take Birth Control Pills?

A woman who has any of the following signs should **not** take oral (or injected) contraceptives:

- A woman whose period is late, who thinks she might be pregnant.
- **Deep or steady pain in one leg or hip.** This may be caused by an inflamed vein (phlebitis or blood clot). Do not use birth control pills. (Women with **varicose veins** that are not inflamed can usually take birth control pills without problems. But they should stop taking them if the veins become inflamed.)

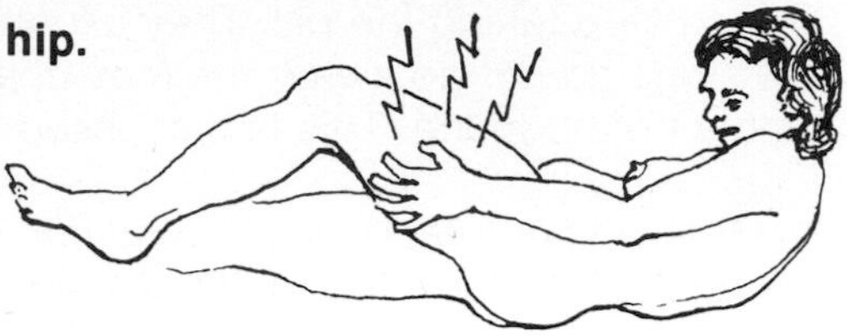

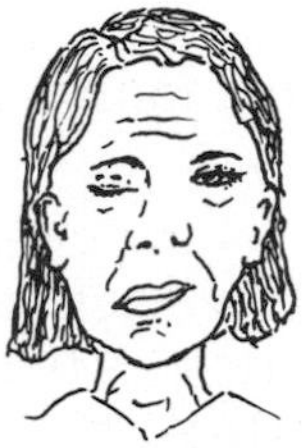

- **Stroke.** A woman who has had any signs of a stroke (p. 327) should not take the pill.

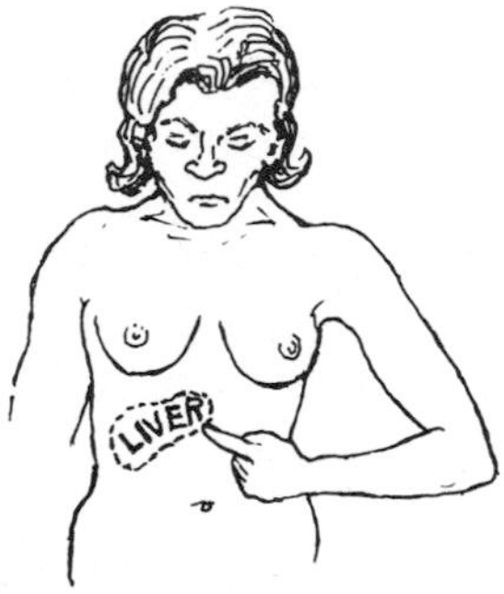

- **Hepatitis (p. 172), cirrhosis (p. 328), or other liver disease.** Women with these problems, or whose eyes had a yellow color during pregnancy, should not take the pill. It is better not to take oral contraceptives for one year after having hepatitis.
- **Cancer.** If you have had or suspect cancer of the breast or womb, do not use oral contraceptives. Before beginning oral contraceptives, examine your breasts carefully (see p. 279). In some health centers you may also be able to get a simple test (Pap smear) to check for cancer of the *cervix* or opening of the womb. Birth control pills have not been proven to cause cancer of the breasts or womb. But if cancer already exists, the pill can make it worse.

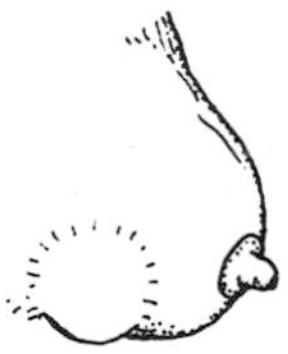

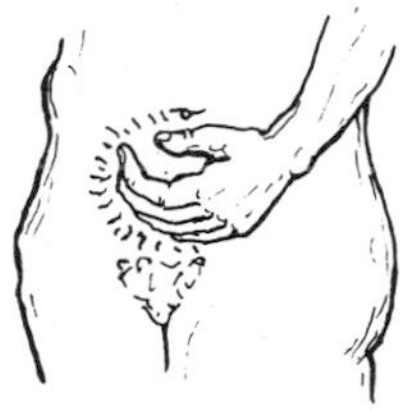

Some health problems may be made worse by oral contraceptives. If you have any of the following problems, it is better to use another method if you can:

- **Migraine** (p. 162). Women who suffer from true migraine should not take oral contraceptives. But simple headache that goes away with aspirin is no reason not to take the pill.
- **Urinary infection with swelling of the feet** (p. 234).
- **Heart disease** (p. 325).
- **High blood pressure** (p. 125).

If you suffer from asthma, tuberculosis, diabetes or epilepsy, it is best to get medical advice before taking birth control pills. However, most women with these diseases can take oral contraceptives without harm.

Precautions Women Should Take when Using Birth Control Pills

1. Do not smoke, especially if you are over 35. It can cause heart problems.

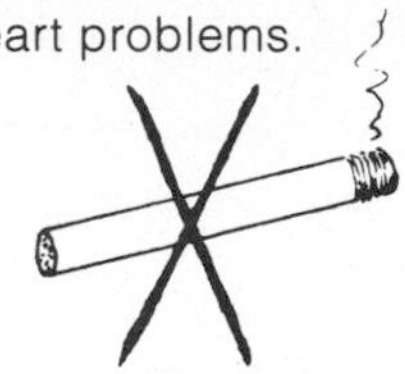

2. Examine the breasts carefully every month for lumps or possible signs of cancer (see page 279).

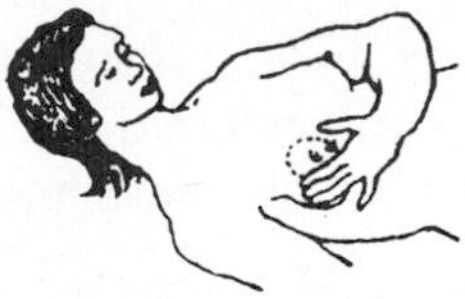

3. If possible, have your blood pressure measured every 6 months.

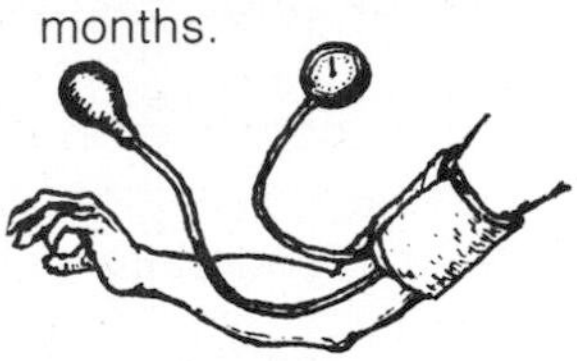

4. Watch for any of the problems mentioned on page 288, especially:

- Severe and frequent migraine headaches (p. 162).
- Dizziness, headache, or loss of consciousness that results in difficulty in seeing, speaking, or moving part of the face or body (see Stroke, p. 327).
- Pain with inflammation in a leg or hip (chance of a blood clot).
- Severe or repeated pain in the chest (see Heart Problems, p. 325).

If one of these problems develops, stop taking the pill and get medical advice. Avoid pregnancy by using another method, as these problems also make pregnancy especially dangerous.

Questions and Answers about Birth Control Pills

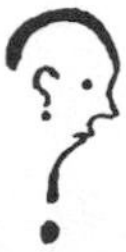	Some people claim birth control pills cause cancer. Is this true?	**No! However, if cancer of the breast or womb already exists, taking the pill may make the tumor grow faster.**
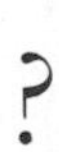	Can a woman have children again if she stops taking the pill?	**Yes. (Sometimes there is a delay of 1 or 2 months before she can become pregnant.)**
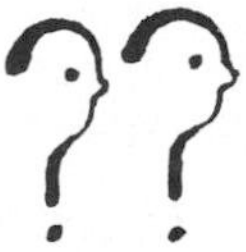	Is the chance of having twins or defective children greater if a woman has used oral contraceptives?	**No. The chances are the same as for women who have not taken the pill.**
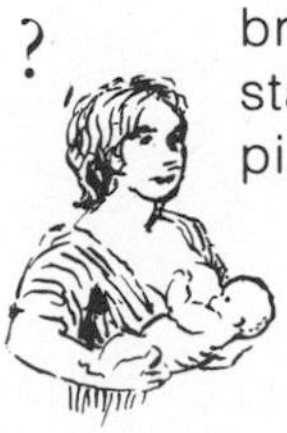	Is it true that a mother's breasts will dry up if she starts taking birth control pills?	**Some women will produce less milk when taking the pill. So it is best to use another method of birth control while nursing, and later change to the pill. Or she can take the 'mini-pill' (p. 395), which contains so little hormone that it usually does not affect the milk.**

For information on the selection of birth control pills, see pages 394 and 395.

OTHER METHODS OF FAMILY PLANNING

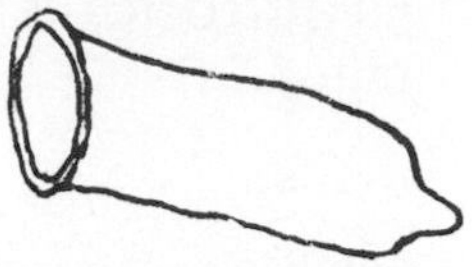

THE CONDOM (also called 'prophylactic', 'rubber', or 'sheath') is a narrow rubber or latex bag that the man wears on his penis while having sex. Usually it works well to prevent pregnancy. **It is also the only effective method for preventing AIDS,** and other sexually transmitted diseases, but is not a complete safeguard.

Put the rolled up condom over the stiff penis. Pinch the tip of the condom to leave a space for sperm. Roll the condom down the penis. The man should hold on to the condom when he pulls out his penis from his partner.

You can buy condoms in most pharmacies. Condoms are sometimes given away free at health clinics or family planning clinics. A condom should be used only once. A re-used condom is less likely to prevent disease or pregnancy. A condom should only be re-used when no other condoms are available. (Make sure to wash it first.)

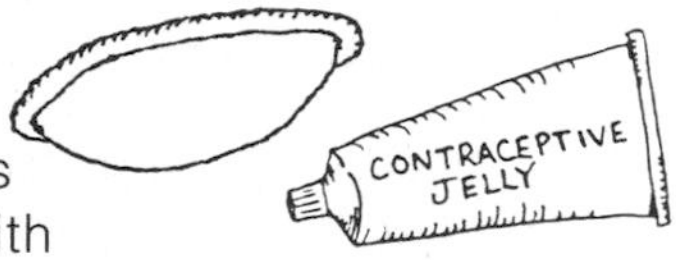

THE DIAPHRAGM is a shallow cup made of soft rubber. A woman wears it in her vagina while having sexual relations. It should be left in for at least 6 hours afterward. It is a fairly sure method if used together with a contraceptive cream or jelly. A health worker or midwife should help fit the diaphragm, as different women need different sizes. Check the diaphragm regularly for holes and cracks by holding it up to the light. If there is even a tiny hole, get a new one. They usually last a year or longer. After use, wash it in warm soapy water, rinse, and dry. Keep in a clean, dry place.

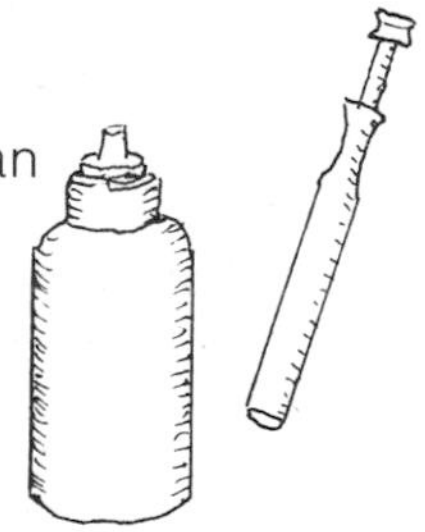

CONTRACEPTIVE FOAM comes in a tube or can. The woman puts it into her vagina with a special applicator. It must be applied no longer than 1 hour before having sex, and left in for at least 6 hours afterward. The application should be repeated before each time the couple has sex, even if this is several times in one night. It is a fairly sure method if used correctly.

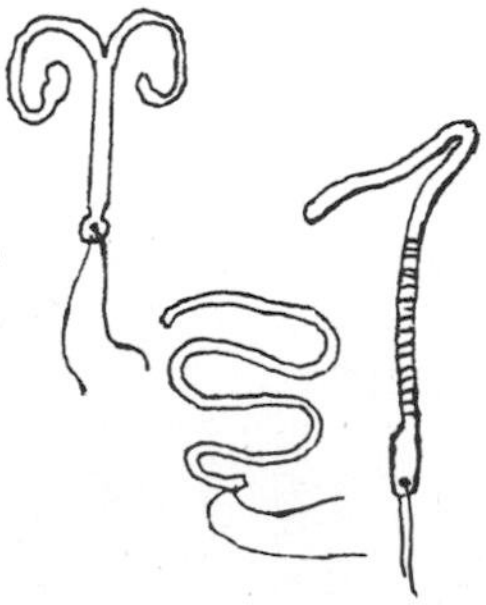

THE INTRAUTERINE DEVICE (IUD) is a plastic (or sometimes metal) object that a specially trained health worker or midwife places inside the womb. While in the womb, it prevents pregnancy. IUDs fall out of some women. In others they cause pain, discomfort, heavy bleeding during periods, and sometimes serious problems, but for some women they give no trouble at all. For these women, the IUD may be the simplest and most economical method. See p. 396 before deciding to use an IUD.

WITHDRAWAL OR PULLING OUT (COITUS INTERRUPTUS) is a method in which the man pulls his penis out of the woman before the sperm comes. This method is perhaps better than none, but may be disturbing to the couple and does not always work, because some men do not pull out in time, especially if they have been drinking. This method is risky because some sperm are present in the first drops of clear liquid that come from a man's penis.

THE RHYTHM METHOD

This method is not very sure to prevent pregnancy, but it has the advantage of not costing anything. **It is more likely to work for a woman whose periods come very regularly, more or less once every 28 days.** Also, the husband and wife must be willing to pass one week out of each month without having sex the regular way.

Usually a woman has a chance of becoming pregnant only during 8 days of her monthly cycle—her 'fertile days'. These 8 days come midway between her periods, beginning 10 days after the first day of menstrual bleeding. To avoid getting pregnant, a woman should not have sex with her man during these 8 days. During the rest of the month, she is not likely to get pregnant.

To avoid confusion the woman should mark on a calendar the 8 days she is not to have sex.

For example: Suppose your period begins on the 5th day of May. Count that as day number 1.

Mark it like this:

Then count 10 days. Starting with the 10th day, put a line under the next 8 days like this:

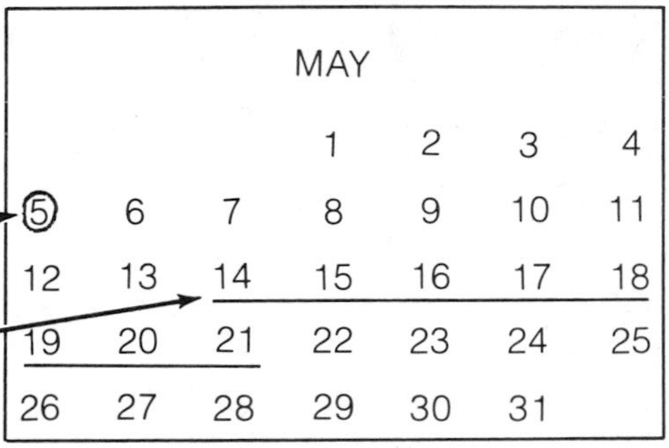
MAY
1 2 3 4
5 6 7 8 9 10 11
12 13 14 15 16 17 18
19 20 21 22 23 24 25
26 27 28 29 30 31

During these 8 'fertile days', do not have sexual relations.

Now suppose your next period begins on the first of June. Mark it the same way, like this:

Once again count off 10 days and underline the following 8 days in which you will not have sexual contact.

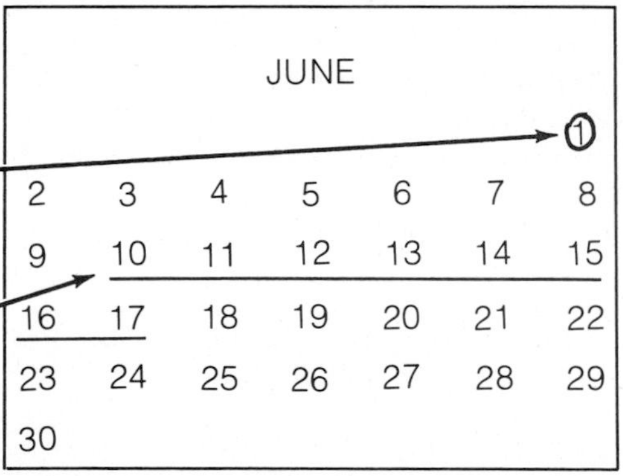
JUNE
1
2 3 4 5 6 7 8
9 10 11 12 13 14 15
16 17 18 19 20 21 22
23 24 25 26 27 28 29
30

If the woman and her husband carefully avoid having sex together during these 8 days of each month, it is possible that they will go years without having another child. However, few couples are successful for very long. This is not a very sure method, unless used in combination with another method such as a diaphragm or condoms, especially during the days from the end of the menstrual period until the fertile days are over.

THE MUCUS METHOD

This is a variation of the rhythm method. A woman finds out when she could become pregnant by checking the mucus in her vagina every day. It works fairly well for some couples but not for others. In general it cannot be considered a very sure way of preventing pregnancy, but it costs nothing and has no risks other than those that come with pregnancy itself. However, it is more difficult to do if the woman has a vaginal infection with a lot of discharge, if her periods are not regular, or if she douches often.

Every day, except during her period, the woman should examine the mucus from her vagina. Take a little mucus out of your vagina with a clean finger and try to make it stretch between your thumb and forefinger, like this:

As long as the mucus is sticky like paste—not slippery or slimy—you probably cannot become pregnant, and can continue to have sexual relations.

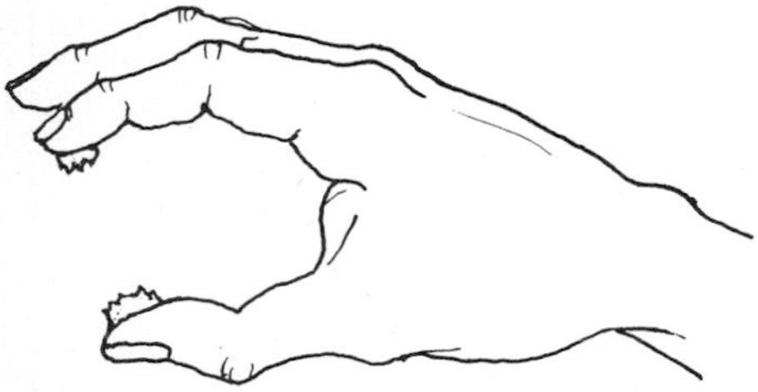

When the mucus begins to get slippery or slimy, like raw egg, or if it stretches between your fingers, you may become pregnant if you have sexual relations. So, **do not have sex when the mucus is slippery or stretches, or until 4 days after it has stopped being slippery or stretchy and has become sticky again.**

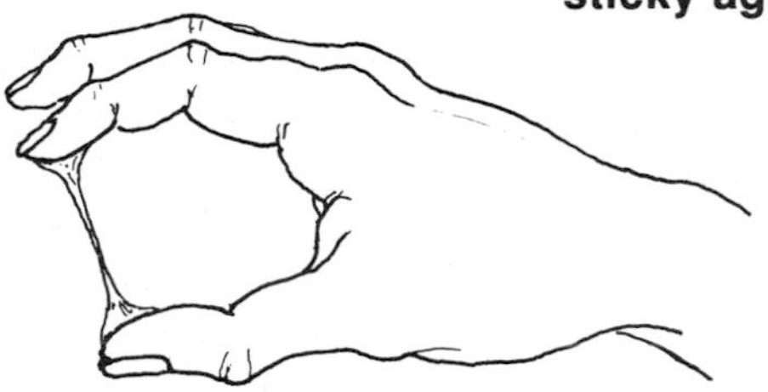

The mucus will usually become slippery during a few days midway between your periods. These are the same days you would not have sex with your man if you were using the rhythm method.

To be more sure, use the mucus and rhythm methods together. To be still more sure, see below.

Combined Methods:

If you want to be more certain not to become pregnant, it often helps to use 2 methods at the same time. The rhythm or mucus method combined with the use of a condom, diaphragm, foam, or sponge is surer than any of these methods alone. Likewise, if a man uses condoms and the woman a diaphragm or foam, the chance of pregnancy is very low.

INJECTIONS. There are special hormone injections to prevent pregnancy. *Depo-Provera* is one. An injection is needed every 3 months. Side effects and precautions are similar to those for birth control pills, but there can be more problems with irregular bleeding. Once side effects begin, they can take months to end, even if the woman stops receiving the injections. Also, it can take a year or more for a woman to become pregnant after she stops getting the injections.

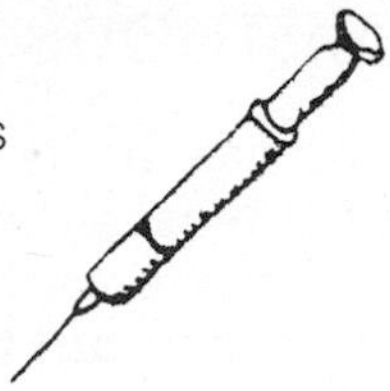

IMPLANTS. With this method, 6 small tubes of the hormone progesterone are put under the skin. If left there, they can prevent pregnancy for up to 5 years. Side effects are similar to those of birth control pills and injections. Irregular bleeding is a common side effect. Menstrual bleeding may be heavy during the first year.

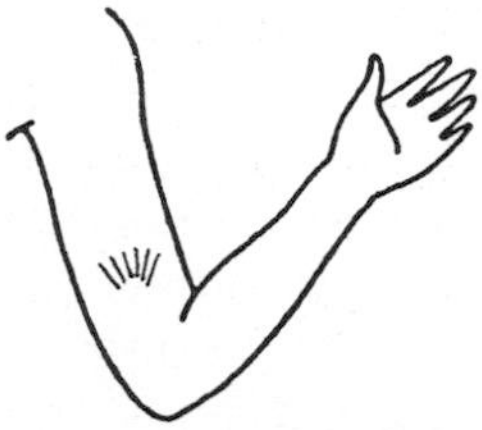

Those who promote these 2 methods say that they are helpful for women who have trouble remembering to take pills, or who have problems using other types of birth control. Those who oppose these methods say that they may not be safe and that they are frequently used on women who are not fully informed of the risks. For more information, see pages 396 and 397.

METHODS FOR THOSE WHO NEVER WANT TO HAVE MORE CHILDREN

STERILIZATION. For those who never want to have more children, there are fairly safe, simple operations for both men and women. In many countries these operations are free. Ask at the health center.

- **For men,** the operation is called a vasectomy. It can be done simply and quickly in a doctor's office or a health center, usually without putting the man to sleep. Small cuts are made here so that the tubes from the man's testicles can be cut and tied. The testicles are not removed.

  The operation has no effect on the man's sexual ability or pleasure. His fluid comes just the same, but has no sperm in it.

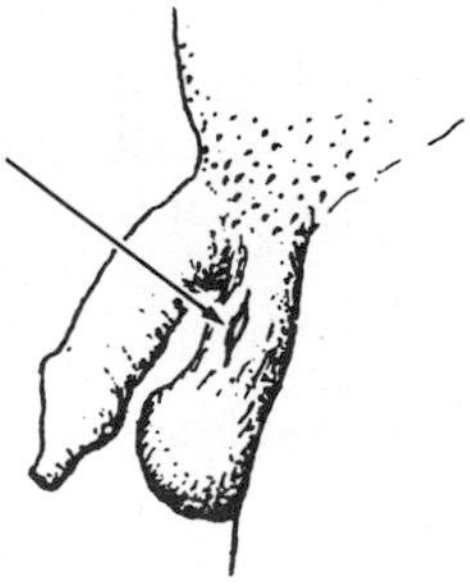

- **For women,** the operation is called a tubal ligation, which means to tie the tubes. One method is to make a small cut in the lower belly so that the tubes coming from the ovaries, or egg-makers, can be cut and tied. It can usually be done in a doctor's office or health center without putting the woman to sleep. Although usually successful, there is a higher risk of infection in the operation for women than for men.

  This operation has no effect on the woman's menstrual periods or sexual ability, and may make having sex more pleasant because she does not have to worry about pregnancy.

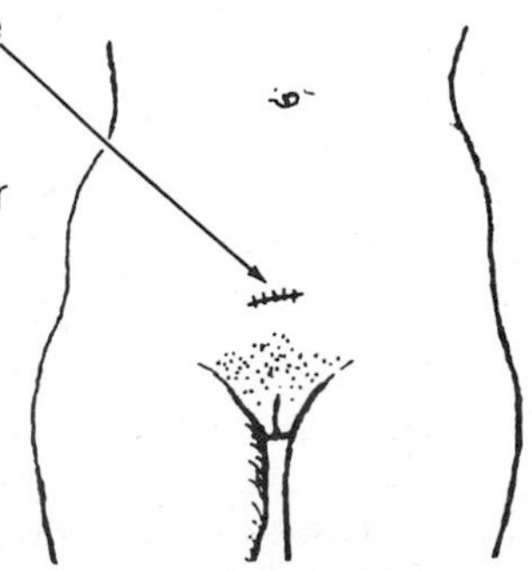

HOME METHODS FOR PREVENTING PREGNANCY

Every land has 'home remedies' for preventing or interrupting pregnancy. Unfortunately, most either do not work or are dangerous. For example, some women think that to wash out the vagina or to urinate after having sex will prevent pregnancy, **but this is not true.**

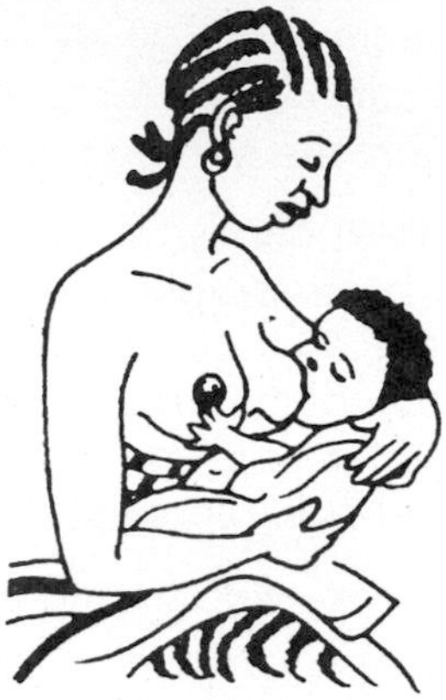

BREAST FEEDING. While a woman is breast feeding her baby she is less likely to become pregnant—especially when breast milk is the only food her baby receives. The chance of her becoming pregnant is much greater after 4 to 6 months, when the baby begins to get other foods in addition to breast milk. Even then, breast feeding can help prevent pregnancy if she breast feeds frequently, both day and night, and gives breast milk as the main food. (But if her periods start, she cannot depend on breast feeding to prevent pregnancy.)

To be more sure she will not become pregnant, the mother who is breast feeding should begin some method of birth control when the baby is 3 to 4 months old. A method other than birth control pills is better because the pills cause some women to produce less milk. (The 'mini-pill' causes less of a problem. See p. 395.)

THE SPONGE METHOD. Here is a home method that is not harmful and sometimes works. You cannot be sure it will prevent pregnancy every time, but it can be used when no other method is available.

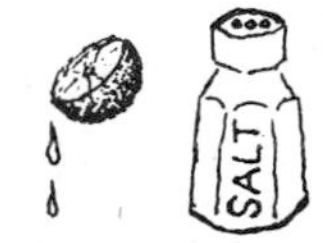

You will need a sponge and either **vinegar, lemons,** or **salt.** Either a sea sponge or an artificial sponge will work. If you do not have a sponge, try a ball of cotton, wild kapok, or soft cloth.

- Mix:

  2 tablespoons vinegar in 1 cup clean water
  or
  1 teaspoon lemon juice in 1 cup clean water
  or
  1 spoon of salt in 4 spoons clean water

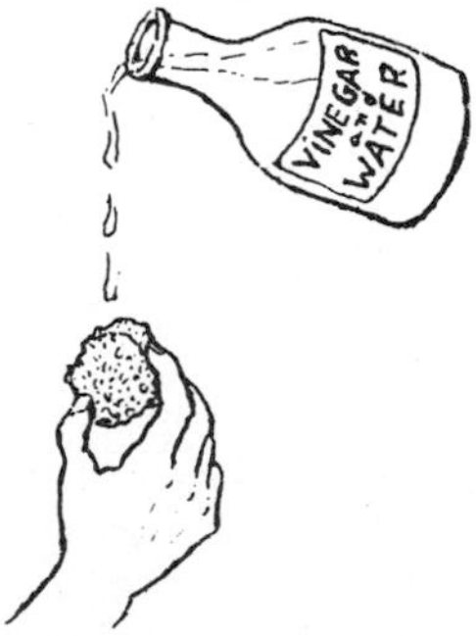

- Wet the sponge with one of these liquids.
- Push the wet sponge deep into your vagina before having sex. You can put it in up to an hour before.
- Leave the sponge in at least 6 hours after having sex. Then take it out. If you have trouble getting it out, next time tie a ribbon or piece of string to it that you can pull.

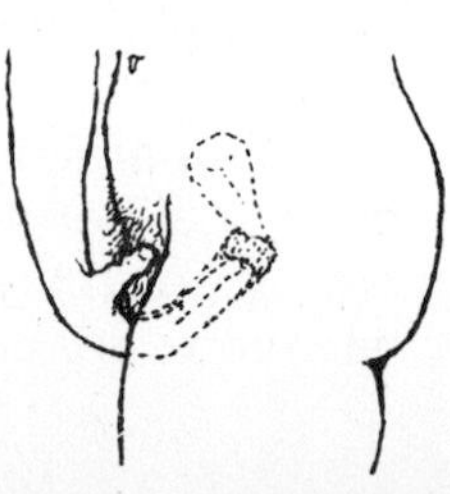

The sponge can be washed and used again, many times. Keep it in a clean place.

You can make up the liquid in advance and keep it in a bottle.

CHAPTER 21

HEALTH AND SICKNESSES OF CHILDREN

WHAT TO DO TO PROTECT CHILDREN'S HEALTH

NUTRITIOUS FOOD, CLEANLINESS, AND VACCINATIONS

ARE THE THREE IMPORTANT 'BODY GUARDS' THAT KEEP CHILDREN HEALTHY AND PROTECT THEM AGAINST MANY SICKNESSES.

Chapters 11 and 12 tell more about the importance of nutritious food, cleanliness, and vaccination. Parents should read these chapters carefully and use them to help care for—and teach—their children. The main points are briefly repeated here.

Nutritious Food

It is important that children eat the most nutritious foods they can get, so that they grow well and do not get sick.

The best foods for children at different ages are:

- in the first 4 to 6 months: **breast milk** and nothing more.
- from 6 months to 1 year: **breast milk** and also **other nutritious foods—**such as boiled cereals, mashed-up beans, eggs, meat, cooked fruits and vegetables.
- from 1 year on: the child should eat the **same foods as adults—**but **more often.** To the main food (rice, maize, wheat, potatoes, or cassava) add 'helper foods' as discussed in Chapter 11.
- Above all, children should get **enough** to eat—several times a day.
- All parents should watch for signs of malnutrition in their children and should give them the best food they can.

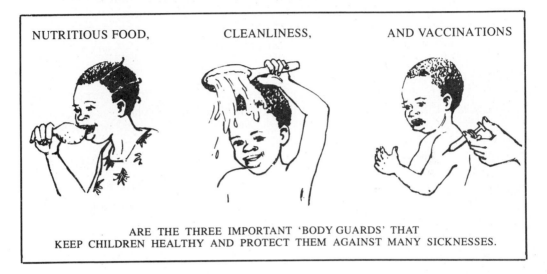

Cleanliness

Children are more likely to be healthy if their village, their homes, and they themselves are kept clean. Follow the Guidelines of Cleanliness explained in Chapter 12. Teach children to follow them—and to understand their importance. Here the most important guidelines are repeated:

- Bathe children and change their clothes often.
- Teach children always to wash their hands when they get up in the morning, after they have a bowel movement, and before they eat or handle food.
- Make latrines or 'outhouses'—and teach children to use them.
- Where hookworm exists, do not let children go barefoot; use sandals or shoes.
- Teach children to brush their teeth; and do not give them a lot of candies, sweets, or carbonated drinks.
- Cut fingernails very short.
- Do not let children who are sick or have sores, scabies, lice, or ringworm sleep with other children or use the same clothing or towels.
- Treat children quickly for scabies, ringworm, intestinal worms, and other infections that spread easily from child to child.
- Do not let children put dirty things in their mouths or let dogs or cats lick their faces.
- Keep pigs, dogs, and chickens out of the house.
- Use only pure, boiled, or filtered water for drinking. This is especially important for babies.
- Do not feed babies from 'baby bottles', because these are hard to keep clean and can cause illness. Feed babies with a cup and spoon.

Vaccinations

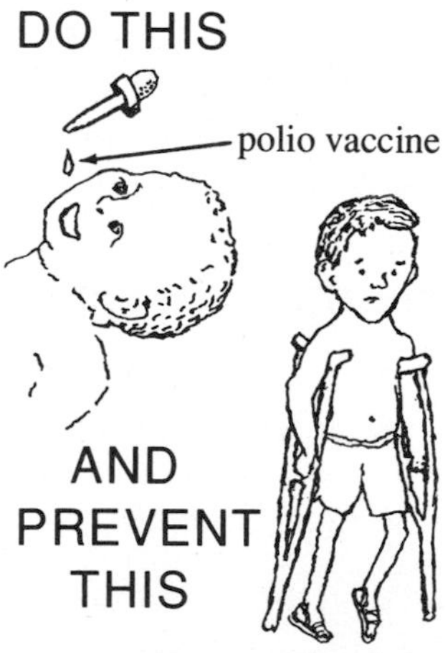
DO THIS
polio vaccine
AND PREVENT THIS

Vaccinations protect children against many of the most dangerous diseases of childhood—whooping cough, diphtheria, tetanus, polio, measles, and tuberculosis.

Children should be given the different vaccinations during the first months of life, as shown on page 147. Polio drops should be first given if possible at birth, but no later than 2 months of age, because the risk of developing infantile paralysis (polio) is highest in babies under 1 year old.

Important: For complete protection, the DPT (diphtheria, whooping cough, tetanus) and polio vaccines should be given once a month for 3 months and once again a year later.

Tetanus of the newborn can be prevented by vaccinating mothers against tetanus during pregnancy (see p. 250).

Be sure your children get all the vaccinations they need.

CHILDREN'S GROWTH—AND THE 'ROAD TO HEALTH'

A healthy child grows steadily. If he eats enough nutritious food, and has no serious illness, a child gains weight each month.

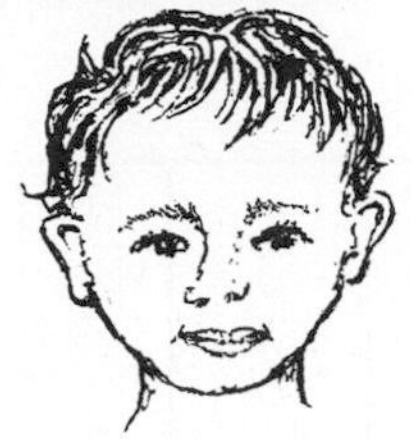

A child who grows well is healthy.

A child who gains weight more slowly than other children, stops gaining weight, or is losing weight is not healthy. He may not be eating enough or he may have a serious illness, or both.

A good way to check whether a child is healthy and is getting enough nutritious food is to weigh him each month and see if he gains weight normally. If a monthly record of the child's weight is kept on a Child Health Chart, it is easy to see at a glance whether the child is gaining weight normally.

When used well, the charts tell mothers and health workers when a child is not growing normally, so they can take early action. They can make sure the child gets more to eat, and can check for and treat any illness the child may have.

On the next page is a typical Child Health Chart showing the 'road to health'. This chart can be cut out and copied. Or larger, ready-made cards can be obtained (in English, French, Spanish, Portuguese, or Arabic) from Teaching Aids at Low Cost (TALC, see p. 429 for address). Similar charts are produced in local languages by the Health Departments in many countries.

It is a good idea for every mother to keep a Child Health Chart for each of her children under 5 years of age. If there is a health center or 'under-fives clinic' nearby, she should take her children, with their charts, to be weighed and to have a 'check-up' each month. The health worker can help explain the Chart and its use. To protect the Chart, keep it in a plastic envelope.

HOMEMADE BEAM SCALE

You can make a beam scale of dry wood or bamboo. Place all hooks as shown and hang scale. To make kg. marks on the beam, fill 2 plastic one-liter bottles with water. Place the first bottle where baby would hang. Hang the second bottle, and where beam balances, make the 1 kg. mark, and so on. With a ruler, measure the distance between the marks, and make marks for 200, 400, 600, and 800 grams.

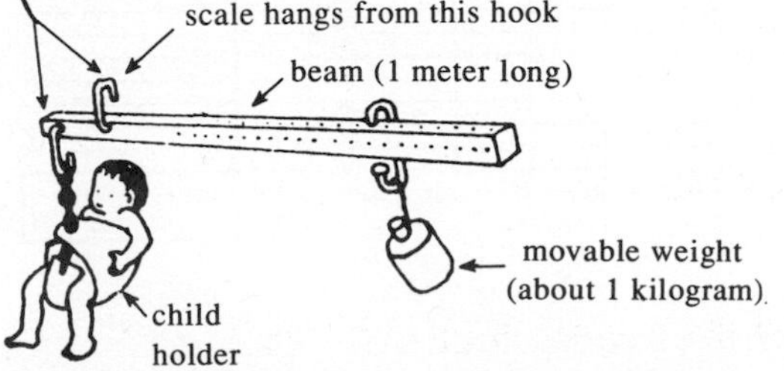

Weight is correct when beam stays horizontal.

DIRECT RECORDING SCALE

available from TALC (see p. 429)

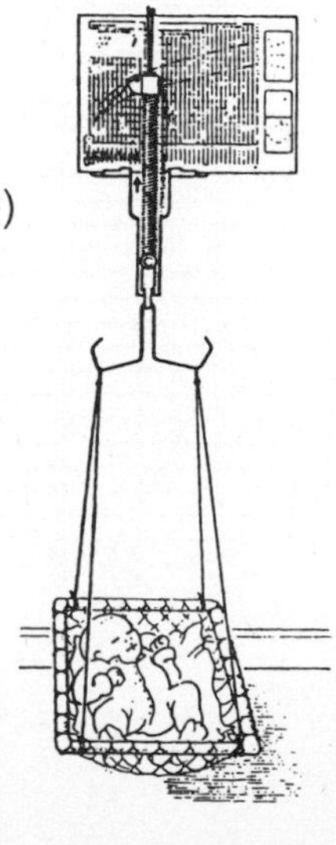

The growth chart slips in behind the scales so you can mark the child's weight directly onto the chart.

It is best to hang this and other scales close to the ground. A baby may be scared of hanging up high.

SIDE ONE

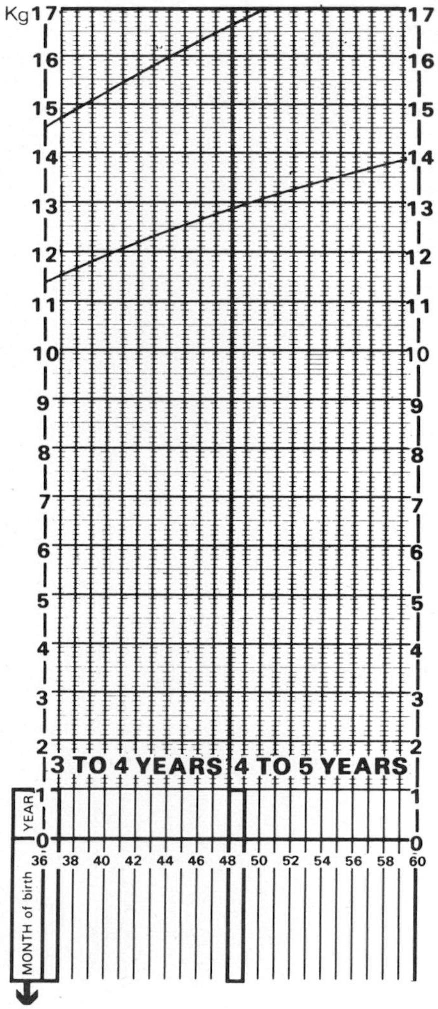

CHILD HEALTH CHART

CLINIC 1 .... No ....

CLINIC 2 .... No ....

CHILD'S NAME		GIRL / BOY
DATE OF BIRTH (day, month, year)	BIRTH WEIGHT	

MOTHER'S NAME
CARETAKER IF NOT THE MOTHER
FATHER'S NAME
WHERE DOES THE CHILD LIVE?

How many children has the mother had? ....
Number alive .... Number dead ....

CARD GIVEN AND MOTHER TAUGHT BY

ASK THE MOTHER ABOUT THESE REASONS FOR GIVING THE CHILD EXTRA CARE (make a circle round the right answer)		TAKE EXTRA CARE
Was the baby **less than 2.5 kg at birth**	no	yes
Is this baby a **twin**	no	yes
Is this baby **bottle fed**	no	yes
Does the mother need more **family support**	no	yes
Are any brothers or sisters **underweight**	no	yes
Are there any other reasons for **taking extra care**?	no	yes

For example – tuberculosis or leprosy or **social problems**

Remember to discuss child spacing

chart produced by
TALC TALC P.O. BOX 49, ST. ALBANS, UK.
Training materials are also available

GROWTH CURVE **Reference values – WHO recommended 1980**
UPPER LINE: 50th CENTILE BOYS LOWER LINE: 3rd CENTILE GIRLS

IMMUNISATIONS			DATE GIVEN
BCG			
POLIO		FIRST DOSE	
		SECOND DOSE	
		THIRD DOSE	
		FOURTH DOSE	
DPT	Diptheria	FIRST DOSE	
	Whooping Cough	SECOND DOSE	
	Tetanus	THIRD DOSE	
MEASLES			
MOTHER'S TETANUS TOXOID (or one booster)		FIRST DOSE	
		SECOND DOSE	
		THIRD DOSE	

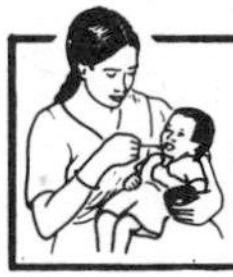

ORAL REHYDRATION

	DATES		
Taught			
Used			

Date of visit

SIDE TWO

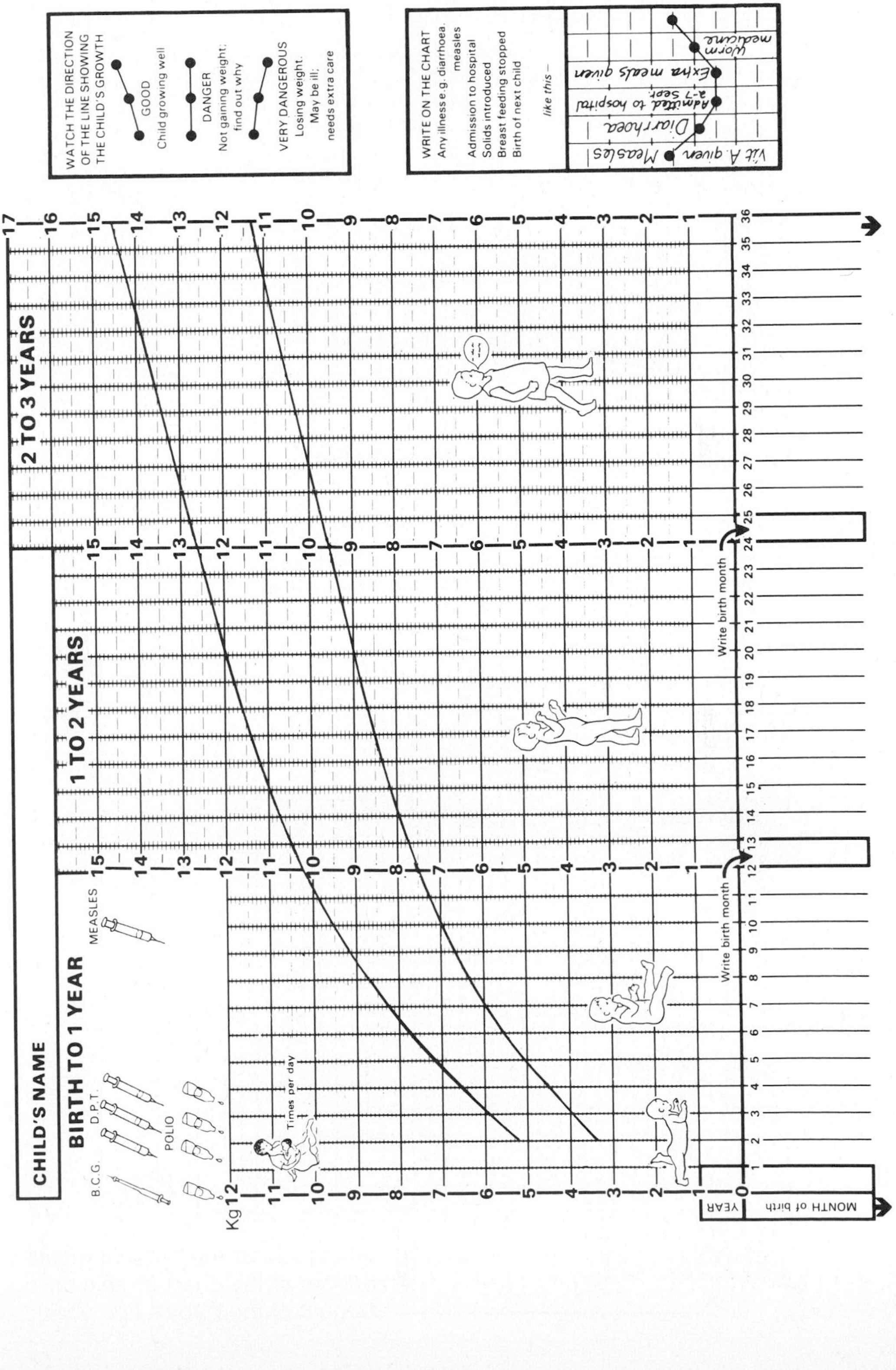

WATCH THE DIRECTION OF THE LINE SHOWING THE CHILD'S GROWTH
GOOD
Child growing well
DANGER
Not gaining weight; find out why
VERY DANGEROUS
Losing weight. May be ill; needs extra care
WRITE ON THE CHART
Any illness e.g. diarrhoea, measles
Admission to hospital
Solids introduced
Breast feeding stopped
Birth of next child
like this—
Vit A given
Measles
Diarrhoea
Admitted to hospital 2-7 Sept.
Extra meals given
Worm medicine
CHILD'S NAME
BIRTH TO 1 YEAR
1 TO 2 YEARS
2 TO 3 YEARS
B.C.G.
D.P.T.
POLIO
MEASLES
Times per day
Kg
Write birth month
Write birth month
YEAR
MONTH of birth

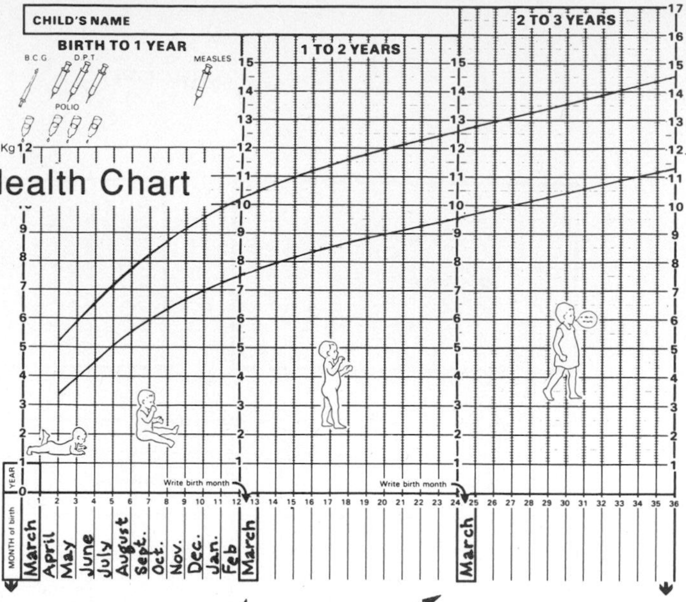

How to Use the Child Health Chart

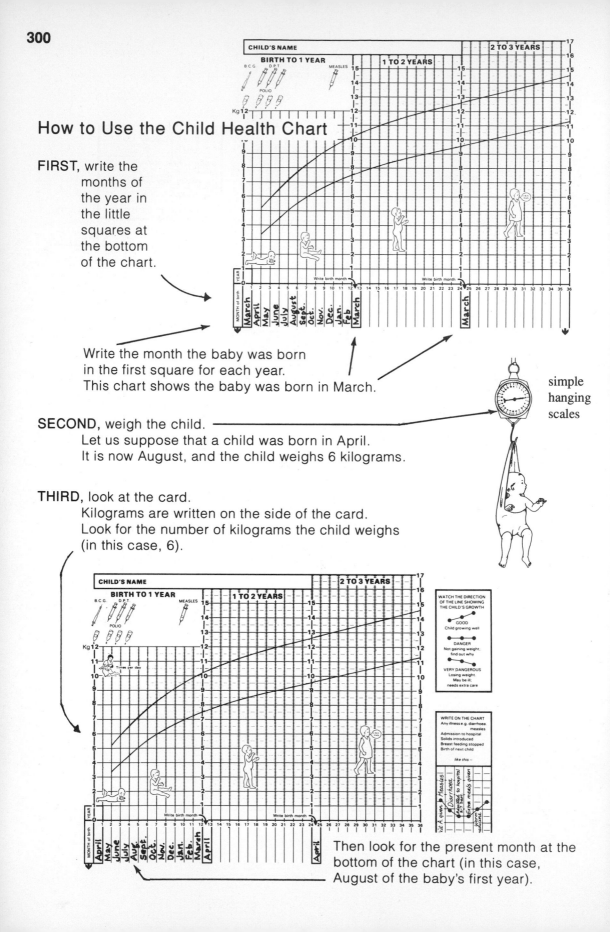

FIRST, write the months of the year in the little squares at the bottom of the chart.

Write the month the baby was born in the first square for each year. This chart shows the baby was born in March.

SECOND, weigh the child.

Let us suppose that a child was born in April. It is now August, and the child weighs 6 kilograms.

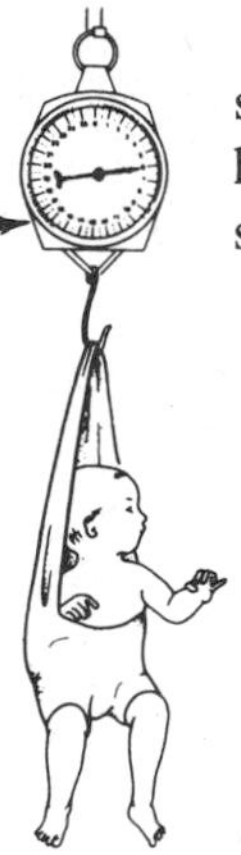

simple hanging scales

THIRD, look at the card.

Kilograms are written on the side of the card. Look for the number of kilograms the child weighs (in this case, 6).

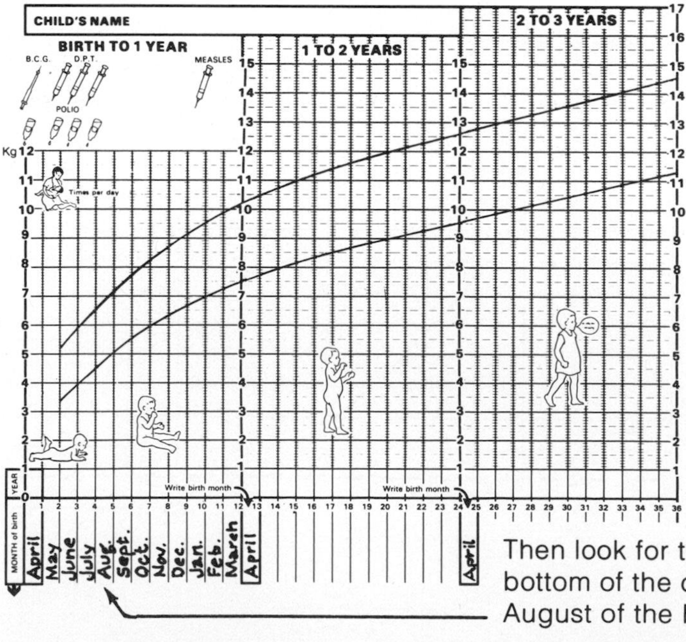

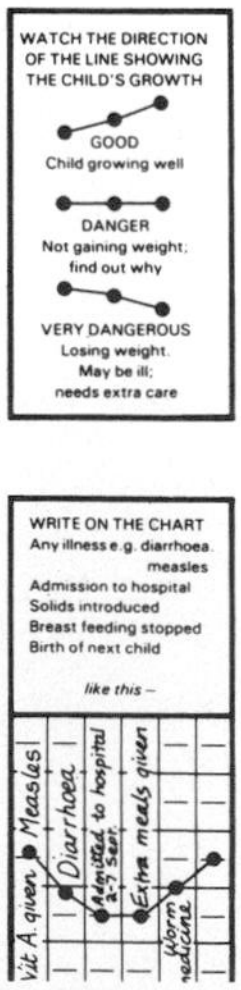

Then look for the present month at the bottom of the chart (in this case, August of the baby's first year).

FOURTH, follow the line that goes out from the 6

and

the lines that go up from August.

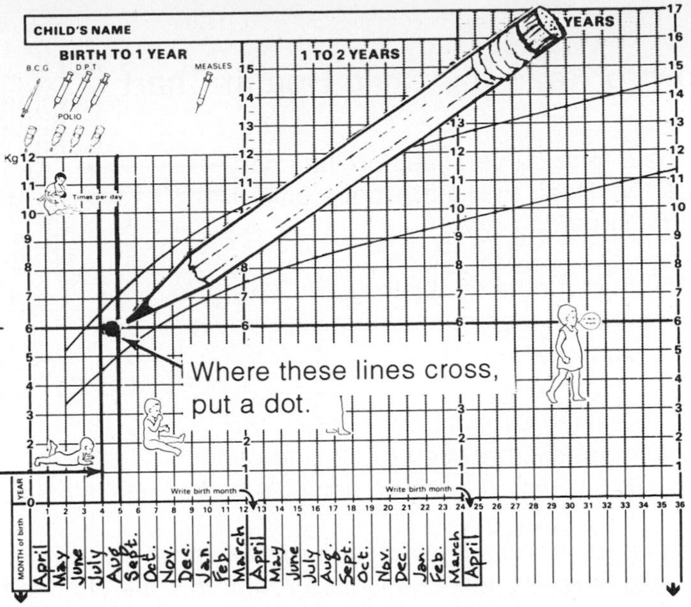

It is easy to know where to put the dot if you hold a square piece of paper against the chart.

1 Line up one edge of the paper with the child's weight.

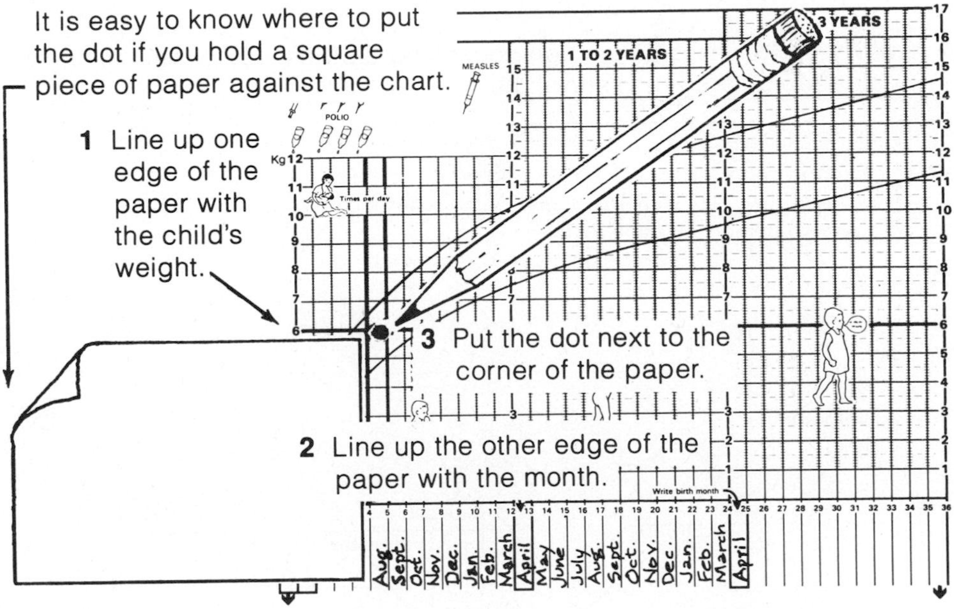

Each month weigh the child and put another dot on the chart.

If the child is healthy, each month the new dot will be higher on the chart than the last.

To see how well the child is growing, join the dots with lines.

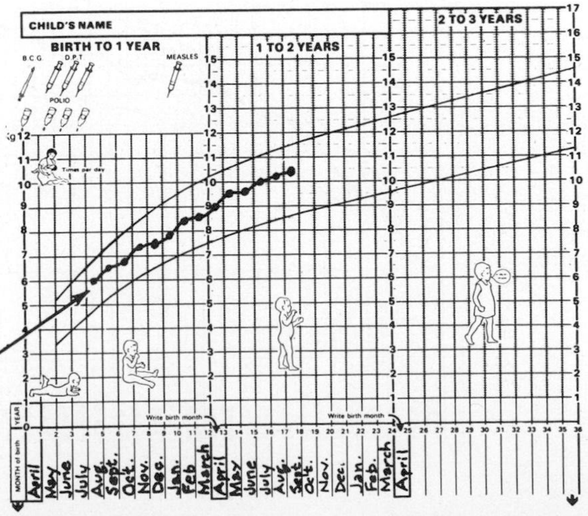

How to Read the Child Health Chart

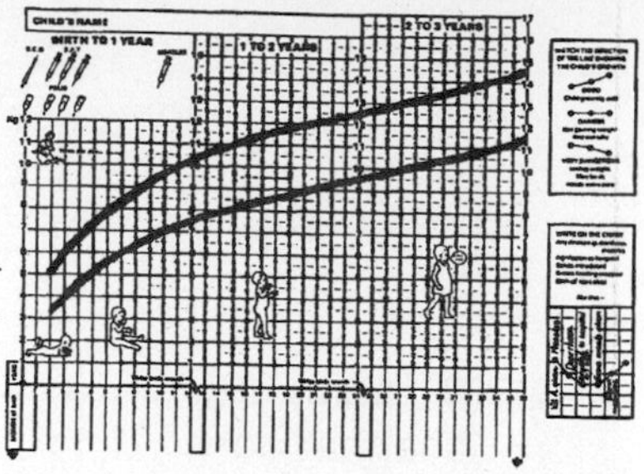

The 2 long curved lines on the chart mark the 'Road to Health' that a child's weight should follow.

The line of dots marks the child's weight from month to month, and from year to year.

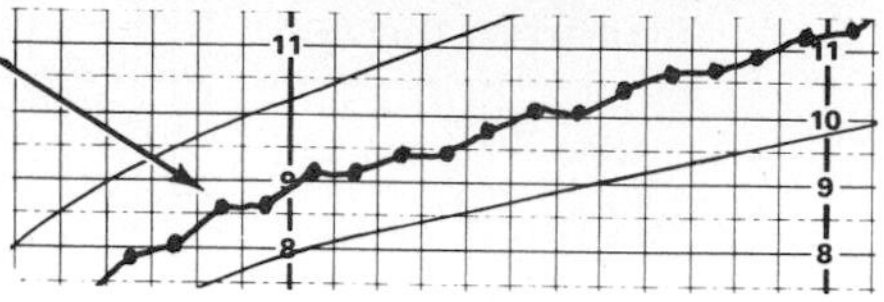

In most normal, healthy children, the line of dots falls between the 2 long curved lines. That is why the space between these lines is called the Road to Health.

If the line of dots rises steadily, month after month, in the same direction as the long curved lines, this is also a sign that the child is healthy.

A healthy child who gets enough nourishing food usually begins to sit, walk, and speak at about the times shown here.

Typical chart of
THE HEALTHY,
WELL-NOURISHED
CHILD

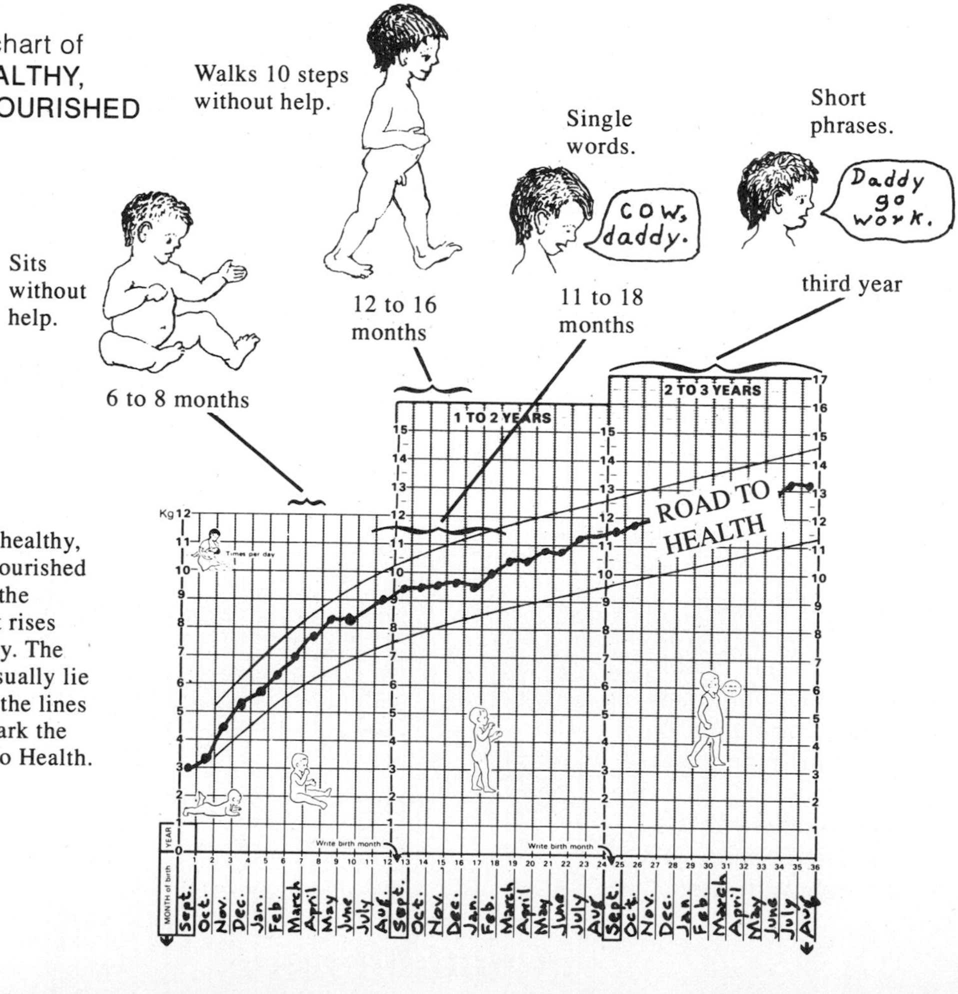

In the healthy, well-nourished child, the weight rises steadily. The dots usually lie inside the lines that mark the Road to Health.

A malnourished, sickly child may have a chart like the one below. Notice that the line of dots (his weight) is below the Road to Health. The line of dots is also irregular and does not rise much. This shows the child is in danger.

Typical chart of
THE UNDERWEIGHT OR MALNOURISHED CHILD

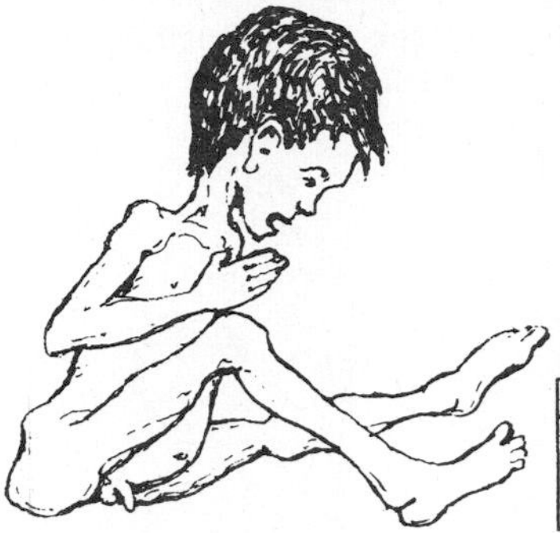

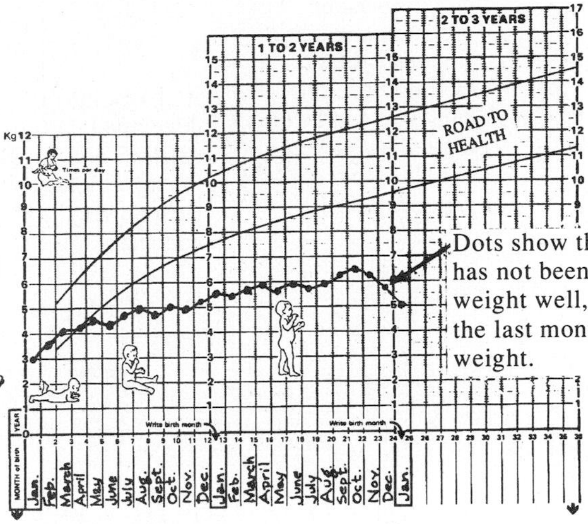

A child with a chart like the one above is seriously underweight. Perhaps he is not getting enough food. Or perhaps he has a disease like tuberculosis or malaria. Or both. He should be given **more energy-rich foods more often.** He should also be checked or tested for possible illnesses, and visit a health worker frequently until his chart shows he is gaining weight well.

IMPORTANT: **Watch the direction of the line of dots.**

The direction of the line of dots tells more about the child's health than whether the dots are inside or below the two curved lines. For example:

DANGER! This child is not gaining weight.

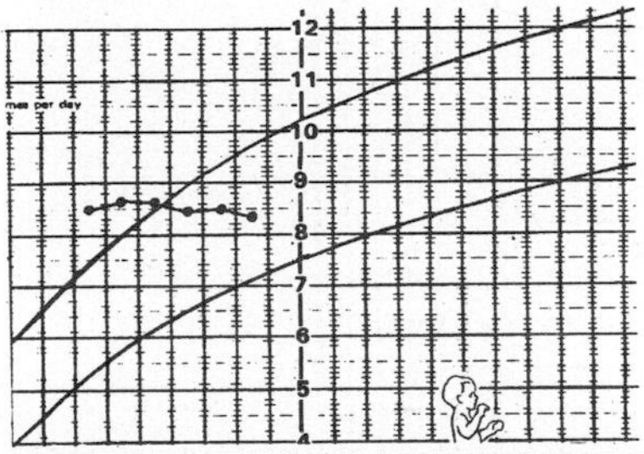

Although the dots for this child are within the curved lines, the child has not been gaining weight well for several months.

GOOD! This child is gaining weight well.

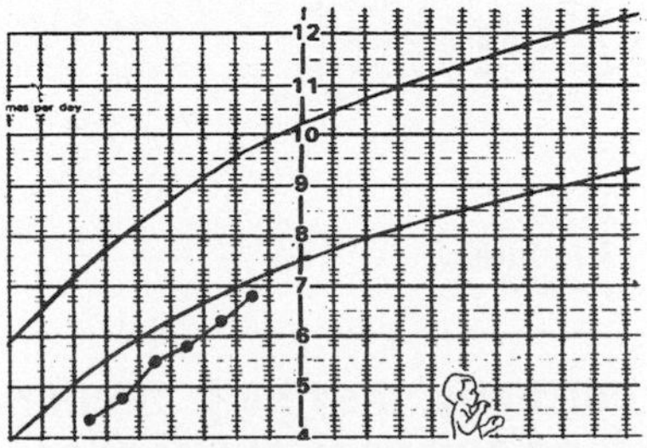

Although the dots for this child are below the 2 curved lines, their upward direction shows the child is growing well. Some children are naturally smaller than others. Perhaps this child's parents are also smaller than average.

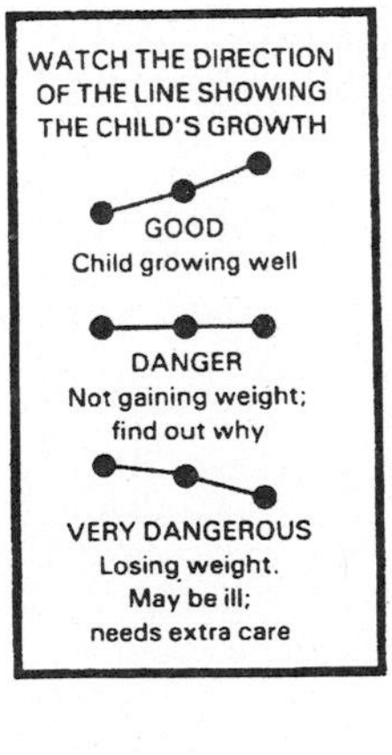

WATCH THE DIRECTION OF THE LINE SHOWING THE CHILD'S GROWTH
GOOD
Child growing well
DANGER
Not gaining weight; find out why
VERY DANGEROUS
Losing weight.
May be ill;
needs extra care

A typical **CHILD HEALTH CHART SHOWING A CHILD'S PROGRESS:**

This baby was healthy and gained weight well for the first 6 months of life, because his mother breast fed him.

At 6 months, the mother became pregnant again and stopped breast feeding him. The baby was fed little more than corn and rice. He stopped gaining weight.

At 10 months he developed chronic diarrhea and began losing weight. He became very thin and sick.

When the child was 13 months old, his mother learned how important it is to give the child enough good food. He began gaining weight fast. By age 2 he was back on the Road to Health.

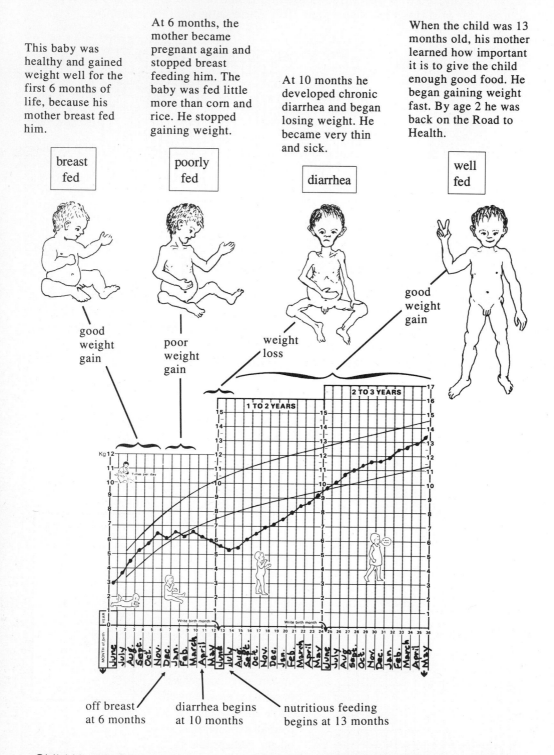

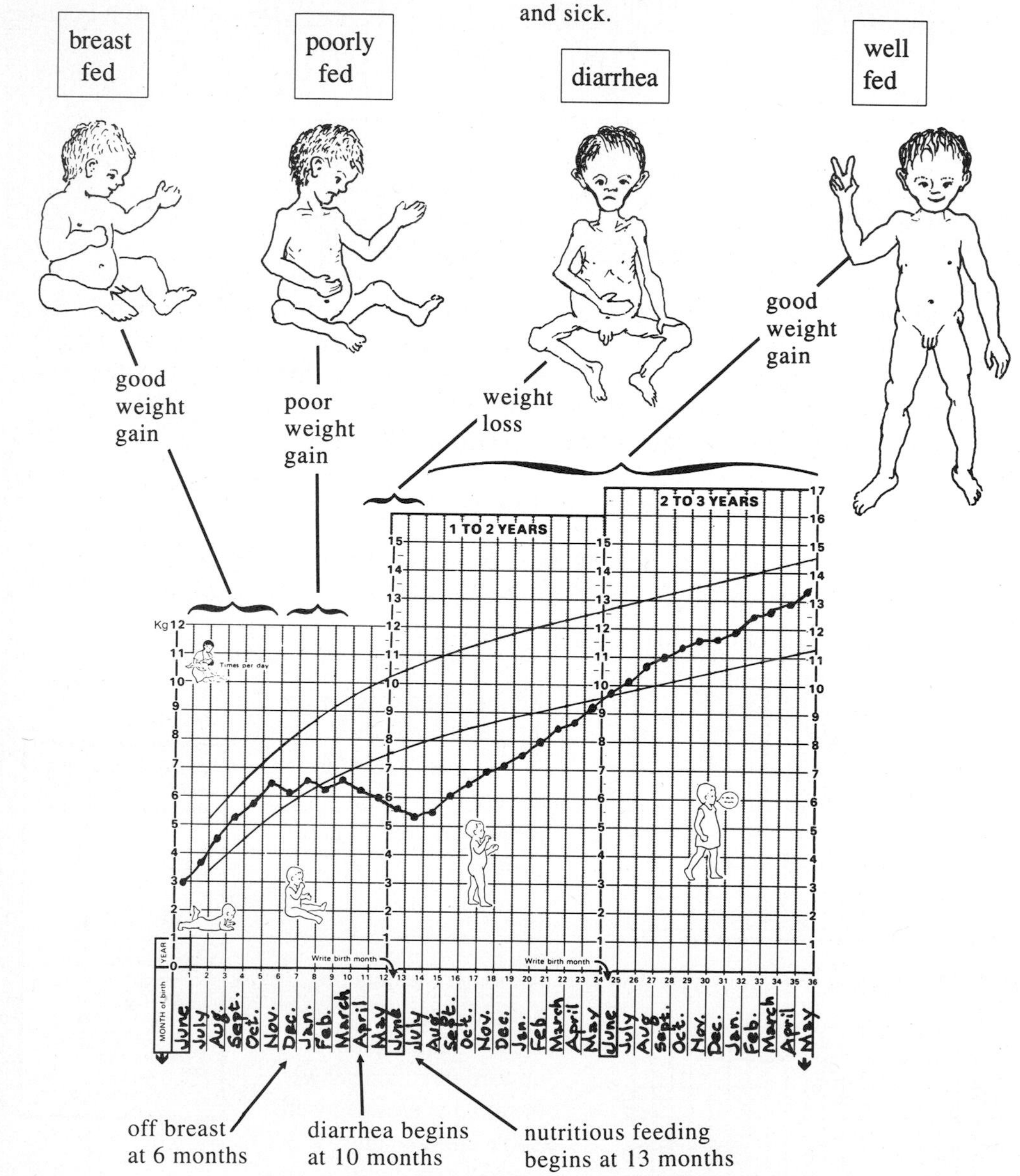

Child Health Charts are important. **When used correctly, they help mothers know when their children need more nutritious food and special attention.** They help health workers better understand the needs of the child and his family. They also let the mother know when she is doing a good job.

REVIEW OF CHILDREN'S HEALTH PROBLEMS DISCUSSED IN OTHER CHAPTERS

Many of the sicknesses discussed in other chapters of this book are found in children. Here some of the more frequent problems are reviewed in brief. For more information on each problem, see the pages indicated.

For special care and problems of newborn babies, see p. 270 to 275, and p. 405.

Remember: In children, sicknesses often become serious very quickly. An illness that takes days or weeks to severely harm or kill an adult may kill a small child in hours. So, it is important to **notice early signs of sickness and attend to them right away.**

Malnourished Children

Many children are malnourished because they do not get enough to eat. Or if they eat mainly foods with a lot of water and fiber in them, like cassava, taro root, or maize gruel, their bellies may get full before they get enough energy food for their bodies' needs. Also, some children may lack certain things in their food, like Vitamin A (see p. 226) or iodine (see p. 130). For a fuller discussion of the foods children need, read Chapter 11, especially pages 120 to 122.

THESE TWO CHILDREN ARE MALNOURISHED

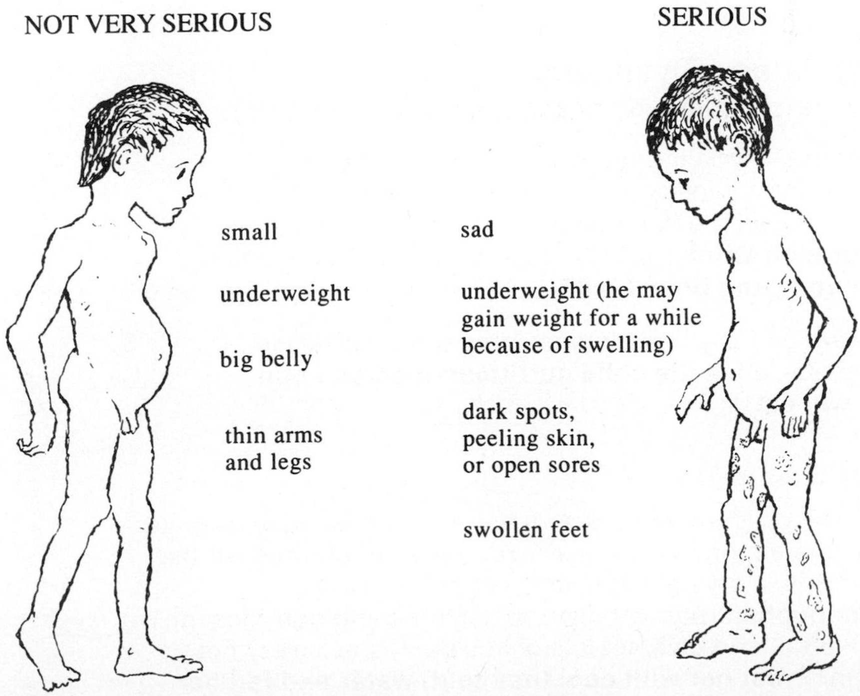

Malnutrition may cause many different problems in children, including:

In mild cases:

- slower growth
- swollen belly
- thin body
- loss of appetite
- loss of energy
- paleness (anemia)
- desire to eat dirt (anemia)
- sores in corners of mouth
- frequent colds and other infections
- night blindness

In more serious cases:

- little or no weight gain
- swelling of feet (sometimes face also)
- dark spots, 'bruises', or open peeling sores
- thinness or loss of hair
- lack of desire to laugh or play
- sores inside mouth
- failure to develop normal intelligence
- 'dry eyes' (xerophthalmia)
- blindness (p. 226)

Severe forms of general malnutrition are 'dry malnutrition' or marasmus, and 'wet malnutrition' or kwashiorkor. Their causes and prevention are discussed on p. 112 and 113.

Signs of malnutrition are often first seen after an acute illness like diarrhea or measles. A child who is sick, or who is getting well after a sickness, has an even greater need for enough good food than a child who is well.

Prevent and treat malnutrition by giving your children ENOUGH TO EAT and by feeding them MORE OFTEN. Add some high energy food, such as oil or fat, to the main food the child eats. Also try to add some body-building and protective foods like beans, lentils, fruits, vegetables, and if possible, milk, eggs, fish, or meat.

Diarrhea and Dysentery

(For more complete information see p. 153 to 160.)

The greatest danger to children with diarrhea is **dehydration,** or losing too much liquid from the body. The danger is even greater if the child is also vomiting. Give **Rehydration Drink** (p. 152). If the child is breast feeding, **continue giving breast milk,** but give Rehydration Drink also.

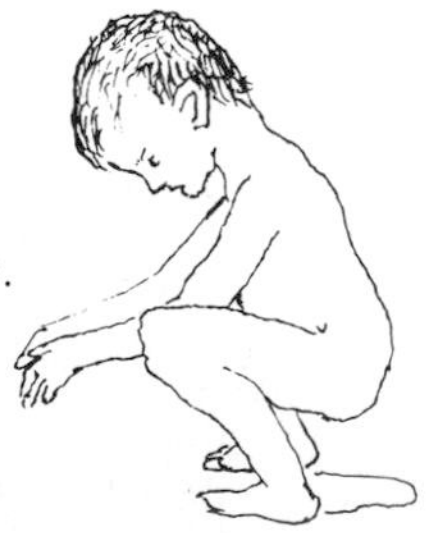

The second big danger to children with diarrhea is malnutrition. **Give the child nutritious food as soon as he will eat.**

Fever (see p. 75)

In small children, high fever (over 39°) can easily cause fits or damage the brain. To lower fever, **take the clothes off** the child. If she is crying and seems unhappy, give her **acetaminophen** (paracetamol) or aspirin in the right dosage (see p. 380), and give her lots of liquids. If she is very hot and shaky, **wet her with cool (not cold) water and fan her.**

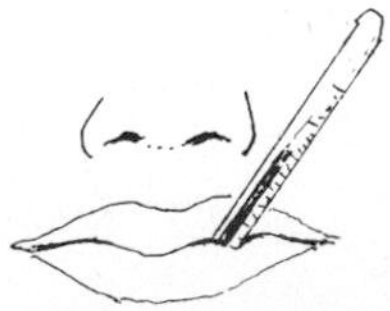

Fits (Convulsions) (see p. 178)

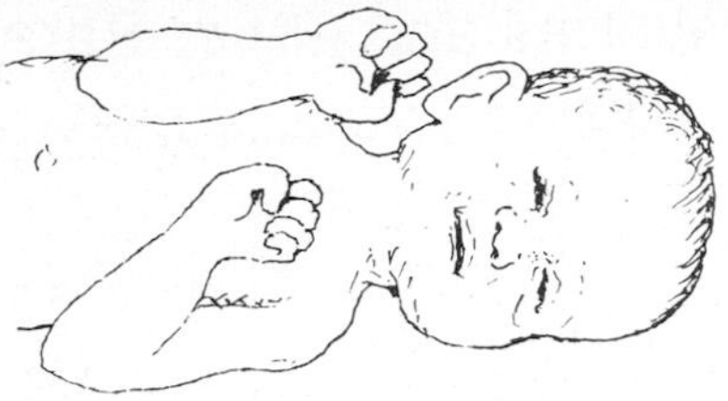

Common causes of fits or convulsions in children are high fever, dehydration, epilepsy, and meningitis. If fever is high, lower it rapidly (see p. 76). Check for signs of dehydration (p. 151) and meningitis (p. 185). Fits that come suddenly without fever or other signs are probably epilepsy (p. 178), especially if the child seems well between them. Fits or spasms in which first the jaw and then the whole body become stiff may be tetanus (p. 182).

Meningitis (see p. 185)

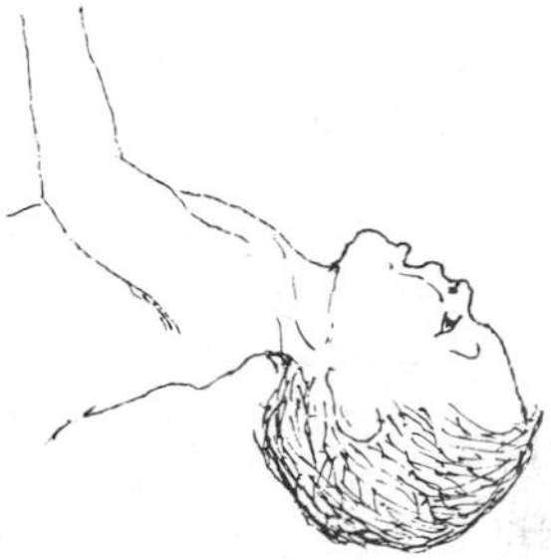

This dangerous disease may come as a complication of measles, mumps, or another serious illness. Children of mothers who have tuberculosis may get tubercular meningitis. A very sick child who lies with his head tilted way back, whose neck is too stiff to bend forward, and whose body makes strange movements (fits) may have meningitis.

Anemia (see p. 124)

Common signs in children:

- pale, especially inside eyelids, gums, and fingernails
- weak, tires easily
- likes to eat dirt

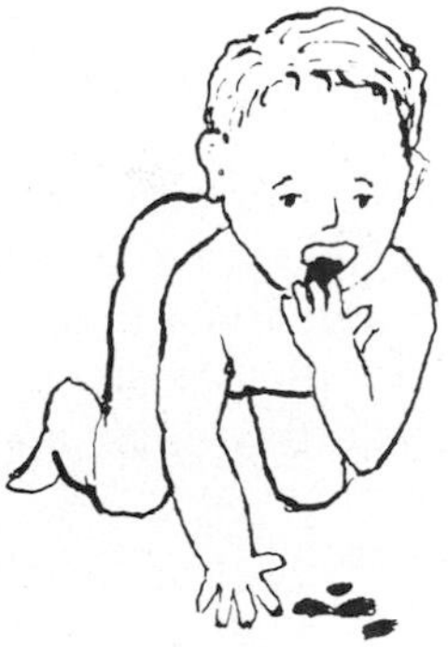

Common causes:

- diet poor in iron (p. 124)
- chronic gut infections (p. 145)
- hookworm (p. 142)
- malaria (p. 186)

Prevention and Treatment:

- ♦ Eat iron-rich foods like meat and eggs. Beans, lentils, groundnuts (peanuts), and dark green vegetables also have some iron.
- ♦ Treat the cause of anemia—and do not go barefoot if hookworm is common.
- ♦ If you suspect hookworm, a health worker may be able to look at the child's stools under a microscope. If hookworm eggs are found, treat for hookworm (p. 374 to 376).
- ♦ If necessary, give iron salts by mouth (ferrous sulfate, p. 393).

CAUTION: **Do not give iron tablets to a baby or small child. They could poison her. Instead, give iron as a liquid. Or crush a tablet into powder and mix it with food.**

Worms and Other Parasites of the Gut (see p. 140)

If one child in the family has worms, all the family should be treated. To prevent worm infections, children should:

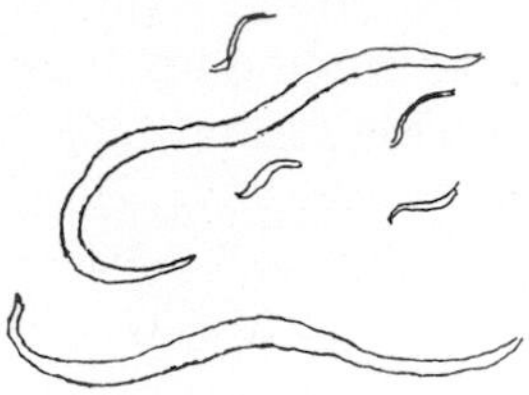

- Observe the Guidelines of Cleanliness (p. 133).
- Use latrines.
- Never go barefoot.
- Never eat raw or partly raw meat or fish.
- Drink only boiled or pure water.

Skin Problems (see Chapter 15)

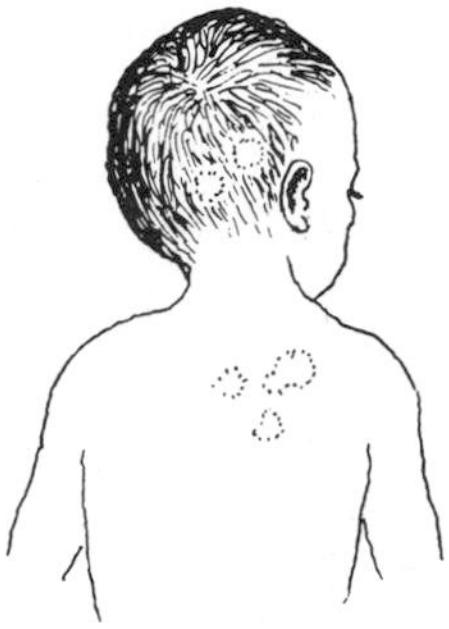

Those most common in children include:

- scabies (p. 199)
- infected sores and impetigo (p. 201 and 202)
- ringworm and other fungus infections (p. 205)

To prevent skin problems, observe the Guidelines of Cleanliness (p. 133).

- Bathe and delouse children often.
- Control bedbugs, lice, and scabies.
- Do not let children with scabies, lice, ringworm, or infected sores play or sleep together with other children. Treat them early.

Pink Eye (Conjunctivitis) (see p. 219)

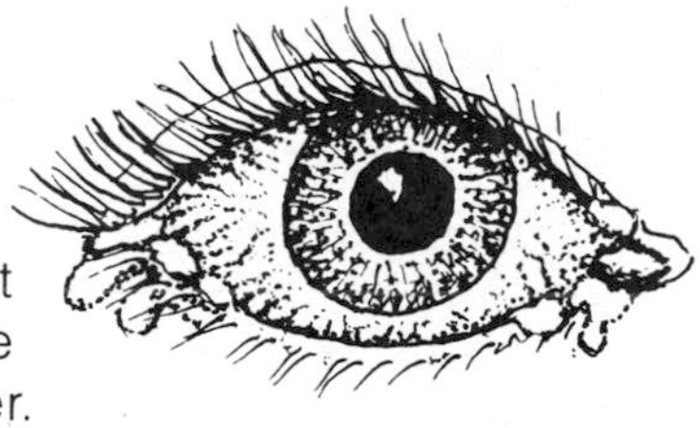

Wipe the eyelids clean with a clean wet cloth several times a day. Put an antibiotic eye ointment (p. 379) **inside** the eyelids 4 times a day. Do not let a child with pink eye play or sleep with others. If he does not get well in a few days, see a health worker.

Colds and the 'Flu' (see p. 163)

The common cold, with runny nose, mild fever, cough, often sore throat, and sometimes diarrhea is a frequent but not a serious problem in children.

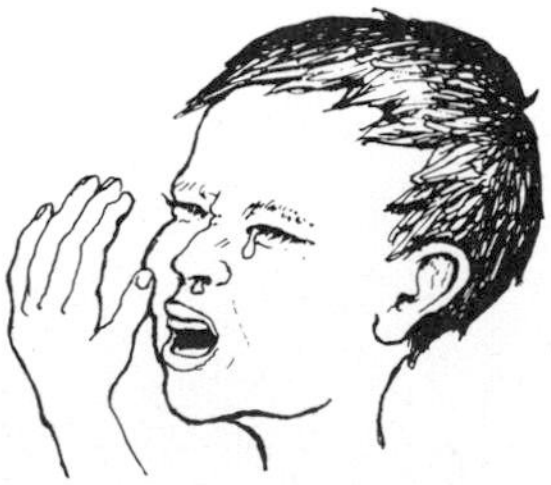

Treat with lots of liquids. Give acetaminophen or perhaps aspirin (see p. 379). Let children who want to stay in bed do so. Good food and lots of fruit help children avoid colds and get well quickly.

Penicillin, tetracycline, and other antibiotics do no good for the common cold or 'flu'. Injections are not needed for colds.

If a child with a cold becomes very ill, with high fever and shallow, rapid breathing, he may be getting **pneumonia** (see p. 171), and antibiotics should be given. Also watch for an ear infection (next page) or 'strep throat' (p. 310).

HEALTH PROBLEMS OF CHILDREN NOT DISCUSSED IN OTHER CHAPTERS

Earache and Ear Infections

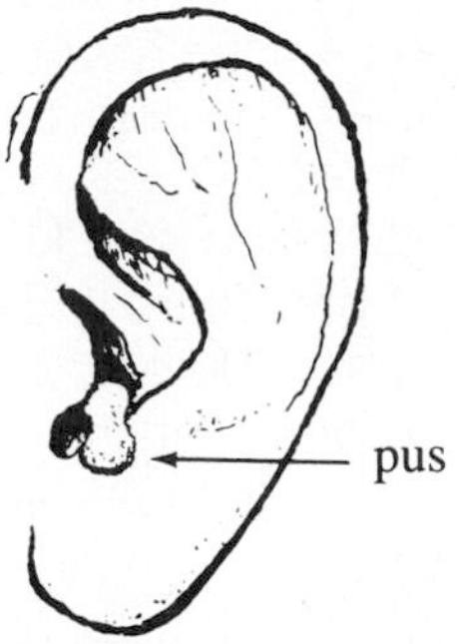

Ear infections are common in small children. The infection often begins after a few days with a cold or a stuffy or plugged nose. The fever may rise, and the child often cries or rubs the side of his head. Sometimes pus can be seen in the ear. In small children an ear infection sometimes causes vomiting or diarrhea. So when a child has diarrhea and fever be sure to check his ears.

Treatment:

- It is important to treat ear infections early. Give an antibiotic like penicillin (p. 351) or co-trimoxazole (p. 358). In children under 3 years of age, ampicillin (p. 353) often works better. Give acetaminophen (p. 380) for pain. Aspirin also works but is less safe (see p. 379).
- Carefully clean pus out of the ear with cotton, but do not put a plug of cotton, a stick, leaves, or anything else in the ear.
- Children with pus coming from an ear should bathe regularly but should not swim or dive for at least 2 weeks after they are well.

Prevention:

- Teach children to wipe but **not** to blow their noses when they have a cold.
- Do not bottle feed babies—or if you do, do not let a baby feed lying on his back, as the milk can go up his nose and lead to an ear infection.
- When children's noses are plugged up, use salt drops and suck the mucus out of the nose as described on p. 164.

Infection in the ear canal:

To find out whether the canal or tube going into the ear is infected, gently pull the ear. If this causes pain, the canal is infected. Put drops of water with vinegar in the ear 3 or 4 times a day. (Mix 1 spoon of vinegar with 1 spoon of boiled water.) If there is fever or pus, also use an antibiotic.

Sore Throat and Inflamed Tonsils

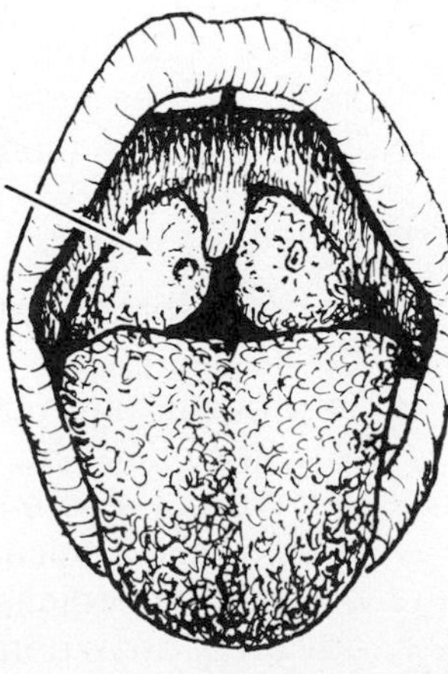

These problems often begin with the common cold. The throat may be red and hurt when the child swallows. The tonsils (two lymph nodes seen as lumps on each side at the back of the throat) may become large and painful or drain pus. Fever may reach 40°.

Treatment:

- Gargle with warm salt water (1 teaspoon of salt in a glass of water).
- Take acetaminophen or aspirin for pain.
- If pain and fever come on suddenly or continue for more than 3 days, see the following page.

Sore throat and the danger of rheumatic fever:

For the sore throat that often comes with the common cold or flu, antibiotics should usually not be used and will do no good. Treat with gargles and acetaminophen (or aspirin).

However, one kind of sore throat—called **strep throat**—should be treated with penicillin. It is most common in children and young adults. It usually begins suddenly with severe sore throat and high fever, often without signs of a cold or cough. The back of the mouth and tonsils become very red, and the lymph nodes under the jaw or in the neck may become swollen and tender.

Give penicillin (p. 351) for 10 days. If penicillin is given early and continued for 10 days, there is less danger of getting rheumatic fever. A child with strep throat should eat and sleep far apart from others, to prevent their getting it also.

Rheumatic Fever

This is a disease of children and young adults. It usually begins 1 to 3 weeks after the person has had a strep throat (see above).

Principal signs (usually only 3 or 4 of these signs are present):

- fever
- joint pain, especially in the wrists and ankles, later the knees and elbows. Joints become swollen, and often hot and red.

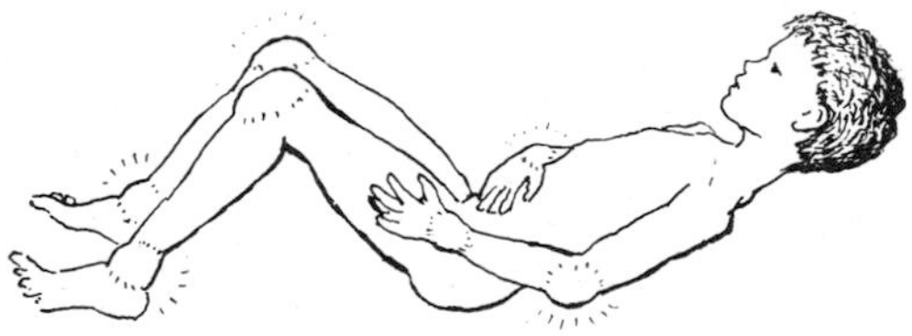

- curved red lines or lumps under the skin
- in more serious cases, weakness, shortness of breath, and perhaps heart pain

Treatment:

- If you suspect rheumatic fever, see a health worker. There is a risk that the heart may become damaged.
- Take aspirin in large doses (p. 380). A 12-year-old can take up to 2 or 3 tablets of 300 mg. 6 times a day. Take them together with milk or food to avoid stomach pain. If the ears begin to ring, take less.
- Give penicillin (see p. 351).

Prevention:

- To prevent rheumatic fever, treat 'strep throat' early with penicillin—for 10 days.
- To prevent return of rheumatic fever, and added heart damage, a child who has once had rheumatic fever should take penicillin for 10 days at the first sign of a sore throat. If he already shows signs of heart damage, he should take penicillin on a regular basis or have monthly injections of benzathine penicillin (p. 353) perhaps for the rest of his life. Follow the advice of an experienced health worker or doctor.

INFECTIOUS DISEASES OF CHILDHOOD

Chickenpox

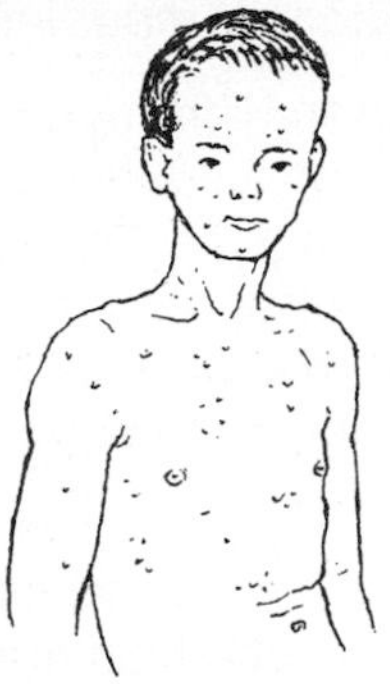

This mild virus infection begins 2 to 3 weeks after a child is exposed to another child who has the disease.

Signs:

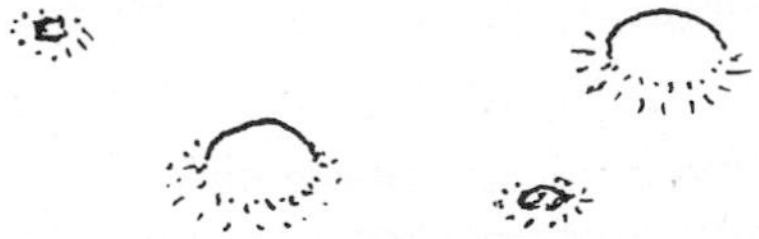

spots, blisters, and scabs

First many small, red, itchy spots appear. These turn into little pimples or blisters that pop and finally form scabs. Usually they begin on the body, and later on the face, arms, and legs. There may be spots, blisters, and scabs, all at the same time. Fever is usually mild.

Treatment:

The infection usually goes away in a week. Bathe the child daily with soap and warm water. To calm itching, apply cool cloths soaked in water from boiled and strained oatmeal. Cut fingernails very short. If the scabs get infected, keep them clean. Apply hot, wet compresses, and put an antibiotic ointment on them. Try to keep the child from scratching.

Measles

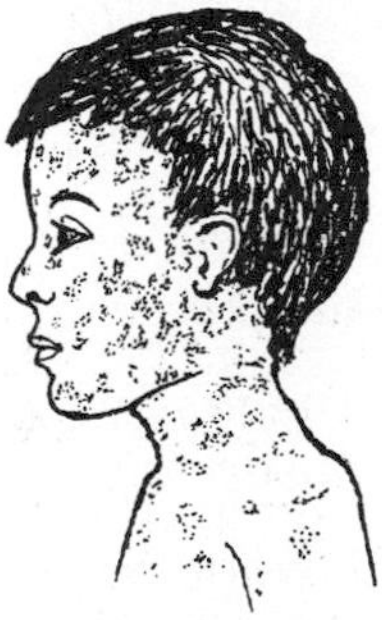

This severe virus infection is **especially dangerous in children** who are **poorly nourished** or have **tuberculosis.** Ten days after being near a person with measles, it begins with signs of a cold—fever, runny nose, red sore eyes, and cough.

The child becomes increasingly ill. The mouth may become very sore and he may develop diarrhea.

After 2 or 3 days a few tiny white spots like salt grains appear in the mouth. A day or 2 later the rash appears—first behind the ears and on the neck, then on the face and body, and last on the arms and legs. After the rash appears, the child usually begins to get better. The rash lasts about 5 days. Sometimes there are scattered black spots caused by bleeding into the skin ('black measles'). This means the attack is very severe. Get medical help.

Treatment:

- The child should stay in bed, drink lots of liquids, and be given nutritious food. If she cannot swallow solid food, give her liquids like soup. If a baby cannot breast feed, give breast milk in a spoon (see p. 120).
- If possible, give vitamin A to prevent eye damage (p. 392).
- For fever and discomfort, give acetaminophen (or aspirin).
- If earache develops, give an antibiotic (p. 351).
- If signs of pneumonia, meningitis, or severe pain in the ear or stomach develop, get medical help.
- If the child has diarrhea, give Rehydration Drink (p. 152).

Prevention of measles:

Children with measles should keep far away from other children, even from brothers and sisters. Especially try to protect children who are poorly nourished or who have tuberculosis or other chronic illnesses. Children from other families should not go into a house where there is measles. If children in a family where there is measles have not yet had measles themselves, they should not go to school or into stores or other public places for 10 days.

To prevent measles from killing children, make sure all children are well nourished. Have your children vaccinated against measles when they are 8 to 14 months of age.

German Measles

German measles are not as severe as regular measles. They last 3 or 4 days. The rash is mild. Often the lymph nodes on the back of the head and neck become swollen and tender.

The child should stay in bed and take acetaminophen or aspirin if necessary.

Women who get German measles in the first 3 months of pregnancy may give birth to a child who is damaged or deformed. For this reason, **pregnant women** who have not yet had German measles—or are not sure—**should keep far away** from children who have this kind of measles. Girls or women who are not pregnant can try to catch German measles before they get pregnant. Vaccine exists for German measles, but is not often available.

Mumps

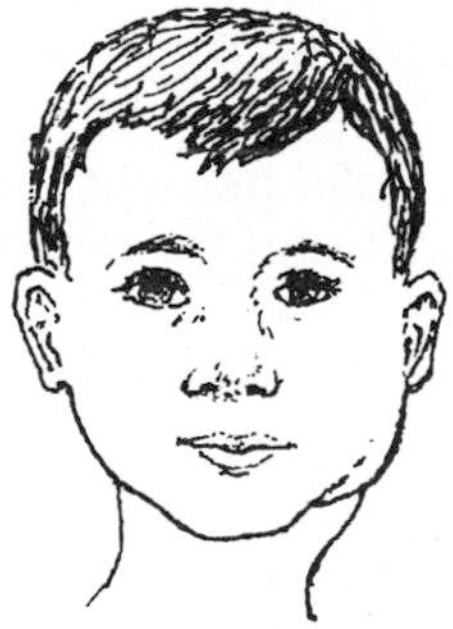

The first symptoms begin 2 or 3 weeks after being exposed to someone with mumps.

Mumps begin with fever and pain on opening the mouth or eating. In 2 days, a soft swelling appears below the ears at the angle of the jaw. Often it comes first on one side, and later on the other side.

Treatment:

The swelling goes away by itself in about 10 days, without need for medicine. Acetaminophen or aspirin can be taken for pain and fever. Feed the child soft, nourishing foods and keep his mouth clean.

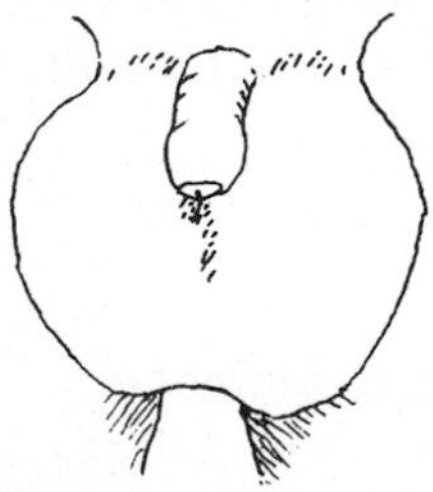

Complications:

In adults and children over 11 years of age, after the first week there may be pain in the belly or a painful swelling of the testicles in men. Persons with such swelling should stay quiet and put ice packs or cold wet cloths on the swollen parts to help reduce the pain and swelling.

If signs of meningitis appear, get medical help (p. 185).

Whooping Cough

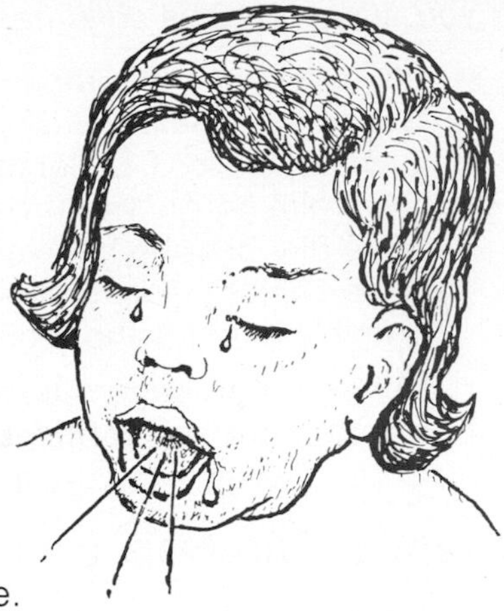

Whooping cough begins a week or two after being exposed to a child who has it. It starts like a cold with fever, a runny nose, and cough.

Two weeks later, the whoop begins. The child coughs rapidly many times without taking a breath, until she coughs up a plug of sticky mucus, and the air rushes back into her lungs with a loud whoop. While she is coughing, her lips and nails may turn blue for lack of air. After the whoop, she may vomit. Between coughing spells the child seems fairly healthy.

Whooping cough often lasts 3 months or more.

Whooping cough is **especially dangerous in babies** under 1 year of age, so vaccinate children early. Small babies do not develop the typical whoop so it is hard to be sure if they have whooping cough or not. If a baby gets fits of coughing and swollen or puffy eyes when there are cases of whooping cough in your area, treat her for whooping cough **at once.**

Treatment:

- Antibiotics are helpful only in the early stage of whooping cough, before the whoop begins. Use erythromycin (p. 355) or ampicillin (p. 353). Chloramphenicol also helps but is more risky. For the dosage for babies, see p. 358. It is especially important to treat babies under 6 months at the first sign.
- In severe cases of whooping cough, phenobarbital (p. 389) may help, especially if the cough does not let the child sleep or causes convulsions.
- If the baby stops breathing after a cough, turn her over and pull the sticky mucus from her mouth with your finger. Then slap her on the back with the flat of your hand.
- To avoid weight loss and malnutrition, be sure the child gets enough nutritious food. Have her eat and drink shortly after she vomits.

Complications:

A bright red hemorrhage (bleeding) inside the white of the eyes may be caused by the coughing. No treatment is necessary (see p. 224). If fits or signs of pneumonia develop (p. 171), get medical help.

Protect all children against whooping cough.
See that they are first vaccinated at 2 months of age.

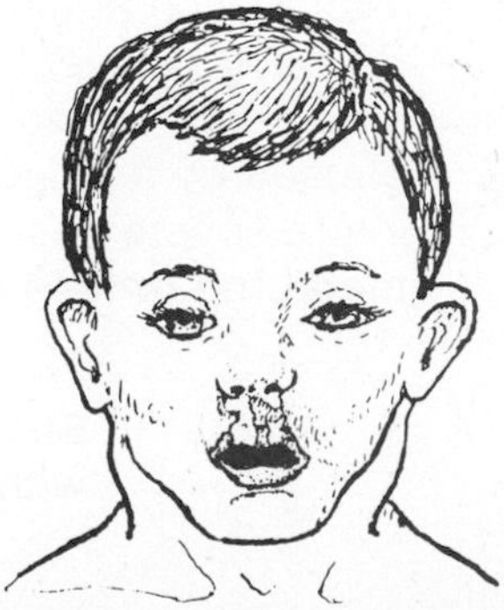

Diphtheria

This begins like a cold with fever, headache, and sore throat. A yellow-gray coating or *membrane* may form in the back of the throat, and sometimes in the nose and on the lips. The child's neck may become swollen. His breath smells very bad.

If you suspect that a child has diphtheria:

- Put him to bed in a room separate from other persons.
- Get medical help quickly. There is special antitoxin for diphtheria.
- Give penicillin, 1 tablet of 400,000 units, 3 times a day for older children.
- Have him gargle warm water with a little salt.
- Have him breathe hot water vapors often or continually (p. 168).
- If the child begins to choke and turn blue, try to remove the membrane from his throat using a cloth wrapped around your finger.

Diphtheria is a dangerous disease that can easily be prevented with the DPT vaccine. **Be sure your children are vaccinated.**

Infantile Paralysis (Polio, Poliomyelitis)

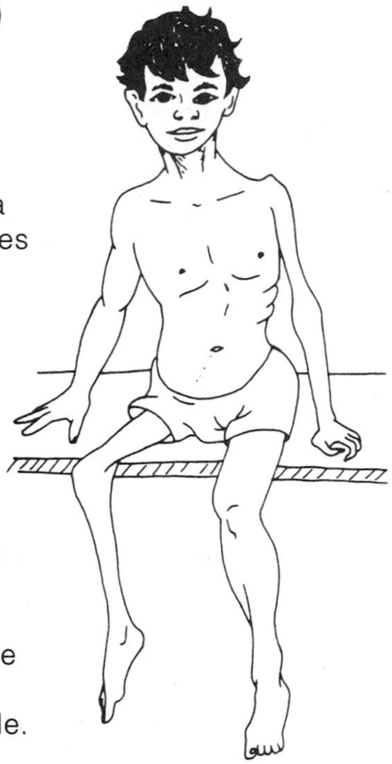

Polio is most common in children under 2 years of age. It is caused by a virus infection similar to a cold, often with fever, vomiting, diarrhea, and sore muscles. Usually the child gets completely well in a few days. But sometimes a part of the body becomes weak or paralyzed. Most often this happens to one or both legs. In time, the weak limb becomes thin and does not grow as fast as the other one.

Treatment:

Once the disease has begun, no medicine will correct the paralysis. (However, sometimes part or all of the lost strength slowly returns.) Antibiotics do not help. For early treatment, calm the pain with acetaminophen or aspirin and put hot soaks on painful muscles. Position the child to be comfortable and avoid ***contractures.*** Gently straighten his arms and legs so that the child lies as straight as possible. Put cushions under his knees, if necessary to reduce pain, but try to keep his knees straight.

Prevention:

- Vaccination against polio is the best protection.
- Do not give injections of any medicine to a child with signs of a cold, fever, or other signs that might be caused by the polio virus. The irritation caused by an injection could turn a mild case of polio without paralysis into a severe case, with paralysis. **Never inject children with any medicine unless it is absolutely necessary.**

See that children are vaccinated against polio, with 'polio drops' at 2, 3, AND 4 months of age.

A child who has been paralyzed by polio should eat nutritious food and do exercises to strengthen remaining muscles.

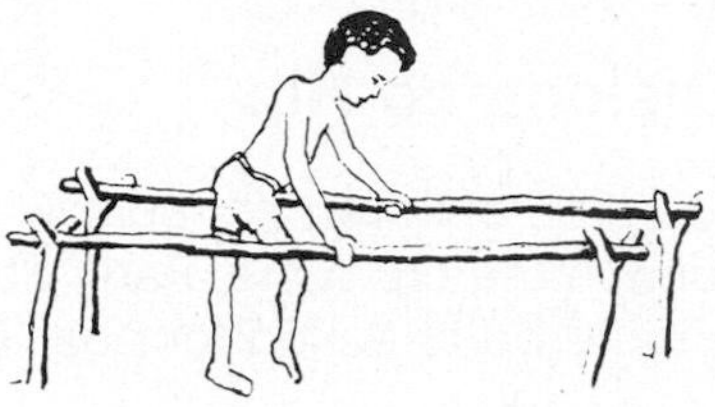

Help the child learn to walk as best he can. Fix 2 poles for support, like these, and later make him some crutches. Leg braces (calipers), crutches, and other aids may help the child to move better and may prevent deformities.

For more information on polio and other childhood disabilities, see *Disabled Village Children,* also published by The Hesperian Foundation.

HOW TO MAKE SIMPLE CRUTCHES

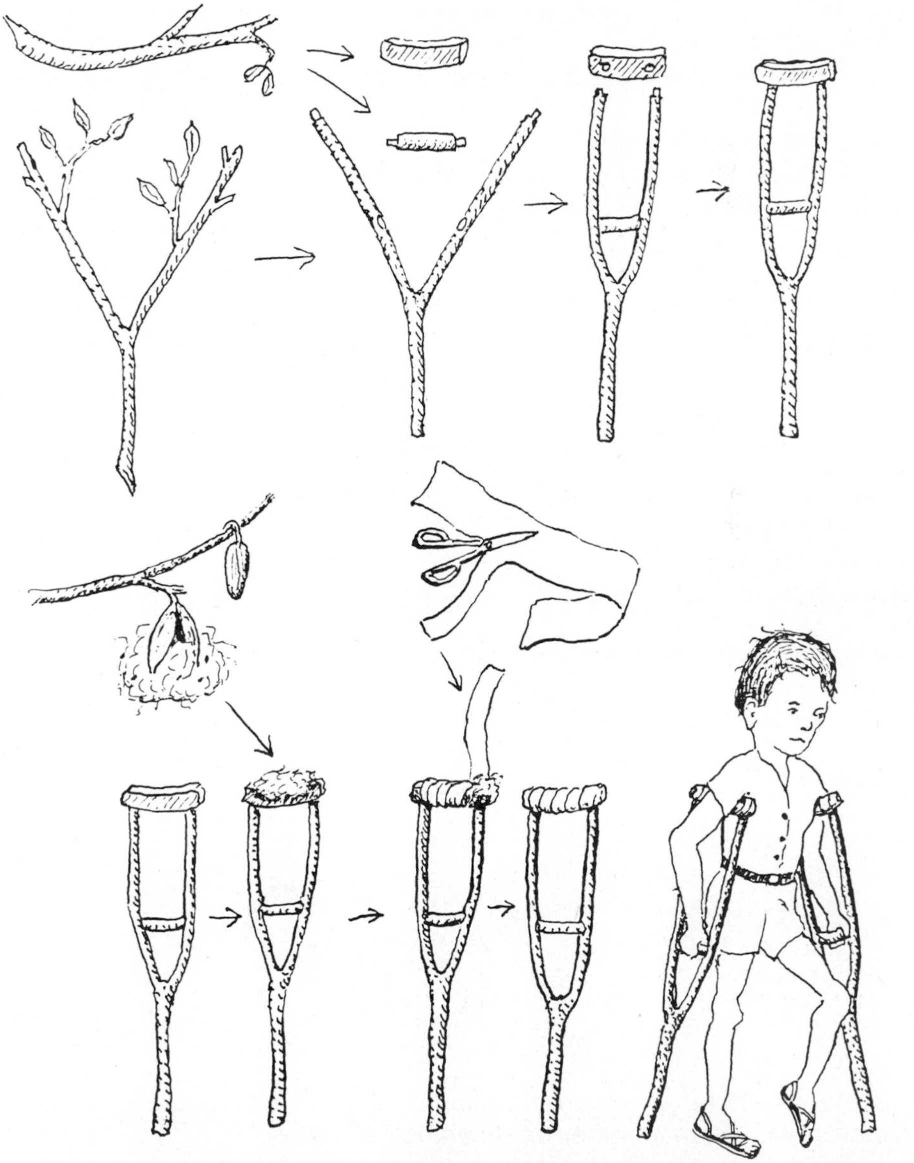

PROBLEMS CHILDREN ARE BORN WITH

Dislocated Hip

Some children are born with a dislocated hip—the leg has slipped out of its joint in the hip bone. Early care can prevent lasting harm and a limp. So babies should be checked for possible hip dislocation at about 10 days after birth.

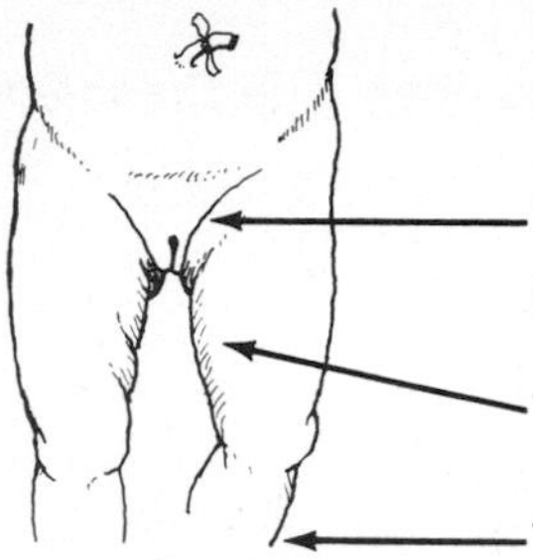

1. Compare the 2 legs. If one hip is dislocated, that side may show:

The upper leg partly covers this part of the body on the dislocated side.

There are fewer folds here.

The leg seems shorter or turns out at a strange angle.

2. Hold both legs with the knees doubled, like this,

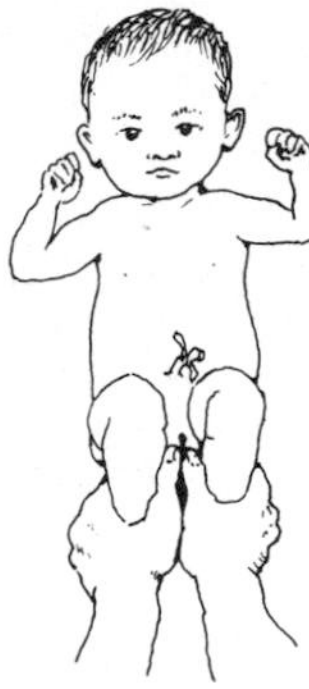

and open them wide like this.

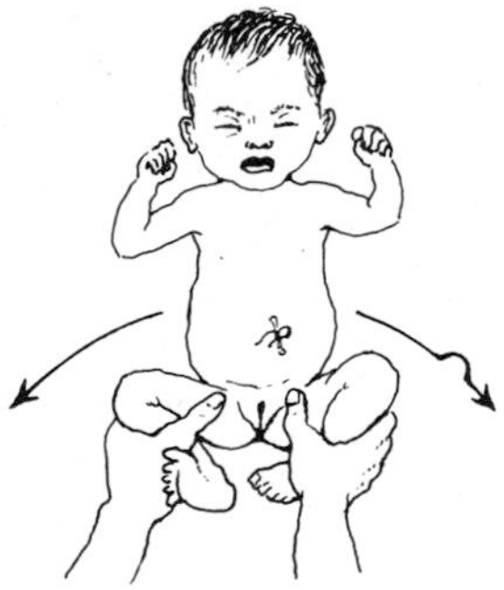

If one leg stops early or makes a jump or click when you open it wide, the hip is dislocated.

Treatment:

Keep the baby with her knees high and wide apart:

by using many thickness of diapers like this,

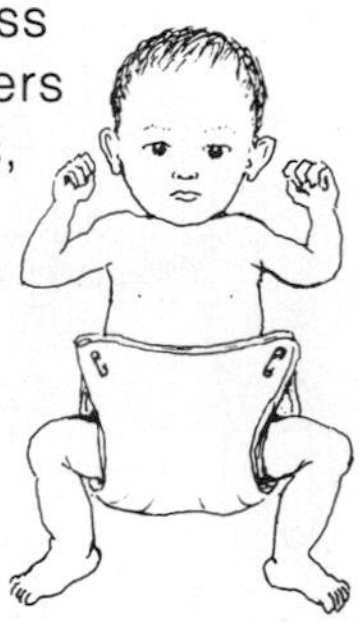

or by pinning her legs like this (when the baby sleeps),

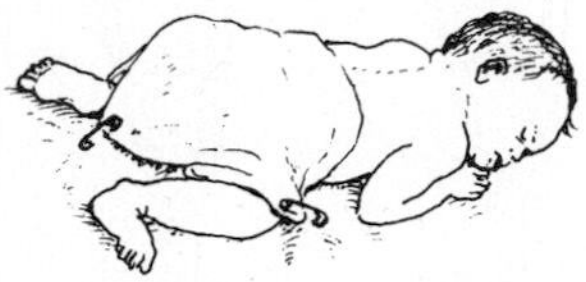

or by doing this.

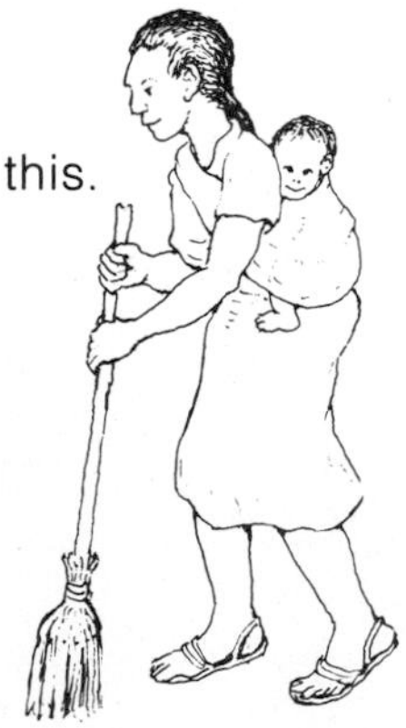

In places where babies are traditionally carried with their legs spread on the woman's hips, often no other treatment is necessary.

Umbilical Hernia (Belly Button that Sticks Out)

A belly button that sticks out like this is no problem. No medicine or treatment is needed. Tying a tight cloth or 'belly band' around the belly will not help.

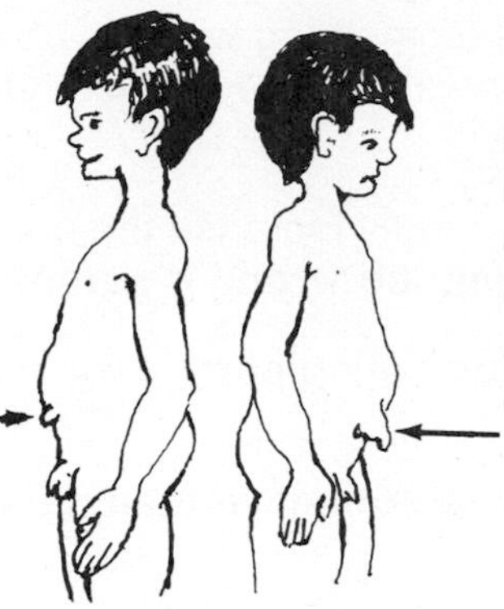

Even a big umbilical hernia like this one is not dangerous and will often go away by itself. If it is still there after age 5, an operation may be needed. Get medical advice.

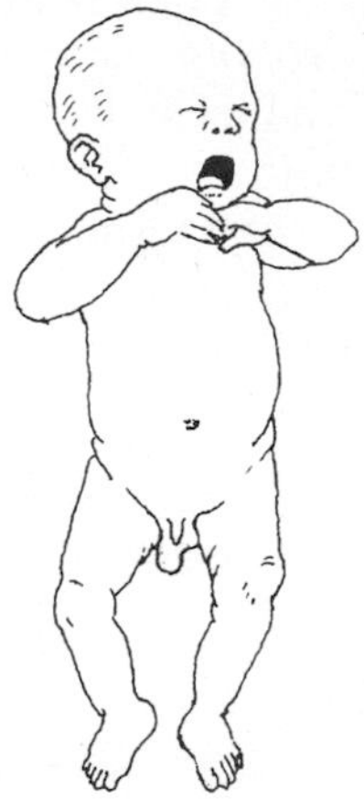

A 'Swollen Testicle' (Hydrocele or Hernia)

If a baby's ***scrotum,*** or bag that holds his testicles, is swollen on one side, this is usually because it is filled with liquid (a hydrocele) or because a loop of gut has slipped into it (a hernia).

To find out which is the cause, shine a light through the swelling.

If light shines through easily, it is probably a **hydrocele.**

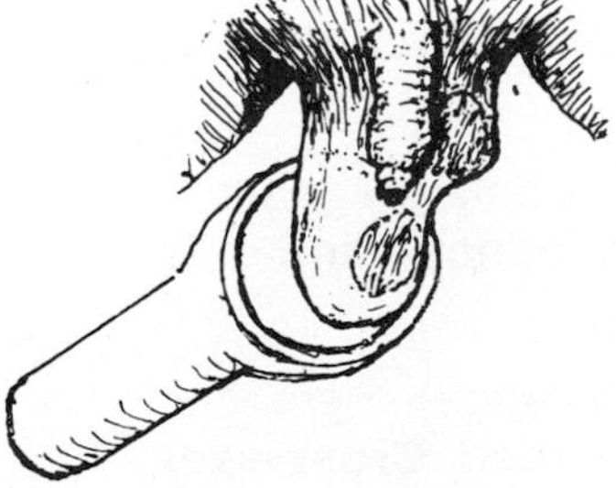

A hydrocele usually goes away in time, without treatment. If it lasts more than a year, get medical advice.

If light does not shine through, and if the swelling gets bigger when the baby coughs or cries, it is a **hernia.**

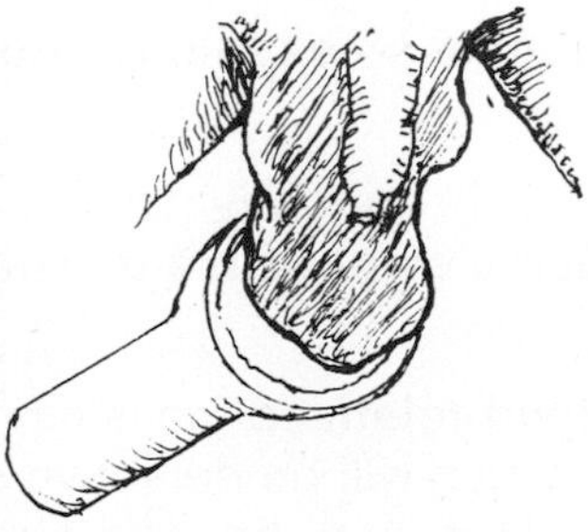

A hernia needs surgery (see p. 177).

Sometimes the **hernia** causes a swelling above and to one side of the baby's scrotum, not in it.

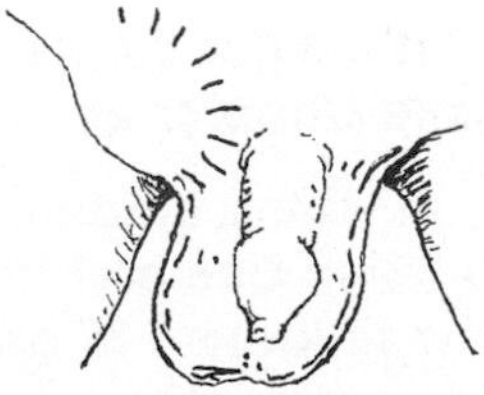

You can tell this from a swollen lymph node (p. 88) because the hernia swells when the baby cries or is held upright and disappears when he lies quietly.

MENTALLY SLOW, DEAF, OR DEFORMED CHILDREN

Sometimes parents will have a child who is born deaf, mentally *retarded* (slow), or with ***birth defects*** (something wrong with part of his body). Often no reason can be found. No one should be blamed. Often it just seems to happen by chance.

However, certain things greatly increase the chance of birth defects. **A baby is less likely to have something wrong if parents take certain precautions.**

1. **Lack of nutritious food** during pregnancy can cause mental slowness or birth defects in babies.

To have healthy babies, pregnant women must eat enough nutritious food (see p. 110).

2. **Lack of iodine** in a pregnant woman's diet can cause *cretinism* in her baby. The baby's face is puffy, and he looks dull. His skin and eyes may remain yellow (jaundiced) for a long time after he is born. His tongue hangs out, and his forehead may be hairy. He is weak, feeds poorly, cries little, and sleeps a lot. He is retarded, may be deaf, and usually has an umbilical hernia. He will begin to walk and talk later than normal babies.

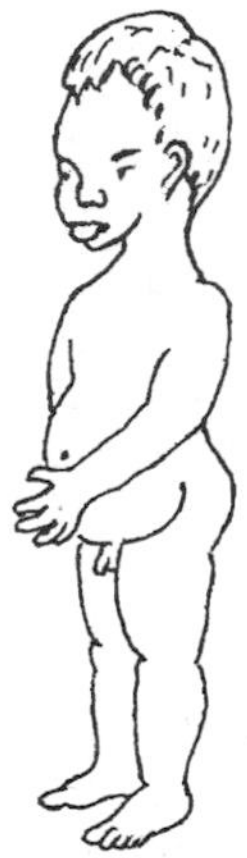
CRETINISM

To help prevent cretinism, pregnant women should use iodized salt instead of ordinary salt (see p. 130).

If you suspect your baby may have cretinism, take him to a health worker or doctor at once. The sooner he gets special medicine (thyroid) the more normal he will be.

3. **Smoking or drinking** of alcoholic drinks during pregnancy causes babies to be born small or to have other problems (see p. 149). **Do not drink or smoke—especially during pregnancy.**

4. **After age 35,** there is more chance that a mother will have a child with defects. *Mongolism* or Down disease, which looks somewhat like cretinism, is more likely to occur in babies of older mothers.

It is wise to plan your family so as to have no more children after age 35 (see Chapter 20).

5. **Many medicines** can harm the baby developing inside a pregnant mother. **Use as little medicine as possible during pregnancy—and only those known to be safe.**

6. **When parents are blood relatives** (cousins, for instance), there is a higher chance that their children will be defective or retarded. **Cross-eyes, extra fingers or toes, club feet, hare lip, and cleft palate** are common defects.

To lower the chance of these and other problems, do not marry a close relative. And if you have more than one child with a birth defect, consider not having more children (see Family Planning, Chapter 20).

If your child is born with a birth defect, take him to a health center. Often something can be done.

- For cross-eyes, see p. 225.

- If an extra finger or toe is very small with no bone in it, tie a string around it very tightly. It will dry up and fall off. If it is larger or has bone in it, either leave it or have it taken off by surgery.

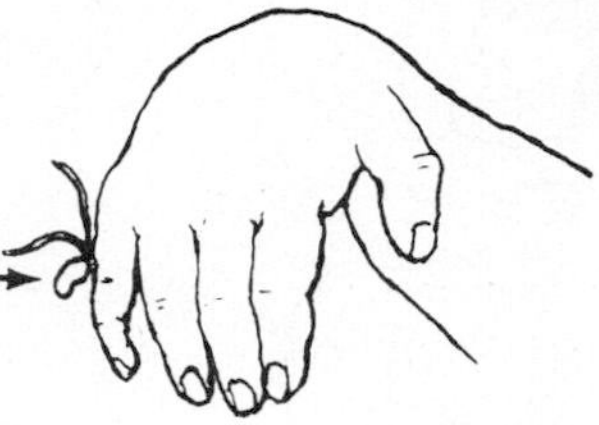

- If a newborn baby's feet are turned inward or have the wrong shape (clubbed), try to bend them to normal shape. If you can do this easily, repeat this several times each day. The feet (or foot) should slowly grow to be normal.

  If you cannot bend the baby's feet to normal, take him **at once** to a health center where his feet can be strapped in a correct position or put in casts. For the best results, it is important to **do this within 2 days after birth.**

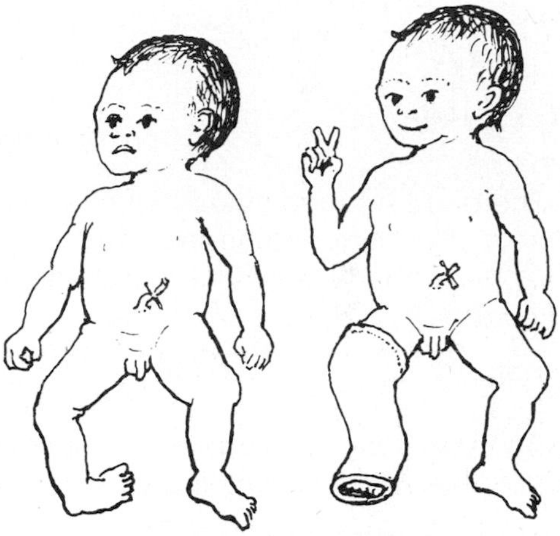

- If a baby's lip or the top of his mouth *(palate)* is divided *(cleft),* he may have trouble breast feeding and need to be fed with a spoon or dropper. With surgery, his lip and palate can be made to look almost normal. The best age for surgery is usually at 4 to 6 months for the lip, and at 18 months for the palate.

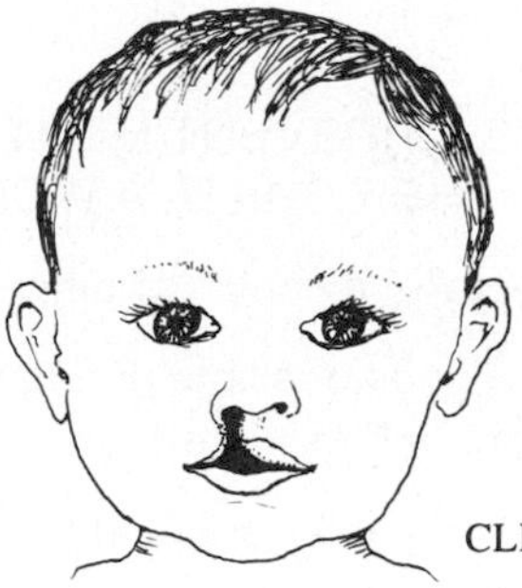
HARE LIP AND CLEFT PALATE

7. **Difficulties before and during birth** sometimes result in **brain damage** that causes a child to be **spastic** or have **fits.** The chance of damage is greater if at birth the baby is slow to breathe, or if the midwife injected the mother with an oxytocic (medicine to speed up the birth or to 'give force' to the mother, p. 266) before the baby was born.

Be careful in your choice of a midwife—and do not let your midwife use an oxytocic before the baby is born.

For more information on children with birth defects, see *Disabled Village Children,* Chapter 12.

The Spastic Child (Cerebral Palsy)

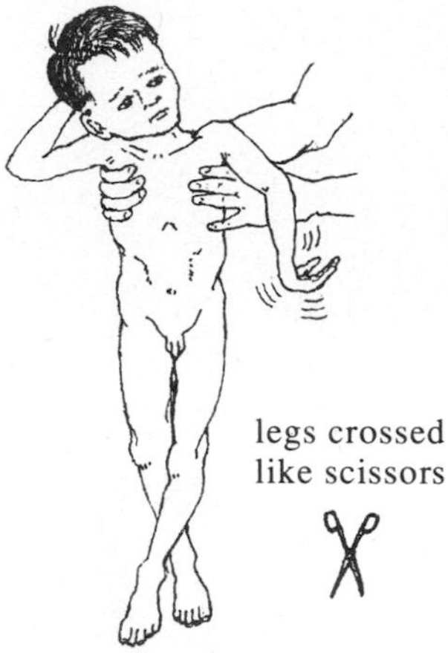

A child who is spastic has tight, stiff muscles that he controls poorly. His face, neck, or body may twist, and his movements may be jerky. Often the tight muscles on the inside of his legs cause them to cross like scissors.

At birth the child may seem normal or perhaps floppy. The stiffness comes as he gets older. He may or may not be mentally slow.

The brain damage that causes cerebral palsy often results from brain damage at birth (when the baby does not breathe soon enough) or from meningitis in early childhood.

There are no medicines that cure the brain damage that makes a child spastic. But the child needs special care. To help prevent tightening of muscles in the legs or in a foot, straighten and bend them **very slowly** several times a day.

Help the child learn to roll over, sit, stand—and if possible to walk (as on p. 314). Encourage him to use both his mind and body as much as he can (see p. 322). Even if he has trouble with speaking he may have a good mind and be able to learn many skills if given a chance. **Help him to help himself.**

For more information on cerebral palsy, see *Disabled Village Children,* Chapter 9.

TO HELP PREVENT MENTAL RETARDATION OR BIRTH DEFECTS IN HER CHILD, A WOMAN SHOULD DO THESE THINGS:

1. Do not marry a cousin or other close relative.
2. Eat as well as possible during pregnancy: as much beans, fruit, vegetables, meat, eggs, and milk products as you can.
3. Use iodized salt instead of regular salt, especially during pregnancy.
4. Do not smoke or drink during pregnancy (see p. 149).
5. While pregnant, avoid medicines whenever possible—use only those known to be safe.
6. While pregnant, keep away from persons with German measles.
7. Be careful in the selection of a midwife—and do not let the midwife use an oxytocic before the child is born (see p. 266).
8. Do not have more children if you have more than one child with the same birth defect (see Family Planning, p. 283).
9. Consider not having more children after age 35.

Retardation in the First Months of Life

Some children who are born healthy do not grow well. Their minds and bodies are slow to develop because they do not eat enough nutritious food. During the first few months of life the brain develops more rapidly than at any other time. For this reason the nutrition of the newborn is of great importance. Breast milk is the best food for a baby (see The Best Diet for Babies, p. 120).

Sickle Cell Disease (Sickle Cell Anemia)

Some children of African origin (or less often from India) are born with a 'weakness of the blood', called sickle cell disease. This disease is passed on from the parents, who often do not know they carry the 'sickle cell' trait. The baby may appear normal for 6 months, then signs may begin to appear.

Signs:

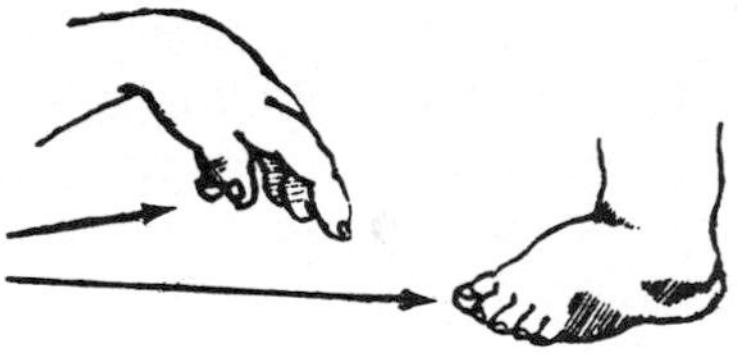

- fever and crying
- occasional swelling of the feet and fingers which lasts for 1 or 2 weeks
- big belly that feels hard at the top
- anemia, and sometimes yellow color in the eyes (jaundice)
- child frequently sick (cough, malaria, diarrhea)
- child grows slowly
- by age 2, bony bumps may appear on the head ('bossing')

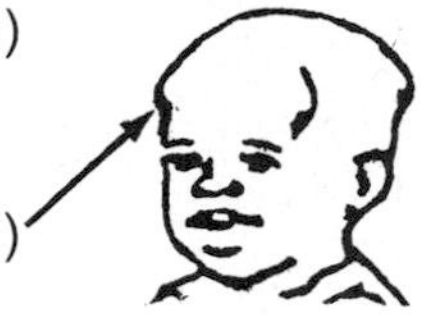

Malaria or other infections can bring on a 'sickle cell crisis' with high fever and severe pain in the arms, legs, or belly. Anemia becomes much worse. Swellings on the bones may discharge pus. The child may die.

Treatment:

There is no way to change the weakness in the blood. Protect the child from malaria and other diseases and infections that can bring on a 'crisis'. Take the child for regular monthly visits to a health worker for an examination and medicines.

- **Malaria.** In areas where malaria is common, the child should have regular malaria medicines to help prevent the disease (see p. 365). Add to this a daily dose of folic acid (p. 393) to help build up the blood. Iron medicine (ferrous sulfate) is not usually necessary.
- **Infections.** The child should be vaccinated against measles, whooping cough, and tuberculosis at the earliest recommended time. If the child shows signs of fever, cough, diarrhea, passing urine too often, or pains in the belly, legs or arms, take him to a health worker as soon as possible. Antibiotics may be necessary. Give plenty of water to drink, and acetaminophen (p. 380) for pain in the bones.
- **Avoid exposure to cold.** Keep warm with a blanket at night when necessary. Use a foam mattress if possible.

HELPING CHILDREN LEARN

As a child grows, she learns partly from what she is taught. Knowledge and skills she learns in school may help her to understand and do more later. School can be important.

But a child does much of her learning at home or in the forest or fields. She learns by watching, listening, and trying for herself what she sees others do. She learns not so much from what people tell her, as from how she sees them act. **Some of the most important things a child can learn—such as kindness, responsibility, and sharing—can only be taught by setting a good example.**

A child learns through adventure. She needs to learn how to do things for herself, even though she makes mistakes. When she is very young, protect a child from danger. But as she grows, help her learn to care for herself. Give her some responsibility. Respect her judgment, even if it differs from your own.

When a child is young, she thinks mostly of filling only her own needs. Later, she discovers the deeper pleasure of helping and doing things for others. Welcome the help of children and let them know how much it means.

Children who are not afraid ask many questions. If parents, teachers, and others take the time to answer their questions clearly and honestly—and to say they do not know when they do not—a child will keep asking questions, and as she grows may look for ways to make her surroundings or her village a better place to live.

Some of the best ideas for helping children learn and become involved in community health care have been developed through the CHILD-to-child Program. This is described in *Helping Health Workers Learn,* Chapter 24.

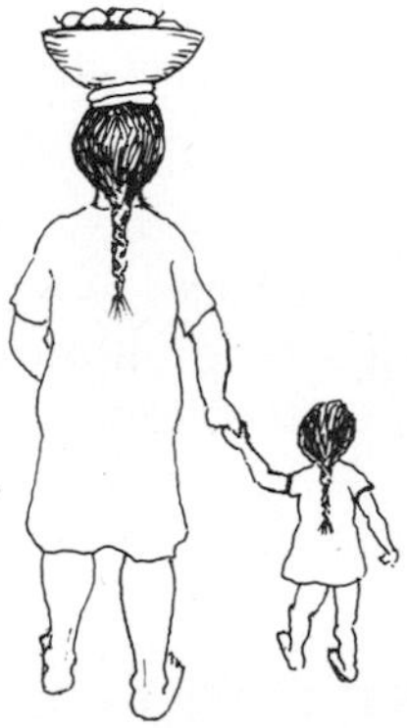

Or write to:

Child-to-child
Institute of Education
20 Bedford Way
London WC1H 0AL
England
Fax: 44-0-207-612-6645
E-mail: c.scotchmer@ioe.ac.uk

CHAPTER

HEALTH AND SICKNESSES OF OLDER PEOPLE

22

This chapter is about the prevention and treatment of problems seen mostly in older persons.

SUMMARY OF HEALTH PROBLEMS DISCUSSED IN OTHER CHAPTERS

Difficulties with Vision (see p. 217)

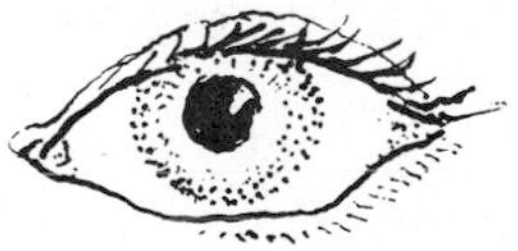

After the age of 40, many people have problems seeing close objects clearly. They are becoming ***farsighted.*** Often glasses will help.

Everyone over age 40 should watch for signs of glaucoma, which can cause blindness if left untreated. Any person with signs of glaucoma (see p. 222) should seek medical help.

Cataracts (see p. 225) and 'flies before the eyes' (tiny moving spots—p. 227) are also common problems of old age.

Weakness, Tiredness, and Eating Habits

Old people understandably have less energy and strength than when they were younger, but they will become even weaker if they do not eat well. Although older people often do not eat very much, they should eat some body-building and protective foods every day (see p. 110 to 111).

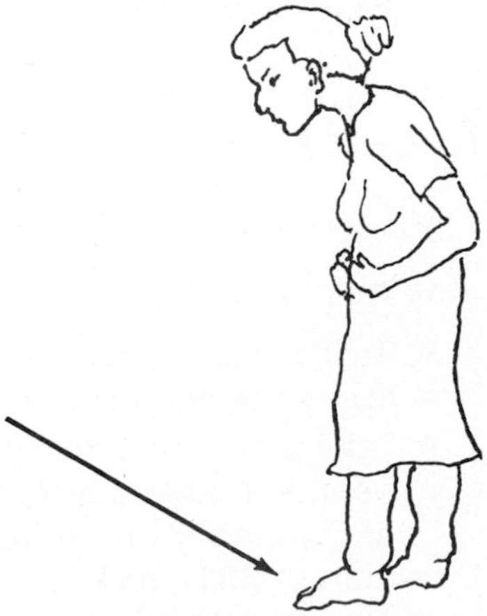

Swelling of the Feet (see p. 176)

This can be caused by many diseases, but in older people it is often caused by poor circulation or heart trouble (see p. 325). Whatever the cause, **keeping the feet up is the best treatment.** Walking helps too—but do not spend much time standing or sitting with the feet down.Keep the feet up whenever possible.

Chronic Sores of the Legs or Feet (see p. 213)

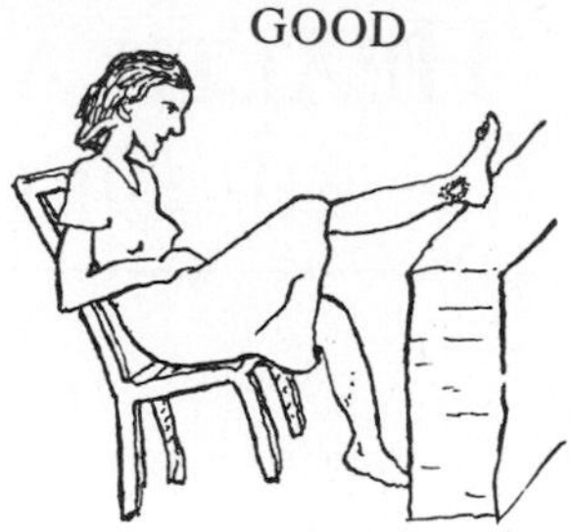

These may result from poor circulation, often because of varicose veins (p. 175). Sometimes diabetes is part of the cause (p. 127). For other possibilities, see page 20.

Sores that result from poor circulation heal very slowly.

Keep the sore as clean as possible. Wash it with boiled water and mild soap and change the bandage often. If signs of infection develop, treat as directed on p. 88.

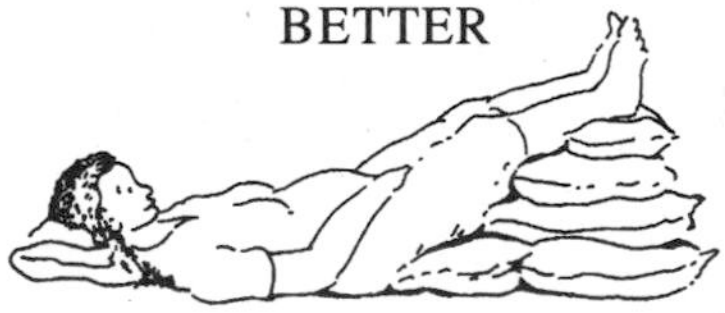

When sitting or sleeping, keep the foot up.

Difficulty Urinating (see p. 235)

Older men who have difficulty urinating or whose urine drips or dribbles are probably suffering from an enlarged prostate gland. Turn to page 235.

Chronic Cough (see p. 168)

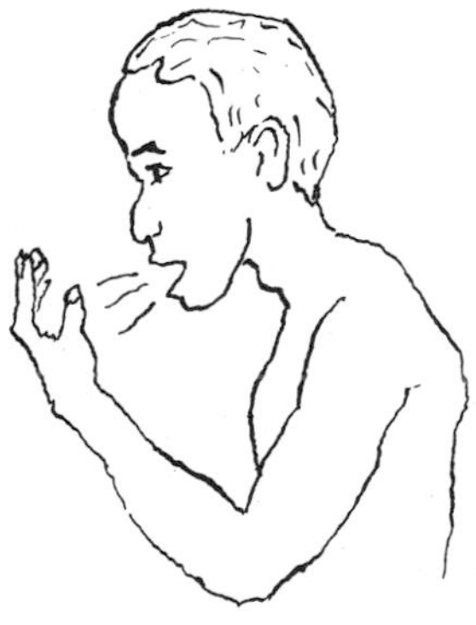

Older people who cough a lot should not smoke and should seek medical advice. If they had symptoms of tuberculosis when they were younger, or have ever coughed up blood, they may have tuberculosis.

If an older person develops a cough with wheezing or trouble breathing (asthma) or if his feet also swell, he may have heart trouble (see the next page).

Rheumatoid Arthritis (painful joints) (see p. 173)

Many older people have arthritis.

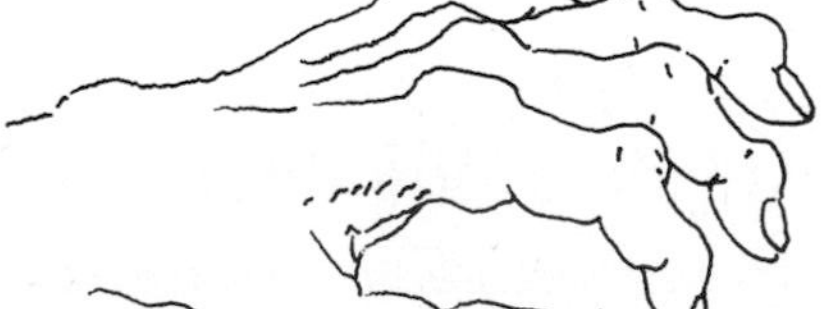

To help arthritis:

- Rest the joints that hurt.
- Apply hot compresses (see p. 195).
- Take a medicine for pain; aspirin is best. For severe arthritis, take 2 to 3 aspirin tablets up to 6 times a day with bicarbonate of soda, an antacid (see p. 381), milk, or a lot of water. (If the ears begin to ring, take less.)
- It is important to do exercises that help maintain as much movement as possible in the painful joints.

OTHER IMPORTANT ILLNESSES OF OLD AGE

Heart Trouble

Heart disease is more frequent in older people, especially in those who are fat, who smoke, or who have high blood pressure.

Signs of heart problems:

- Anxiety and difficulty in breathing after exercise; asthma-like attacks that get worse when the person lies down (cardiac asthma).
- A rapid, weak, or irregular pulse.
- Swelling of the feet—worse in the afternoons.

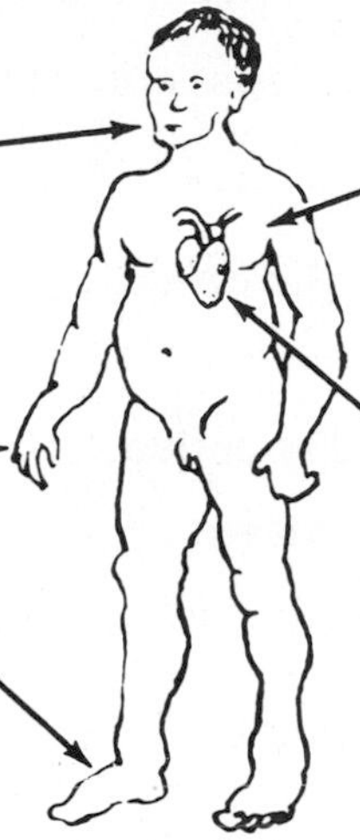

- Sudden, painful attacks in the chest, left shoulder, or arm that occur when exercising and go away after resting for a few minutes (angina pectoris).
- A sharp pain like a great weight crushing the chest; does not go away with rest (heart attack).

Treatment:

- ♦ Different heart diseases may require different specific medicines, which must be used with great care. If you think a person has heart trouble, seek medical help. It is important that he have the right medicine when he needs it.
- ♦ People with heart trouble should not work so hard that they get chest pain or have trouble breathing. However, regular exercise helps prevent a heart attack.
- ♦ Persons with heart problems should not eat greasy food and should lose weight if they are overweight. Also, they should not smoke or drink alcohol.
- ♦ If an older person begins having attacks of difficult breathing or swelling of the feet, he should not use salt or eat food that contains salt. For the rest of his life he should eat little or no salt.
- ♦ Also, taking one aspirin tablet a day may help prevent a heart attack or a stroke.
- ♦ If a person has angina pectoris or heart attack, she should rest very quietly in a cool place until the pain goes away.

If the chest pain is very strong and does not go away with rest, or if the person shows signs of **shock** (see p. 77), the heart has probably been severely damaged. The person should stay in bed for at least a week or as long as she is in pain or shock. Then she can begin to sit up or move slowly, but should stay very quiet for a month or more. Consider getting medical help.

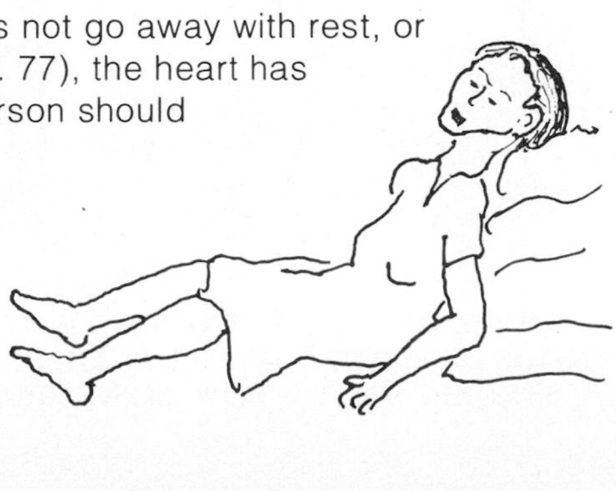

Prevention: See the next page.

Words to Younger Persons Who Want to Stay Healthy When They Are Older

Many of the health problems of middle and old age, including high blood pressure, hardening of the arteries, heart disease, and stroke, result from the way a person has lived and what he ate, drank, and smoked when younger. Your chances for living and staying healthy longer are greater if you:

1. **Eat well**—enough nutritious foods, but not too much rich, greasy, or salty food. Avoid getting overweight or fat. Use vegetable oil rather than animal fat for cooking.
2. **Do not drink a lot of alcoholic drinks.**
3. **Do not smoke.**
4. **Keep physically and mentally active.**
5. **Try to get enough rest and sleep.**
6. **Learn how to relax** and deal positively with things that worry or upset you.

High blood pressure (p. 125) and hardening of the arteries (arteriosclerosis), which are the main causes of heart disease and stroke, can usually be prevented—or reduced—by doing the things recommended above. The lowering of high blood pressure is important in the prevention of heart disease and stroke. Persons who have high blood pressure should have it checked from time to time and take measures to lower it. For those who are not successful in lowering their blood pressure by eating less (if they are overweight), giving up smoking, getting more exercise, and learning to relax, taking medicines to lower blood pressure (antihypertensives) may help.

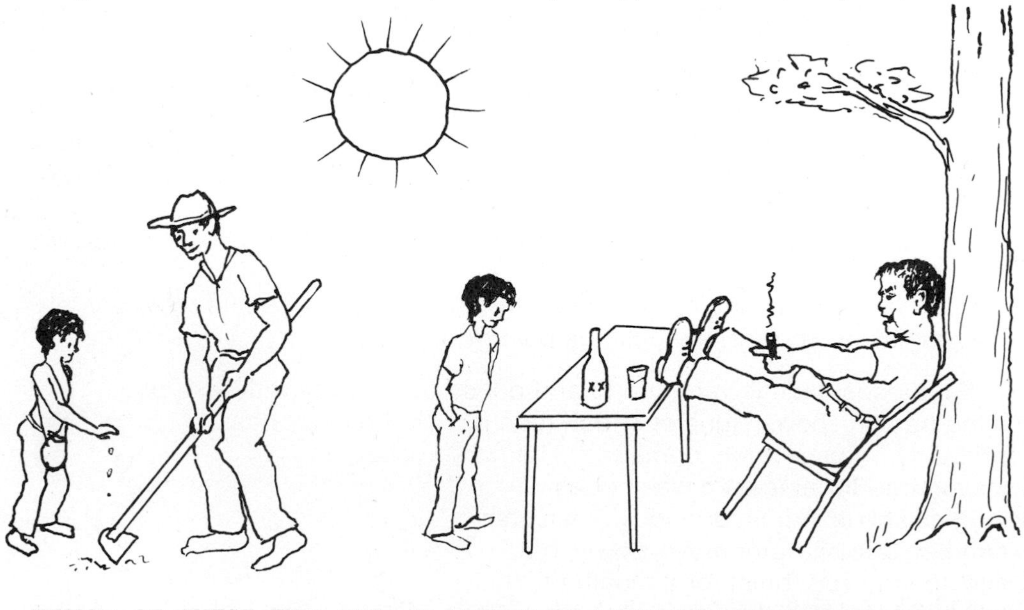

WHICH OF THESE TWO MEN IS LIKELY TO LIVE LONGER AND BE HEALTHY IN HIS OLD AGE? WHICH IS MORE LIKELY TO DIE OF A HEART ATTACK OR A STROKE? WHY? HOW MANY REASONS CAN YOU COUNT?

Stroke (Apoplexy, Cerebro-Vascular Accident, CVA)

In older people ***stroke*** or ***cerebro-vascular accident*** (CVA) commonly results from a blood clot or from bleeding inside the brain. The word ***stroke*** is used because this condition often strikes without warning. The person may suddenly fall down, unconscious. Her face is often reddish, her breathing hoarse and noisy, her pulse strong and slow. She may remain in a coma (unconscious) for hours or days.

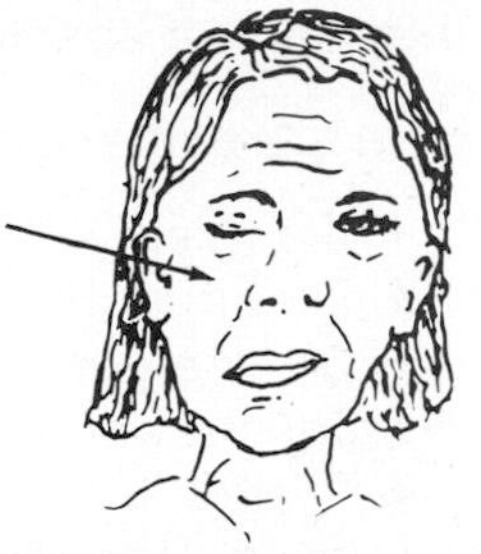

If she lives, she may have trouble speaking, seeing, or thinking, or one side of her face and body may be paralyzed. In minor strokes, some of these same problems may result without loss of consciousness. The difficulties caused by stroke sometimes get better with time.

Treatment:

Put the person in bed with her head a little higher than her feet. If she is unconscious, roll her head back and to one side so her saliva (or vomit) runs out of her mouth, rather than into her lungs. While she is unconscious, give no food, drink, or medicines by mouth (see the Unconscious Person, p. 78). If possible, seek medical help.

After the stroke, if the person remains partly paralyzed, help her to walk with a cane and to use her good hand to care for herself. She should avoid heavy exercise and anger.

Prevention: See the page before this one.

Note: If a younger or middle-aged person suddenly develops paralysis on one side of his face, with no other signs of stroke, this is probably a ***temporary paralysis of the face nerve (Bell's Palsy).*** It will usually go away by itself in a few weeks or months. The cause is usually not known. No treatment is needed but hot soaks may help. If one eye does not close all the way, bandage it shut at night to prevent damage from dryness.

Deafness

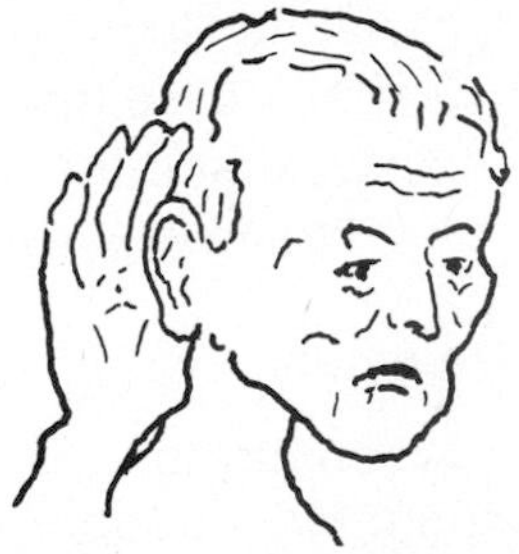

Deafness that comes on gradually without pain or other symptoms occurs most often in men over 40. It is usually incurable, though a hearing aid may help. Sometimes deafness results from ear infections (see p. 309), a head injury, or a plug of dry wax. For information on how to remove ear wax, see p. 405.

DEAFNESS WITH RINGING OF THE EARS AND DIZZINESS

If an older person loses hearing in one or both ears—occasionally with severe dizziness—and hears a loud 'ringing' or buzzing, he probably has Ménière's disease. He may also feel nauseous, or vomit, and may sweat a lot. He should take an antihistamine, such as dimenhydrinate (***Dramamine,*** p. 387) and go to bed until the signs go away. He should have no salt in his food. If he does not get better soon, or if the problem returns, he should seek medical advice.

Loss of Sleep (Insomnia)

It is normal for older people to need less sleep than younger people. And they wake up more often at night. During long winter nights, older people may spend hours without being able to sleep.

Certain medicines may help bring sleep, but it is better not to use them if they are not absolutely necessary.

Here are some suggestions for sleeping:

- Get plenty of exercise during the day.
- Do not drink coffee or black tea, especially in the afternoon or evening.
- Drink a glass of warm milk or milk with honey before going to bed.
- Take a warm bath before going to bed.
- In bed, try to relax each part of your body—then your whole body and mind. Remember good times.
- If you still cannot sleep, try taking an antihistamine like promethazine (*Phenergan,* p. 386) or dimenhydrinate (*Dramamine,* p. 387) half an hour before going to bed. These are less habit-forming than stronger drugs.

DISEASES FOUND MORE OFTEN IN PEOPLE OVER 40 YEARS OLD

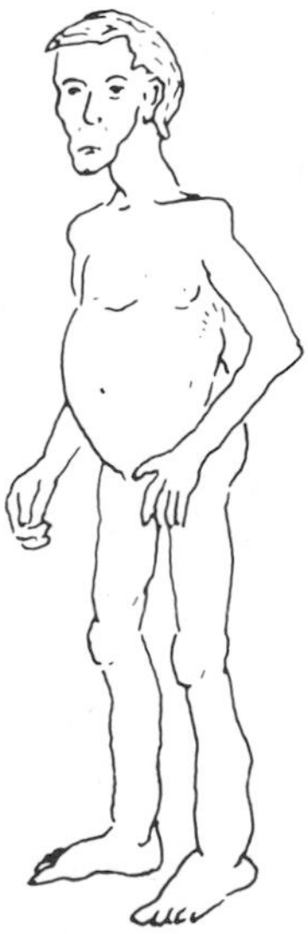

Cirrhosis of the Liver

Cirrhosis usually occurs in men over 40 who for years have been drinking a lot of liquor (alcohol) and eating poorly.

Signs:

- Cirrhosis starts like hepatitis, with weakness, loss of appetite, upset stomach, and pain on the person's right side below the ribs.
- As the illness gets worse, the person gets thinner and thinner. He may vomit blood. In serious cases the feet swell, and the stomach swells with liquid until it looks like a drum. The eyes and skin may turn yellowish (jaundice).

Treatment:

When cirrhosis is severe, it is hard to cure. There are no medicines that help much. Most people with severe cirrhosis die from it. If you want to stay alive, **at the first sign of cirrhosis** do the following:

- Never drink alcohol again! Alcohol poisons the liver.
- Eat as well as possible: vegetables, fruit, and some protein (p. 110 and 111). But do not eat a lot of protein (meat, eggs, fish, etc.) because this makes the damaged liver work too hard.
- If a person with cirrhosis has swelling, he should not use any salt in his food.

Prevention of this disease is easy: **DO NOT DRINK SO MUCH.**

Gallbladder Problems

The gallbladder is a small sac attached to the liver. It collects a bitter, green juice called bile, which helps digest fatty foods. Gallbladder disease occurs most commonly in women over 40 who are overweight and still having menstrual periods.

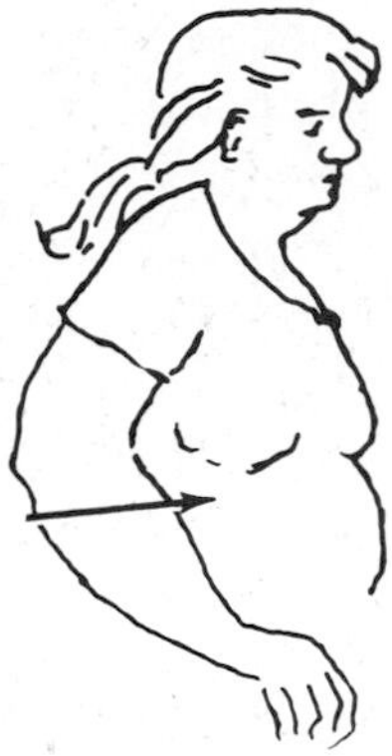

Signs:

- Sharp pain in the stomach at the edge of the right rib cage: This pain sometimes reaches up to the right side of the upper back.
- The pain may come an hour or more after eating rich or fatty foods. Severe pain may cause vomiting.
- Belching or burping with a bad taste.
- Sometimes there is fever.
- Occasionally the eyes may become yellow (jaundice).

Treatment:

- Do not eat greasy food. Overweight (fat) people should eat small meals and lose weight.
- Take an antispasmodic to calm the pain (see p. 381). Strong painkillers are often needed. (Aspirin will probably not help.)
- If the person has a fever, she should take tetracycline (p. 356) or ampicillin (p. 353).
- In severe or chronic cases, seek medical help. Sometimes surgery is needed.

Prevention:

Women (and men) who are overweight should try to lose weight (see p. 126). Avoid rich, sweet, and greasy food, do not eat too much, and get some exercise.

BILIOUSNESS

In many countries and in different languages, bad-tempered persons are said to be 'bilious'. Some people believe that fits of anger come when a person has too much bile.

In truth, most bad-tempered persons have nothing wrong with their gallbladders or bile. However, persons who do suffer from gallbladder disease often live in fear of a return of this severe pain and perhaps for this reason are sometimes short-tempered or continually worried about their health. (In fact, the term 'hypochondria', which means to worry continually about one's own health, comes from 'hypo', meaning under, and 'chondrium', meaning rib—referring to the position of the gallbladder!)

ACCEPTING DEATH

Old people are often more ready to accept their own approaching death than are those who love them. Persons who have lived fully are not usually afraid to die. Death is, after all, the natural end of life.

We often make the mistake of trying to keep a dying person alive as long as possible, no matter what the cost. Sometimes this adds to the suffering and strain for both the person and his family. There are many occasions when the kindest thing to do is not to hunt for 'better medicine' or a 'better doctor' but to be close to and supporting of the person who is dying. Let him know that you are glad for all the time, the joy and the sorrow you have shared, and that you, too, are able to accept his death. In the last hours, love and acceptance will do far more good than medicines.

Old or chronically ill persons would often prefer to be at home, in familiar surroundings with those they love, than to be in a hospital. At times this may mean that the person will die earlier. But this is not necessarily bad. We must be sensitive to the person's feelings and needs, and to our own. Sometimes a person who is dying suffers more knowing that the cost of keeping him barely alive causes his family to go into debt or children to hunger. He may ask simply to be allowed to die—and there are times when this may be the wise decision.

Yet some people fear death. Even if they are suffering, the known world may be hard to leave behind. Every culture has a system of beliefs about death and ideas about life after death. These ideas, beliefs, and traditions may offer some comfort in facing death.

Death may come upon a person suddenly and unexpectedly or may be long-awaited. How to help someone we love accept and prepare for his approaching death is not an easy matter. Often the most we can do is offer support, kindness, and understanding.

The death of a younger person or child is never easy. Both kindness and honesty are important. A child—or anyone—who is dying often knows it, partly by what her own body tells her and partly by the fear or despair she sees in those who love her. Whether young or old, if a person who is dying asks for the truth, tell her, but tell her gently, and leave some room for hope. Weep if you must, but let her know that even as you love her, and because you love her, you have the strength to let her leave you. This will give her the strength and courage to accept leaving you. To let her know these things you need not say them. You need to feel and show them.

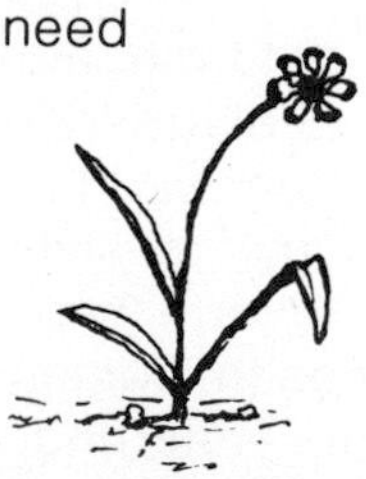

We must all die. Perhaps the most important job of the healer is to help people accept death when it can or should no longer be avoided, and to help ease the suffering of those who still live.

CHAPTER

THE MEDICINE KIT 23

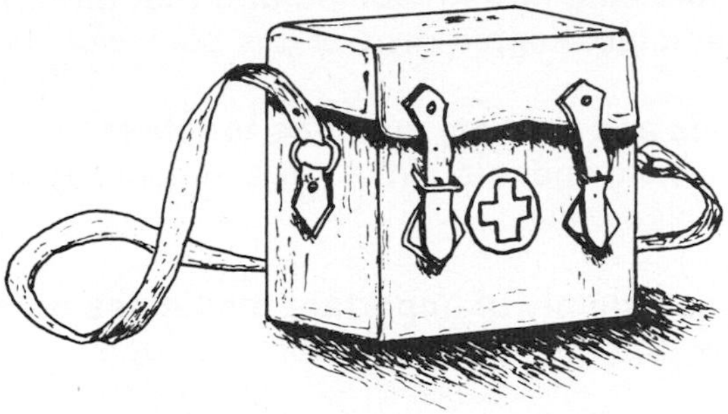

Every family and every village should have certain medical supplies ready in case of emergency:

- The family should have a HOME MEDICINE KIT (see p. 334) with the necessary medicines for first aid, simple infections, and the most common health problems.
- The village should have a more complete medical kit (see VILLAGE MEDICINE KIT, p. 336) with supplies necessary to care for day-to-day problems as well as to meet a serious illness or an emergency. A responsible person should be in charge of it—a health worker, teacher, parent, storekeeper, or anyone who can be trusted by the community. If possible, all members of the village should take part in setting up and paying for the medical kit. Those who can afford more should contribute more. But everyone should understand that **the medicine kit is for the benefit of all**—those who can pay and those who cannot.

On the following pages you will find suggestions for what the medicine kits might contain. You will want to change these lists to best meet the needs and resources in your area. Although the list includes mostly modern medicines, important home remedies known to be safe and to work well can also be included.

How much of each medicine should you have?

The amounts of medicines recommended for the medicine kits are the smallest amounts that should be kept on hand. In some cases there will be just enough to **begin** treatment. It may be necessary to take the sick person to a hospital or go for more medicine at once.

The amount of medicine you keep in your kit will depend on how many people it is intended to serve and how far you have to go to get more when some are used up. It will also depend on cost and how much the family or village can afford. Some of the medicines for your kit will be expensive, but it is wise to have enough of the important medicines on hand to meet emergencies.

Note: **Supplies for birth kits**—the things midwives and pregnant mothers need to have ready for a birth—are listed on pages 254 to 255.

HOW TO CARE FOR YOUR MEDICINE KIT

1. *CAUTION:* **Keep all medicines out of the reach of children.** Any medicine taken in large doses can be poisonous.

2. **Be sure that all medicine is well labeled and that directions for use are kept with each medicine.** Keep a copy of this book with the medicine kit.

3. **Keep all medicines and medical supplies together in a clean, dry, cool place** free from cockroaches and rats. Protect instruments, gauze, and cotton by wrapping them in sealed plastic bags.

4. **Keep an emergency supply of important medicines on hand at all times.** Each time one is used, replace it as soon as possible.

5. **Notice the DATE OF EXPIRATION on each medicine.** If the date has passed or the medicine looks spoiled, destroy it and get new medicine.

Note: Some medicines, especially tetracyclines, may be very dangerous if they have passed their expiration date. However, penicillins in dry form (tablets or powder for syrup or injection) can be used for as long as a year after the expiration date if they have been stored in a clean, dry, and fairly cool place. Old penicillin may lose some of its strength so you may want to increase the dose. (*CAUTION:* While this is safe with penicillin, with other medicines it is often too dangerous to give more than the recommended dose.)

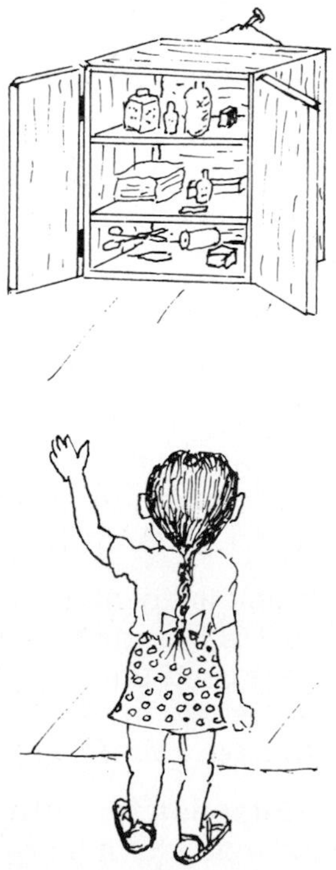

Keep medicines out of reach of children.

BUYING SUPPLIES FOR THE MEDICINE KIT

Most of the medicines recommended in this book can be bought in the pharmacies of larger towns. If several families or the village get together to buy what they need at once, often the pharmacist may sell them supplies at lower cost. Or if medicines and supplies can be bought from a wholesaler, prices will be cheaper still.

If the pharmacy does not supply a brand of medicine you want, buy another brand, but be sure that it is the same medicine and check the dosage.

When buying medicines, compare prices. Some brands are much more expensive than others even though the medicine is the same. More expensive medicines are usually no better. When possible, **buy generic medicines rather than brand-name products,** as the generic ones are often much cheaper. Sometimes you can save money by buying larger quantities. For example, a 600,000-unit vial of penicillin often costs only a little more than a 300,000-unit vial—so buy the large vial and use it for two doses.

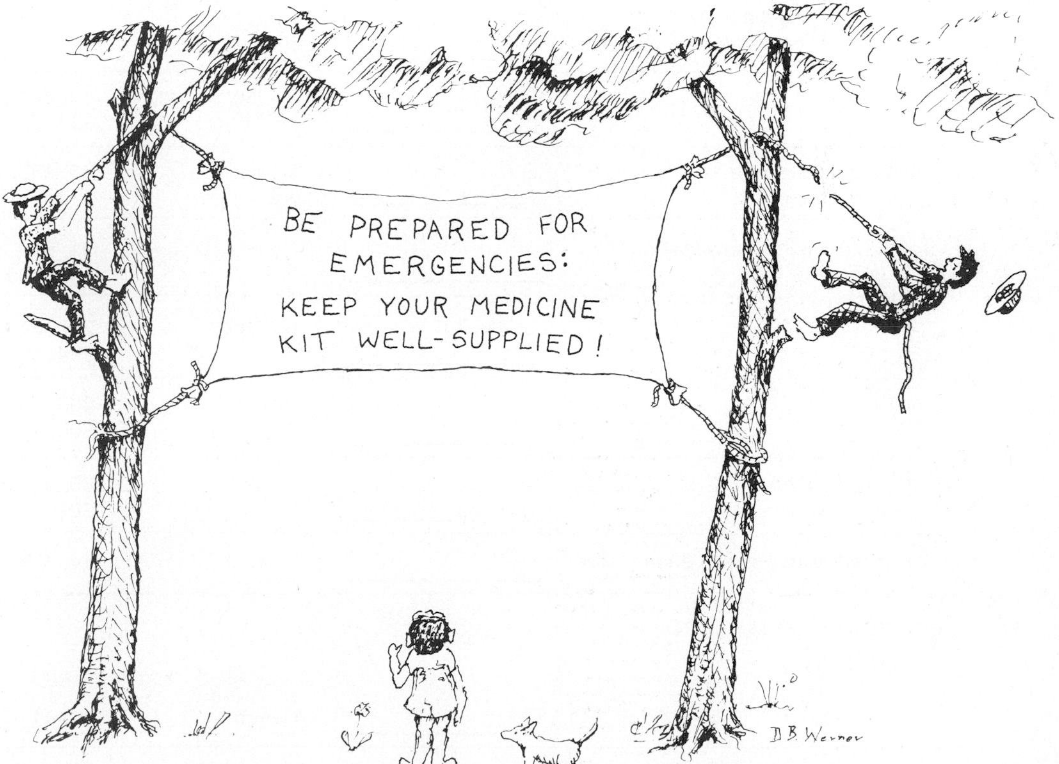
BE PREPARED FOR
EMERGENCIES:
KEEP YOUR MEDICINE
KIT WELL-SUPPLIED!
D.B. Werner

THE HOME MEDICINE KIT

Each family should have the following things in their medicine kit. These supplies should be enough to treat many common problems in rural areas.

Also include useful home remedies in your medicine kit.

SUPPLIES

Use	Supply	Price (write in)	Amount recommended	See page
FOR WOUNDS AND SKIN PROBLEMS:				
	sterile gauze pads in individual sealed envelopes	______	20	97, 218, 263
	1-, 2-, and 3-inch gauze bandage rolls	______	2 each	87
	clean cotton	______	1 small package	14, 72, 83, 254
	adhesive tape (adhesive plaster), 1-inch wide roll	______	2 rolls	85, 218
	soap—if possible a disinfectant soap like ***Betadine***	______	1 bar or small bottle	371
	70% alcohol	______	1/4 liter	72, 201, 211, 254
	hydrogen peroxide, in a dark bottle	______	1 small bottle	83, 183, 213
	petroleum jelly ***(Vaseline)*** in a jar or tube	______	1	91, 97, 141, 199
	white vinegar	______	1/2 liter	200, 241, 294, 309
	sulfur	______	100 gm.	200, 205, 206, 211
	scissors (clean, not rusty)	______	1 pair	85, 254, 262
	tweezers with pointed ends	______	1 pair	84, 175
FOR MEASURING TEMPERATURE:				
	thermometers for mouth for rectum	______	1 each	30, 41
FOR KEEPING SUPPLIES CLEAN:				
	plastic bags	______	several	195, 332

MEDICINES

Use	Medicine (generic name)	Local brand (write in)	Price (write in)	Amount recommended	See page
FOR BACTERIAL INFECTIONS:					
	1. Penicillin, 250 mg. tablets	____	____	40	351
	2. Co-trimoxazole (sulfamethoxazole, 400 mg., with trimethoprim, 80 mg.)	____	____	100	358
	3. Ampicillin, 250 mg. capsules	____	____	24	353
FOR WORMS:					
	4. Mebendazole tablets	____	____	40 tablets of 100 mg. or 2 bottles	374
FOR FEVER AND PAIN:					
	5. Aspirin, 300 mg. (5 grain) tablets	____	____	50	379
	6. Acetaminophen, 500 mg. tablets	____	____	50	380
FOR ANEMIA:					
	7. Iron (ferrous sulfate), 200 mg. pills (best if pills also contain vitamin C and folic acid)	____	____	100	393
FOR SCABIES AND LICE:					
	8. Lindane (gamma benzene hexachloride) and/or sulfur powder	____	____	1 bottle 20 gm.	373
FOR ITCHING AND VOMITING:					
	9. Promethazine, 25 mg. tablets	____	____	12	386
FOR MILD SKIN INFECTIONS:					
	10. Gentian violet, small bottle; or an antibiotic ointment	____	____	1 bottle 1 tube	371
FOR EYE INFECTIONS:					
	11. Antibiotic eye ointment	____	____	1 tube	378

THE VILLAGE MEDICINE KIT

This should have all the medicines and supplies mentioned in the Home Medicine Kit, but in larger amounts, depending on the size of your village and distance from a supply center. The Village Kit should also include the things listed here; many of them are for treatment of more dangerous illnesses. You will have to change or add to the list depending on the diseases in your area.

ADDITIONAL SUPPLIES

Use	Supply	Price	Amount	Page
FOR INJECTING:	syringes, 5 ml.		2	65
	needles #22, 3 cm. long		3–6	
	#25, 1 1/2 cm. long	____	2–4	
FOR TROUBLE URINATING:	catheter (rubber or plastic #16 French)	____	2	239
FOR SPRAINS AND SWOLLEN VEINS:	elastic bandages, 2 and 3 inches wide	____	3–6	102, 175 213
FOR SUCKING OUT MUCUS:	suction bulb	____	1–2	84, 255, 262
FOR LOOKING IN EARS, ETC.:	penlight (small flashlight)	____	1	34, 255, 309

ADDITIONAL MEDICINES

Use	Medicine	Local Brand	Price	Amount	Page
FOR SEVERE INFECTIONS:					
	1. Penicillin, injectable; if only one, procaine penicillin 600,000 U. per ml.	________	____	20–40	352
	2. Ampicillin, injectable 250 mg. ampules			20–40	353
	and/or streptomycin 1 gm. vials for combined use with penicillin (if ampicillin is too expensive)	________	____	20–40	354
	3. Tetracycline, capsules or tablets 250 mg.	________	____	40–80	356
FOR AMEBA AND GIARDIA INFECTIONS:					
	4. Metronidazole, 250 mg. tablets	________	____	40–80	369
FOR FITS, TETANUS, AND SEVERE WHOOPING COUGH:					
	5. Phenobarbital 15 mg. tablets			40–80	
	and 200 mg. injections	________	____	15–30	389

Use	Medicine	Local Brand	Price	Amount	Page
FOR SEVERE ALLERGIC REACTIONS AND SEVERE ASTHMA:					
	6. Epinephrine *(Adrenalin)* injections, ampules with 1 mg.			5–10	385
FOR ASTHMA:					
	7. Ephedrine, 15 mg. tablets			20–100	385
FOR SEVERE BLEEDING AFTER CHILDBIRTH:					
	8. Ergonovine, injections of 0.2 mg.			6–12	391

OTHER MEDICINES NEEDED IN MANY BUT NOT ALL AREAS

Use	Medicine	Local Brand	Price	Amount	Page
WHERE DRY EYES (XEROPHTHALMIA) IS A PROBLEM:					
	Vitamin A, 200,000 U. capsules			10–100	392
WHERE TETANUS IS A PROBLEM:					
	Tetanus antitoxin, 50,000 units (Lyophilized if possible)			2–4 bottles	389
WHERE SNAKEBITE OR SCORPION STING IS A PROBLEM:					
	Specific antivenom			2–6	388
WHERE MALARIA IS A PROBLEM:					
	Chloroquine tablets with 150 mg. of base			50–200	365
	(or whatever medicine works best in your area)				365
TO PREVENT OR TREAT BLEEDING IN UNDERWEIGHT NEWBORNS:					
	Vitamin K, injections of 1 mg.			3–6	394

MEDICINES FOR CHRONIC DISEASES

It may or may not be wise to have medicines for chronic diseases such as **tuberculosis, leprosy,** and **schistosomiasis** in the Village Medicine Kit. To be sure a person has one of these diseases, often special tests must be made in a health center, where the necessary medicine can usually be obtained. Whether these and other medicines are included in the village medical supplies will depend on the local situation and the medical ability of those responsible.

VACCINES

Vaccines have not been included in the Village Medicine Kit because they are usually provided by the Health Department. However, a great effort should be made to see that all children are vaccinated as soon as they are old enough for the different vaccines (see p. 147). Therefore, if refrigeration is available, vaccines should be part of the village medical supplies—especially the DPT, polio, and measles vaccines.

WORDS TO THE VILLAGE STOREKEEPER (OR PHARMACIST)

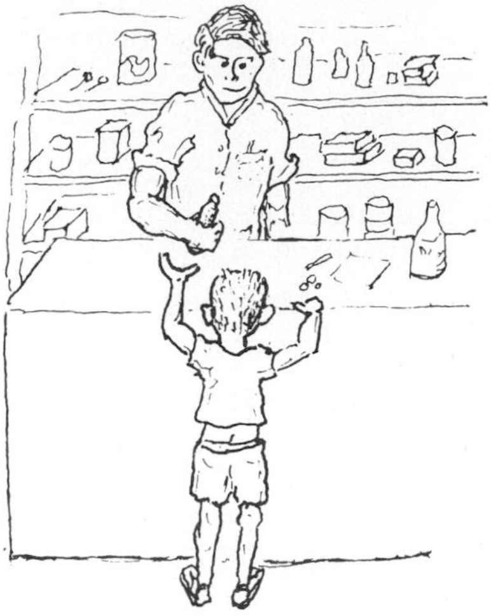

Dear friend,

If you sell medicines in your store, people probably ask you about which medicines to buy and when or how to use them. You are in a position to have an important effect on people's knowledge and health.

This book can help you to give correct advice and to see that your customers buy only those medicines they really need.

As you know, people too often spend the little money they have for medicines that do not help them. But **you** can help them understand their health needs more clearly and spend their money more wisely. For example:

- If people come asking for cough syrups, for a diarrhea-thickener like ***Kaopectate,*** for vitamin B_{12} or liver extract to treat simple anemia, for penicillin to treat a sprain or ache, or for tetracycline when they have a cold, explain to them that these medicines are not needed and may do more harm than good. Discuss with them what to do instead.
- If someone wants to buy a vitamin tonic, encourage him to buy eggs, fruit, or vegetables instead. Help him understand that these have more vitamins and nutritional value for the money.
- If people ask for an injection when medicine by mouth would work as well and be safer—which is usually the case—tell them so.
- If someone wants to buy 'cold tablets' or some other form of 'expensive aspirin' for a cold, encourage him to save money by buying plain aspirin (or acetaminophen) tablets and taking them with lots of liquids.

You may find it easier to tell people these things if you look up the information in this book, and read it together with them.

Above all, sell only useful medicines. Stock your store with the medicines and supplies listed for the Home and Village Medicine Kits, as well as other medicines and supplies that are important for common illnesses in your area. Try to stock low-cost generic products or the least expensive brands. And never sell medicines that are expired, damaged, or useless.

Your store can become a place where people learn about caring for their own health. If you can help people use medicines intelligently, making sure that anyone who purchases a medicine is well informed as to its correct use and dosage, as well as the risks and precautions, you will provide an outstanding service to your community.

Good luck!

Sincerely,

David Werner

THE GREEN PAGES

THE USES, DOSAGE, AND PRECAUTIONS FOR THE MEDICINES REFERRED TO IN THIS BOOK

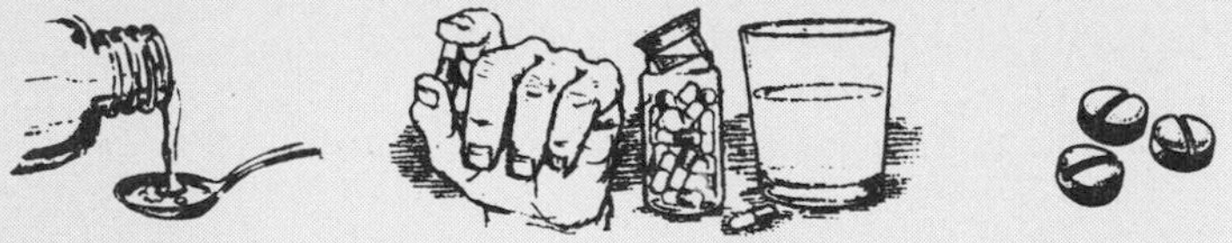

The medicines in this section are grouped according to their uses. For example, all the medicines used to treat infections caused by worms are listed under the heading FOR WORMS.

If you want information on a medicine, look for the name of that medicine in the LIST OF MEDICINES beginning on page 341. Or look for the medicine in the INDEX OF MEDICINES beginning on page 345. When you find the name you are looking for, turn to the page number shown.

Medicines are listed according to their *generic* (scientific) names rather than their *brand names* (names given by the companies that make them). This is because generic names are similar everywhere, but brand names differ from place to place. Also, **medicines are often much cheaper when you buy generic rather than brand-name products.**

In a few cases, well-known brand names are given after the generic name. In this book brand names are written in *italics* and begin with a capital letter. For example, *Phenergan* is a brand name for an antihistamine called **promethazine** (promethazine is the generic name).

With the information on each medicine, blank spaces __________ have been left for you to **write in** the name and price of the most common or least expensive product in your area. For example, if the cheapest or only available form of tetracycline in your area is *Terramycin,* you would write in the blank spaces as follows:

Tetracycline (tetracycline HCl, oxytetracycline, etc.)

Name: Terramycin price: $1.25 for 6 capsules

If, however, you find you can buy generic **tetracycline** more cheaply than *Terramycin,* write instead:

Name: tetracycline price: $1.00 for 60 capsules

Note: Not all the medicines listed in the Green Pages are needed in your Home or Village Medicine kit. Because different medicines are available in different countries, information has sometimes been given for a number of medicines that do the same job. However, it is wise to

KEEP AND USE ONLY A SMALL NUMBER OF MEDICINES.

Dosage Information:

HOW FRACTIONS ARE SOMETIMES WRITTEN

1 tablet = one tablet = 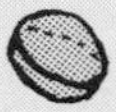

1/2 tablet = half a tablet = 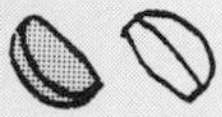

1 1/2 tablets = one and a half tablets = 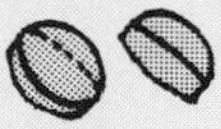

1/4 tablet = one quarter or one fourth of a tablet = 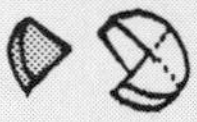

1/8 tablet = one eighth of a tablet (dividing it into 8 equal pieces and taking 1 piece) = 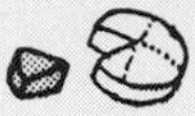

DECIDING DOSAGE BY HOW MUCH A PERSON WEIGHS

In these pages most instructions for dosage are given according to the age of a person—so that children get smaller doses than adults. However, it is more exact to determine dosage according to a person's weight. Information for doing this is sometimes included briefly in parentheses ( ), for use of health workers who have scales. If you read . . .

(100 mg./kg./day),

this means 100 mg. per kilogram of body weight per day. In other words, during a 24 hour period you give 100 mg. of the medicine for each kilogram the person weighs.

For example, suppose you want to give aspirin to a boy with rheumatic fever who weighs 36 kilograms. The recommended dose of aspirin for rheumatic fever is 100 mg./kg./day. So multiply:

100 mg. x 36 = 3600 mg.

The boy should get 3600 mg. of aspirin a day. One aspirin tablet contains 300 mg. of aspirin. 3600 mg. comes to 12 tablets. So give the boy 2 tablets 6 times a day (or 2 tablets every 4 hours).

This is one way to figure the dosages for different medicines. For more information on measuring and deciding on dosages, see Chapter 8.

Note to educators and planners of health care programs and to local distributors of this book:

If this book is to be used in training programs for village health workers or is distributed by a local health care program, **information about local names and prices of medicines should accompany the book.**

Local distributors are encouraged to duplicate a sheet with this information, so that it can be copied into the book by the user. Wherever possible, include local sources for **generic or low-cost medicines and supplies.** (See "Buying Supplies for the Medicine Kit," page 333.)

LIST OF MEDICINES IN THE GREEN PAGES

Listed in the order in which they appear

ANTIBIOTICS

The Penicillins:

Very Important Antibiotics

See page

Penicillin by Mouth
Penicillin G or V 351

Injectable Penicillin
Short-acting penicillin: crystalline penicillin, benzylpenicillin, penicillin G, aqueous penicillin, soluble penicillin, sodium penicillin, potassium penicillin 352
Intermediate-acting penicillin: procaine penicillin, procaine penicillin aluminum monostearate (PAM) 352
Long-acting penicillin: benzathine penicillin 353

Ampicillin and Amoxicillin: Wide-Range (Broad-Spectrum) Penicillins 353

Penicillin with Streptomycin 354

Erythromycin:

An Alternative to Penicillin . . 355

Tetracyclines:

Wide-range Antibiotics

Tetracycline, tetracycline HCl, oxytetracycline, etc. 356
Doxycycline 356

Chloramphenicol:

An Antibiotic for Certain Severe Infections 357

The Sulfas or Sulfonamides:

Inexpensive Medicine for Common Infections

Sulfadiazine, sulfisoxazole, sulfadimidine, triple sulfa 358
Co-trimoxazole (sulfamethoxazole with trimethoprim) 358

Kanamycin and Gentamicin . . 359

Cephalosporins 359

Medicines

For Gonorrhea and Chlamydia . 360

Medicines

For Tuberculosis

Isoniazid (INH) 361
Rifampin (rifampicin, rifamycin) 362
Pyrazinamide 362
Ethambutol 362
Streptomycin 363
Thiacetazone 363

Medicines

For Leprosy

Dapsone (diaminodiphenylsulfone, DDS) . . 364
Rifampin (rifampicin, rifamycin) 364
Clofazimine *(Lamprene)* 364

OTHER MEDICINES

For Malaria

Chloroquine 365
Quinine 366
Mefloquine 367
Pyrimethamine with sulfadoxine *(Fansidar)* . 368
Proguanil 368
Primaquine 368
Tetracycline 368

For Amebas and Giardia

Metronidazole 369
Diloxanide furoate 369
Tetracycline 356
Chloroquine 365
Quinacrine 370
Hydroxyquinolines (clioquinol, iodoquinol) . 370

For Vaginal Infections

White vinegar 370
Metronidazole 370
Nystatin or miconazole—tablets, cream, and vaginal inserts 370
Gentian violet (crystal violet) 370
Povidone iodine 371

For Skin Problems

Soap 371
Sulfur 371
Gentian violet (crystal violet) 371
Antibiotic ointments 371
Cortico-steroid ointment or lotion 371
Petroleum jelly (Petrolatum, *Vaseline*) 371

For Ringworm And Other Fungus Infections

Ointments with undecylenic, benzoic, or salicylic acid 372
Sulfur and vinegar 372
Sodium thiosulfate (hypo) 372
Selenium sulfide *(Selsun, Exsel)* 372
Tolnaftate *(Tinactin)* 372
Griseofulvin 372
Gentian violet—for yeast infections (thrush) . 373
Nystatin or miconazole 373

For Scabies and Lice

Gamma benzene hexachloride (lindane, *Kwell*) 373
Benzyl benzoate, cream or lotion 373
Sulfur in *Vaseline* or lard 373
Pyrethrins with piperonyl *(RID)* 373
Crotamiton *(Eurax)* 373

For Genital Warts

Podophyllin 374
Bichloroacetic or Trichloroacetic acid . . . 374

For Worms

Mebendazole *(Vermox)*—for many kinds of worms 374
Albendazole *(Zentel)*—for many kinds of worms 374
Piperazine—for roundworm and pinworm (threadworm) 375
Thiabendazole—for many kinds of worms . 375
Pyrantel—for pinworm, hookworm, and roundworm 376
Niclosamide *(Yomesan)*—for tapeworm . . . 376
Praziquantel *(Biltricide, Droncit)*—for tapeworm 376

For Schistosomiasis

Praziquantel *(Biltricide, Droncit)* 377
Metrifonate *(Bilarcil)* 377
Oxamniquine *(Vansil, Mansil)* 377

For River Blindness (Onchocerciasis)

Ivermectin ***(Mectizan)*** 378
Diethylcarbamazine 378
Suramin 378

For The Eyes

Antibiotic eye ointment—for conjunctivitis and newborn babies' eyes 378
Silver nitrate drops, 1%—for newborn babies' eyes 379

For Pain:

Analgesics

Aspirin 379
Child's aspirin 380
Acetaminophen (paracetamol) 380
Ibuprofen 380
Ergotamine with caffeine—for migraine headache 380
Codeine 384

For Stopping Pain When Closing Wounds:

Anesthetics

Lidocaine (xylocaine) 380

For Gut Cramps:

Antispasmodics

Belladonna (with or without phenobarbital) 381

For Acid Indigestion, Heartburn, And Stomach Ulcers

Aluminum hydroxide or magnesium hydroxide 381
Sodium bicarbonate (bicarbonate of soda, baking soda) 381
Calcium carbonate 382
Cimetidine *(Tagamet)* 382
Ranitidine *(Zantac)* 382

For Dehydration

Rehydration Mix 382

For Hard Stools (Constipation):

Laxatives

Milk of magnesia (magnesium hydroxide) . . 383
Epsom salts (magnesium sulfate) 383
Mineral oil 383
Glycerin suppositories *(Dulcolax)* 383

For Mild Diarrhea

Kaolin with pectin 384

For Stuffy Nose

Nose drops with ephedrine or phenylephrine 384

For Cough

Codeine 384

For Asthma

Ephedrine 385
Theophylline or aminophylline 385
Salbutamol (Albuterol) 385
Epinephrine (Adrenaline, ***Adrenalin***) 385

For Allergic Reactions and Vomiting: The Antihistamines

Promethazine *(Phenergan)* 386
Diphenhydramine *(Benadryl)* 387
Chlorpheniramine 387
Dimenhydrinate *(Dramamine)* 387

Antitoxins

Scorpion antitoxin or antivenom 388
Snakebite antitoxin or antivenom 388
Antitoxins for tetanus 389

For Swallowed Poisons

Syrup of Ipecac 389
Powdered or activated charcoal 389

For Fits (Convulsions)

Phenobarbital (phenobarbitone) 389
Phenytoin (diphenylhydantoin, *Dilantin*) . . . 390
Diazepam *(Valium)* 390

For Severe Bleeding After Birth (Postpartum Hemorrhage)

Ergonovine or ergometrine maleate *(Ergotrate, Methergine)* 391
Oxytocin *(Pitocin)* 391

For Piles (Hemorrhoids)

Suppositories for hemorrhoids 392

For Malnutrition and Anemia

Powdered milk (dried milk) 392
Mixed (or multi) vitamins 392
Vitamin A—for night blindness and xerophthalmia 392
Iron sulfate (ferrous sulfate)—for anemia . . 393
Folic acid—for anemia 393
Vitamin B_{12} (cyanocobalamin)—for pernicious anemia **only** 393
Vitamin K (phytomenadione)—for bleeding in the newborn 394
Vitamin B_6 (pyridoxine)—for persons taking INH 394

Family Planning Methods

Oral contraceptives (birth control pills) . . . 394
Condoms 396
Diaphragm 396
Contraceptive foam 396
Contraceptive suppositories *(Neo Sampoon)* 396
Intrauterine device (IUD) 396
Injectable contraceptives 396
Contraceptive implants *(Norplant)* 396

Blank sheets for writing information about other medicines or home remedies . . . 397

Index Of Medicines In The Green Pages

Listed in this order: A B C D E F G H I J K L M N O P Q R S T U V W X Y Z

Note: Medicines not listed in the GREEN PAGES, but mentioned in the book, are listed in the main Index (yellow pages).

A

Acetaminophen (paracetamol) 380
Acetylsalicylic acid (aspirin) 379
Activated charcoal 389
Adrenalin (epinephrine) 385
Adrenaline 385
Alacramyn (antivenom) 388
Albendazole 374
Albuterol 385
Alka-Seltzer (sodium bicarbonate) 381
Allergic reactions, medicines for 386
Aluminum hydroxide 381
Amebas, medicines for 368
Amicline 370
Aminophylline 385
Amoxicillin 353
Ampicillin 353
Analgesics 379
Anemia, medicines for 393
Anesthetics 380
Antacids 381
Antibiotics 351
Antihistamines 386
Antiminth (pyrantel) 376
Antispasmodics 381
Antitoxins 388
Antivenoms 388
Antivip-DL (antivenom) 388
Antrypol (suramin) 378
Aralen (chloroquine) 366
Aspirin 379
Asthma, medicines for 385
Atabrine 370
Atropine 381

B

Bactrim (co-trimoxazole) 358
Banocide (diethylcarbamazine) 378
Bayer 205 (suramin) 378
Belladonna 381
Benadryl (diphenhydramine) 387
Benzathine 353
Benzoic acid 372
Benzyl benzoate 373
Betadine (povidone iodine) 371
Bicarbonate of soda 381
Bichloroacetic acid 374
Bilarcil (metrifonate) 377
Biltricide (praziquantel) 376, 377
Birth control 394
Bleeding, medicines for 391
Brevicon (birth control pills) 395
Brevicon 1 + 35 (birth control pills) 394
Brevinor (birth control pills) 395
Broxyquinoline 370

C

Cafergot (ergotamine with caffeine) 380
Calcium carbonate 382
Ceftriaxone 360
Cephalosporins 359
Charcoal, powdered or activated 389
Chlamydia, medicines for 360
Chlorambin 370
Chloramphenicol 357
Chloromycetin (chloramphenicol) 357
Chloroquine 365
Chlorpheniramine 387
Chlortetracycline 356
Cimetidine 382
Ciprofloxacin 360
Clavulanic acid 360
Clioquinol 370
Clofazimine 364
Cloxacillin 351
Cobrantril (pyrantel) 376
Codeine 384
Condoms 396
Contraceptive foam 396
Contraceptive suppositories 396
Contraceptives, oral 394
Convulsions (fits), medicines for 389
Copper T (IUD) 396
Copper 7 (IUD) 396
Cortico-steroid 371
Cortisone 392
Co-trimoxazole 358
Cough medicines 384
Cramps of the gut, medicines for 381
Crotamiton 373
Crystal violet 371
Cyanocobalamin (vitamin B12) 393

D

Dapsone (diaminodiphenylsulfone, DDS) . . 364
Dehydration, medicines for 382
Delfen (contraceptive foam) 396
Demulen (birth control pills) 395
Depo-Provera (birth control injection) 396
Diaphragm 396
Diarrhea, medicines for 384
Diazepam 390
Dicloxacillin 351
Diethylcarbamazine 378
Diiodohydroxyquin 370
Dilantin (phenytoin) 390
Diloxanide furoate 369
Dimenhydrinate 387
Diodoquin (diiodohydroxyquin) 370
Diphenhydramine 387
Diphenylhydantoin (phenytoin) 390
Doxycycline 356
Dramamine (dimenhydrinate) 387
Droncit (praziquantel) 376, 377
Dulcolax (glycerin suppositories) 383

E

Emko (contraceptive foam) 396
Enteroquinol 370
Entero-Vioform 370
Ephedrine 385
Epinephrine 385
Epsom salts 383
Ergometrine 391
Ergonovine 391
Ergotamine with caffeine 380
Ergotrate (ergotamine tartrate) 390
Erythromycin 355
Ethambutol 362
Eugynon (birth control pills) 395
Eurax (crotamiton) 373
Expectorants 384
Exsel (selenium sulfide) 372
Eyes, medicines for 378

F

Family planning methods 394
Fansidar (pyrimethamine with sulfadoxine) . 368
Femenal (birth control pills) 395
Femulen (birth control pills) 395
Ferrous sulfate 393
Fits (convulsions), medicines for 389
Flagyl (metronidazole) 369
Floraquin 370
Folic acid 393
Fungus infections, medicines for 372
Furamide (diloxanide furoate) 369

G

Gamma benzene hexachloride (lindane) . . 373
Gammezane (lindane) 373
Garamycin (gentamicin) 359
Gentamicin 359
Gentian violet 371
Germanin (suramin) 378
Giardia, medicines for 368
Glycerin suppositories 383
Gonorrhea, medicines for 360
Griseofulvin 372

H

Halquinol 370
Headache, medicines for 379
Helmex (pyrantel) 376
Hemorrhage, medicines for 391
Hemorrhoids, medicines for 392
Hetrazan (diethylcarbamazine) 378
Hydroxyquinolines 370
Hyoscyamine (atropine) 381
Hyper-tet (tetanus immune globulin) 389

I

Ibuprofen 380
Infections, medicines for 351
Injectable contraceptives 396
Insecticides for scabies and lice 373
Intrauterine device (IUD) 396
Iodochlorhydroxyquin 370
Iodoquinol 370
Ipecac syrup 389
Iron sulfate 393
Isoniazid (INH) 361
Ivermectin 378

K

Kanamycin 359
Kantrex 359
Kaolin with pectin 384
Kaopectate (kaolin with pectin) 384
Kwell (lindane) 373

L

Lamprene (clofazimine) 364
Lariam (mefloquine) 367
Laxatives 383
Lempko (contraceptive foam) 396
Leprosy, medicines for 363
Lice, medicines for 373
Lidocaine 380
Lindane 373
Lippes Loop (IUD) 396
Loestrin 1/20 (birth control pills) 395
Lo-Femenal (birth control pills) 395
Logynon (birth control pills) 394
Lo-ovral (birth control pills) 395
Luminal (phenobarbital) 389

M

Magnesium hydroxide 383
Magnesium sulfate 383
Malaria, medicines for 365
Mansil (oxamniquine) 377
Mebendazole *(Vermox)* 374
Mectizan (ivermectin) 378
Mefloquine 367
Mepacrine 370
Methergine (methylergonovine maleate) . . 391
Methicillin 351
Metrifonate 377
Metronidazole 369
Miconazole 370
Microgynon 30 (birth control pills) 395
Microlut (birth control pills) 395
Microvlar (birth control pills) 395
Micronor (birth control pills) 395
Micronovum (birth control pills) 395
Milk of magnesia 383
Milk, powdered 392
Mineral oil 383
Mini-pill 395
Minovlar (birth control pills) 395
Modicon (birth control pills) 395
Myambutol (ethambutol) 362

N

Nafcillin 351
Naphuride (suramin) 378
Neo Sampoon (contraceptive suppositories) 396
Neocon (birth control pills) 394
Neogynon (birth control pills) 395
Neomycin 371
Neosporin (antibiotic ointment) 371
Neo-Synephrine (phenylephrine) 384
Net-En (injectable contraceptive) 396
Niclosamide 376
Nivembin 370
Nordette (birth control pills) 395
Nordiol (birth control pills) 395
Noriday 1 + 50 (birth control pills) 394
Norimin (birth control pills) 394
Nor-QD (birth control pills) 395
Norlestrin (birth control pills) 395
Norplant (contraceptive implant) 396
Nose, medicines for 384
Nystatin 373

O

Onchocerciasis, medicines for 378
Oral contraceptives 394
Oral rehydration salts 382
Ortho-Novum 1/35 (birth control pills) . . . 394
Ortho-Novum 1/50 (birth control pills) . . . 394
Ovcon (birth control pills) 395
Ovral (birth control pills) 395
Ovrette (birth control pills) 395
Ovulen (birth control pills) 395
Ovum 50 (birth control pills) 395
Ovysmen (birth control pills) 395
Ovysmen 1/35 (birth control pills) 394
Oxacillin 351
Oxamniquine 377
Oxytetracycline 356
Oxytocin 391

P

Pain, medicines for 379
Paludrine (proguanil) 368
Paracetamol 380
Penicillins 351
    Amoxicillin 353
    Ampicillin 353
    Benzathine 353
    Benzylpenicillin (penicillin G) 352
    Crystalline 352
    For resistance to penicillin 351
    PAM (procaine penicillin aluminum
        monostearate) 352
    Phenoxymethyl (penicillin V) 351
    Procaine 352
    With streptomycin 354

Perle . . . 394
Perle LD . . . 395
Petroleum jelly (petrolatum, *Vaseline*) . . . 371
Phenergan (promethazine) . . . 386
Phenobarbital . . . 389
Phenobarbitone . . . 389
Phenoxymethyl (penicillin V) . . . 351
Phenytoin . . . 390
Phytomenadione (vitamin K) . . . 394
Phytonadione . . . 394
Piperazine . . . 375
Pitocin (oxytocin) . . . 391
Pituitrin . . . 391
Podophyllin . . . 374
Poisoning, medicines for . . . 389
Polymyxin . . . 371
Polysporin (polymyxin) . . . 371
Polyvalent Crotalid Antivenin
(for snakebites) . . . 388
Povidone iodine . . . 371
Powdered charcoal . . . 389
Praziquantel for schistosomiasis . . . 377
Praziquantel for tapeworm . . . 376
Primaquine . . . 368
Primovlar (birth control pills) . . . 395
Probenecid . . . 360
Proguanil . . . 368
Promethazine . . . 386
Pyrantel . . . 376
Pyrazinamide . . . 362
Pyrethrins with piperonyl . . . 373
Pyridoxine (vitamin B_6) . . . 394
Pyrimethamine with sulfadoxine . . . 368

Q

Quinacrine . . . 370
Quinine . . . 366
Quogyl . . . 370

R

Ranitidine . . . 382
Rehydration Drink . . . 382
Retinol . . . 392
RID (pyrethrins with piperonyl) . . . 373
Rifampin (rifampicin, rifamycin) for TB . . . 362
Rifampin (rifampicin, rifamycin) for leprosy . 364
Ringworm, medicines for . . . 372
River blindness, medicines for . . . 378

S

Safety Coil (IUD) . . . 396
Salbutamol . . . 385
Salicylic acid . . . 372
Scabies, medicines for . . . 373
Scorpion sting, antivenoms for . . . 388
Selenium sulfide . . . 372
Selsun (selenium sulfide) . . . 372
Septra (co-trimoxazole) . . . 358
Silver nitrate . . . 379
Simethicone . . . 381
Skin problems, medicines for . . . 371
Snakebite, antivenoms for . . . 388
Soaps . . . 371
Sodium bicarbonate . . . 381
Sodium thiosulfate . . . 372
Spectinomycin . . . 360
Streptomycin . . . 363
Suero Anticrotalico (snakebite antivenom) . 388
Sulfas (sulfonamides) . . . 358
Co-trimoxazole . . . 358
Sulfadiazine . . . 358
Sulfadimidine . . . 358
Sulfamethazine . . . 358
Sulfisoxazole . . . 358
Trimethoprim with sulfamethoxazole
(co-trimoxazole) . . . 358
Triple sulfa . . . 358
Sulfones (dapsone, DDS) . . . 364
Sulfur . . . 371
Suramin . . . 378
Synophase (birth control pills) . . . 394
Syrup of Ipecac . . . 389

T

Tagamet (cimetidine) . . . 382
Terramycin (tetracycline) . . . 356
Tetanus antitoxin . . . 389
Tetanus immune globulin . . . 389
Tetracycline . . . 356
Doxycycline . . . 356
Oxytetracycline . . . 356
Tetracycline HCl . . . 356
Theophylline . . . 385
Thiabendazole . . . 375
Thiacetazone . . . 363
Tinactin (tolnaftate) . . . 372
Tolnaftate . . . 372
Trinordiol (birth control pills) . . . 394
Trinovum (birth control pills) . . . 394
Triphasil (birth control pills) . . . 394
Triquilar (birth control pills) . . . 394
Tuberculosis, medicines for . . . 361
Typhoid, medicines for . . . 357

U

Ulcers, medicines for 381
Undecylenic acid 372

V

Vaginal infections, medicines for 370
Valium (diazepam) 390
Vansil (oxamniquine) 377
Vaseline (petroleum jelly) 371
Vermox (mebendazole) 374
Vibramycin (doxycycline) 356
Vinegar 372
Vitamins 392
Vomiting, medicines for 386

W

Warts on the genitals, medicines for 374
Water as a medicine 384
White vinegar 372
Whitfield's Ointment 372
Worms, medicines for 374

X

Xylocaine (lidocaine) 380
Xerophthalmia, vitamins for 392

Y

Yomesan (niclosamide) 376

Z

Zentel (albendazole) 374
Zantac (ranitidine) 382

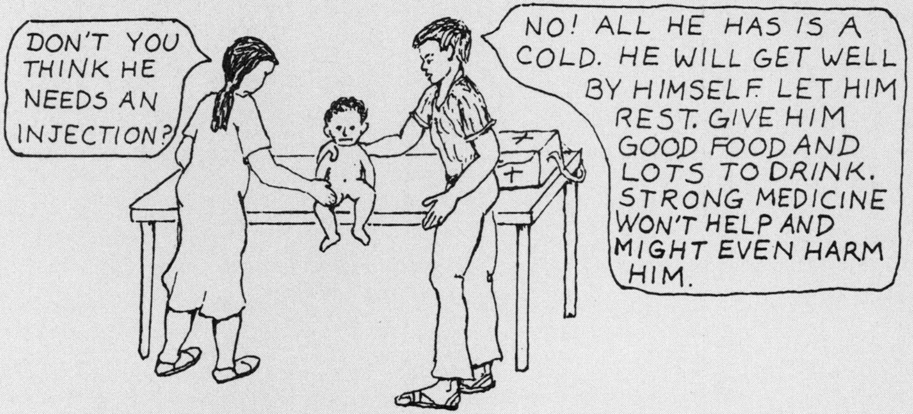
DON'T YOU THINK HE NEEDS AN INJECTION?
NO! ALL HE HAS IS A COLD. HE WILL GET WELL BY HIMSELF. LET HIM REST. GIVE HIM GOOD FOOD AND LOTS TO DRINK. STRONG MEDICINE WON'T HELP AND MIGHT EVEN HARM HIM.

ONLY USE A MEDICINE WHEN YOU ARE SURE IT IS NEEDED AND WHEN YOU ARE SURE HOW TO USE IT

Note: Some medicines can cause bad reactions if taken together. Before taking two or more medicines at the same time, consult a health worker, if possible. Also, read the information on the package of any medicine before using it.

INFORMATION ON MEDICINES

ANTIBIOTICS

THE PENICILLINS: VERY IMPORTANT ANTIBIOTICS

Penicillin is one of the most useful antibiotics. It fights certain kinds of infections, including many that produce pus. It does no good for diarrhea, most urinary infections, backache, bruises, the common cold, chickenpox, or other virus infections (see p. 18 and 19).

Penicillin is measured in milligrams (mg.) or units (U.). For penicillin G, 250 mg. = 400,000 U.

Risks and precautions for all kinds of penicillin (including ampicillin and amoxicillin):

For most people penicillin is one of the safest medicines. Too much does no harm and only wastes money. Too little does not completely stop the infection and may make the bacteria *resistant* (more difficult to kill).

In certain persons penicillin causes **allergic reactions.** Mild allergic reactions include itchy raised spots or rashes. Often these come several hours or days after taking penicillin and may last for days. Antihistamines (p. 386) help calm the itching.

Rarely, penicillin causes a dangerous reaction called **allergic shock.** Soon after penicillin is injected (or swallowed), the person suddenly gets pale, has trouble breathing, and goes into the state of shock (see p. 70). **Epinephrine** *(Adrenalin)* **must be injected at once.**

Always have epinephrine ready when you inject penicillin (see p. 385).

A person who has once had **any** allergic reaction to penicillin should **never** be given any kind of penicillin, ampicillin or amoxicillin again, either by mouth or by injection. This is because the next time the reaction would likely be far worse and might kill him. (But stomach upset from taking penicillin is not an allergic reaction, and no cause to stop taking it.)

Persons who cannot take penicillin can sometimes be treated with tetracycline or erythromycin by mouth (see pages 355 and 356 for uses and precautions).

Most infections that can be treated with penicillin can be treated quite well with penicillin taken by mouth. Injected forms of penicillin are more dangerous than those taken by mouth.

Use injectable penicillin only for severe or dangerous infections.

Before injecting penicillin or any medicine that contains it, take the precautions given on page 70.

Resistance to penicillin:

Sometimes penicillin does not work against an infection it would normally control. This may be because the bacteria have become resistant, so that penicillin no longer harms them (see p. 58).

Nowadays, infections that are at times resistant to penicillin include impetigo, sores on the skin with pus, respiratory infections, breast infections (mastitis) and infections of the bone (osteomyelitis). If one of these infections does not respond to ordinary penicillin, another antibiotic may be tried. Or special forms of penicillin (methicillin, nafcillin, oxacillin, cloxacillin, dicloxacillin) may work. Consult a health worker for dosage and precautions.

In many parts of the world, gonorrhea is now resistant to penicillin; see p. 360 for other antibiotics. Pneumonia is also sometimes resistant to penicillin—try co-trimoxazole (p. 358) or erythromycin (p. 355).

PENICILLIN BY MOUTH

<u>**Penicillin G or Penicillin V**</u>

Name:__________________ price:______ for______

Often comes in: 250 mg. (400,000 U.) tablets
also: suspensions or powders for suspension, 125 or 250 mg. per teaspoon

(Penicillin V is used by the body more easily than penicillin G, but is more expensive.)

Penicillin by mouth (rather than injections) should be used for mild and moderately severe infections, including:

- abscessed or infected teeth
- infected wounds or many infected sores
- widespread impetigo
- erysipelas
- ear infections
- sinusitis
- sore throat with sudden, high fever (strep throat)
- some cases of bronchitis
- prevention of tetanus in persons who have not been vaccinated and who have deep or dirty wounds
- rheumatic fever
- pneumonia

If infection is severe, it may be best to start with injections of penicillin, but often penicillin by mouth can be given instead once improvement begins.

If improvement does not begin within 2 or 3 days, consider using another antibiotic and try to get medical advice.

Dosage of penicillin by mouth—using tablets of 250 mg. (20 to 60 mg./kg./day):

For mild infections:

- adults: 1 or 2 tablets (250 to 500 mg.) 4 times a day
- children 7 to 12: 1 tablet (250 mg.) 4 times a day
- children 2 to 6: 1/2 tablet (125 mg.) 3 or 4 times a day
- children under 2: 1/4 tablet (63 mg.) 3 or 4 times a day

For more serious infections: double the above dosage.

Important: Keep taking the penicillin for at least 5 days, and for 2 or 3 days after fever and other signs of infection are gone.

To help the body make better use of the medicine, **always take penicillin on an empty stomach,** an hour before meals. (This is more important for penicillin G than for penicillin V.)

INJECTABLE PENICILLIN

Injectable penicillin should be used for certain severe infections, including:

- meningitis
- septicemia (bacteria in the blood)
- tetanus
- severe pneumonia
- badly infected wounds
- gangrene
- infected bones and to prevent infection when a bone pokes through the skin
- gonorrhea
- syphilis
- pelvic inflammatory disease

Injectable penicillin comes in many different preparations. Before you inject any penicillin, be sure to check the **amount** and the **kind.**

Choosing the right kind of penicillin for injection:

Some kinds of penicillin do their job quickly but do not last long. Others work more slowly but last longer. There are times when it is better to use one kind than another.

Short-acting penicillin: These are known by many names, including crystalline penicillin, benzylpenicillin, aqueous penicillin, soluble penicillin, sodium penicillin, potassium penicillin, and penicillin G injections. These penicillins act quickly but only stay in the body a short time, so that they must be injected every 6 hours (4 times a day). A short-acting penicillin is the best choice for very severe infections when high doses of penicillin are needed. For example, for gas gangrene or when a broken bone pokes through the skin, or meningitis.

Intermediate-acting penicillin: Procaine penicillin or procaine penicillin aluminum monostearate (PAM). These work more slowly and last about a day in the body, so injections should be given once daily. Procaine penicillin, or a combination of procaine and a short-acting penicillin, is the best choice for most infections when injectable penicillin is needed.

Long-acting penicillin: Benzathine penicillin. This penicillin goes into the blood slowly and lasts up to a month. Its main use is in the treatment of strep throat and syphilis, and for prevention of rheumatic fever. It is useful when a person lives far away from someone who injects or cannot be counted upon to take penicillin by mouth. For mild infections a single injection may be enough. Benzathine penicillin often comes combined with faster-acting penicillins.

Crystalline penicillin (a short-acting penicillin)

Name:__________________ price:______ for_____

Often comes in: vials of 1 million U. (625 mg.) or 5 million U. (3125 mg.)

Dosage of crystalline penicillin or any short-acting penicillin—for severe infections:

Give an injection every 4 to 6 hours.

In each injection give:

adults and children over age 8: 1 million U.
children age 3 to 8: 500,000 U.
children under 3: 250,000 U.

For meningitis and some other very severe infections, higher doses should be given.

Procaine penicillin (intermediate-acting)

Name:__________________ price:______ for_____

Often comes in: vials of 300,000 U., 400,000 U., and more

Dosage of procaine penicillin—for moderately severe infections:

Give **1** injection a day.

With each injection give:

adults: 600,000 to 1,200,000 U.
children age 8 to 12: 600,000 U.
children age 3 to 7: 300,000 U.
children under 3: 150,000 U.
newborn babies: DO NOT USE unless no other penicillin or ampicillin is available. In emergencies, 75,000 U.

For very severe infections, give twice the above dose. However, it is better to use a short-acting penicillin.

The dosage for procaine penicillin combined with a short-acting penicillin is the same as for procaine penicillin alone.

For treatment of gonorrhea that is not resistant to penicillin, procaine penicillin is best. Very high doses are needed. For dosage, see page 360. For pelvic inflammatory disease, the dosages are the same as for gonorrhea.

Benzathine penicillin (long-acting)

Name:__________________ price:______ for_____

Often comes in: vials of 1,200,000 or 2,400,000 U.

Dosage of benzathine penicillin—for mild to moderately severe infections:

Give 1 injection every 4 days. For mild infections, 1 injection may be enough.

adults: 1,200,000 U. to 2,400,000 U.
children age 8 to 12: 900,000 U.
children age 1 to 7: 300,000 U. to 600,000 U.

For strep throat, give one injection of the above dose.

To prevent return infection in persons who have had rheumatic fever, give the above dose every 4 weeks (see p. 310).

For treatment of syphilis, benzathine penicillin is best. For dosage, see page 238.

AMPICILLIN AND AMOXICILLIN: WIDE-RANGE (BROAD-SPECTRUM) PENICILLINS

Ampicillin

Often comes in:
solutions,
125 or 250 mg./tsp. price: ________ for _____
capsules, 250 mg. price: ________ for _____
injections, 500 mg. price: ________ for _____

Amoxicillin

Often comes in:

capsules or tablets:
250 or 500 mg. price: _______ for _____

mixture:
125 mg. in 5 ml. price: _______ for _____
or 250 mg. in 5 ml. price: _______ for _____

These *broad-spectrum* (wide-range) penicillins kill many more kinds of bacteria than other penicillins. They are safer than other broad-spectrum antibiotics and are especially useful for babies and small children.

Ampicillin and amoxicillin are often interchangeable. When you see a recommendation for ampicillin in this book, you will often be able to use amoxicillin in its place, in the correct dose (see below). But **do not take amoxicillin by mouth when injected ampicillin is recommended** (amoxicillin does not come in injectable form). Also note that amoxicillin may be less effective against Shigella infections. Use ampicillin or another antibiotic (see p. 158).

Ampicillin and amoxicillin are more expensive than penicillin and they can cause diarrhea or 'thrush'. Therefore, they should not be used for infections that could be treated with penicillin just as effectively (see p. 58).

Ampicillin works well when taken by mouth. Injections should only be used for severe illnesses such as meningitis, peritonitis, and appendicitis, or when the sick person vomits or cannot swallow the medicine.

Ampicillin and amoxicillin are often useful in treating pneumonia or ear infections of children under 6 years, severe urinary tract infections, gonorrhea, and typhoid fever (if it is resistant to chloramphenicol). Ampicillin is also useful in treating septicemia and unexplained illness in the newborn, meningitis, peritonitis, and appendicitis.

Persons allergic to penicillin should not take ampicillin or amoxicillin. See *Risks and Precautions* for all types of penicillin, page 351.

Dosage for ampicillin and amoxicillin:

By mouth—(25 to 50 mg./kg./day):
capsules of 250 mg.; syrup with 125 mg. per teaspoon (5 ml.)

Ampicillin: Give 4 doses a day.

Amoxicillin: Give 3 doses a day.

In each dose give:

adults: 2 capsules or 4 teaspoons (500 mg.)
children age 8 to 12: 1 capsule or 2 teaspoons (250 mg.)
children 3 to 7: 1/2 capsule or 1 teaspoon (125 mg.)
children under 3: 1/4 capsule or 1/2 teaspoon (62 mg.)
newborn babies: same as for children under 3 years

For typhoid fever that is resistant to chloramphenicol, if you do not have injectable ampicillin, give 200 mg./kg./day of ampicillin by mouth or 100 mg./kg./day of amoxicillin.

For gonorrhea, see doses on p. 360.

Dosage for ampicillin:

By injection, for severe infections—(50 to 100 mg./kg./day—up to 300 mg./kg./day for meningitis):
vials of 500 mg.

Give 4 doses a day, once every 6 hours.

In each dose give:

adults: 500 to 1000 mg. (one to two 500 mg. vials)
children age 8 to 12: 250 mg. (1/2 of a 500 mg. vial)
children age 3 to 7: 125 mg. (1/4 of a 500 mg. vial)
children under 3: 62 mg. (1/8 of a 500 mg. vial)
newborn babies: 125 mg. (1/4 of a 500 mg. vial) **twice** a day only

Keep giving the ampicillin for at least 2 days after signs of infection have gone.

PENICILLIN WITH STREPTOMYCIN

Products that combine penicillin with streptomycin are found in most countries and are often used more than they should be. If one of these products is widely used in your area, write down its name, contents, and price:

Name: ________________ mg. of penicillin: ____

mg. of streptomycin: ____ price:________ for_____

Penicillin and streptomycin should be used together only in special cases, as an alternative to ampicillin, when ampicillin cannot be obtained or is too expensive. They should not be used for minor infections or for the common cold or 'flu'.

Frequent use of streptomycin for illnesses other than tuberculosis makes the tuberculosis bacteria in a community resistant to streptomycin, and therefore harder to treat. Also, streptomycin may cause deafness.

Streptomycin with penicillin can be used for most of the illnesses for which ampicillin is recommended (see p. 353), but ampicillin is safer, especially for babies.

Usually, it is cheaper, as well as easier to figure the correct dosage, if streptomycin and penicillin are injected separately, rather than in a combination.

Dosage of penicillin with streptomycin—**for severe infections:**

Give short-acting penicillin, at least 25,000 U./kg. 4 times a day, and streptomycin, no more than 30 to 50 mg./kg./day.

In newborns, give short-acting penicillin, 50,000 U./kg. twice a day together with streptomycin, 20 mg./kg. once a day.

	Give this much short-acting penicillin	with this much streptomycin
adults	1,000,000 U. 4 to 6 times a day	1 gm. (usually 2 ml.) once a day
children 8 to 12 years	500,000 U. 4 to 6 times a day	750 mg. (1 1/2 ml.) once a day
children 3 to 7 years	250,000 U. 4 to 6 times a day	500 mg. (1 ml.) once a day
children under 3	125,000 U. 4 to 6 times a day	250 mg. (1/2 ml.) once a day
newborn babies	150,000 U. twice a day	60 mg. (1/8 ml.) once a day

For very severe infections, such as peritonitis, appendicitis, meningitis, or an acute infection of the bone (osteomyelitis), even higher doses of penicillin may be given, but **the dosage of streptomycin must never be higher than what is suggested here.**

For less severe infections calling for penicillin with streptomycin, procaine penicillin can be used with streptomycin. For the dosage of procaine penicillin, see page 353. The dosage for streptomycin is the same as that given above.

Be sure to read the *Risks and Precautions* for both penicillin and streptomycin, pages 351 and 363.

ERYTHROMYCIN: AN ALTERNATIVE TO PENICILLIN

Erythromycin

Name: ____________________

Often comes in:
tablets or capsules of 250 mg. Price: _____ for ___
syrups with 125 or 200 mg. in 5 ml. Price: _____ for ___
eye ointment at 1% or 3% Price: _____ for ___

Erythromycin works against many of the same infections as penicillin and tetracycline, but is more expensive. In many parts of the world, erythromycin now works better than penicillin for some cases of pneumonia and certain skin infections.

Erythromycin may be used instead of penicillin by persons allergic to penicillin. Also, it may often be used by persons allergic to tetracycline, and by pregnant women and children, who should not take tetracycline. In some cases, erythromycin is not a good substitute for tetracycline. See the sections of the book which discuss each illness.

Erythromycin is fairly safe, but care should be taken not to give more than the recommended dose. Do not use for more than 2 weeks, as it may cause jaundice.

Dosage of erythromycin:

Take erythromycin with meals to avoid stomach upset.

Give 1 dose 4 times a day.

In each dose give:

adults: 500 mg. (2 tablets or 4 teaspoons)
children 8 to 12 years: 250 mg. (1 tablet or 2 teaspoons)
children 3 to 7 years: 150 mg. (1/2 tablet or 1 teaspoon)
children under 3 years: 75 to 150 mg. (1/4 to 1/2 tablet or 1/2 to 1 teaspoon)

TETRACYCLINES: WIDE-RANGE ANTIBIOTICS

Tetracycline (tetracycline HCl, oxytetracycline, etc.)
(Familiar but expensive brand: *Terramycin*)

Name: ______________________________

Often comes in:

capsules of 250 mg.	Price: _____ for ___
mixture, 125 mg. in 5 ml.	Price: _____ for ___
eye ointment at 1% or 3%	Price: _____ for ___

Tetracyclines are *broad-spectrum* antibiotics; that is, they fight a wide range of different kinds of bacteria.

Tetracycline should be taken by mouth, as this works as well and causes fewer problems than when it is injected.

Tetracycline can be used for:

- diarrhea or dysentery caused by bacteria or amebas
- sinusitis
- respiratory infections (bronchitis, etc.)
- infections of the urinary tract
- typhus
- brucellosis
- cholera
- trachoma
- gallbladder infections
- chlamydia
- gonorrhea
- pelvic inflammatory disease
- malaria (chloroquine resistant)

Tetracycline does no good for the common cold. For many common infections it does not work as well as penicillin or sulfas. It is also more expensive. Its use should be limited.

Risks and Precautions:

1. Pregnant women should not take tetracycline, as it can damage or stain the baby's teeth and bones. For the same reason, children under 8 years old should take tetracycline only when absolutely necessary, and for short periods only. Use erythromycin instead.

2. Tetracycline may cause diarrhea or upset stomach, especially if taken for a long time.

3. It is dangerous to use tetracycline that is 'old' or has passed the expiration date.

4. For the body to make the best use of tetracycline, milk or antacids should not be taken within 1 hour before or after taking the medicine.

5. Some people may develop a skin rash after spending time in the sun while taking tetracycline.

Dosage for tetracycline—(20 to 40 mg./kg./day):
—capsules of 250 mg. and mixture of 125 mg. in 5 ml.—

Give tetracycline by mouth 4 times a day.

In each dose give:

adults: 250 mg. (1 capsule)
children 8 to 12 years: 125 mg. (1/2 capsule or 1 teaspoon)
children under 8 years: As a general rule, **do not use tetracycline**—instead use co-trimoxazole or erythromycin. If there is no other choice, give:
children 4 to 7 years: 80 mg. (1/3 capsule or 2/3 teaspoon)
children 1 to 3 years: 60 mg. (1/4 capsule or 1/2 teaspoon)
babies under 1 year: 25 mg. (1/10 capsule or 1/5 teaspoon)
newborn babies (when other antibiotics are not available): 8 mg. (1/30 capsule or 6 drops of the mixture)

In severe cases, and for infections like gonorrhea, chlamydia, pelvic inflammatory disease, cholera, typhus, and brucellosis, twice the above dose should be given (except to small children).

For most infections, tetracycline should be continued for 1 or 2 days after the signs of infection are gone (usually 7 days altogether). For some illnesses, longer treatment is needed: typhus 6 to 10 days; brucellosis 2 to 3 weeks; gonorrhea and chlamydia 7 to 10 days; pelvic inflammatory disease 10 to 14 days. Cholera usually requires a shorter treatment: 3 to 5 days.

Doxycycline (familiar brand name: *Vibramycin*)

Name: ______________________________

Often comes in:
capsules or tablets of 100 mg.
Price: _____ for ___
ampules with 100 mg. for injection
Price: _____ for ___

Doxycycline is an expensive form of tetracycline that is taken twice a day instead of 4 times a day. When available, it can be used for the same illnesses as tetracycline. Doxycycline can be taken with food or milk. Otherwise, **the risks and precautions are the same as for tetracycline (see p. 356).**

Dosage of doxycycline:
—tablets of 100 mg.—

Give doxycycline by mouth twice a day.

In each dose give:

adults: 100 mg. (1 tablet)
children 8 to 12: 50 mg. (1/2 tablet)
children under 8: **Do not use doxycycline.**

CHLORAMPHENICOL: AN ANTIBIOTIC FOR CERTAIN SEVERE INFECTIONS

Chloramphenicol *(Chloromycetin)*

Name: ______________________

Often comes in:

capsules of 250 mg.	Price: _____ for ___
mixture, 125 mg. in 5 ml.	Price: _____ for ___
injections, 1000 mg. per vial	Price: _____ for ___
eye ointment at 1% or 3%	Price: _____ for ___

This broad-spectrum antibiotic fights a wide range of different bacteria. It is cheap, but there is some danger in using it. For this reason, its use must be very limited.

Chloramphenicol should be used only for typhoid and for very serious infections that are not cured by sulfas, penicillin, tetracycline, or ampicillin. For life-threatening illnesses such as meningitis, peritonitis, deep gut wounds, septicemia, or severe childbirth fever, chloramphenicol may be used when less dangerous medicines (like cephalosporins) are not available.

Ampicillin usually works as well as or better than chloramphenicol, and is much safer. Unfortunately, ampicillin is expensive, so there are times when chloramphenicol must be used instead.

WARNING: Chloramphenicol harms the blood of some persons. It is even more dangerous for newborn babies, especially premature babies. **To newborn babies with serious infections, give ampicillin rather than chloramphenicol** if this is at all possible. As a rule, except for eye ointment, **do not give chloramphenicol to babies under 1 month of age.**

Take care not to give more than the recommended dose of chloramphenicol. **For babies, the dose is very small** (see below).

Avoid long or repeated use.

In treating typhoid, change from chloramphenicol to ampicillin as soon as the illness is under control. (In regions where typhoid is known to be resistant to chloramphenicol, the entire treatment should be with ampicillin or co-trimoxazole.)

In some areas of Central and South America, typhoid has become resistant to both chloramphenicol and ampicillin and is no longer cured by them. Try using co-trimoxazole (see p. 358).

Chloramphenicol taken by mouth often does more good than when it is injected, and is less dangerous. Except in rare cases when the person cannot swallow, **do not inject chloramphenicol.**

Dosage for chloramphenicol—(50 to 100 mg./kg./day):—capsules of 250 mg., or a mixture of 125 mg. in 5 ml.—

Give by mouth 4 times a day.

In each dose give:

adults: 500 to 750 mg. (2 to 3 capsules). For typhoid, peritonitis, and other dangerous infections the higher dose should be given. (3 capsules 4 times a day is 12 capsules a day.)

children 8 to 12 years: 250 mg. (1 capsule or 2 teaspoons of mixture)

children 3 to 7 years: 125 mg. (1/2 capsule or 1 teaspoon)

babies 1 month to 2 years: give 12 mg. (1/2 ml. of the mixture or 1/20 part of a capsule) for *each* kg. of body weight. (This way, a 5 kg. baby would get 60 mg., which is 1/2 teaspoon of mixture, or 1/4 capsule, at each dose. With 4 doses, this means the 5 kg. baby will get 1 capsule, or 2 teaspoons of mixture, a day.)

newborn babies: *As a general rule, do not use chloramphenicol.* If there is no other choice, give 5 mg. (1/4 ml. or 5 drops of the mixture) for each kg. of body weight. Give a 3 kg. baby 15 mg. (15 drops of the mixture) 4 times a day, or about 1/4 capsule a day. Do not give more.

THE SULFAS (OR SULFONAMIDES): INEXPENSIVE MEDICINE FOR COMMON INFECTIONS

Sulfadiazine, sulfisoxazole, sulfadimidine, or 'triple sulfa'

Name: ______________________________

Often comes in:

tablets of 500 mg. Price:_____ for___

mixture, 500 mg. in 5 ml. Price:_____ for___

The sulfas or sulfonamides fight many kinds of bacteria, but they are weaker than many antibiotics and more likely to cause allergic reactions (itching) and other problems. Because they are cheap and can be taken by mouth, they are still useful.

The most important use of sulfas is for urinary infections. They may also be used for some ear infections and for impetigo and other skin infections with pus.

Not all the sulfas are used the same way or have the same dosage. If you have a sulfonamide other than one of those listed above, be sure of the correct use and dosage before you use it. Sulfathiazole is similar to the sulfas named above, and is very cheap, but is not recommended because it is more likely to cause side effects.

The sulfas do not work as well for diarrhea as they used to, because many of the microbes that cause diarrhea have become resistant to them. Also, giving sulfas to a person dehydrated from diarrhea can cause dangerous kidney damage.

WARNING:

It is important to **drink lots of water,** at least 8 glasses a day, when taking sulfa, to prevent harm to the kidneys.

If the sulfa causes a rash, blisters, itching, joint pain, fever, lower back pain or blood in the urine, **stop taking it and drink lots of water.**

Never give sulfa to a person who is dehydrated, or to babies under 1 year old.

Note: To do any good, these sulfas must be taken in the right dose, which is large. Be sure to take enough—but not too much!

Dosage for sulfadiazine, sulfisoxazole, sulfadimidine, or triple sulfa (200 mg./kg./day):
—tablets of 500 mg., or a mixture with 500 mg. in 5 ml.—

Give 4 doses a day—**with lots of water!**

In each dose give:

adults and children over 10 years: 3 to 4 gm. (6 to 8 tablets) for the first dose; then 1 gm. (2 tablets) for the other doses

children 6 to 10 years: 750 mg. (1 1/2 tablets or teaspoons) in each dose

children 1 to 5 years: 500 mg. (1 tablet or 1 teaspoon) in each dose

babies under 1 year: **Do not give sulfa.** If you have no choice, give 250 mg. (1/2 tablet or teaspoon) 4 times a day

Co-trimoxazole (sulfamethoxazole with trimethoprim)
(familiar brand names: *Bactrim, Septra*)

Name: ______________________________

Often comes in:

tablets of 100 mg. sulfamethoxazole with 20 mg. trimethoprim Price:_____ for__

tablets of 400 mg. sulfamethoxazole with 80 mg. trimethoprim Price:_____ for__

mixture of 200 mg. sulfamethoxazole with 40 mg. trimethoprim in 5 ml. Price:_____ for__

Note: This medicine also comes in double strength tablets *(Bactrim DS* and *Septra DS)* with 800 mg. sulfamethoxazole and 160 mg. trimethoprim. Use half the number of tablets given below if the medicine you have is double strength.

This combination medicine fights a wide range of bacteria, and is less expensive than ampicillin.

Women in the last 3 months of pregnancy should not use co-trimoxazole.

Co-trimoxazole can be used to treat:

- urinary infections
- diarrhea with blood and fever (shigella)
- typhoid
- cholera
- brucellosis
- respiratory infections (pneumonia)
- impetigo
- ear infections
- chancroid and gonorrhea

Dosage of co-trimoxazole:

—using tablets of 400 mg. sulfamethoxazole with 80 mg. trimethoprim, or teaspoons of mixture as described above—

Give 2 doses a day—**with lots of water!**

In each dose give:

adults and children over 12 years: 2 tablets or 4 teaspoons
children 9 to 12 years: 1 1/2 tablets or 3 teaspoons
children 4 to 8 years: 1 tablet or 2 teaspoons
children 1 to 3 years: 1/2 tablet or 1 teaspoon
babies under 1 year: **Do not give.** If you have no choice, give 1/4 tablet or 1/2 teaspoon 2 times a day.

For urinary infections, give the above dose for 10 to 14 days. For acute bronchitis and typhoid, give for 14 days. For chancroid, give for 7 days. For shigella, give for 5 to 10 days.

For gonorrhea, very high doses must be used (see p. 360).

KANAMYCIN AND GENTAMICIN

Kanamycin and gentamicin are injectable antibiotics that are greatly overused in some countries. Use of these dangerous medicines should be **very** limited, because they can cause deafness and damage to the kidneys. Also, bacteria quickly become resistant to them and they lose their effectiveness. (Streptomycin is another medicine from this same group, but it is generally used only for tuberculosis—see p. 363.)

They should be given by experienced health workers only for certain severe infections when other, safer medicines are not available or are too expensive. Kanamycin is sometimes used to treat gonorrhea (see next page), or eye infections (conjunctivitis) in newborn babies (p. 221).

Kanamycin *(Kantrex)*

Name:________________ price:______ for_____

Often comes in:

vials for injection with 75 mg., 500 mg., or 1000 mg.

Risks and Precautions:

Too much kanamycin for too long may cause deafness. If ringing of the ears or hearing loss begins, stop taking the medicine and see a health worker. **Kanamycin should not be taken by pregnant women** or persons with kidney problems.

Dosage of kanamycin (15 mg./kg./day):

—vials of liquid; or powder for mixing with water to give 1 gm. of kanamycin in 2 ml.—

Give twice a day.

With each injection give:

adults: 500 mg.
children 8 to 12: 250 mg.
children 3 to 7: 125 mg.
children under 3: 63 mg.
babies: give 8 for each kg. of body weight; thus a 3 kg. baby gets 24 mg.

For gonorrhea, larger amounts are given in a single dose: for eye infection in newborn babies, give one injection of 25 mg. for each kg. the baby weighs. (Thus, a 3 kg. baby would get 75 mg.) For gonorrhea in adults, see p. 360.

Gentamicin *(Garamycin)*

In many countries today, gentamicin is used instead of kanamycin. Its action and the risks and precautions are similar, but the dosage is smaller (2 to 5 mg./kg./day). This dosage is divided, and usually given 3 times a day.

CEPHALOSPORINS

These are powerful new antibiotics that work against many different kinds of bacteria. They are often very expensive and not widely available. For that reason, we have not recommended them as first choice treatments in this book. However, they generally have fewer risks and side effects than many other antibiotics and, when obtainable, can be useful in treating certain serious diseases.

There are many different types, including cefazolin *(Ancef)*, cephalexin *(Keflex)*, cephradine *(Velosef)*, cefurazine *(Ceftin)*, cefoxitin *(Mefoxin)*, ceftriaxone *(Rocephin)*, cefotaxime *(Claforan)*, and ceftazidime *(Fortaz, Taxidime, Tazicef)*. Various cephalosporins can be used for pneumonia, urinary infections, typhoid, gut or pelvic infections, bone infections, and meningitis. Some, like ceftriaxone, can be useful for treating sexually transmitted diseases such as chancroid, eye infections in newborns, or gonorrhea that is resistant to penicillin.

Get advice on dosages and side effects before using these medicines. Also, do not use them for mild illnesses or diseases that can be treated equally well with less expensive antibiotics.

MEDICINES FOR GONORRHEA AND CHLAMYDIA

In most parts of the world, penicillin no longer works against gonorrhea, because the bacteria have become resistant to it. So other antibiotics must usually be used. Seek local advice about which medicines are effective in your area. Here we list some possible treatments that might be recommended, depending on what is available and affordable.

If the pain and drip are not gone 3 days after treating for gonorrhea, the disease may be resistant to the medicine, or the person may have chlamydia. These diseases have the same early signs, and often occur together (see p. 236). If both gonorrhea and chlamydia are common in your area, it is probably a good idea to treat both diseases at the same time. (Be sure to use a condom until you are certain you and your partner are fully treated.)

Some of the medicines listed here can have serious side effects when given for long periods of time, or to babies, children, or pregnant women. Before treating, be sure to check the Green Pages warnings and information about these medicines. The dosages listed here are for adults.

For gonorrhea, use one of the following:

1. **Co-trimoxazole** (p. 358) can be used to treat gonorrhea. Using tablets with 400 mg. sulfamethoxazole and 80 mg. trimethoprim: Give 5 tablets twice each day for 2 or 3 days.

2. One injection of 2 grams of **kanamycin** (p. 359).

3. **Tetracycline** (p. 356) or **erythromycin** (p. 355) tablets can be used to treat both gonorrhea and chlamydia at the same time, but sometimes gonorrhea is resistant to tetracycline. Give 500 mg. 4 times a day for 7 to 10 days.

4. Give one injection of 2 grams of **streptomycin** (p. 363). But only use streptomycin for gonorrhea that is resistant to penicillin when no other medicines are available. Too much use of streptomycin for diseases other than tuberculosis reduces its usefulness for that illness.

5. If gonorrhea in your area is not resistant to penicillin, inject 4.8 million units of **procaine penicillin,** or 5 million units of **crystalline penicillin,** all at once. Put half the dose in each buttock, and give 1 gram of **probenecid** by mouth at the same time. Or give by mouth 3500 mg. **ampicillin** (or 3000 mg. **amoxicillin**) and 1 gram probenecid at one time.

   If **clavulanic acid** is added to one of these penicillin treatments, it will make the treatment effective against most gonorrhea resistant to penicillin. If available, give 125 to 250 mg. clavulanic acid along with the penicillin, ampicillin or amoxicillin. (*Augmentin* is a combination tablet of clavulanic acid and a kind of penicillin.)

6. There may be other very expensive but effective medicines **(ceftriaxone, ciprofloxacin, spectinomycin, thiamphenicol)** for gonorrhea in your area. Seek experienced medical advice before using these medicines.

For chlamydia, use one of the following:

1. Give **tetracycline** (p. 356) or **erythromycin** (p. 355): 500 mg. 4 times a day for 7 to 10 days.

2. Or, give **doxycycline** (p. 356): 100 mg. twice a day for 7 to 10 days.

3. **Sulfa drugs** (p. 358) can also be used. For example, give 500 mg. of sulfisoxazole by mouth 4 times a day for 10 days.

MEDICINES FOR TUBERCULOSIS

In treating tuberculosis (TB), it is very important to **always use 2, 3, or even 4 anti-tuberculosis medicines at the same time.** If only 1 medicine is used, the TB bacteria become resistant to it and make the disease harder to treat.

Tuberculosis must be treated for a long time, usually 6 to 9 months, or longer. The length of treatment depends on what combination of medicines is used. To keep tuberculosis from coming back again, the **full, long-term treatment is extremely important.**

Some medicines for tuberculosis are expensive (rifampin, pyrazinamide, ethambutol) if you buy them in a pharmacy. But many governments have programs that test for tuberculosis and give medicine free or at low cost.

Experienced local advice is important, because treatments change, bacteria become resistant, and new medicines may become available. Also, some programs give medicines only twice a week, in higher doses.

Isoniazid (INH) should always be used in the treatment of TB. **Rifampin** is a very effective medicine that should be used whenever possible, especially until a 'sputum test' comes out negative. **Ethambutol** and **streptomycin** are also often used to treat TB. Taking **pyrazinamide** with INH and rifampin can shorten the time of treatment. **Thiacetazone** is an inexpensive TB medicine, but it causes side effects so often that many persons cannot use it.

If the medicines cause itching, yellowing of the skin and eyes (jaundice), or stomach pains, see a health worker about possibly changing the dosage or medicines. If blisters occur, stop taking medicines until you can see a health worker. Avoid alcohol when taking TB medicines, especially INH.

Recommended treatments

Use one of the following combinations of medicines, depending on which are available, affordable, and recommended in your area:

1. Give isoniazid, rifampin, ethambutol, and pyrazinamide for 2 months. Then stop taking pyrazinamide, but continue using rifampin, isoniazid, and ethambutol for another 4 months.

2. Give isoniazid, rifampin, and ethambutol for 9 months.

3. Combine isoniazid, rifampin, streptomycin, and pyrazinamide for 2 months. Then give isoniazid with ethambutol, streptomycin, or possibly thiacetazone for 6 months. This treatment has the advantage of being cheaper, because less rifampin is needed.

4. If rifampin is not available or is too expensive, give isoniazid, ethambutol, and streptomycin for 2 months, or until a test shows the sputum is negative. Then continue to give streptomycin for 2 more months, and to give INH and ethambutol for 1 year.

5. Pregnant women with TB should seek experienced medical advice. Otherwise, give isoniazid and either ethambutol, rifampin, or thiacetazone for 18 months. Also give 50 mg. of vitamin B_6 (pyridoxine) a day. Do not give pyrazinamide or streptomycin during pregnancy.

Isoniazid (INH)

Name:__________________ price:______ for_____

Often comes in: tablets of 100 or 300 mg.

This is the most basic anti-TB medicine. To treat TB, it must always be given with at least 1 other anti-TB medicine whenever possible. For prevention it can be given alone.

Risks and Precautions:

Rarely, isoniazid causes anemia, nerve pains in the hands and feet, muscle twitching, or even fits, especially in malnourished persons. These side effects can usually be treated by giving 50 mg. of pyridoxine (vitamin B_6) daily, by mouth (p. 394).

Sometimes isoniazid can damage the liver. Persons who develop the signs of hepatitis (yellow color of skin and eyes, itching, loss of appetite, pain in the belly, see p. 172) while taking isoniazid should stop taking the medicine.

Dosage for isoniazid—(5 to 10 mg./kg./day):
—using tablets of 100 mg.—

Give isoniazid once a day.

In each dose give:

adults: 300 mg. (3 tablets)
children: 50 mg. (1/2 tablet) for each 5 kg. the child weighs.

For children with severe TB, or persons with tubercular meningitis, double the above dose until improvement takes place.

For prevention of TB in family members of persons with TB, it is often recommended to give the above dose of INH for 6 to 9 months.

Rifampin (rifampicin, rifamycin)

Name:__________________ price:______ for_____

Often comes in: tablets or capsules of 150 or 300 mg.

This antibiotic is expensive, but is powerful in fighting TB. It is never taken alone or the TB will become ***resistant*** to it. When combined with isoniazid and at least one other TB medicine, it can shorten treatment by several months. (Rifampin is also used to treat leprosy— see p. 364.)

It is important to keep taking rifampin regularly, without interruption. Be sure to get more before your supply runs out.

Risks and Precautions:

Rifampin can cause serious damage to the liver. A person who has liver problems or is pregnant should take this medicine under medical supervision.

Side effects: Urine, tears, feces (shit), saliva, mucus from coughing (sputum), and sweat are colored red-orange by rifampin. Rarely, rifampin can cause fever, loss or increase of appetite, vomiting, nausea, confusion, skin rash, and menstrual problems.

Rifampin reduces the effectiveness of oral contraceptives. So women taking birth control pills should get medical advice about increasing the dose. Or, use another method such as condoms, IUD, or a diaphragm while taking this medicine.

Dosage of rifampin for TB—(10 mg./kg./day):
—tablets or capsules of 150 mg. or 300 mg.—

Give rifampin once a day, either 1 hour before or 2 hours after eating.

In each dose give:

adults: 600 mg. (two 300 mg. tablets or four 150 mg. tablets)
children 8 to 12 years: 450 mg.
children 3 to 7 years: 300 mg.
children under 3 years: 150 mg.

Pyrazinamide

Name:__________________ price:______ for_____

Often comes in: tablets of 500 mg.

Risks and Precautions:

Pregnant women should not take pyrazinamide.

Side effects: May cause swollen and painful joints, loss of appetite, nausea and vomiting, painful urination, fatigue, and fever.

Dosage for pyrazinamide—(20 to 30 mg./kg./day):
—using tablets of 500 mg.—

Give 1 dose daily for 2 months, together with other TB medicines. In each dose give:

adults: 1500 or 2000 mg. (3 or 4 tablets)
children 8 to 12 years: 1000 mg. (2 tablets)
children 3 to 7 years: 500 mg. (1 tablet)
children under 3 years: 250 mg. (1/2 tablet)

Ethambutol (familiar brand name: *Myambutol*)

Name:__________________ price:______ for_____

Often comes in: tablets of 100 or 400 mg.

Risks and Precautions:

Ethambutol may cause eye pain or damage if taken in large doses for a long time. The medicine should be stopped if eye problems or vision changes develop. Eye damage caused by ethambutol usually slowly gets better after the medicine is stopped.

Dosage of ethambutol—(25 mg./kg./day for the first 2 months, then 15 mg./kg./day):
—100 mg. tablets or 400 mg. tablets—

Give once a day.

For the first two months, in each dose give:

adults: 1200 mg. (three 400 mg. tablets or twelve 100 mg. tablets)
children: Give 15 mg. for each kg. the child weighs. But for tubercular meningitis give 25 mg. for each kg. the child weighs.

After the first two months give:

adults: 800 mg. (two 400 mg. tablets or eight 100 mg. tablets)
children: Give 15 mg. for each kg. the child weighs.

Streptomycin

Name:__________________ price:______ for_____

Often comes in: vials for injection with 500 mg. in each ml.

Streptomycin is still a very useful medicine for treating tuberculosis. It is somewhat less effective but much cheaper than rifampin.

Risks and Precautions:

Great care must be taken not to give more than the correct dose. Too much streptomycin for too long may cause deafness. If ringing of the ears or deafness begins, stop taking the medicine and see a health worker.

Streptomycin should not be taken by pregnant women or persons with kidney problems.

Dosage for streptomycin (15 mg./kg./day):
—vials of liquid; or powder for mixing with water to give 1 gm. of streptomycin in 2 ml.—

For treatment of tuberculosis:

very severe cases, give 1 injection daily for 3 to 8 weeks
for mild cases, give 1 injection 2 or 3 times a week for 2 months

With each injection give:

adults: 1 gm. (or 2 ml.)
adults over age 50: 500 mg. (1 ml.)
children 8 to 12 years: 750 mg. (1 1/2 ml.)
children 3 to 7 years: 500 mg. (1 ml.)
children under 3 years: 250 mg. (1/2 ml.)
newborn babies: give 20 mg. for each kg. of body weight; thus a 3 kg. baby gets 60 mg. (1/8 ml.)

Use of streptomycin for other than TB:

In emergencies, streptomycin and penicillin together can be used to treat certain severe infections (see PENICILLIN WITH STREPTOMYCIN, p. 354). However, the use of streptomycin for infections other than tuberculosis should be very limited, because frequent use of streptomycin for other illnesses makes tuberculosis resistant to it, and therefore harder to treat. Streptomycin is sometimes used to treat gonorrhea that is resistant to penicillin—a single high dose is needed (see p. 360).

Thiacetazone

Name:__________________ price:______ for_____

Often comes in: tablets with 50 mg. of thiacetazone (often in combination with 100 or 133 mg. of isoniazid)

Side effects: May cause rashes, vomiting, dizziness, or loss of appetite. **People with HIV/AIDS must not use this drug. It can cause severe, even deadly allergic reactions, and can make the skin peel off.**

Dosage for thiacetazone—(2.5 mg./kg./day):
—tablets with 50 mg. thiacetazone, with or without isoniazid—

Give once a day.

In each dose give:

adults: 3 tablets (150 mg.)
children 8 to 12 years: 2 tablets (100 mg.)
children 3 to 7 years: 1 tablet (50 mg.)
children under 3 years: 1/2 tablet (25 mg.)

MEDICINES FOR LEPROSY

When treating leprosy, it is important to know which of the two main types of leprosy the person has. If there are light-colored skin patches with loss of sensation but no lumps or thickened skin, then the person probably has **tuberculoid** leprosy and only 2 medicines are required. If there are lumps, then the person probably has **lepromatous** leprosy and it is best to use 3 medicines. **If possible, medicines for leprosy should be taken with the guidance of an experienced health worker or doctor, according to the national plan.**

Treatment of leprosy must usually continue for at least 6 months and sometimes for life. To prevent the bacteria (bacilli) that cause leprosy from becoming resistant, it is important to keep taking the medicines regularly, without interruption. Be sure to get more medicine before your supply runs out.

Recommended treatment:

For tuberculoid leprosy take both of these for at least 6 months:

Dapsone daily
Rifampin each month

For lepromatous leprosy take all of these for 2 to 5 years:

Dapsone daily
Clofazimine daily and a larger dose each month
Rifampin each month

Note: Although the cure of leprosy is quicker using dapsone together with other medicines, sometimes only dapsone is available. When taken alone, it often gives good results, but more slowly, so treatment must continue for at least 2 years and sometimes for life for lepromatous leprosy.

Occasionally, a person may develop a serious problem called 'lepra reaction' while taking leprosy medicines. There may be lumpy and inflamed spots, fever, and swollen, tender nerves. It may also cause joint pains, tender lymph nodes and testicles, swelling of the hands and feet, or red and painful eyes which may lead to loss of vision.

In case of a severe 'lepra reaction' (pain along the nerves, numbness or weakness, eye irritation, or painful testicles), it is usually best to keep taking the leprosy treatment, but to also take an anti-inflammatory medicine (cortico-steroid). Seek experienced medical advice about this because the cortico-steroid can also cause serious problems.

Dapsone (diaminodiphenylsulfone, DDS)

Name:__________________ price:______ for_____

Often comes in: tablets of 50 and 100 mg.

Dapsone sometimes causes anemia or skin rashes, which can be severe. If severe skin peeling occurs, stop taking the medicine.

WARNING: DDS is a dangerous drug. Keep it where children cannot reach it.

Dosage for DDS—(2 mg./kg./day):
—using tablets of 100 mg.—

Take once a day.

adults: 100 mg. (one 100 mg. tablet)
children 13 to 18 years: 50 mg. (half of a 100 mg. tablet)
children 6 to 12 years: 25 mg. (a quarter of a 100 mg. tablet)
children 2 to 5 years: 25 mg. (a quarter of a 100 mg. tablet) **3 times a week only.**

Rifampin (rifampicin, rifamycin)

Name:__________________ price:______ for_____

Often comes in: tablets or capsules of 150 and 300 mg.

Rifampin is a very expensive medicine, but only a small amount is needed to treat leprosy, so the total cost is not great. See p. 362 for side effects and risks. Take rifampin only with the advice of an experienced health worker or doctor:

Dosage of rifampin for leprosy—(10 to 20 mg./kg.):
—using tablets of 300 mg.—

For leprosy, give rifampin once a month. It should be taken either 1 hour before or 2 hours after eating.

In each monthly dose give:

adults: 600 mg. (two 300 mg. tablets)
children 8 to 12 years: 450 mg. (one and a half 300 mg. tablets)
children 3 to 7 years: 300 mg. (one 300 mg. tablet)
children under 3 years: 150 mg. (half a 300 mg. tablet)

Clofazimine *(Lamprene)*

Name:__________________ price:______ for_____

Often comes in: capsules of 50 and 100 mg.

Clofazimine is also an expensive medicine. Although it is less effective in killing leprosy bacteria than rifampin, it has the advantage that it also helps to control lepra reaction to some extent, particularly in persons with lepromatous leprosy.

Side effects: Causes the skin to become a red-purple color. This is only temporary and will disappear 1 to 2 years after stopping the medicine. May cause stomach or digestive problems. Not recommended for pregnant women.

Dosage for clofazimine—(1 mg./kg./day):
—using capsules of 50 mg.—

Give one dose of clofazimine each day and a second, larger dose once a month.

In each daily dose give:

adults: 50 mg. (one 50 mg. capsule)
children 8 to 12 years: 37 mg. (3/4 of a 50 mg. capsule)
children 3 to 7 years: 25 mg. (1/2 of a 50 mg. capsule)
children under 3 years: 12 mg. (1/4 of a 50 mg. capsule)

In each monthly dose give:

adults: 300 mg. (six 50 mg. capsules)
children 8 to 12 years: 225 mg. (four and a half 50 mg. capsules)
children 3 to 7 years: 150 mg. (three 50 mg. capsules)
children under 3 years: 75 mg. (one and a half 50 mg. capsules)

Note: The larger dose of clofazimine, which can also be used daily to control lepra reaction, is best given with the advice of an experienced health worker or doctor.

OTHER MEDICINES

MEDICINES FOR MALARIA

There are several medicines that fight malaria. Unfortunately, in many parts of the world, malaria parasites have become resistant to the best malaria medicines. This is especially true for the most serious type of malaria (*falciparum* malaria).

It is important to learn from the Health Department or at a health center what medicines work best in your area. New medicines are being developed, but these are likely to be effective for a limited time before resistance to them develops.

IMPORTANT: Malaria can quickly kill persons who have not developed immunity. Children, and also people who visit areas with malaria, must be treated immediately.

Medicines for malaria can be used in two ways:

1. TREATMENT of the person who is ill with malaria. Medicine is given daily for just a few days.

2. PREVENTION: To keep any malaria parasites that may be in the blood from doing harm. Prevention is used in areas where malaria is common, especially to protect children who are weak or sick for other reasons. It is also used by persons visiting a malaria area who have no defenses against the disease. Medicines are usually given weekly. To prevent malaria, also be sure to follow the advice on p. 187 to avoid mosquito bites.

Certain malaria medicines are used only to treat attacks of malaria, while some only work for prevention. Others can be used for both.

As of the beginning of 1996, **chloroquine** is still the most useful medicine to prevent and treat malaria in Mexico, Central America, and Haiti, but resistance is likely to develop as it has in other parts of the world. Chloroquine resistance is widespread in South America, East Africa, and especially Southeast Asia. **Quinine** is usually the best medicine to treat severe malaria in an area where resistance is likely, or to treat malaria affecting the brain.

Mefloquine is a new medicine used to prevent and treat malaria that is resistant to chloroquine. *Fansidar* is another medicine for treatment of malaria resistant to chloroquine. **Proguanil** is used with chloroquine for prevention. **Primaquine** is sometimes taken after treatment with another malaria medicine to keep the disease from coming back. **Tetracycline** is now also used occasionally in malaria treatment and prevention.

Chloroquine

Chloroquine comes in two forms, chloroquine phosphate and chloroquine sulfate. The doses are different, so be sure you know which type of chloroquine you have and the amount of medicine (chloroquine base) in the tablet.

In some areas and for some forms of malaria, other medicines are needed in addition to chloroquine for a complete cure. Seek local advice.

CHLOROQUINE PHOSPHATE (familiar brand names: *Aralen, Resochin, Avlochlor*)

Name:__________________ price:______ for_____

Often comes in: 250 mg. tablets (which have 150 mg. of chloroquine) or 500 mg. (which have 300 mg. of chloroquine)

Dosage for chloroquine phosphate by mouth:
—using 250 mg. tablets—

For treatment of acute attacks of malaria:

For the first dose give:

adults: 4 tablets (1000 mg.)
children 10 to 15 years: 3 tablets (750 mg.)
children 6 to 9 years: 2 tablets (500 mg.)
children 3 to 5 years: 1 tablet (250 mg.)
children 1 to 2 years: 1/2 tablet (125 mg.)
babies under 1 year: 1/4 tablet (63 mg.)

Then give the following dose 6 hours after the first dose, 1 day after the first dose, and 2 days after the first dose:

adults: 2 tablets (500 mg.)
children 10 to 15 years: 1 1/2 tablets (375 mg.)
children 6 to 9 years: 1 tablet (250 mg.)
children 3 to 5 years: 1/2 tablet (125 mg.)
children 1 to 2 years: 1/4 tablet (63 mg.)
babies under 1 year: 1/8 tablet (32 mg.)

For prevention of malaria (where it is not resistant to chloroquine):

Give once a week beginning 1 week before and continuing for 4 weeks after leaving malaria area.

adults: 2 tablets (500 mg.)
children 10 to 15 years: 1 1/2 tablets (375 mg.)
children 6 to 9 years: 1 tablet (250 mg.)
children 3 to 5 years: 1/2 tablet (125 mg.)
children 1 to 2 years: 1/4 tablet (63 mg.)
babies under 1 year: 1/8 tablet (32 mg.)

CHLOROQUINE SULFATE (familiar brand name: *Nivaquine*)

Name:__________________ price:______ for_____

Often comes in: 200 mg. tablets (which have 150 mg. of chloroquine)

Dosage of chloroquine sulfate by mouth:
—200 mg. tablets—

For treatment of acute attacks of malaria:

For the first dose give:

adults: 4 tablets (800 mg.)
children 10 to 15 years: 3 tablets (600 mg.)
children 6 to 9 years: 2 tablets (400 mg.)
children 3 to 5 years: 1 tablet (200 mg.)
children 1 to 2 years: 1/2 tablet (100 mg.)
babies under 1 year: 1/4 tablet (50 mg.)

Then give the following dose 6 hours after the first dose, 1 day after the first dose, and 2 days after the first dose:

adults: 2 tablets (400 mg.)
children 10 to 15 years: 1 1/2 tablets (300 mg.)
children 6 to 9 years: 1 tablet (200 mg.)
children 3 to 5 years: 1/2 tablet (100 mg.)
children 1 to 2 years: 1/4 tablet (50 mg.)
babies under 1 year: 1/8 tablet (25 mg.)

For prevention of malaria:

Give once a week beginning 1 week before and continuing for 4 weeks after leaving a malaria area.

adults: 2 tablets (400 mg.)
children 10 to 15 years: 1 1/2 tablet (300 mg.)
children 6 to 9 years: 1 tablet (200 mg.)
children 3 to 5 years: 1/2 tablet (100 mg.)
children 1 to 2 years: 1/4 tablet (50 mg.)
babies under 1 year: 1/8 tablet (25 mg.)

For treatment of liver abscess caused by amebas:
—using tablets of 250 mg. chloroquine phosphate or 200 mg. chloroquine sulfate—

adults: 3 or 4 tablets twice daily for 2 days and then 1 1/2 or 2 tablets daily for 3 weeks.
Give children less, according to age or weight.

Quinine (quinine sulfate or quinine bisulfate)

Name:__________________ price:______ for_____

Often comes in: tablets of 300 mg. or 650 mg.

Quinine is used to treat resistant malaria (malaria that does not get better with other medicines) and severe malaria, including malaria that affects the brain. It is best given by mouth. If vomiting is a problem when giving quinine by mouth, a medicine such as promethazine may help.

Side effects: Quinine sometimes causes sweaty skin, ringing of the ears or impaired hearing, blurred vision, dizziness, nausea and vomiting, and diarrhea.

Dosage of quinine for treating acute attacks of malaria:
—using tablets of 300 mg.—

Give 3 times a day for 3 days:

adults: 2 tablets (600 mg.)
children 10 to 15 years: 1 1/2 tablets (450 mg.)
children 6 to 9 years: 1 tablet (300 mg.)
children 3 to 5 years: 1/2 tablet (150 mg.)
children 1 to 2 years: 1/4 tablet (75 mg.)
babies under 1 year: 1/8 tablet (38 mg.)

Note: In some parts of the world, such as Southeast Asia, it is necessary to take quinine for 7 days.

Injections of quinine or chloroquine: when to give them:

Injections of quinine or chloroquine should be given only rarely, in cases of great emergency. If a person who shows signs of malaria, or lives in an area where there is a lot of malaria, is vomiting, having fits (convulsions), or showing other signs of meningitis (see p. 185), he may have cerebral malaria (malaria in the brain). **Inject quinine at once.** (Or, if you have no other medicine available, try injecting chloroquine.) Great care must be taken to **be sure the dose is right. Seek medical help.**

QUININE DIHYDROCHLORIDE INJECTIONS, 300 mg. in 2 ml.:

Quinine injections should be given very slowly, and never directly into the vein—this can be dangerous to the heart. Take great care with children.

Inject half this dose slowly into each buttock. Before injecting, draw back on the plunger; if blood appears, inject in another site. Repeat same dose 12 hours later:

adults: 600 mg. (2 ampules of 2 ml.)
children: .07 ml. (1/15 ml., or 10 mg.) for each kg. the child weighs. (A one-year-old baby who weighs 10 kg. would get 0.70 ml.)

CHLOROQUINE INJECTIONS, 200 mg. in 5 ml.:

Give the dose once only (inject 1/2 into each buttock):

adults: 200 mg. (the entire ampule of 5 ml.)
children: inject 0.1 ml. (1/10 ml.) for each kg. the child weighs. (A one-year-old baby who weighs 10 kg. would get 1 ml.)

The dose may be repeated 1 day later if improvement has not taken place.

Mefloquine (familiar brand name: *Lariam*)

Name:__________________ price:______ for_____

Often comes in: tablets of 250 mg.

Mefloquine can prevent and stop acute attacks of malaria that is resistant to chloroquine.

Precautions and side effects: Mefloquine should not be taken by persons with epilepsy or mental illness. Pregnant women should take mefloquine only if they are not able to get another medicine. Persons with heart problems should get experienced medical advice before taking this medicine. Take with a large meal. Mefloquine sometimes causes strange behavior, confusion, anxiety, fits or unconsciousness. **If any of these signs develop, stop taking mefloquine immediately.** Other side effects include dizziness, stomach upset, headache, and vision problems. Side effects are more frequent and severe with higher doses used for treatment.

Dosage of mefloquine:

For treatment of acute attacks of malaria:

Give one time:

adults: 5 tablets (1250 mg.)
children 12 to 15 years: 4 tablets (1000 mg.)
children 8 to 11 years: 3 tablets (750 mg.)
children 5 to 7 years: 2 tablets (500 mg.)
children 1 to 4 years: 1 tablet (250 mg.)
babies under 1 year: 1/2 tablet (125 mg.)

For prevention of malaria:

Give once a week continuing until 4 weeks after leaving malaria area.

adults: 1 tablet (250 mg.)
children over 45 kg.: 1 tablet (250 mg.)
children 31 to 45 kg.: 3/4 tablet (188 mg.)
children 20 to 30 kg.: 1/2 tablet (125 mg.)
children 15 to 19 kg.: 1/4 tablet (63 mg.)
children under 15 kg.: not recommended

Pyrimethamine with sulfadoxine *(Fansidar)*

Name:__________________ price:______ for_____

Comes in: combination tablet with 25 mg. pyrimethamine and 500 mg. sulfadoxine

Fansidar is used to treat resistant malaria.

WARNING: Fansidar should not be taken by anyone who has ever had a reaction to a sulfa medicine. If the medicine causes a rash or itching, **drink lots of water and do not take it again.**

Dosage to treat acute attacks of malaria:

Give one time:

adults: 3 tablets
children 9 to 14 years: 2 tablets
children 4 to 8 years: 1 tablet
children 1 to 3 years: 1/2 tablet
babies under 1 year: 1/4 tablet

Proguanil *(Paludrine)*

Name:__________________ price:______ for_____

Often comes in: tablets of 100 mg.

Proguanil is taken with chloroquine for prevention of chloroquine resistant malaria. Proguanil is not used to treat acute attacks of malaria.

Dosage of proguanil for prevention:

Give medicine each day, starting the day entering a malaria area until 28 days after leaving the area.

adults: 2 tablets (200 mg.)
children 9 to 14 years: 1 1/2 tablets (150 mg.)
children 3 to 6 years: 1 tablet (100 mg.)
children 1 to 2 years: 1/2 tablet (50 mg.)
babies under 1 year: 1/4 tablet (25 mg.)

Primaquine

Name:__________________ price:______ for_____

Often comes in: tablets of 26.3 mg. of primaquine phosphate, which contains 15 mg. of primaquine base.

Primaquine is usually used after treatment with chloroquine or another malaria medicine to keep some kinds of malaria from coming back. Primaquine does not work by itself for acute attacks.

Side effects: Pregnant women should not take primaquine. In certain persons, especially some black people, this medicine causes anemia. Seek local advice.

Dosage of primaquine:

Give once a day for 14 days.

In each dose give:

adults: 1 tablet (15 mg. base)
children 8 to 12 years: 1/2 tablet (7 mg. base)
children 3 to 7 years: 1/4 tablet (4 mg. base)

Tetracycline

Tetracycline can be used to treat acute attacks of malaria in Southeast Asia and some other areas where there is much chloroquine-resistant malaria. But because it works slowly, it should be given with another medicine (usually quinine). Visitors to these areas sometimes take doxycycline daily for prevention. See p. 356 for tetracycline and doxycycline doses, risks, and precautions.

FOR AMEBAS AND GIARDIA

In diarrhea or dysentery caused by amebas there are usually frequent stools with much mucus and sometimes blood. Often there are gut cramps, but little or no fever. Amebic dysentery is best treated with **metronidazole** together with **diloxanide furoate** or **tetracycline. Chloroquine** is sometimes used when metronidazole is not available, or in cases of amebic abscess. **Iodoquinol** is another medicine used to treat amebic dysentery, but it may have dangerous side effects.

In order to kill all the amebas in the gut, very long (2 to 3 weeks) and expensive treatment is necessary. It often makes more sense to stop giving medicines when the person has no more symptoms and then let the body defend itself against the few amebas that are left. This is especially true in areas where the chance of getting a new infection is high.

In diarrhea caused by giardia the stools are often yellow and frothy, but without blood or mucus. Metronidazole is often used, but quinacrine is cheaper.

Metronidazole (familiar brand name: *Flagyl*)

Name: ________________________________

Often comes in:
tablets of 200, 250, or 500 mg. Price:____ for__
vaginal inserts, 500 mg. Price:____ for__

Metronidazole is useful for gut infections caused by amebas and giardia, and sometimes for diarrhea that comes from taking 'wide-range' antibiotics (such as ampicillin). It is also useful for vaginal infections caused by Trichomonas, or by certain bacteria. It can also help to treat the symptoms of guinea worm.

CAUTION: Do not drink alcoholic drinks when taking metronidazole, as this causes severe nausea.

WARNING: Metronidazole may cause birth defects. Pregnant women should avoid using this medicine if possible, especially during the first 3 months of pregnancy. Breast feeding women using large doses should not give their babies breast milk for 24 hours after taking metronidazole. Persons with liver problems should not use metronidazole.

Dosage for **giardia** infection:

Give metronidazole 3 times a day for 5 days.

In each dose give:

adults: 250 mg. (1 tablet)
children 8 to 12 years: 250 mg. (1 tablet)
children 3 to 7 years: 125 mg. (1/2 tablet)
children under 3 years: 62 mg. (1/4 tablet)

Dosage for **guinea worm:**

Give the same dose as for giardia, 3 times a day for 10 days.

Dosage for **Trichomonas** infections of the vagina:

The woman should take 8 tablets (2 gm.) by mouth in one single dose. Or, if the infection is not very severe, she can use a vaginal insert twice a day for 10 days. Both the woman and man should be treated for Trichomonas at the same time. (He should do this even if he has no symptoms or he will pass it back to the woman.)

Dosage for **bacterial** infections of the vagina:

The woman should take 2 tablets (500 mg.) of metronidazole twice a day for 5 days. If the infection returns, both the woman and man should take the same treatment, at the same time.

Dosage for **amebic dysentery**—(25 to 50 mg./kg./day):—using 250 mg. tablets—

Give metronidazole 3 times a day for 5 to 10 days.

In each dose give:

adults: 750 mg. (3 tablets)
children 8 to 12 years: 500 mg. (2 tablets)
children 4 to 7 years: 375 mg. (1 1/2 tablets)
children 2 to 3 years: 250 mg. (1 tablet)
children under 2 years: 80 to 125 mg. (1/3 to 1/2 tablet)

For amebic dysentery, metronidazole should be taken together with diloxanide furoate or tetracycline.

Diloxanide furoate *(Furamide)*

Name:__________________ price:______ for_____

Often comes in: 500 mg. tablets
also, syrup with 125 mg. in 5 ml.

Side effects: Occasionally causes gas, stomach pain, or nausea.

Dosage for diloxanide furoate—(20 mg./kg./day) —tablets of 500 mg.—

Give 3 times a day with meals. For complete treatment take for 10 days.

In each dose give:

adults: 1 tablet (500 mg.)
children 8 to 12 years: 1/2 tablet (250 mg.)
children 3 to 7 years: 1/4 tablet (125 mg.)
children under 3 years: 1/8 tablet (62 mg.) or less, depending on weight

Tetracycline (see p. 356)

Chloroquine (It is sometimes used when metronidazole is not available or when amebas have formed abscesses—see p. 365)

Quinacrine (mepacrine)
(familiar brand name: *Atabrine*)

Name:__________________ price:______ for_____

Often comes in: 100 mg. tablets

Quinacrine can be used in treating giardia, malaria, and tapeworm, but is not the best medicine for any of these. It is used because it is cheap. Quinacrine often causes headache, dizziness, and vomiting.

Dosage of quinacrine for treating **giardia:**

Give quinacrine 3 times a day for a week.

In each dose give:

adults: one 100 mg. tablet
children under 10 years: 50 mg. (1/2 tablet)

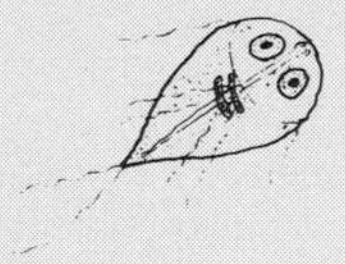

Dosage of quinacrine for treating **tapeworm:**

(Half an hour before giving quinacrine, give an antihistamine like **promethazine** to help prevent vomiting.)

Give 1 large dose only:

adults: 1 gm. (10 tablets)
children 8 to 12 years: 600 mg. (6 tablets)
children 3 to 7 years: 400 mg. (4 tablets)

DANGER! DO NOT USE!

↓

Hydroxyquinolines (clioquinol, iodoquinol, di-iodohydroxyquinoline, halquinol, broxyquinoline) (familiar brand names: *Diodoquin, Amicline, Floraquin, Enteroquinol, Chlorambin, Nivembin, Quogyl, Entero-Vioform,* and many other brands)

These medicines were commonly used in the past to treat diarrhea. They are now known to sometimes cause permanent paralysis, blindness, and even death. Do not use these dangerous medicines. (See p. 51.)

FOR VAGINAL INFECTIONS

Vaginal discharge, itching, and discomfort can be caused by different infections, the most common of which are **Trichomonas, yeast** (Candida, moniliasis), and **bacteria.** Cleanliness and vinegar-and-water douches (vaginal washes) help many vaginal infections. Specific medicines are also listed below.

White vinegar for vaginal douches (washes):

Price:________ for____

Mix 2 or 3 tablespoons of white vinegar in a liter of boiled water. As shown on page 241, give 1 to 3 douches a day for a week, then 1 every other day. This works especially well for bacterial infections of the vagina.

Metronidazole, tablets to be taken by mouth and vaginal inserts (see p. 369):

For Trichomonas and bacterial infections of the vagina. (Only use metronidazole for bacterial infections if vinegar and water douches do not work.)

Nystatin or **Miconazole,** tablets, cream, and vaginal inserts (see p. 373):

For yeast infection (Candida, moniliasis) of the vagina.

Gentian violet (crystal violet) 1 percent solution (see p. 371):

Price:________ for____

For treatment of yeast infection (Candida, moniliasis) and other infections of the vulva and vagina.

Paint on gentian violet once daily for 3 weeks.

Povidone iodine ***(Betadine)***

Price:_______ for___

For treatment of bacterial infections of the vagina.

Mix 2 tablespoons of povidone iodine in a liter of warm water that has been boiled. As shown on page 241, give 1 douche a day for 10 to 14 days.

FOR SKIN PROBLEMS

Washing the hands and bathing frequently with soap and water help prevent many infections, both of the skin and of the gut. Wounds should be carefully washed with soap and boiled water before they are closed or bandaged.

Frequent scrubbing with soap and water is often the only treatment necessary for dandruff, cradle cap (seborrhea), pimples, mild impetigo, as well as for minor ringworm, tinea, and other fungus infections of the skin or scalp. For these purposes it is better if the soap has in it an antiseptic like iodine, such as povidone iodine ***(Betadine).*** But ***Betadine*** can be irritating to tissue and should not be used on open skin.

Sulfur

Often comes as a yellow powder.

Price:____ for__

Also comes in many skin lotions and ointments.

Sulfur is useful for many skin problems:

1. To avoid or discourage ticks, mites, chiggers, jiggers, and fleas. Before going into fields or forests where these are common, dust the skin—especially legs or ankles, wrists, waist, and neck—with sulfur.

2. To help treat scabies, burrowing fleas, mites, and tiny ticks in or on the skin. Make an ointment: Mix 1 part of sulfur with 10 parts of petrolatum ***(Vaseline)*** or lard, and smear this on the skin (see p. 200).

3. For ringworm, tinea, and other fungus infections, use the same ointment, 3 or 4 times a day, or a lotion of sulfur and vinegar (see p. 205).

4. For cradle cap (seborrhea) and severe dandruff, the same ointment can be used, or the scalp can be dusted with sulfur.

Gentian violet (crystal violet)

Often comes as dark blue crystals.

Price:____ for__

Gentian violet helps fight certain skin infections, including impetigo and sores with pus. It can also be used to treat yeast infections (Candida, moniliasis) in the mouth (thrush) or in the vulva or skin folds.

Dissolve a teaspoon of gentian violet in half a liter of water. This makes a 2 percent solution. Paint it on the skin or in the mouth or the vulva.

Antibiotic ointments

Name:__________________ price:______ for_____

These are expensive and often do no more good than gentian violet. However, they do not color the skin or clothes and are of use in treating minor skin infections like impetigo. A good ointment is one that contains a neomycin/polymyxin combination (for example ***Neosporin*** or ***Polysporin***). An ointment of tetracycline can also be used.

Cortico-steroid ointments or lotions

Name:__________________ price:______ for_____

These can be used for 'weeping' or severely itchy skin irritations caused by insect bites, by touching certain 'poisonous' plants, and other things. They are also useful in treating severe eczema (see p. 216) and psoriasis (p. 216). Use 3 or 4 times a day. Avoid using for long periods of time, or on large areas of skin.

Petroleum jelly (petrolatum, ***Vaseline*****)**

Price:____ for__

Useful for preparing ointments or dressings in the treatment of: scabies (see p. 199 and 373)
ringworm (p. 372)
itching from pinworm (p. 141)
burns (p. 96 and 97)
chest wounds (p. 91)

FOR RINGWORM AND OTHER FUNGUS INFECTIONS

Many fungus infections are very difficult to get rid of. For complete control, treatment must be continued for days or weeks after the signs disappear. Bathing and cleanliness are also important.

Ointments with undecylenic, benzoic, or salicylic acid

Name:__________________ price:______ for_____

Ointments with these acids can be used to treat ringworm, tinea of the scalp, and other fungus infections of the skin. Often they are (or can be) combined with sulfur. Ointments with salicylic acid and sulfur can also be used for cradle cap (seborrhea).

Whitfield's Ointment is a combination of salicylic and benzoic acid. It is useful for many fungal infections, including tinea versicolor. Apply twice daily for 2 to 4 weeks.

Ointments and lotions are cheaper if you make them yourself. Mix 3 parts of salicylic acid and/or 6 parts of benzoic acid with 100 parts of *Vaseline,* petrolatum, mineral oil, lard, or 40 percent alcohol (or rum). Rub onto skin 3 or 4 times a day.

Sulfur and vinegar

A lotion of 5 parts of sulfur to 100 parts vinegar helps fight fungus infections of the skin. Let dry on skin. Also, an ointment can be made using 1 part sulfur to 10 parts of lard.

Sodium thiosulfate ('hypo')

Comes as white crystals, sold in photographic supply stores as 'hypo'. Price:____ for__

Used for **tinea versicolor** infections of the skin (see p. 206).

Dissolve a tablespoon of 'hypo' in 1/2 cup of water and spread it on the skin with a piece of cotton or cloth. Then rub the skin with a piece of cotton soaked in vinegar. Do this twice daily until the 'spots' go away and then once again every 2 weeks to keep them from coming back.

Selenium sulfide *(Selsun, Exsel)*

Name:__________________ price:______ for_____

Often comes as lotion containing 1 or 2.5 percent selenium sulfide.

Lotions with selenium sulfide are useful for treating tinea versicolor. Apply to the affected area, and wash off 30 minutes later. Use daily for one week.

Tolnaftate *(Tinactin)*

Name:__________________ price:______ for_____

Often comes in: cream, powder, and solution of 1 percent tolnaftate.

This may be used for fungus infections caused by tinea on the feet, groin, scalp, hands, and body. Apply twice daily until 2 weeks after symptoms are gone.

Griseofulvin

Name:__________________ price:______ for_____

Often comes in: tablets or capsules of 250 or 500 mg.

Preparations in 'microsized' particles are best.

This is very expensive and should be used only for severe fungus infections of the skin and deep tinea infections of the scalp. It is also used for fungal infections of the nails, but this may take months and does not always work. Pregnant women should avoid taking griseofulvin.

Dosage of griseofulvin—(15 mg./kg./day):
—for microsized particle form, 250 mg. capsules–

Give once a day for at least a month.

- adults: 500 to 1000 mg. (2 to 4 capsules)
- children 8 to 12 years: 250 to 500 mg. (1 to 2 capsules)
- children 3 to 7 years: 125 to 250 mg. (1/2 to 1 capsule)
- children under 3 years: 125 mg. (1/2 capsule)

Gentian violet—for yeast infections (see p. 371)

Nystatin or Miconazole

Name:__________________ price:______ for_____

Comes in: solutions, dusting powders, vaginal tablets, ointments, and creams

Used for treating yeast infections (Candida, moniliasis) in the mouth (thrush), the vagina, or in the folds of the skin. Nystatin only works for infections caused by yeast, but miconazole works against other fungus infections as well.

Dosage for nystatin and miconazole—the same for children and adults:

Thrush in the mouth: put 1 ml. of solution in the mouth and hold it there for at least 1 minute before swallowing. Do this 3 or 4 times a day.

Yeast infection on the skin: keep as dry as possible and use nystatin or miconazole dusting powder or ointment 3 or 4 times a day.

Yeast infection in the vulva or vagina: put cream inside the vagina twice daily or a vaginal tablet inside the vagina nightly for 10 to 14 days.

FOR SCABIES AND LICE: INSECTICIDES

Gamma benzene hexachloride (lindane)
(familiar brand names: *Kwell, Gammezane*)

Name:__________________ price:______ for_____

This comes in expensive preparations for people and cheap preparations for animals which work just as well for people. Lindane for a sheep or cattle dip is quite cheap, but it often comes concentrated in a 15 percent solution and must be diluted to 1 percent. Mix 1 part of 15 percent lindane concentrate with 15 parts of water or *Vaseline,* and use on the skin for scabies following the instructions on page 199. For head lice, see page 200.

CAUTION: Lindane is a poison and can cause dangerous side effects, including fits, especially in babies. Do not overuse. Make only one application; if necessary repeat once more a week later.

Benzyl benzoate, cream or lotion

Name:__________________ price:______ for_____

Use the same as gamma benzene hexachloride (lindane) cream or lotion.

Sulfur in petroleum jelly *(Vaseline)* or lard

Use this for scabies if you cannot get the above.

Mix 1 part of sulfur in 20 parts of *Vaseline,* mineral oil, or lard to form a 5 percent sulfur ointment.

Pyrethrins with piperonyl *(RID)*

Name:__________________ price:______ for_____

Often comes as a liquid solution containing pyrethrins and piperonyl butoxide.

Works well for all kinds of lice and is safer than gamma benzene hexachloride (lindane). Without adding any water, apply the liquid to dry hair until it is completely wet. (Do not use on eyebrows or eyelashes.) Wait 10 minutes, no longer. Wash the hair with warm water and soap or shampoo. Repeat in 1 week. Change clothing and bedding after treatment. To get rid of nits (lice eggs), see p. 200.

Crotamiton *(Eurax)*

Name:__________________ price:______ for_____

This often comes as a cream or lotion containing 10 percent crotamiton.

Crotamiton is used for treatment of scabies only, not lice. After bathing, apply over the whole body, from the chin to the toes—don't miss the folds and creases in the skin! A second application may be used the next day. Take a bath or shower 2 days after the last application to clean off all the cream or lotion. Clothing and bedding should be changed at this time.

FOR GENITAL WARTS

Podophyllin

Name:__________________ price:______ for_____

Often comes as a solution containing 10 to 25 percent podophyllin mixed with benzoin.

This is used to shrink genital warts. Podophyllin is very irritating to healthy skin, so it should be used with care. Before applying, it helps to protect the area around the warts with petroleum jelly *(Vaseline)* or some other greasy ointment. Apply solution to warts and let dry completely. (This is especially important in areas where normal skin may touch the wart, such as the foreskin of the penis.) Wash off thoroughly in 4 to 6 hours. Treatment can be repeated in one week. Usually several weekly treatments are needed.

CAUTION: If severe skin irritation develops, do not use again. Podophyllin should not be used on bleeding warts. Women who are pregnant or breast feeding should not use podophyllin.

Bichloroacetic acid or Trichloroacetic acid

Name:__________________ price:______ for_____

Comes as a clear liquid.

If podophyllin is not available, bichloroacetic acid or trichloroacetic acid can be used to shrink warts. It also dissolves healthy skin, so it must be used with care. Protect the skin around the wart with ***Vaseline*** or some other greasy ointment. Carefully trim off dead tissue from large or thick warts. with a toothpick, apply a small drop of acid to the wart. Gently work the acid into the wart with the point of the toothpick. Several treatments are usually needed and can be repeated weekly.

CAUTION: This acid can cause severe burns. Protect hands and other healthy skin from the acid, and wash immediately in case of contact.

FOR WORMS

Medicines by themselves are not enough to get rid of worm infections for very long. Guidelines of personal and public cleanliness must also be followed. When 1 person in the family has worms, it is wise to treat the whole family.

Mebendazole *(Vermox)*—for many different worm infections

Name:__________________ price:______ for_____

Often comes in: tablets of 100 mg.

This medicine works against hookworm, whipworm, roundworm, pinworm (threadworm), and another worm called Strongyloides. Works well for mixed infections. It may do some good in cases of trichinosis. When treating heavy worm infections there may be some gut pain or diarrhea, but side effects are not common.

WARNING: Do not give mebendazole to pregnant women or children under 2 years old.

Dosage of mebendazole—using 100 mg. tablets—

Give the same amount to children and adults.

For pinworm: one tablet once a week for 3 weeks.

For roundworm (Ascaris), whipworm (Trichuris), hookworm, and Strongyloides: one tablet twice a day (morning and evening) for 3 days (6 tablets in all).

Albendazole *(Zentel)*—for many different worm infections

Name:__________________ price:______ for_____

Often comes in: tablets of 200 and 400 mg.

This medicine is similar to mebendazole, but often more expensive. It works against hookworm, whipworm, Strongyloides, roundworm, and pinworm. Side effects are rare.

WARNING: Do not give albendazole to pregnant women or children under 2 years.

Dosage of albendazole—using 200 mg. tablets—

Give the same amount to children and adults.

For pinworm, roundworm (Ascaris), whipworm (Trichuris), and hookworm: 400 mg. (2 tablets) one time.

For Strongyloides: 400 mg. (2 tablets) twice a day for 3 days, and then repeat one week later.

Piperazine—for roundworm (Ascaris) and pinworm (threadworm, Enterobius)

Name: ______________________________

Comes as piperazine citrate, tartrate, hydrate, adipate, or phosphate

Often comes in:

500 mg. tablets Price:_____ for___

Mixture, 500 mg. in 5 ml. Price:_____ for___

A large dose is given for 2 days to treat roundworm. Smaller doses every day for a week are given for pinworm. There are few side effects.

Dosage of piperazine for **roundworm** (Ascaris)—(75 mg./kg./day)

—500 mg. tablets or mixture with 500 mg. in 5 ml.—

Give once daily for 2 days.

- adults: 3500 mg. (7 tablets or 7 teaspoons)
- children 8 to 12 years: 2500 mg. (5 tablets or 5 teaspoons)
- children 3 to 7 years: 1500 mg. (3 tablets or 3 teaspoons)
- children 1 to 3 years: 1000 mg. (2 tablets or 2 teaspoons)
- babies under 1 year: 500 mg. (1 tablet or 1 teaspoon)

Dosage of piperazine for **pinworm** (Enterobius)—(40 mg./kg./day):

Give 2 doses daily for a week.

- adults: 1000 mg. (2 tablets or 2 teaspoons)
- children 8 to 12 years: 750 mg. (1 1/2 tablets or 1 1/2 teaspoons)
- children 3 to 7 years: 500 mg. (1 tablet or 1 teaspoon)
- children under 3 years: 250 mg. (1/2 tablet or 1/2 teaspoon)

Thiabendazole—for many different worm infections

Name:________________ price:_____ for_____

Often comes as: 500 mg. tablets or mixture with 1 gm. in 5 ml.

Because thiabendazole causes more side effects than mebendazole or albendazole, it should only be used for worms when these medicines are not available, or for worm infections that are not inside the gut.

It can be used to treat hookworm, whipworm (Trichuris), and another worm called Strongyloides. It also works for roundworm and pinworm, but piperazine has fewer side effects. It can be helpful in treating guinea worm, and may do some good in cases of trichinosis.

CAUTION: Thiabendazole may cause roundworm (Ascaris) to crawl up the throat. This can block breathing. Therefore, if you suspect a person has roundworm in addition to other worms, it is wise to treat first with piperazine before giving thiabendazole.

Side effects: Thiabendazole often causes tiredness, a sick feeling, and sometimes vomiting.

Dosage for thiabendazole—(25 mg./kg./day):

—500 mg. tablets or mixture with 1 gm. in 5 ml.—

Give twice a day for 3 days. Tablets should be chewed.

In each dose give:

- adults: 1500 mg. (3 tablets or 1 1/2 teaspoons)
- children 8 to 12 years: 1000 mg. (2 tablets or 1 teaspoon)
- children 3 to 7 years: 500 mg. (1 tablet or 1/2 teaspoon)
- children under 3 years: 250 mg. (1/2 tablet or 1/4 teaspoon)

Pyrantel *(Antiminth, Cobrantril, Helmex)*

Name: ____________________________________

Comes as pamoate or embonate

Often comes in:

250 mg. tablets Price:_____ for___
Mixture, 250 mg. in 5 ml. Price:_____ for___

This medicine works for pinworm, hookworm, and roundworm (Ascaris), but it may be expensive. Pyrantel occasionally causes vomiting, dizziness, or headache.

Dosage for pyrantel—(10 mg./kg.):
—using 250 mg. tablets—

For hookworm and roundworm, give one time. For pinworm, repeat dose after 2 weeks.

In each dose give:

adults: 750 mg. (3 tablets)
children 10 to 14 years: 500 mg. (2 tablets)
children 6 to 9 years: 250 mg. (1 tablet)
children 2 to 5 years: 125 mg. (1/2 tablet)
children under 2 years: 62 mg. (1/4 tablet)

FOR TAPEWORM

There are several types of tapeworms. Niclosamide works best for most types and praziquantel is the next best treatment.

Niclosamide *(Yomesan)*—for tapeworm infection

Name:__________________ price:______ for_____

Often comes in: chewable tablets of 500 mg.

Niclosamide is probably the best medicine for tapeworm. It works against most kinds of tapeworm in the gut, but not against cysts outside the gut.

Dosage of niclosamide for tapeworm—500 mg. tablets:

Chew well and swallow 1 dose only. Do not eat before or until 2 hours after taking the medicine. Giving a purge may help get rid of the tapeworm.

adults and children over 8 years: 2 gm. (4 tablets)
children 2 to 8 years: 1 gm. (2 tablets)
children under 2 years: 500 mg. (1 tablet)

Praziquantel *(Biltricide, Droncit)*

Name:__________________ price:______ for_____

Often comes in: tablets of 150 mg. and 600 mg.

Praziquantel is effective in treating most types of tapeworms, but is more expensive than niclosamide.

WARNING: Pregnant women and children under 4 years old should not take praziquantel. Women who are breast feeding should stop giving their babies breast milk while taking praziquantel and for 72 hours after taking it (squeeze out the milk and throw it away).

Side effects: Praziquantel may cause tiredness, dizziness, headache, and loss of appetite, but these side effects are rare at the low dosages used to treat tapeworm.

Dosage of praziquantel for **most kinds of tapeworm,** including beef and pork tapeworm—(10 to 20 mg./kg.):
—using 600 mg. tablets—

Take once only.

adults: 600 mg. (1 tablet)
children 8 to 12 years: 300 mg. (1/2 tablet)
children 4 to 7 years: 150 mg. (1/4 tablet)

Treatment of dwarf tapeworm *(H. nana)* requires a larger dosage:

Take once only.

adults: 1500 mg. (2 1/2 tablets)
children 8 to 12 years: 600 to 1200 mg. (1 to 2 tablets)
children 4 to 7 years: 300 to 600 mg. (1/2 to 1 tablet)

Quinacrine (mepacrine, ***Atabrine*****)** for tapeworm, see p. 370.

FOR SCHISTOSOMIASIS (BLOOD FLUKES, BILHARZIA)

In different parts of the world there are several types of schistosomiasis, which require different treatments. Praziquantel is a medicine that works against all forms of the disease. Metrifonate and oxamniquine are effective against some kinds of schistosomiasis. Medicines should be given under direction of an experienced health worker.

Praziquantel *(Biltricide, Droncit)*

Name:__________________ price:______ for_____

Often comes in: tablets of 150 mg. or 600 mg.

WARNING: Pregnant women should not take praziquantel. Women who are breast feeding should stop giving their babies breast milk while taking praziquantel and for 72 hours after taking it (squeeze out the milk and throw it away). Do not give praziquantel to children under 4 years old.

Side effects: Praziquantel frequently causes tiredness, headache, dizziness, and loss of appetite, but treatment need not be stopped if these side effects occur. To lessen side effects, praziquantel is best taken with a large meal.

Dosage of praziquantel for schistosomiasis—(40 mg./kg.): —using 600 mg. tablets—

To treat schistosomiasis that causes blood in the urine ***(S. hematobium)***, give in a single dose:

adults: 2400 to 3000 mg. (4 or 5 tablets)
children 8 to 12 years: 1200 to 1800 mg. (2 or 3 tablets)
children 4 to 7 years: 600 mg. (1 tablet)

The above doses will also treat one kind of schistosomiasis found in East and Central Africa and South America that causes blood in the stool ***(S. mansoni)***. But in Eastern Asia, schistosomiasis causing blood in the stool ***(S. japonicum)*** requires a larger dose (60 mg./kg.):

Give in one day:

adults: 3600 to 4200 mg. (6 or 7 tablets)
children 8 to 12 years: 1800 to 2400 mg. (3 or 4 tablets)
children 4 to 7 years: 900 mg. (1 1/2 tablets)

(To reduce side effects, this larger amount can be divided into 3 smaller doses, given in one day.)

Metrifonate *(Metriphonate, Bilarcil)*

Metrifonate is a much cheaper medicine that can be used to treat schistosomiasis that causes blood in the urine ***(S. hematobium)***. Pregnant women should not take this medicine.

Name:__________________ price:______ for_____

Comes in: 100 mg. tablets

Dosage of metrifonate for schistosomiasis—(7.5 to 10 mg./kg. per dose):
—100 mg. tablets—

Give 3 doses at 2 week intervals.

In each dose give:

adults: 400 to 600 mg. (4 to 6 tablets)
children 6 to 12 years: 300 mg. (3 tablets)
children 3 to 5 years: 100 mg. (1 tablet)

Oxamniquine *(Vansil, Mansil)*

Name: ______________________________________

Often comes in:
capsules with 250 mg. Price:____ for__
syrup with 250 mg. in 5 ml. Price:____ for__

Oxamniquine is used to treat schistosomiasis causing blood in the stools in South and Central America ***(S. mansoni)***. (To treat ***S. mansoni*** found in Africa, larger doses than those given here are needed. Seek local advice.) This medicine is best taken after a meal.

WARNING: Pregnant women should not take oxamniquine. This medicine may cause dizziness, drowsiness, and, rarely, fits. Persons with epilepsy should use oxamniquine only when also taking epilepsy medicine.

Dosage of oxamniquine—(adults: 15 mg./kg./day. children: 10 mg./kg./twice a day):
—250 mg. capsules—

Give for one day only:

For adults, give 750 to 1000 mg. (3 or 4 capsules) in one dose.

For children, give the following dose twice in one day:

children 8 to 12 years: 250 mg. (1 capsule)
children 4 to 7 years: 125 mg. (1/2 capsule)
children 1 to 3 years: 63 mg. (1/4 capsule)

FOR RIVER BLINDNESS (ONCHOCERCIASIS)

The best medicine for treating river blindness is ivermectin. This new medicine kills the baby worms slowly and does not cause the dangerous reaction of other treatments. If ivermectin is not available, an experienced health worker can give diethylcarbamazine first and then also suramin.

Ivermectin *(Mectizan)*

Name:__________________ price:______ for_____

Often comes in: 6 mg. tablets

To determine the correct dose, if possible weigh the person first. Give one dose. Another dose is sometimes needed 6 months to 1 year later.

CAUTION: Do not give to children who weigh less than 15 kg. (or children who are under 5 years old), to pregnant or breast feeding women, or to persons with meningitis or other serious illness.

Dosage of ivermectin:

Give one time:

heavy adults (over 64 kg.): 2 tablets (12 mg.)
average adults (45 to 63 kg.): 1 1/2 tablets (9 mg.)
light adults and youths (26 to 44 kg.): 1 tablet (6 mg.)
children (15 to 25 kg): 1/2 tablet (3 mg.)

Diethylcarbamazine *(Hetrazan, Banocide)*

Name:__________________ price:______ for_____

Often comes in: tablets of 50 mg.

Diethylcarbamazine kills the young worms, but not the adults. The medicine should be used only under the direction of an experienced health care worker.

To avoid severe damage to the eyes, it is important to start with a low dose. Take the medicine like this:

First day: ½ mg./kg., 1 time only
Second day: ½ mg./kg., 2 times
Third day: 1 mg./kg., 3 times

Continue taking 1mg./kg/3 times a day for 13 more days. (Example: a person who weighs 60 kg. would take 1 single dose of 30 mg. the first day; 60 mg. in 2 doses (of 30 mg. each) the second day, and 3 doses of 60 mg. each, per day, for 14 days.) Take the medicine after meals.

Diethylcarbamazine may cause severe allergic reactions, which can partly be controlled with antihistamines—or cortico-steroids, given by a health worker.

Side effects: Diethylcarbamazine sometimes causes headache, tiredness, weakness, loss of appetite, stomach upset, cough, chest pains, muscle or joint pain, fever and rash.

Suramin *(Naphuride, Bayer 205, Antrypol, Germanin)*

Name:__________________ price:______ for_____

This is more effective than diethylcarbamazine in killing adult worms and should be used after treatment with diethylcarbamazine, when reactions have nearly stopped. Suramin sometimes poisons the kidneys. If swelling of the feet or other signs of urinary poisoning occur, stop using this medicine. Persons with kidney problems should not use it.

Suramin must be given intravenously and should only be used with the assistance of an experienced health worker. For adults inject 1 gm. of suramin in 10 ml. of distilled water **once a week** for 5 to 7 weeks. Start with a small test dose of 200 mg. Treat allergic reactions with antihistamines.

FOR THE EYES

Antibiotic eye ointment—
for 'pink eye' (conjunctivitis)

Useful examples: oxytetracycline or chlortetracycline eye ointments

Name:__________________ price:______ for_____

These eye ointments can be used for 'pink eye' caused by bacteria and for trachoma. For complete cure of trachoma, tetracycline (p. 356) or erythromycin (p. 355) should be taken by mouth also.

For an eye ointment to do any good, it must be put **inside** the eyelid, not outside. Use it 3 or 4 times a day.

Use 1% tetracycline, erythromycin or chloramphenicol eye ointment to protect newborn babies' eyes from gonorrhea and chlamydia. At birth, put a little ointment in the inner corner of each eye and do not wipe or rinse out. If antibiotic eye ointment is not available, use silver nitrate eye drops.

To treat these diseases in the newborn, see p. 221.

Silver nitrate eye drops, 1 percent—to protect eyes of newborn babies

Name:__________________ price:______ for_____

At birth, put a drop of 1 percent silver nitrate in each eye. This will protect the baby's eyes against gonorrhea (but not chlamydia).

WARNING: Do not use silver nitrate drops that may have become too concentrated because of evaporation—they can burn babies' eyes.

FOR PAIN: ANALGESICS

Note: There are many different kinds of pain medicine, many of which are dangerous (especially those containing **dipyrone**). Use only those you are sure are relatively safe like **aspirin, acetaminophen (paracetamol),** or **ibuprofen** (p. 380). For a stronger painkiller see **codeine** (p. 384).

Aspirin (acetylsalicylic acid)

Often comes in:
300 mg. (5 grain) tablets Price:_____ for__
75 mg. (1 1/4 grain) tablets for children (or 'child's aspirin') Price:_____ for__

Aspirin is a very useful, low-cost 'painkiller' or analgesic. It helps to calm pain, lower fever, and reduce inflammation. It also helps a little to calm cough and reduce itching.

Many different medicines sold for pain, arthritis, or colds contain aspirin, but they are more expensive and often do not do any more good than aspirin alone.

Risks and Precautions:

1. Do not use aspirin for stomach pain or indigestion. Aspirin is acid and may make the problem worse. For the same reason, **persons with stomach ulcers should never use aspirin.**

2. Aspirin causes stomach pain or 'heartburn' in some persons. To avoid this, take aspirin with milk, a little bicarbonate of soda, or a lot of water—or together with meals.

3. Do not give more than 1 dose of aspirin to a dehydrated person until he begins to urinate well.

4. It is better not to give aspirin to children under 12 years and especially not to babies (acetaminophen is safer) or to persons with asthma (this may bring on an attack).

5. Keep aspirin where children cannot reach it. Large amounts can poison them.

6. Do not give to pregnant women.

Dosage of aspirin—for pain or fever:
—tablets of 300 mg. (5 grains)—

Take once every 4 to 6 hours (or 4 to 6 times a day), but do not give to children more than 4 times a day.

adults: 1 or 2 tablets (300 to 600 mg.)
children 8 to 12 years: 1 tablet (300 mg.)
children 3 to 7 years: 1/2 tablet (150 mg.)
children 1 to 2 years old: 1/4 tablet (75 mg.)

(Dose may be doubled for severe menstrual pain, severe arthritis or rheumatic fever. Or give 100 mg./kg./day. If ringing of the ears develops, lower the dose.)

—75 mg. 'child's aspirin' tablets—

Give children aspirin 4 times a day:

children 8 to 12 years: 4 tablets (300 mg.)
children 3 to 7 years: 2 to 3 tablets (150 to 225 mg.)
children 1 to 2 years: 1 tablet (75 mg.)
do not give aspirin to children under 1 year old

Acetaminophen (paracetamol)—for pain and fever

Name:__________________ price:______ for_____

Often comes in: 500 mg. tablets
Also comes in syrups

Acetaminophen (paracetamol) is safer for children than aspirin. It does not cause stomach irritation and so can be used instead of aspirin by persons with stomach ulcers. It can also be used by pregnant women.

Dosage of acetaminophen—for pain and fever:
—500 mg. tablets—

Give acetaminophen by mouth 4 times a day.

In each dose give:

adults: 500 mg. to 1 gm. (1 or 2 tablets)
children 8 to 12 years: 500 mg. (1 tablet)
children 3 to 7 years: 250 mg. (1/2 tablet)
children 1 year to 2 years: 125 mg. (1/4 tablet)
babies under 1 year: 62 mg. (1/8 tablet)

Ibuprofen

Name:__________________ price:______ for_____

Often comes in: 200 mg. tablets

Ibuprofen works for muscle swelling and pain, joint pain from arthritis, menstrual pain, headache, and to lower fever. It is more expensive than aspirin.

WARNING: Ibuprofen should not be taken by persons who are allergic to aspirin. Pregnant women should not use ibuprofen.

Dosage of ibuprofen—for pain and fever:
—200 mg. tablets—

Give ibuprofen by mouth every 4 to 6 hours.

In each dose give:

adults and children 12 years and older: 200 mg. (1 tablet)
children under 12 years: Do not give.

If one tablet does not relieve pain or fever, two tablets may be used. Do not take more than six tablets in 24 hours.

Ergotamine with caffeine *(Cafergot)*—for migraine headache

Name:__________________ price:______ for_____

Often comes in: tablets with 1 mg. of ergotamine

Dosage of ergotamine with caffeine for migraine:

adults: Take 2 tablets at the first sign of a migraine, then 1 tablet every half hour until the pain goes. But do not take more than 6 tablets in all.

WARNING: Do not take this medicine often. Do not take when pregnant.

Codeine—for severe pain—see p. 384.

FOR STOPPING PAIN WHEN CLOSING WOUNDS: ANESTHETICS

Lidocaine *(Xylocaine)*
2 percent (with or without epinephrine)

Name:__________________ price:______ for_____

Often comes in: ampules or bottles for injection

Lidocaine can be injected around the edges of a wound before sewing it, to make the area ***anesthetic*** or numb so it will not hurt.

Inject both into and under the skin at points about 1 cm. apart. Be sure to pull back on the plunger before injecting (see p. 73). Inject slowly. Use about 1 ml. of anesthetic for each 2 cm. of skin. (Do not use more than 20 mls. altogether.) If the wound is clean, you can inject into the sides of the wound itself. If the wound is dirty, inject through the skin (after cleaning it) around the wound and then **clean the wound with great care** before closing it.

Use lidocaine with epinephrine for sewing most wounds. The epinephrine makes the numbness last longer and helps control bleeding.

Use lidocaine without epinephrine for wounds on fingers, toes, penis, ears, and nose. This is important because the epinephrine can stop the flow of blood to these areas and cause great damage.

Another use of lidocaine with epinephrine: **For severe nosebleed,** soak a little into some cotton and pack it into the nose. The epinephrine will cause the veins to squeeze shut and help control bleeding.

FOR GUT CRAMPS: ANTISPASMODICS

Belladonna (with or without phenobarbital)

Name:__________________ price:______ for_____

Often comes in: tablets with 8 mg. belladonna

There are many different antispasmodic preparations. Most contain belladonna or something like it (atropine, hyoscyamine) and often phenobarbital (phenobarbitone). These medicines should not be used on a regular basis, but can be used occasionally for treatment of pain or cramps (colic) in the stomach or gut. They may help calm the pain of a bladder infection or inflamed gallbladder. They are sometimes useful in the treatment of ulcers.

Dosage for belladonna—for gut cramps:
—tablets with 8 mg. belladonna—

adults: 1 tablet, 3 to 6 times a day
children 8 to 12 years: 1 tablet, 2 or 3 times a day
children 5 to 7 years: 1/2 tablet, 2 or 3 times a day
do not give to children under 5 years

WARNING: These medicines are poisonous if too much is taken. Keep out of reach of children.

Persons with glaucoma should not take medicines that contain belladonna or atropine.

FOR ACID INDIGESTION, HEARTBURN, AND STOMACH ULCERS

Aluminum hydroxide or magnesium hydroxide *(Milk of Magnesia)*

Name:__________________ price:______ for_____

Often comes in tablets of 500 to 750 mg., or in mixtures with 300 to 500 mg. in 5 ml.

Sometimes these are mixed together or with magnesium trisilicate. If simethicone is added, it helps control gas.

These antacids can be used occasionally for acid indigestion or heartburn or as a regular part of treatment of a stomach (peptic) ulcer. The most important time to take antacids is 1 hour after meals and at bedtime. Chew 2 or 3 tablets. For severe stomach ulcers, it may be necessary to take 3 to 6 tablets (or teaspoons) every hour.

CAUTION: Do not use these medicines if you are also taking tetracycline. Antacids with magnesium sometimes cause diarrhea, and those with aluminum may cause constipation.

Sodium bicarbonate (bicarbonate of soda, baking soda)

Comes as a white powder Price:________ for____

As an antacid, this should be used in a very limited way, when someone has an occasional stomach upset, with 'heartburn' or acid indigestion. **It should not be used in treating chronic indigestion or stomach (peptic) ulcers.** Although it seems to help at first, it causes the stomach to produce more acid, which soon makes things worse. 'Soda' is also useful for the 'hangover' of a person who has drunk too much alcohol the night before. For this purpose (but not for acid indigestion) it can be taken with acetaminophen or aspirin. *Alka-Seltzer* is a combination of sodium bicarbonate and aspirin. As an **occasional** antacid, mix 1/2 teaspoon of sodium bicarbonate with water and drink it. Do not use often.

For cleaning teeth, baking soda or a mixture of 'soda' and salt can be used instead of toothpaste (see p. 230).

WARNING: **Persons with certain heart problems (failure) or with swelling of the feet or face should not take sodium bicarbonate or other products high in sodium (like salt).**

Calcium carbonate

Name:__________________ price:______ for_____

Often comes in tablets of 350 to 850 mg.

This works more slowly than sodium bicarbonate. It is very effective for occasional acid indigestion or heartburn, but should not be used long term or for treatment of ulcers. Chew one 850 mg. tablet or two 350 mg. tablets when symptoms occur. Take another dose in 2 hours if necessary.

Cimetidine *(Tagamet)*

Name:__________________ price:______ for_____

Often comes in: tablets of 200 mg., and injections of 200 mg. in 2 ml.

Cimetidine is an expensive but effective treatment for ulcers of the stomach and the gut. It calms the pain and helps healing. Long-term use can help prevent the most common type of ulcer (ulcer of the gut) from returning. But to keep any ulcer from coming back, it is important to also follow the special diet and other advice for care of an ulcer on p. 128 and 129.

Precautions: Cimetidine should not be taken by women who are pregnant or breast feeding, or children.

Side effects: Occasionally causes mild diarrhea, dizziness, rash, and sleepiness.

Dosage for an active ulcer of the gut:

400 mg. (two 200 mg. tablets) twice a day, or 800 mg. (four 200 mg. tablets) at bedtime, for 6 to 8 months.

Dosage for an active stomach ulcer:

300 mg. (one and a half 200 mg. tablets), 4 times a day, for 6 to 8 weeks.

Dosage to help prevent an ulcer of the gut from coming back:

400 mg. (two 200 mg. tablets) at bedtime, for up to 1 year.

Ranitidine *(Zantac)*

Name:__________________ price:______ for_____

Often comes in: tablets of 150 mg. or 300 mg.

Ranitidine is similar to cimetidine, but more expensive. It can calm pain and help an ulcer to heal. But be sure to also follow the advice on p. 128 and 129 to treat and prevent ulcers.

Dosage of ranitidine for treatment of ulcers:

150 mg. twice a day, or 300 mg. at dinnertime, for 6 to 8 weeks.

Dosage to help prevent an ulcer of the gut from coming back:

150 mg. (one 150 mg. tablet) at bedtime for 6 to 8 weeks.

FOR DEHYDRATION: REHYDRATION DRINKS AND 'ORS'

Instructions for making Rehydration Drink with cereal or ordinary sugar are on page 152.

In some countries packets of a simple sugar (glucose) and salts for making a rehydration drink are sold in stores or are available at health posts. While these packets are sometimes convenient, a homemade mix using cereal, as described on page 152, combats diarrhea as well or better. A home mix using sugar and a little salt also works well. It is better to make a home mix and spend the money you save on more and better food. Be sure to **continue giving breast milk** to a baby with diarrhea. And **start giving food as soon as the sick child will accept it.** Giving food together with rehydration drink combats dehydration more effectively and protects the child from becoming weaker.

WARNING: In some countries, packets of 'ORS' (oral rehydration salts) are sold in a variety of preparations, which require different amounts of water for correct preparation. **If you use ORS packets, be sure you know how much water to mix with it.** Too little water can be dangerous.

CAUTION: If you plan to take a child with diarrhea to the health post or hospital, always give her lots of liquids, and if possible a homemade rehydration drink, before you leave home. And if you can, take some of the drink (or if nothing else, plain water) with you, to give to the child on the way to the health post and while you wait your turn. Give the child the drink often as much as she will take. If the child is vomiting, give small quantities every minute. Some of the drink will stay inside, and it will also help reduce vomiting.

FOR HARD STOOLS (CONSTIPATION): LAXATIVES

A discussion of the use and misuse of different laxatives and purges is found on page 15. Laxatives are used far too much. They should be used only **occasionally** to help soften hard, painful stools (constipation). **Never give laxatives to anyone who has diarrhea or gut pain or who is dehydrated.** Do not give laxatives to small children under 2 years old.

Generally the best stool softeners are foods high in roughage or fiber, like bran or cassava. Drinking a lot of liquid (at least 8 glasses of water a day) and eating lots of fruit also help.

Milk of magnesia (magnesium hydroxide)—laxative and antacid

Name:________________ price:______ for______

Often comes as a milky solution

Shake well before using. Drink some water each time you take it.

Dosage for milk of magnesia:

As an antacid:
adults and children over 12 years: 1 to 3 teaspoons 3 or 4 times a day
children 1 to 12 years: 1/2 to 1 teaspoon 3 or 4 times a day

As a mild laxative give 1 dose at bedtime:
adults and children over 12 years: 2 to 4 tablespoons
children 6 to 11 years: 1 to 2 tablespoons
children 2 to 5 years: 1/3 to 1 tablespoon
do not give to children under 2 years old

Epsom salts (magnesium sulfate)—as a laxative and for itching

Name:________________ price:______ for______

Often comes in white powder or crystals

Dosage for Epsom salts:

As a mild laxative—mix the following amount of Epsom salts in a glass of water and drink (best taken on an empty stomach):
adults: 2 teaspoons
children 6 to 12 years: 1/2 to 1 teaspoon
children 2 to 6 years: 1/4 to 1/2 teaspoon
do not give to children under 2 years old

To help stop itching—mix 8 teaspoons of Epsom salts in a liter of water and put on itching skin as cool soaks or compresses.

Mineral oil—as a laxative

Name:________________ price:______ for______

This is sometimes taken by persons with piles (hemorrhoids) who have hard, painful stools. However, it does not really soften the stools, but merely greases them. Foods high in fiber, like bran or cassava, are far better.

Dosage of mineral oil as a laxative:

adults and children 12 years and over: 1 to 3 tablespoons by mouth at least 1 hour after the evening meal. Do not take with meals because the oil will rob some of the vitamins from the food.

CAUTION: Do not give to children under 12 years old, women who are pregnant or breast feeding, to persons who cannot get out of bed, or to persons who have trouble swallowing.

Glycerine suppositories ***(Dulcolax)***

Name:________________ price:______ for______

These are bullet-shaped pills that are pushed into the anus. They stimulate the bowel and cause it to push out the stool (shit).

Dosage for glycerin suppositories:

adults and children over 12 years: push 1 suppository well up the anus and let it stay there for 15 to 30 minutes (it helps to lie down). The longer you let the suppository stay inside the anus, the better it will work.

FOR MILD DIARRHEA: ANTI-DIARRHEA MEDICINE

Kaolin with pectin *(Kaopectate)*

Name:__________________ price:______ for_____

Often comes as a milky mixture

This can be used to make mild diarrhea thicker (less watery) and less troublesome. **It does not cure the cause of the diarrhea and does not help prevent or cure dehydration.** It is never necessary in the treatment of diarrhea, and its common use is a great waste of money. **It should not be given to persons who are very ill or to small children. WE INCLUDE IT HERE MAINLY TO WARN AGAINST ITS USE.**

Dosage of kaolin with pectin, for **mild diarrhea only:**
—using a standard mixture such as *Kaopectate*—

Give 1 dose after each stool, or 4 or 5 times a day.

In each dose give:

adults: 2 to 8 tablespoons
children 6 to 12 years: 1 to 2 tablespoons
children under 6 years: DO NOT GIVE

FOR STUFFY NOSE

To help open a stuffy nose, often all that is needed is to sniff water with a little salt in it, as described on page 164. Occasionally, decongestant drops may be used, as follows:

Nose drops with ephedrine or phenylephrine *(Neo-Synephrine)*

Name:__________________ price:______ for_____

These may be used for stuffy or 'runny' nose, especially if a person has (or often gets) infection of the inner ear.

Dosage for decongestant nose drops:

Put 1 or 2 drops in each nostril as shown on page 164. Do this 4 times a day. **Do not use for more than 3 days** or make a habit of using these drops.

For nose drops made from ephedrine tablets, see page 385.

FOR COUGH

Cough is the body's method for cleaning the air tubes that go to the lungs and preventing germs and mucus in these tubes from getting into the lungs. Because cough is part of the body's defense, medicines that stop or calm cough sometimes do more harm than good. These **cough-calmers** (or cough *suppressants*) should be used only for irritating, dry coughs that do not let a person sleep. There are other medicines, called **cough-helpers** (or *expectorants*), that are supposed to make it easier to cough up the mucus.

In truth, both kinds of cough syrups (cough-calmers and cough-helpers) are used far more than they need to be. Most popular cough syrups do little or no good and are a waste of money.

The best and most important cough medicine is water. Drinking a lot of water and breathing hot water vapors loosen mucus and help calm cough far better than most cough syrups. For instructions, see page 168. Also, instructions for a homemade cough syrup are given on page 169.

Cough-calmers (cough suppressants): codeine

Name:__________________ price:______ for_____

Often comes in: cough syrups or liquid. Also in tablets of 30 mg. or 60 mg, with or without aspirin or acetaminophen.

Codeine is a strong painkiller and also one of the most powerful cough-calmers, but because it is habit-forming (narcotic), it may be hard to get. It often comes in cough syrup combinations or in tablet form. For dosage, follow the instructions that come with the preparation. Less is needed to calm cough than to control pain. **To calm cough** in adults, 7 to 15 mg. of codeine is usually enough. Children should be given less, according to age or weight (see p. 62). **For severe pain,** adults can take 30 to 60 mg. of codeine every 4 hours.

WARNING: Codeine is habit-forming (narcotic). Use only for a few days.

FOR ASTHMA

To help prevent and manage asthma correctly, see page 167. Persons who suffer from asthma should keep asthma medicines at home. Start using them at the first sign of wheeze or chest tightness.

Ephedrine

Name:__________________ price:______ for_____

Often comes in: tablets of 15 mg. (also 25 mg.)

Ephedrine is useful to control mild attacks of asthma and between severe attacks to prevent them. It works by helping open the tubes that lead into the lungs, so that air can pass more easily. It can also be used when there is difficulty breathing due to pneumonia or bronchitis.

Ephedrine often comes in combination with **theophylline** or **aminophylline,** and sometimes **phenobarbital.** Avoid these combinations except when a single asthma medicine is not available.

Dosage of ephedrine for asthma—
(1 mg./kg./3 times a day when symptoms occur):
—using 15 mg. tablets—

Give by mouth 3 times a day.

In each dose give:

adults: 15 to 60 mg. (1 to 4 tablets)
children 5 to 10 years: 15 to 30 mg. (1 or 2 tablets)
children 1 to 4 years: 15 mg. (1 tablet)
children under 1 year: DO NOT GIVE

For stuffy nose, nose drops with ephedrine can be used. They can be made by dissolving 1 tablet in a teaspoon of water.

Theophylline or Aminophylline

Name:__________________ price:______ for_____

Often comes in: tablets and syrups of different strengths

For controlling asthma and preventing attacks

Dosage—(3 to 5 mg./kg. every 6 hours):
—using 100 mg. tablets—

Give every 6 hours:

adults: 2 tablets
children 7 to 12 years: 1 tablet
children under 7 years: 1/2 tablet
babies: DO NOT GIVE

In severe cases or if asthma is not controlled with the above dosage, double this dosage may be given, but no more. If the patient cannot talk, seek medical help fast.

Salbutamol (Albuterol)

Name:__________________ price:______ for_____

Often comes in: tablets of 4 mg., and syrup with 2 mg. in 5 ml.

For controlling asthma and preventing attacks. Salbutamol can be used alone, or with theophylline.

Dosage for salbutamol—(0.1 mg./kg. every 6 to 8 hours):
—using 4 mg. tablets or syrup with 2 mg. in 1 teaspoon—

Give every 6 to 8 hours:

adults: 1 tablet or 2 teaspoons
children 6 to 12 years: 1/2 tablet or 1 teaspoon
children 2 to 5: 1/4 to 1/2 tablet or 1/2 to 1 teaspoon
babies: DO NOT GIVE

For severe asthma or if asthma is not controlled, these doses can be gradually increased until doubled.

Epinephrine (adrenaline, *Adrenalin*)

Name:__________________ price:______ for_____

Often comes in: ampules of 1 mg. in 1 ml.

Epinephrine should be used for:

1. **severe attacks of asthma** when there is trouble breathing
2. **severe allergic reactions** or allergic shock due to penicillin injections, tetanus antitoxin, or other antitoxins made from horse serum (see p. 70).

Dosage of epinephrine for **asthma:**
—using ampules of 1 mg. in 1 ml. of liquid—

First count the pulse. Then inject just under the skin (see p. 167):

adults: 1/3 ml.
children 7 to 12 years: 1/5 ml.
children 1 to 6 years: 1/10 ml.
children under 1 year: DO NOT GIVE

Dosage of epinephrine for **allergic shock:**
—using ampules of 1 mg. in 1 ml. of liquid—

Inject into the muscle:

adults: 1/2 ml.
children 7 to 12 years: 1/3 ml.
children 1 to 6 years: 1/4 ml.
children under 1 year: DO NOT GIVE

If needed, a second dose can be given after half an hour, and a third dose in another half hour. Do not give more than 3 doses. If the pulse goes up by more than 30 beats per minute after the first injection, do not give another dose.

In using epinephrine, be careful never to give more than the recommended amount.

FOR ALLERGIC REACTIONS AND VOMITING: THE ANTIHISTAMINES

Antihistamines are medicines that affect the body in several ways:

1. They help calm or prevent allergic reactions, such as itchy rashes or lumps on the skin, hives, 'hay fever', and allergic shock.
2. They help prevent or control motion sickness or vomiting.
3. They often cause sleepiness (sedation). Avoid doing dangerous work, operating machines, or drinking alcohol when taking antihistamines.

Promethazine *(Phenergan)* and **diphenhydramine** *(Benadryl)* are strong antihistamines that cause a lot of sleepiness. **Dimenhydrinate** *(Dramamine)* is similar to diphenhydramine and is most used for motion sickness. However, for vomiting due to other causes, promethazine often works better.

Chlorpheniramine is a less expensive antihistamine and causes less sleepiness. For this reason, it is sometimes best to use chlorpheniramine to calm itching in the daytime. Promethazine is useful at night because it encourages sleep at the same time that it calms the itching.

There is no proof that the antihistamines do any good for the common cold. They are often used more than they need to be. They should not be used much.

Antihistamines should **not** be used for asthma, because they make the mucus thicker and can make breathing more difficult.

One antihistamine is all that is usually needed in a medical kit. Promethazine is a good choice. Because it is not always available, doses for other antihistamines are also given.

As a general rule, **antihistamines are best given by mouth.** Injections should be used only to help control severe vomiting or before giving antitoxins (for tetanus, snakebite, etc.) when there is special danger of allergic shock. For children, it is often best to give a rectal suppository.

Promethazine *(Phenergan)*

Name: ______________________________

Often comes in:
tablets of 12.5 mg. Price:______ for____
injections—ampules of 25 mg. in 1 ml. Price:______ for____
suppositories of 12.5 mg., 25 mg., and 50 mg. Price:______ for____

CAUTION: Pregnant women should only use promethazine if it is absolutely necessary.

Dosage of promethazine—(1 mg./kg./day):
—using tablets of 12.5 mg.—

Give by mouth 2 times a day.

In each dose give:

adults: 25 to 50 mg. (2 to 4 tablets)
children 7 to 12 years: 12.5 to 25 mg. (1 or 2 tablets)
children 2 to 6 years: 6 to 12 mg. (1/2 to 1 tablet)
babies 1 year old: 4 mg. (1/3 tablet)
babies under 1 year: 3 mg. (1/4 tablet)

—using intramuscular (IM) injections, 25 mg. in a ml.—

Inject once, and again in 2 to 4 hours, if necessary.

In 1 dose inject:

adults: 25 to 50 mg. (1 to 2 ml.)
children 7 to 12 years: 12.5 to 25 mg. (1/2 to 1 ml.)
children under 7 years: 6 to 12 mg. (1/4 to 1/2 ml.)
babies under 1 year: 2.5 mg. (0.1 ml.)

—using rectal suppositories of 25 mg.—

Put high up the rectum (anus) and repeat in 4 to 6 hours if necessary.

In each dose insert:

adults and children over 12 years: 25 mg. (1 suppository)
children 7 to 12 years: 12.5 mg. (1/2 suppository)
children 2 to 6 years: 6 mg. (1/4 suppository)

Diphenhydramine *(Benadryl)*

Name: ____________________

Often comes in:
capsules of 25 mg. and 50 mg. Price:______ for____
injections—ampules with 10 mg. or 50 mg. in each ml. Price:______ for____

CAUTION: Do not give diphenhydramine to newborn babies or to women who are breast feeding. It is best not to use diphenhydramine in pregnancy unless absolutely necessary.

Dosage of diphenhydramine—(5 mg./kg./day):
—using capsules of 25 mg.—

Give 3 or 4 times a day:

adults: 25 to 50 mg. (1 or 2 capsules)
children 8 to 12 years: 25 mg. (1 capsule)
children 2 to 7 years: 12.5 mg. (1/2 capsule)
babies: 6 mg. (1/4 capsule)

—using intramuscular (IM) injections, 50 mg. in each ml.—

Diphenhydramine should be injected only in the case of allergic shock. Inject once, and again in 2 to 4 hours if necessary:

adults: 25 to 50 mg. (1/2 to 1 ml.)
children: 10 to 25 mg., depending on size (1/5 to 1/2 ml.)
babies: 5 mg. (1/10 ml.)

Chlorpheniramine

Name:__________________ price:______ for_____

Often comes in: 4 mg. tablets (also tablets of other sizes, syrups, etc.)

Dosage for chlorpheniramine:

Take 1 dose 3 or 4 times a day.

In each dose give:

adults: 4 mg. (1 tablet)
children under 12: 2 mg. (1/2 tablet)
babies: 1 mg. (1/4 tablet)

Dimenhydrinate *(Dramamine)*

Name:__________________ price:______ for_____

Often comes in: 50 mg. tablets; also syrups with 12.5 mg. in a teaspoon; also suppositories to put up the anus

This is sold mostly for motion sickness, but can be used like other antihistamines to calm allergic reactions and to encourage sleep.

Dosage of dimenhydrinate:

Take up to 4 times a day.

In each dose give:

adults: 50 to 100 mg. (1 or 2 tablets)
children 7 to 12 years of age: 25 to 50 mg. (1/2 to 1 tablet)
children 2 to 6 years: 12 to 25 mg. (1/4 to 1/2 tablet)
children under 2 years: 6 to 12 mg. (1/8 to 1/4 tablet)

ANTITOXINS

WARNING: Many antitoxins are made from horse serum, such as some tetanus antitoxins and the antivenoms for snakebite and scorpion sting. With these there is a risk of causing a dangerous allergic reaction (allergic shock, see p. 70). Before you inject a horse serum antitoxin, **always have epinephrine ready in case of an emergency.** In persons who are allergic, or who have been given any kind of antitoxin made of horse serum before, it is a good idea to inject an antihistamine like promethazine *(Phenergan)* or diphenhydramine *(Benadryl)* 15 minutes before giving the antitoxin.

Scorpion antitoxin or antivenom

Name:__________________ price:______ for_____

Often comes *lyophilized* (in powdered form) for injection

Different antivenoms are produced for scorpion sting in different parts of the world. In Mexico, Laboratories BIOCLON produces *Alacramyn.*

Antivenoms for scorpion sting should be used only in those areas where there are dangerous or deadly kinds of scorpions. Antivenoms are usually needed only when a small child is stung, especially if stung on the main upper part of the body or head. To do most good, the antivenom should be injected as soon as possible after the child has been stung.

Antivenoms usually come with full instructions. Follow them carefully. Small children often need **more** antivenom than larger children. Two or 3 vials may be necessary.

Most scorpions are not dangerous to adults. Because the antivenom itself has some danger in its use, it is usually better not to give it to adults.

Snakebite antivenom or antitoxin

Name:__________________ price:______ for_____

Often comes in: bottles or kits for injection

Antivenoms, or medicines that protect the body against poisons, have been developed for the bites of poisonous snakes in many parts of the world. If you live where people are sometimes bitten or killed by poisonous snakes, find out what antivenoms are available, **get them ahead of time,** and keep them on hand. Some antivenoms—those in dried or 'lyophilized' form—can be kept without refrigeration. Others need to be kept cold.

The following are a few of the products sold in different parts of the world:

North America: *Polyvalent Crotalid Antivenom.* Through Wyeth Laboratories. For rattlesnakes and other pit vipers.

Mexico, Central America, and South America: *Antivip-DL: suero antiofídico polivalente liofilizado* (for different snakes including rattlesnakes and other pit vipers, as well as *nauyaca, terciopelo, mapana, toboba, jacaranda, cuatro narices, cola de hueso, baraba amarilla* and *palanca.*) Through Laboratorios BIOCLON, Mexico, D.F.; telephone: (5) 6-65-41-11. Antivenoms are also available from the Instituto Clodomiro Picado in San Jose, Costa Rica, and through the Instituto Butantan, in Brazil (telephone: (11) 813-72-22).

Thailand: Specific antivenoms for different snakes. Through the Red Cross Pasteur Institute, Bangkok.

India: A polyvalent antivenom (for different snakes). Through Hoffkins Institute, Bombay.

Ethiopia: Polyvalent antivenom. From Behringwerke Laboratories.

Egypt: Polyvalent antivenom. Available only through government.

West Africa: Polyvalent antivenom against Echis-Bitis-Naja (carpet viper, gaboon viper, and cobra) is usually provided by the government. Antivenom against carpet viper (Echis) alone may be advisable in some areas.

Instructions for the use of snakebite antivenoms usually come with the kit. Study them **before** you need to use them. The bigger the snake, or the smaller the person, the larger the amount of antivenom needed. Often 2 or more vials are necessary. To be most helpful, antivenom should be injected as soon as possible after the bite.

Be sure to take the necessary precautions to avoid allergic shock (see p. 70).

Antitoxins for tetanus

Tetanus Immune Globulin (human) often comes in:
vials of 250 units

Tetanus antitoxin (horse) often comes in: vials of 1,500, 20,000, 40,000, and 50,000 units

In areas where there are people who have not been vaccinated against tetanus, the medical kit should have an antitoxin for tetanus. There are 2 forms, one made from human serum (tetanus immune globulin, *Hyper-tet*), and one made from horse serum (tetanus antitoxin). **If available, use tetanus immune globulin, as it is less likely to cause a severe allergic reaction.**

But if you use horse serum tetanus antitoxin, take precautions against allergic reaction: If the person suffers from asthma or other allergies, or has ever received any kind of antitoxin made from horse serum, give an injection of antihistamine such as promethazine 15 minutes before injecting the antitoxin.

If a person who is not fully vaccinated against tetanus has a severe wound likely to cause tetanus (see p. 89), **before he develops the signs of tetanus,** inject 250 units (1 vial) of tetanus immune globulin. If using tetanus antitoxin, inject 1,500 to 3,000 units. Inject babies with 750 units of tetanus antitoxin.

If a person develops the signs of tetanus, inject 5,000 units of tetanus immune globulin, or 50,000 units of tetanus antitoxin. Give it in many intramuscular injections in the large muscles of the body (buttocks and thighs). Or, half the amount can be given intravenously if someone knows how.

The signs of tetanus usually continue to get worse in spite of treatment with antitoxin. **The other measures of treatment described on pages 183 and 184 are equally or more important.** Begin treatment at once and get medical help fast.

FOR SWALLOWED POISONS

Syrup of Ipecac—to cause vomiting

Name:________________ price:_____ for_____

Often comes in: syrup **(Do not use the elixir.)**

To cause vomiting when a person has swallowed a poison. **Do not use if the person has swallowed strong acid, lye, gasoline, or kerosene.**

Dosage of Ipecac:

1 tablespoon for any age. Repeat in half an hour if the person has not vomited.

Powdered charcoal (or activated charcoal)—for swallowed poison

Price:________ for______

Charcoal soaks up swallowed poisons and makes them less harmful.

Dosage of powdered charcoal:

1 tablespoon mixed in water or fruit juice.

Dosage of activated charcoal:

1 cupful mixed with an equal amount of water or fruit juice.

FOR FITS (CONVULSIONS)

Phenobarbital and phenytoin are common medicines used to prevent fits or convulsions of epilepsy. Other, more expensive medicines are sometimes available, and doctors often prescribe two or more medicines. However, usually a single medicine works as well or better, with fewer side effects. Medicines to prevent fits are best taken at bedtime, because they often cause sleepiness. Diazepam can be given to stop a long-lasting epileptic fit, but it is not usually taken daily to prevent fits.

Phenobarbital (phenobarbitone, *Luminal*)

Name: ______________________________

Often comes in:
tablets of 15 mg., 30 mg., 50 mg. and 100 mg.
Price:______ for___
ampules of 65 mg., 130 mg., or 200 mg. in 1 ml.
Price:______ for___
syrup of 15 mg. in 1 ml.
Price:______ for___

Phenobarbital can be taken by mouth to help prevent fits or convulsions (epilepsy), and the spasms of tetanus. For epilepsy, it is often necessary to continue the medicine for life. The lowest dose that prevents fits should be used. Low doses of phenobarbital can also be used to help lessen the cough of whooping cough or to help control severe vomiting.

WARNING: Too much phenobarbital can slow down or stop breathing. Its action begins slowly and lasts a long time (up to 24 hours, or longer if the person is not urinating). **Be careful not to give too much!**

Dosage of phenobarbital—(3 to 6 mg./kg./day):
—using tablets of 100 mg.—

Give 1 dose by mouth (at bedtime for epilepsy).

In each dose give:

adults and children over 12 years: 100 to 300 mg. (1 to 3 tablets)
children from 7 to 12 years: 50 to 100 mg. (1/2 to 1 tablet)
children under 7 years: 20 to 50 mg. (1/4 to 1/2 tablet)

Phenobarbital injections can be given to stop an epileptic fit or the spasms of advanced tetanus.

Dosage for phenobarbital injections:
—using ampules with 200 mg. in 1 ml.—

Give 1 injection, intramuscular

adults: 200 mg. (1 ml.)
children 7 to 12 years: 150 mg. (3/4 ml.)
children 2 to 6 years: 100 mg. (1/2 ml.)
children under 2 years: 50 mg. (1/4 ml.)

If the fit does not stop, 1 more dose can be given after 15 minutes, but then give no more. For tetanus repeat the dose 3 times a day, and if the spasms are controlled, begin to lower the dose a little at a time.

Phenytoin (diphenylhydantoin, *Dilantin*)

Name: ____________________

Often comes in: capsules of 25 mg., 30 mg., and 100 mg. Price:______ for___
syrup with 125 mg. in 5 ml. (1 teaspoon) Price:______ for___

This helps prevent the fits of epilepsy. The medicine must often be taken for life. The lowest dosage that prevents fits should be used.

Side effects: Swelling and abnormal growth of the gums often occur with long-time use of phenytoin. If this is severe, another medicine should be used instead. Gum problems can be partly prevented by keeping the mouth clean and brushing or cleaning the teeth and gums well after eating.

Dosage of phenytoin for fits—(5 mg./kg./day):
—using capsules of 100 mg.—

Start with the following dose once a day at bedtime:

In each dose take:

adults and children over 12 years: 100 to 300 mg. (1 to 3 capsules)
children 7 to 12 years: 100 mg. (1 capsule)
children under 7 years: 50 mg. (1/2 capsule)

If fits are not completely prevented with this dose, up to twice this dose can be given but not more.

If fits are prevented, try lowering the dose a little at a time, until you find the lowest dose that prevents the fits.

Diazepam (*Valium*)

Name:__________________ price:______ for_____

Often comes in: injections of 5 mg. in 1 ml. of liquid and of 10 mg. in 2 ml. of liquid; also tablets of 5 mg. and 10 mg.

The uses of diazepam are similar to those of phenobarbital, but it is more expensive.

For stopping long-lasting epileptic fits the adult dose is 5 to 10 mg. Repeat in 2 hours if necessary.

Or, 'suppositories' of diazepam or phenobarbital can be put up the anus (asshole). If you only have liquid medicine for taking by mouth, put it up the anus with a plastic syringe without a needle. Or grind up a pill of diazepam or phenobarbital, mix with water, and put up the anus.

For tetanus give enough to control most of the spasms. Start with 5 mg. (less in children) and give more as needed, but not more than 10 mg. at a time or 50 mg. a day. If necessary, diazepam can be given together with phenobarbital, but care must be taken not to give too much.

For relaxing muscles and calming pain, 15 minutes before **setting broken bones,** inject up to 10 mg. (in an adult) or give 10 mg. by mouth 30 minutes before.

Diazepam may also be useful in cases of extreme fright (hysteria) or anxiety, but its use for these should be very limited.

Dosage for injectable diazepam
—using ampules with 10 mg. in 2 ml.—

adults and children over 12 years: 5 to 10 mg. (1 to 2 ml.)
children 7 to 12 years: 3 to 5 mg. (2/3 to 1 ml.)
children 1 to 6 years: 1 to 5 mg. (1/5 to 1 ml.)
children under 1 year: DO NOT USE

Repeat dosage in 3 to 4 hours if necessary.

WARNINGS: (1) Although it is safer to inject diazepam in the muscle (IM) than the vein (IV), it does not work as well or as fast. If you inject in the vein, pick a large vein and inject very slowly.
(2) Too much diazepam can slow down or stop breathing. Be careful not to give too much!
(3) Diazepam is a habit-forming (addictive) drug. Avoid long or common use. Keep under lock and key.

FOR SEVERE BLEEDING AFTER BIRTH (POSTPARTUM HEMORRHAGE)

For information on the right and wrong use of medicines to control bleeding after a woman gives birth, see page 266. As a general rule, **oxytocics (ergonovine, oxytocin, etc.) should only be used to control bleeding after the baby is born.** Their use to speed up labor or to give strength to the mother in labor can be dangerous both to the mother and child. These medicines should never be given until the baby is born, and better, not until the placenta or afterbirth has come out, too. If there is much bleeding before the afterbirth comes out (but after the child has been born), 1/2 ml. (5 units) of oxytocin can be given by intramuscular injection. **Do not use ergonovine before the afterbirth comes out,** as this may prevent it from coming out.

Pituitrin is similar to oxytocin, but more dangerous, and should never be used except in a case of emergency bleeding when oxytocin and ergonovine are not available.

For bleeding in the newborn child, use **vitamin K** (see p. 394). Vitamin K is of no use for bleeding of the woman from childbirth, miscarriage, or abortion.

Ergonovine or ergometrine maleate *(Ergotrate, Methergine)*

Name: ______________________________

Often comes in:
injections of 0.2 mg. in a 1 ml. ampule Price:______ for___
tablets of 0.2 mg. Price:______ for___

To prevent or control severe bleeding **after** the placenta has come out.

Dosage of injectable ergonovine:

For severe bleeding (more than 2 cups) after the afterbirth (placenta) has come out, give 1 or 2 ampules (0.2 to 0.4 mg.) of ergonovine by intramuscular injection (or 1 ampule by intravenous injection in extreme emergencies). Dose may be repeated if necessary in half an hour to an hour. Change to ergonovine tablets as soon as bleeding is under control.

Dosage for ergonovine by mouth—using tablets of 0.2 mg.:

To prevent severe bleeding after giving birth or to lessen the amount of blood loss (especially in mothers who are anemic) give 1 tablet 3 or 4 times daily, beginning when the afterbirth comes out. If bleeding is heavy, 2 tablets can be given in each dose.

Oxytocin *(Pitocin)*

Name:__________________ price:______ for_____

Often comes in: ampules of 10 units in 1 ml.

To help stop severe bleeding of the mother **after** the baby is born and **before** the afterbirth comes out. (Also helps bring the afterbirth out, but should not be used for this unless there is severe bleeding or great delay.)

Dosage of oxytocin for the mother after the baby is born:

Inject 1/2 ml. (5 units). If severe bleeding continues, inject another 1/2 ml. in 15 minutes.

FOR PILES (HEMORRHOIDS)

Suppositories for hemorrhoids

Name:__________________ price:______ for_____

These are special bullet-shaped tablets to be put up the anus. They help make hemorrhoids smaller and less painful. There are many different preparations. Those that are often most helpful, but are more expensive, contain **cortisone** or a **cortico-steroid.** Special ointments are also available. Diets to soften stools are important (see p. 126).

Dosage:

Put a suppository up the anus after the daily bowel movement, and another on going to bed.

FOR MALNUTRITION AND ANEMIA

Powdered milk (dried milk)

Name:__________________ price:______ for_____

For babies, **mother's milk is best.** It is rich in body-building vitamins and minerals. When breast milk is not available, other milk products—including powdered milk—can be used. To allow a baby to make full use of its food value, mix the powdered milk with some sugar and cooking oil (see p. 120).

In 1 cup of boiled water, put:
12 level teaspoons of powdered milk,
2 level teaspoons of sugar,
and 3 teaspoons of oil

Mixed (or multi) vitamins

Name:__________________ price:______ for_____

These come in many forms, but tablets are usually cheapest and work well. Injections of vitamins are rarely necessary, are a waste of money, cause unnecessary pain and sometimes abscesses. Tonics and elixirs often do not have the most important vitamins and are usually too expensive for the good they do.

Nutritious food is the best source of vitamins. If additional vitamins are needed, use vitamin tablets.

In some cases of poor nutrition added vitamins may help. Be sure the tablets used contain the important vitamins the person needs (see p. 118).

Using standard tablets of mixed vitamins, 1 tablet daily is usually enough.

Vitamin A (retinol)—for night blindness and xerophthalmia

Name:__________________ price:______ for_____

Often comes as: capsules of 200,000 units,
60 mg. of retinol
(also in smaller doses)

injections of 100,000 units

WARNING: Too much vitamin A can cause fits. Do not give too much, and keep out of the reach of children.

For prevention: In areas where night blindness and xerophthalmia are common problems in children, they should eat more yellow fruits and vegetables and dark green leafy foods as well as animal foods, such as eggs and liver. Fish liver oil is high in vitamin A. Or vitamin A capsules can be given. Give 1 capsule once every 4 to 6 months—no more for prevention.

Mothers can help prevent these eye problems in their babies by taking 1 vitamin A capsule (200,000 units) by mouth when their baby is born or within 1 month after giving birth.

Children with measles are at especially high risk of xerophthalmia, and should be given vitamin A when the illness begins.

In areas where children do not get enough vitamin A, added foods or capsules with vitamin A often help children survive measles and other serious illnesses.

For treatment: Give 1 vitamin A capsule (200,000 units) by mouth, or an injection of 100,000 units. The next day give 1 vitamin A capsule (200,000 units) by mouth, and another capsule 1 to 2 weeks later.

For children less than 1 year old, reduce all doses by one-half.

Iron sulfate (ferrous sulfate)—for anemia

Name:__________________ price:______ for_____

Often comes in: tablets of 200, 300, or 500 mg.
(also in drops, mixtures, and elixirs for children)

Ferrous sulfate is useful in the treatment or prevention of most anemias. Treatment with ferrous sulfate by mouth usually takes at least 3 months. If improvement does not take place, the anemia is probably caused by something other than lack of iron. Get medical help. If this is difficult, try treating with folic acid.

Ferrous sulfate is especially important for pregnant women who may be anemic or malnourished.

Iron may work best if it is taken with some vitamin C (either fruits and vegetables, or a vitamin C tablet).

Ferrous sulfate sometimes upsets the stomach and is best taken with meals. Also, it can cause constipation, and it may make the stools (shit) look black. For children under 3 years, a piece of a tablet can be ground up very fine and mixed with the food.

WARNING: Be sure the dose is right. Too much ferrous sulfate is poisonous. Keep tablets out of the reach of children. Do not give ferrous sulfate to severely malnourished persons.

Dosage of ferrous sulfate for anemia:
—using tablets of 200 mg.—

Give 3 times a day, with meals.

In each dose give:

adults: 200 to 400 mg. (1 or 2 tablets)
children over 6 years old: 200 mg. (1 tablet)
children 3 to 6 years: 100 mg. (1/2 tablet)
children under 3 years: 25 to 50 mg. (1/8 to 1/4 tablet) ground up fine and mixed with food.

Folic acid—for some kinds of anemia

Name:__________________ price:______ for_____

Often comes in: tablets of 5 mg.

Folic acid can be important in the treatment of kinds of anemia in which blood cells have been destroyed in the veins, as is the case with malaria. An anemic person who has a large spleen or looks yellow may need folic acid, especially if his anemia does not get much better with ferrous sulfate. Babies who are fed goat's milk and pregnant women who are anemic or malnourished often need folic acid as well as iron.

Folic acid can be obtained by eating dark green leafy foods, meat, and liver, or by taking folic acid tablets. Usually 2 weeks treatment is enough for children, although in some areas children with ***sickle cell disease,*** or a kind of anemia called ***thalassemia*** may need it for years. Pregnant women who are anemic and malnourished would be helped by taking folic acid and iron tablets daily throughout pregnancy.

Dosage of folic acid for anemia:
—using 5 mg. tablets—

Give by mouth once a day.

adults and children over 3 years: 1 tablet (5 mg.)
children under 3 years: 1/2 tablet (2 1/2 mg.)

Vitamin B_{12} (cyanocobalamin)—for pernicious anemia **only**

This is mentioned only to discourage its use. Vitamin B_{12} is useful only for a rare type of anemia that is almost never found except in some persons over 35 years whose ancestors are from northern Europe. Many doctors prescribe it when it is not needed, just to be giving their patients something. **Do not waste your money on vitamin B_{12}** or let a doctor or health worker give it to you unless a blood analysis has been done, and it has been shown that you have ***pernicious anemia.***

Vitamin K (phytomenadione, phytonadione)

Name:__________________ price:______ for_____

Often comes in: ampules of 1 mg. in 2.5 ml. of milky solution.

If a newborn child begins to bleed from any part of his body (mouth, cord, anus), this may be caused by a lack of vitamin K. Inject 1 mg. (1 ampule) of vitamin K into the outer part of the thigh. Do not inject more, even if the bleeding continues. In babies who are born very small (under 2 kg.) an injection of vitamin K may be given to reduce the risk of bleeding.

Vitamin K is of no use to control bleeding of the mother after childbirth.

Vitamin B_6 (pyridoxine)

Often comes in: 25 mg. tablets

Price:______ for___

Persons with tuberculosis being treated with **isoniazid** sometimes develop a lack of vitamin B_6. To prevent this 50 mg. of vitamin B_6 (pyridoxine) may be taken daily while taking isoniazid. Or the vitamin can be given only to persons who develop problems because of its lack. Signs include pain or tingling in the hands or feet, muscle twitching, nervousness, and being unable to sleep.

Dosage of vitamin B_6—while taking isoniazid:

Take two 25 mg. tablets daily.

FAMILY PLANNING METHODS

Oral contraceptives (Birth Control Pills)

Information about the use, risks, and precautions for birth control pills can be found on pages 286 to 289. The following information is about choosing the right pill for individual women. (In January 2002, we changed the groups of birth control pills in this section. If someone you are working with has an older version of the book, be careful not to confuse the different kinds of pills!)

Most birth control pills contain 2 hormones similar to those produced in a woman's body to control her monthly bleeding. These hormones are called estrogen and progesterone (progestin). The pills come under many different brand names with different strengths and combinations for the 2 hormones. A few of the brand names are listed in the groups below.

Usually, brands that contain a smaller amount of both hormones are the safest and work best for most women. These "low-dose" pills are found in Groups 1, 2, and 3.

Group 1 - Triphasic pills

These contain low amounts of both estrogen and progestin in a mix that changes throughout the month. Since the amounts change, it is important to take the pills in order.

Common brand names:

Logynon *Synophase* *Tricyclen* *Trinordiol* *Trinovum* *Triquilar* *Triphasal*

Group 2 - Low dose pills

These contain low amounts of estrogen (35 micrograms of the estrogen "ethinyl estradiol" or 50 micrograms of the estrogen "mestranol") and progestin in a mix that stays the same throughout the month.

Common brand names:

Brevicon 1 + 35
Noriday 1 + 50
Norinyl 1 + 35, 1 + 50
Ortho-Novum 1/35, 1/50
Ovysmen 1/35
Neocon
Norimin
Perle

Group 3 - Low dose pills

These pills are high in progestin and low in estrogen (30 or 35 micrograms of the estrogen "ethinyl estradiol").

Common brand names:

Lo-Femenal
Lo-Ovral
Microgynon 30
Microvlar
Nordette

To assure effectiveness and minimize spotting (small amounts of bleeding at other times than your normal monthly bleeding), take the pill at the same time each day, especially with pills that have low amounts of hormones. If spotting continues after 3 or 4 months, try one of the brands in Group 3. If there is still spotting after 3 months, try a brand from Group 4.

As a rule, women who take birth control pills have less heavy monthly bleeding. This may be a good thing, especially for women who are anemic. But if a woman misses her monthly bleeding for months or is disturbed by the very light monthly bleeding, she can change to a brand with more estrogen from Group 4.

For a woman who has very heavy monthly bleeding or whose breasts become painful before her monthly bleeding begins, a brand low in estrogen but high in progestin may be better. These pills are found in Group 3.

Women who continue to have spotting or miss their monthly bleeding when using a brand from Group 3, or who became pregnant before while using another type of pill, can change to a pill that has a little more estrogen. These "high dose" pills are found in Group 4.

Group 4 - High dose pills

These pills are higher in estrogen (50 micrograms of the estrogen "ethinyl estradiol") and most are also higher in progestin.

Common brand names:

Eugynon	*Norlestrin*
Femenal	*Ovcon 50*
Minovlar	*Ovral*
Neogynon	*Primovlar*
Nordiol	

If spotting continues even when taking pills from Group 4, the brands Ovulen and Demulen will often stop it. But these are very strong in estrogen and so are rarely recommended. They are sometimes useful for women with severe acne.

Women who are disturbed by morning sickness or other side effects after 2 or 3 months of taking birth control pills, and women who have a higher risk for blood clots, should try a Triphasic birth control pill, low in both estrogen and progestin, from Group 1.

Women who are breastfeeding, or who should not use regular pills because of headaches or mild high blood pressure, may want to use a pill with only progestin. These pills in Group 5 are also called "mini-pills."

Group 5 - Progestin only pills

These pills, also known as "mini-pills," contain only progestin.

These pills should be taken at the same time every day, even during the monthly bleeding. Menstrual bleeding is often irregular. There is also an increased chance of pregnancy if even a single pill is forgotten.

Common brand names:

Femulen	*Microlut*	these brands can also be used for Emergency Family Planning— see the next section
Micronor	*Microval*	
Micronovum	*Neogest*	
Nor-Q D	*Neogeston*	
	Ovrette	

EMERGENCY FAMILY PLANNING
(Emergency Pills)

Emergency pills are special doses of certain birth control pills for a woman who has had unprotected sex and wants to avoid pregnancy. Using birth control pills this way is safe, even for many women who should not use pills all the time.

Dose: Emergency pills must be taken within 3 days of unprotected sex. The sooner you take the pills after unprotected sex, the more likely you will not get pregnant. For emergency family planning, carefully follow these instructions:

Take 2 "high-dose" birth control pills from GROUP 4 within 3 days of unprotected sex, followed by 2 more GROUP 4 pills 12 hours later.

OR

Take 4 "low-dose" birth control pills from GROUP 2 or GROUP 3 within 3 days of unprotected sex, followed by 4 more GROUP 2 or GROUP 3 pills 12 hours later.

OR

Take 25 progestin-only pills or "mini-pills" from the brand names marked in GROUP 5 within 3 days of unprotected sex, followed by 20 more GROUP 5 pills 12 hours later.

New emergency pills have been developed just for emergency family planning and may be available where you live. Some brand names include: ***Norlevo, Plan B, Postinor-2, Schering-PC-4 and Tetragynon.*** With ***Postinor-2,*** for example, which contains only progestin, you take 1 pill within 3 days of unprotected sex, followed by 1 more pill 12 hours later.

Side effects:

More than half of all women who use emergency pills will have nausea and even vomiting. If vomiting occurs within 3 hours after taking the pills, another dose must be taken. If vomiting is a problem for you, you can take 25 mg of promethazine by mouth 2 times a day. Or, instead of taking the emergency pills by mouth you can place them high in the vagina. This method works just as well to prevent pregnancy. It does not reduce the side effects of nausea or vomiting, but it does prevent you from vomiting the pills.

Progestin-only pills cause less nausea and vomiting than combined pills. Women who have heart problems, blood clots or strokes should use progestin-only pills.

Condoms (Rubbers, Prophylactics, Sheaths)

Name:__________________ price:______ for_____

Often come in packages of 3.

There are many different brands of condoms. Some are lubricated, some come in different colors, and some have spermicide.

In addition to helping prevent pregnancy, condoms (especially those with spermicide) can also help to prevent the spread of sexually transmitted (venereal) diseases, including AIDS. Many people use condoms along with another form of birth control.

Use and care of condoms is described on page 290.

Diaphragm

Name:______________________ price:________

To be effective, the diaphragm should be used with a spermicide cream or jelly. Put some inside the diaphragm, and also perhaps spread some on the rim before putting it in the vagina (see p. 290).

Name of jelly or cream:___________ price:______

Contraceptive Foam (Well-known brands: *Emko, Lempko, Delfen*)

Name:______________________ price:________

For discussion of the use of foam, see page 290.

Contraceptive suppositories
(Common brand: *Neo Sampoon*)

Name:______________________ price:________

This is a tablet containing spermicide that a woman puts deep in her vagina near her cervix. The suppository should be put in 15 minutes before having sex. (Follow instructions on the package.) It is a fairly effective method of birth control, especially if the couple also uses a condom.

Intrauterine Device (IUD)

Name:______________________ price:________

fee for putting it in:_________

For information on IUDs, see page 290. There are several different kinds: **Copper T, Copper 7, Lippes Loop,** and the **Safety Coil.** Another kind, called **Progestasert,** must be replaced more often than others. One kind of IUD, **the Dalkon Shield,** causes more problems than others and should not be used.

Because infection and other problems can occur with IUDs, only women who live close to a health center should use them. IUDs can be used by women who have never had a child, but if infection occurs it may be harder for a woman to get pregnant later on.

The best time to have an IUD put in is while the woman is having her period or just after.

Injectable Contraceptives
(Common brands: *Depo-Provera, Perlutal, Net-En*)

Name:______________________ price:________

Injectable contraceptives contain a chemical hormone called progesterone. This is the same chemical hormone used in birth control pills. Injectable contraceptives are being used in many countries, but there are still arguments over their safety. Many people now believe they are safe, except for women who for medical reasons cannot use birth control pills (see p. 288).

The most frequent problem is that they can cause irregular bleeding from the vagina. A woman may have heavy bleeding all month long or she may not have any bleeding at all. Older women who stop having their periods after receiving an injectable contraceptive may mistake this for the menopause, stop getting more injections, and become pregnant.

Sometimes the injections cause infertility. It is common for a woman to be unable to become pregnant for a year or more after she has stopped getting the injections. Also, if the injection is given when the woman is pregnant, there is a greater risk that her baby will have a birth defect.

As with birth control pills, there is not enough known about chemical hormones to be sure that injectable contraceptives increase the risk of womb and breast cancer (see p. 288).

Contraceptive Implants
(Common brand: *Norplant*)

Name:______________________ price:________

fee for putting them in:________

As with all birth control methods, there are advantages and disadvantages to using this method.

Implants are a very convenient and highly effective form of birth control. A specially trained health worker puts six small tubes containing the chemical hormone progesterone under the skin in a woman's upper arm. The tubes prevent pregnancy for 5 years, the woman does not have to remember to take birth control pills, or to return to a clinic every 3 months for an injectable contraceptive.

Possible side effects include irregular bleeding from the vagina, headaches, hair loss, weight gain, pimples, mood swings, depression, dizziness, cramps, and pain or infection in the area of the implant.

The biggest disadvantage of the implants is that once they are inserted, a woman may have little control over when they are removed. The removal of the implants requires the help of someone who is trained to do it. Removing the implants can be more painful than having them put in. It is sometimes difficult to find someone willing to remove them. Often those in charge of providing the implants say that they must stay in the woman for 5 years to justify the cost of the implant.

As with all form of birth control, a woman has a right to know about the advantages and disadvantages of each method, and its side effects and risks, so that she can make a thoughtful decision about whether or not she wants to use it.

WRITE HERE INFORMATION ABOUT OTHER MEDICINES OR HOME REMEDIES USEFUL IN YOUR AREA.

New Information — Blue Pages

In this revised edition of Where There Is No Doctor, *we have added several new topics to bring the book up to date and make it more complete. One of the topics, HIV/AIDS, is a disease which is rapidly spreading over most of the world. Likewise, complications from unsafe abortions, pesticide poisoning, and drug addiction are problems which have come to affect much larger numbers of people in the last few years. Other topics we have included because we have had many requests. We have added the section on measuring blood pressure because the book is widely used by health workers, some of whom have equipment for taking blood pressure.*

HIV/AIDS
(Human Immunodeficiency Virus/ Acquired Immune Deficiency Syndrome)

AIDS is a new and dangerous disease spread from person to person through the HIV virus. It is now found in most countries around the world, and in many has become a leading cause of death.

HIV/AIDS reduces the body's ability to fight disease. A person with HIV/AIDS can get sick very easily — from many different illnesses such as diarrhea, pneumonia, tuberculosis, or a serious type of skin cancer. Most persons with AIDS die from diseases their bodies are no longer strong enough to fight.

HIV/AIDS is spread when blood, semen (sperm), or vaginal juice of someone with the HIV virus enters the body of another person. It can be spread through:

Sex with someone who has the HIV virus.

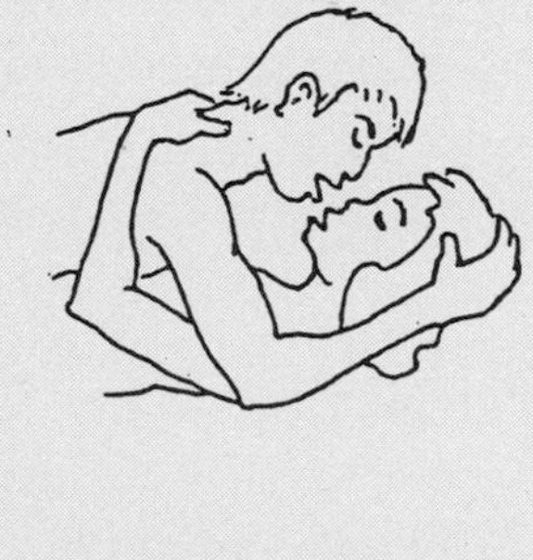

A person who has sex with more than one person has a higher risk of getting HIV/AIDS.

Using the same needle or syringe (or any instrument that cuts the skin) without sterilizing it.

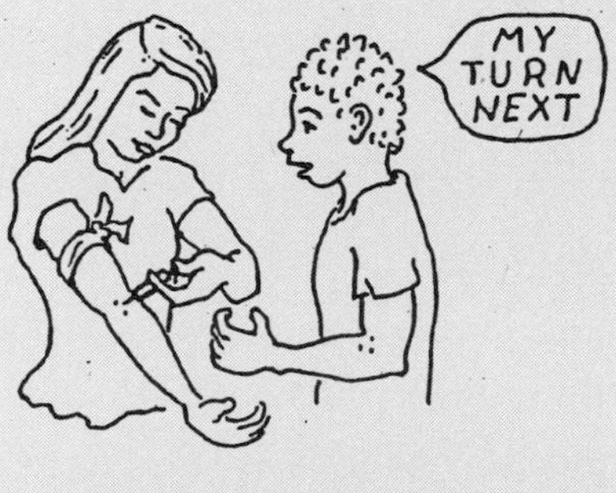

Drug users and others who share needles have a very high risk.

An **infected mother** to her unborn child.

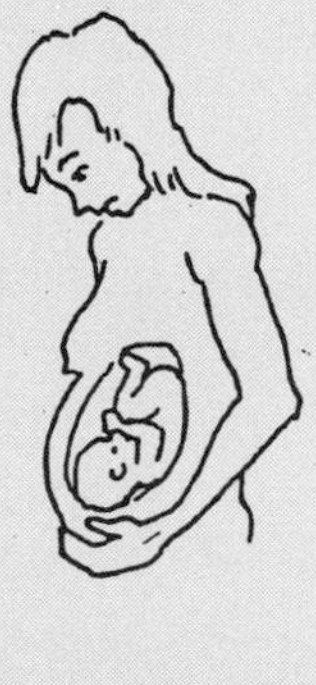

About one third of the babies of mothers with the HIV virus will get HIV/AIDS.

IMPORTANT: **You can get HIV/AIDS from someone who looks completely healthy.** Often it takes months or years after the virus enters the body for the first signs to appear**-but the person can still spread HIV/AIDS to others through sex or sharing needles.**

HIV is not spread through everyday contact such as shaking hands, or living, playing, or eating together. Also, it is not spread by food, water, insects, toilet seats, or communion cups.

Signs: The signs of AIDS are different in different persons. Often they are the typical signs of other common illnesses, but are more severe and last longer.

If a combination of these 3 signs appears and the person gets sick more and more often, he or she may have AIDS (but you cannot be sure without a HIV test to detect the virus):

- gradual weight loss. The person becomes thinner and thinner.
- diarrhea for more than 1 month.
- a fever for more than 1 month, sometimes with chills or soaking night sweats.

The person may also have one or more of these signs:

- a bad cough that lasts for more than 1 month.
- yeast infection in the mouth ('thrush,' see p. 232).
- swollen lymph nodes, anywhere in the body (see p. 88).
- rashes or painless dark patches on the skin.
- warts or sores that keep growing and do not go away with treatment, especially around the genital area and buttocks.
- feels tired all the time.

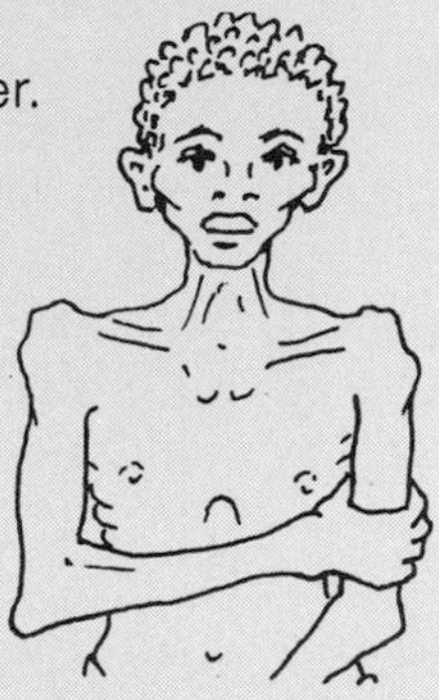

In Africa, AIDS is often called 'slim disease' because people with AIDS lose so much weight.

Persons with HIV/AIDS are more likely to get tuberculosis (p. 179) or shingles (p. 204).

Treatment:

There is still no medicine to cure AIDS. But because people with AIDS have difficulty fighting infections, they should be sure to treat them:

- for diarrhea, give Rehydration Drink (see p. 152).
- For thrush, use gentian violet, nystatin, or miconazole (see p. 232 and 373).
- For warts, use bichloroacetic acid or trichloroacetic acid or podophyllin (see p. 374 and 402).
- For fever give lots of fluids, aspirin and lower high fever with a cool bath (see p. 75 and 76).
- Treat cough and pneumonia with antibiotics (see p. 170 and 171). If cough and fever last long, try to take a TB test. Seek local advice about TB prevention and treatment for people with the HIV virus.
- For itchy skin, give antihistamines (p. 386) and treat any infection (p. 202).
- Stay as healthy as possible: eat well (see Chapter 11); do not drink alcohol, smoke or chew tobacco or use drugs; get enough rest and sleep; and use a condom when having sex.

New medicines called "anti-retrovirals" (ARVs), such as zidovudine (AZT), nevirapine, and "triple therapy" combinations of drugs can help people with HIV/AIDS stay healthy and live longer. They do not kill HIV or cure AIDS, but they make the sickness easier to live with. Unfortunately, these medicines are often expensive and difficult to get in poor countries. Get advice from a health worker experienced with HIV/AIDS to see if these medicines are available in your community. See page 249 for information on using nevirapine to prevent HIV from passing from a mother to her baby.

There is no need for people with HIV/AIDS to live or sleep alone. Their skin or breathing does not spread the infection.

At home, family and friends can give love and support to help the person prepare for his or her approaching death (see p. 330).

Prevention of AIDS:

- Have sex only with one faithful partner.
- Use a condom if you or your partner have had other sexual partners (see p. 290). **Using a condom reduces the risk of getting or giving HIV/AIDS.**
- Do not have sex with persons who have many sex partners, such as prostitutes (female or male), or with persons who inject illegal drugs.
- Treat sexually transmitted infections early — especially those that cause sores.
- Do not have an injection unless you are sure the instruments are sterilized first. **Health workers should NEVER re-use a needle or syringe without sterilizing it first (see p. 74).**
- Do not inject illegal drugs. If you do, do not share the same needle or syringe with someone else unless it is first sterilized with bleach or boiled for 20 minutes (see p. 74).
- Make sure instruments for circumcision, ear piercing, acupuncture, and traditional practices such as scarring, are boiled.
- If possible, do not accept a transfusion of blood that has not first been tested. Avoid transfusions except when absolutely necessary.
- Look for ways to protect and educate 'street children,' migrant workers, drug users, sex workers and others at 'high risk,' about how not to get or give HIV/AIDS.
- In the long run, AIDS can best be prevented by fighting for fairer social and economic conditions, so that families do not need to separate to find work, and so that people need not sell their bodies for sex.

Persons with AIDS who have a lot of fever, diarrhea, or pain need special care. This can usually be done without risk. But to prevent spreading the virus, some things should be remembered:

- Blood, open sores, bloody diarrhea, or bloody vomit can spread the virus. To prevent touching these, if possible wear rubber latex or plastic gloves, or plastic bags on your hands. Wash your hands often.
- Soiled or bloody clothes, bedding, or towels should be handled with care. Wash them in hot soapy water, or add some chlorine bleach.

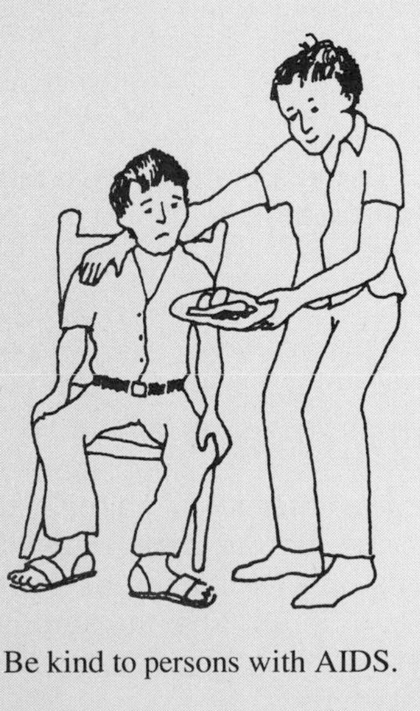

Be kind to persons with AIDS.

SORES ON THE GENITALS

A single, painless sore on the genitals may be a sign of syphilis (see p. 237). But several sores are likely to be a sign of other sexually transmitted diseases: genital warts, genital herpes, or chancroid.

Genital Warts (Venereal warts, Condylomata acuminata)

These warts are caused by a virus that is spread by sexual contact. They look like warts on other parts of the body (see p. 210) but there are usually more of them.

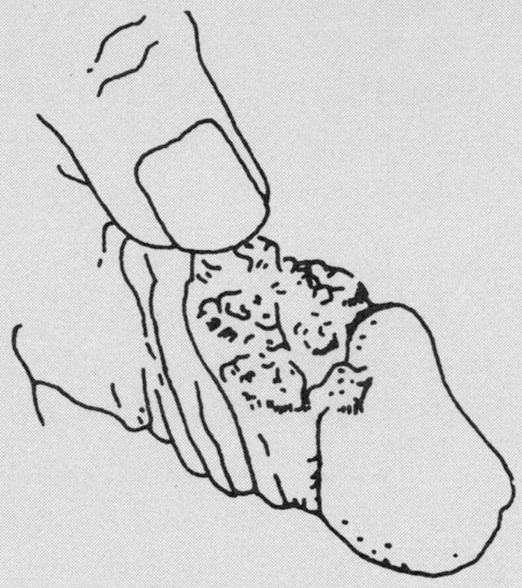

Signs:

Small, hard, whitish or brownish skin growths that have a rough surface. In men they usually grow on the penis but can also grow on the *scrotum* or anus (asshole). In women they grow on the lips of the vagina, inside the vagina, or around the anus.

Treatment:

Apply a small amount of bichloroacetic acid or podophyllin (see p. 374) to each wart. (If possible, first apply some *Vaseline* or other greasy ointment to the skin around each wart to protect the healthy skin.) Podophyllin must be washed off 6 hours later. Several treatments are usually necessary. The warts will slowly shrink and go away, but often return.

Prevention:

The man should wear a condom (see p. 290) during sex if either he or his partner has genital warts.

Using a condom each time you have sex helps prevent the spread of warts, herpes, chancroid, AIDS, and other sexually transmitted diseases.

Genital Herpes

Genital herpes is a painful skin infection caused by a virus. Small blisters appear on the sex parts. Genital herpes is spread from person to person during sex. Genital herpes occasionally appears on the mouth from oral sex. But it is different from the kind of herpes that commonly occurs on the mouth, which is often not spread by sex (see Cold Sores, p. 232).

Signs:

- One or more small very painful blisters, like drops of water on the skin, appear on the sex organs (penis and vagina), anus, buttocks, or thighs.
- Blisters burst and form small, open sores.
- These dry up and become scabs.

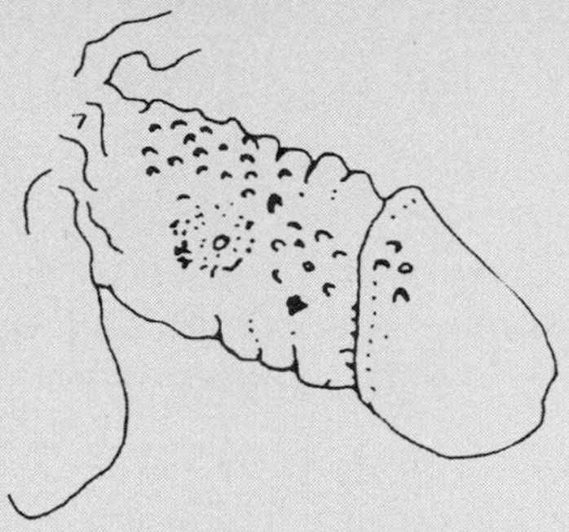

The herpes sores can last for 3 weeks or more, with fever, aches, chills, and swollen lymph nodes in the groin. Women may have trouble urinating.

The virus stays in the body after all signs disappear. New blisters can appear at any time, from weeks to years later. Usually the new sores appear in the same place, but are fewer, not as painful, and heal more quickly.

Treatment:

There is no medicine that cures herpes. Keep the area clean. Do not have sex while the blisters or sores are present—not even with a condom.

Wash hands often and try not to touch the sores. The infection can spread to the eyes if a person rubs them after touching the sores.

CAUTION: If a woman has herpes sores when she gives birth, her baby can get it. This is very dangerous. Let your health worker or midwife know if you have ever had genital herpes.

Chancroid

Signs:

- soft, **painful** sores on the genitals or anus
- enlarged lymph nodes (bubos) may develop in the groin

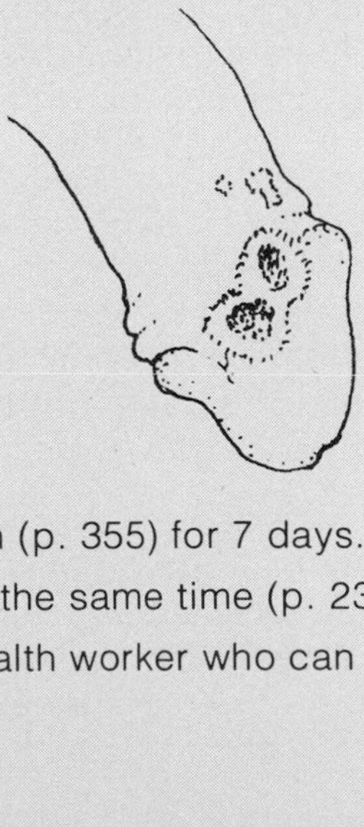

Treatment:

- Give co-trimoxazole (p. 358) or erythromycin (p. 355) for 7 days.
- It is often a good idea to treat for syphilis at the same time (p. 237).
- If there are enlarged lymph nodes, see a health worker who can drain them.

CIRCUMCISION AND EXCISION (CUTTING AWAY SKIN FROM THE SEX PARTS)

In many communities, boy children are circumcised—and in some parts of the world, also girls—as a traditional 'practice' or 'custom'. For health reasons, circumcision is not necessary. To boys it usually does no harm. **But for girls, this practice—sometimes called 'excision', 'infibulation', or 'female genital cutting'—is very dangerous and should be strongly discouraged.**

BOYS

A baby boy is born with a tube of skin (foreskin) covering the 'head' of his penis. As long as urine comes out of the hole at the tip, there should be no problem. The foreskin will usually not pull back completely over the head of the penis until the boy is about 4 years old. This is normal and **circumcision is not necessary.** Do not try to pull the foreskin back by force.

However, if the foreskin becomes red, swollen, and so tight that the baby cannot pass urine without pain, this is not normal. Take him to a health worker for a circumcision as soon as possible.

As a family ritual, simple circumcision of a healthy baby boy may be done by a midwife or person with experience. Using a new razor, she cuts off a little of the foreskin beyond the head of the penis. After the cut, there is some bleeding. Hold the penis firmly with a clean cloth, or gauze, for 5 minutes, until the bleeding stops. Some healers use the juice of a plant to help stop the bleeding (see p. 13).

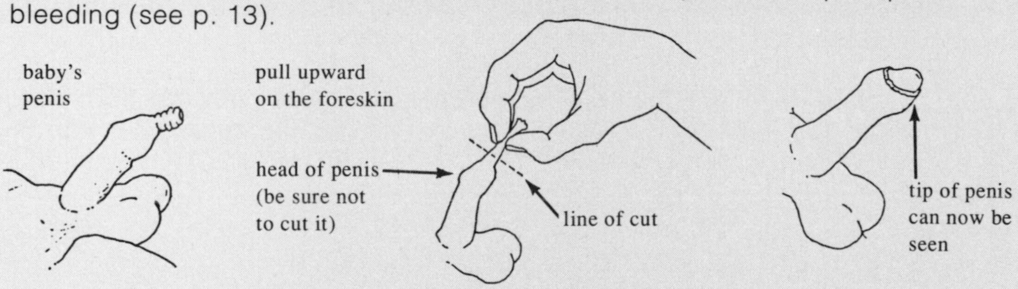

If the bleeding does not stop, wash away the clots of blood with clean water, and pinch the end of the foreskin between the fingers with a piece of clean cloth for as long as it takes the bleeding to stop. No medicine is needed.

GIRLS

In circumcision of girls, or 'excision', the soft knob of flesh (clitoris) at the front end of the vagina is cut out. Sometimes, part of the vaginal lips is also cut away. Removing the clitoris is as bad as cutting off the head of a boy's penis. **Excision should not be done.** Girls who have been excised may have frequent urinary and vaginal infections, and difficulty during childbirth.

There is also danger of severe bleeding during excision. **The child can die** in a few minutes. **Act quickly.** Wash away the clots to find the exact point where the blood is coming from and press on it firmly for 5 minutes. If bleeding continues, keep pressing the bleeding spot while you carry the child to a health worker or doctor for help.

SPECIAL CARE FOR SMALL, EARLY, AND UNDERWEIGHT BABIES—'KANGAROOING'

A baby who is born very small (weighs less than 2 1/2 kilos or 5 pounds) will need special care. If possible, take the baby to a health post or hospital. In the hospital, these babies are often kept warm and protected in a special temperature-controlled box called an incubator. However, for a baby who is basically healthy, a mother can often provide similar warmth and protection by 'kangarooing' the baby:

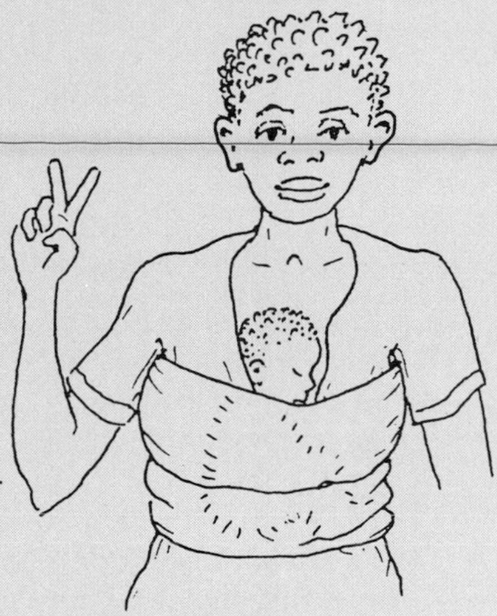

- Place the baby naked, with or without a diaper or nappy, upright inside your clothing against your skin, between your breasts. (It helps to wear a loose blouse, sweater, or wrap tied at the waist.)
- Let the baby suck at your breast as often as he wants, but at least every 2 hours.
- Sleep propped up so that the baby stays upright.
- Wash the baby's face and bottom each day.
- **Make sure the baby stays warm at all times.** If it is cool, dress the baby with extra clothing, and cover his head.
- While you bathe or rest, ask the father, or another family member, to 'kangaroo' the baby.
- Take the baby to a health worker regularly. Be sure that he gets all his vaccinations (see p. 147).
- Give the baby iron and vitamin supplements—especially vitamin D (see p. 392).

EAR WAX

A little wax in the ears is normal. But some people have too much wax, or it dries into a hard lump close to the ear drum. This can block the ear canal so that the person cannot hear well.

Treatment:

To remove the wax, first soften it by putting several drops of warm vegetable oil into the person's ear. Then have her lie down on her side with the ear up for 15 minutes. Next, wash the ear out well by pouring several cups of warm (not hot) water into it.

If this does not work, remove the needle from a syringe and fill the syringe with warm water and squirt it into the ear canal. Repeat this several times, or until the wax comes out. Stop if the person starts to feel dizzy. If the wax still will not come out, seek medical advice.

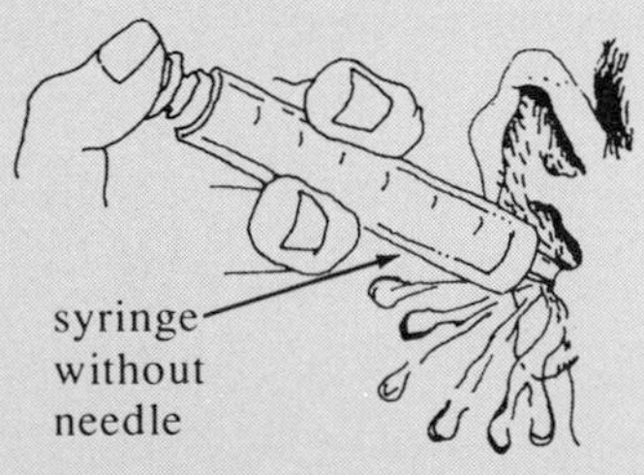

LEISHMANIASIS

This disease is found in Africa, India, and the Middle East, and in southern Mexico, Central America and South America. The infection is carried from person to person by a small sand fly which infects a person when it bites.

Some forms of the disease cause damage inside the body (visceral leishmaniasis, kala-azar, dumdum fever). These are very difficult to recognize and the treatment is very complicated and expensive. If possible, seek medical help.

Other forms affect mainly the skin (cutaneous leishmaniasis, tropical sore, Delhi boil, espundia, forest yaws, uta, chiclero ulcer). These are easier to treat.

Signs of leishmaniasis of the skin:

- 2 to 8 weeks after being bitten, swelling appears where the fly bit.
- The swelling becomes an open sore, usually with pus.
- Sores can heal by themselves, but may take several weeks to 2 years.
- Sores become infected (with bacteria) very easily.

Treatment:

- ♦ Clean the sore with cool, boiled water.
- ♦ Apply a hot, moist cloth to the sore (not so hot that it burns the skin) for 10 to 15 minutes.
- ♦ Do this 2 times a day for 10 days. This 'heat treatment' often brings a complete cure.
- ♦ If the sore looks infected (red and painful), also give antibiotics (see p. 351).

GUINEA WORM

Guinea worm is a long, thin worm that lives under the skin and makes a painful sore on the ankle, leg, or elsewhere on the body. The worm, which looks like a white thread, can be over a meter long. Guinea worm is found in parts of Africa, India, and the Middle East.

Guinea worm is spread from person to person, like this:

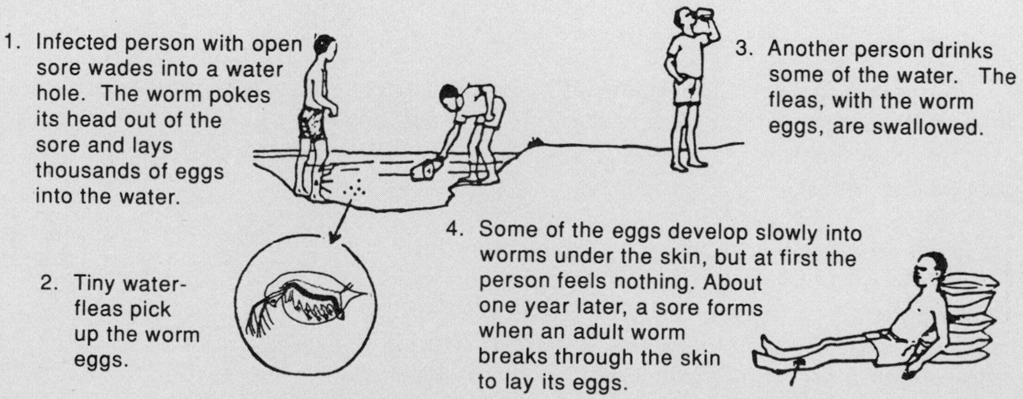

1. Infected person with open sore wades into a water hole. The worm pokes its head out of the sore and lays thousands of eggs into the water.
2. Tiny water-fleas pick up the worm eggs.
3. Another person drinks some of the water. The fleas, with the worm eggs, are swallowed.
4. Some of the eggs develop slowly into worms under the skin, but at first the person feels nothing. About one year later, a sore forms when an adult worm breaks through the skin to lay its eggs.

Signs:

- A painful swelling develops on the ankle, leg, testicles or elsewhere on the body.
- After a week a blister forms, which soon bursts open forming a sore. This often happens when standing in water, or bathing. The end of a white thread-like Guinea worm can be seen poking out of the sore.
- If the sore gets dirty and infected, the pain and swelling spread, and walking becomes impossible. Sometimes tetanus occurs (see p. 182).

Treatment:

- Keep the sore clean. Soak the sore in cold water until the worm's head pokes out.
- Attach a thread to the worm, or roll it round a thin stick, and pull gently, a little more each day. This may take a week or more. The worm can be more than a meter long! Try not to break it, because this can cause severe infection.
- Give metronidazole or thiabendazole to help reduce discomfort and make it easier to slowly pull out the worm. (The medicines do not kill the worms. For dosages and precautions, see p. 369 and 375.)
- Give anti-tetanus vaccination (p. 147).
- If sores become infected (spreading pain, redness, swelling, and fever), give penicillin or dicloxicillin or a similar antibiotic (see p. 351).

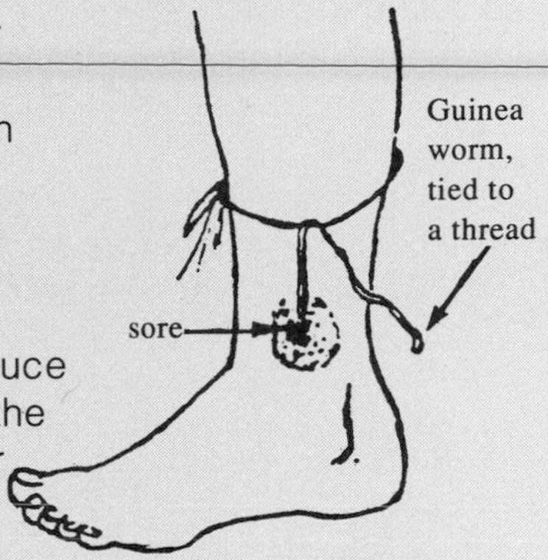

Prevention:

- Use tap water for drinking, if available. If a water hole is the only supply, then do not drink from it directly. Pour the water into a special drinking water pot, through a clean cloth tied over the top. The cloth will filter out the infected water-fleas.

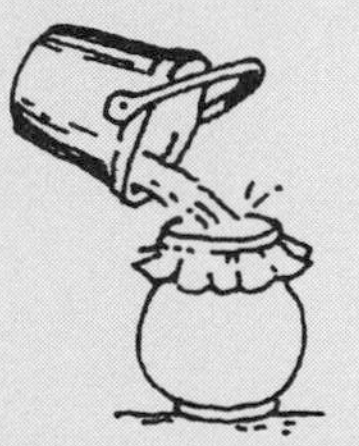

- If the community can build stone steps into the water hole, people can scoop water from the last dry step without getting wet.

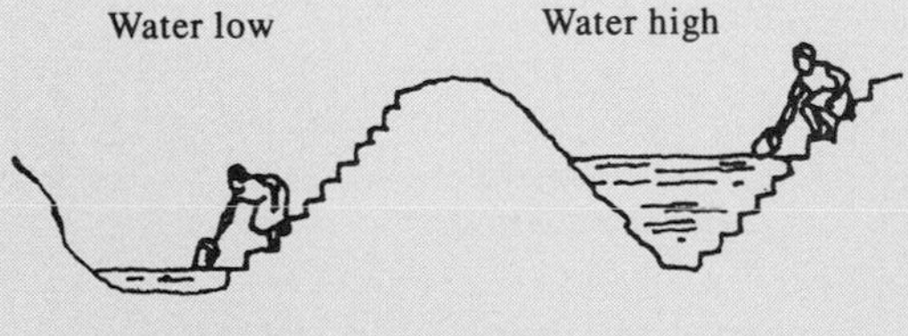

ALWAYS USE THE LAST DRY STEP.
NEVER STEP INTO THE WATER.

- Or turn the water hole into a well, so that people can draw water with a rope and bucket.

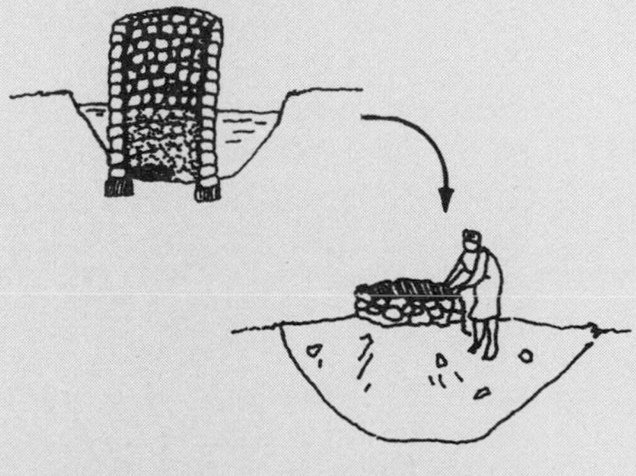

If nobody wades or bathes in water used for drinking, the infection cannot be passed on, and will eventually disappear from the area.

EMERGENCIES CAUSED BY COLD

Loss of Body Heat (Hypothermia)

In cold climates, or cold, wet or windy weather, persons who are not wearing enough warm clothes can lose the heat from their bodies. **This is very dangerous.** Often the person does not realize what is happening to him. He can become so confused that he will not ask for help and may die.

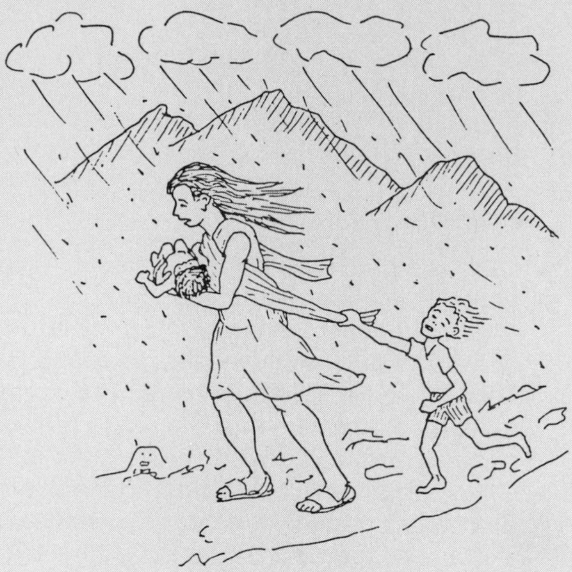

Signs:

- Uncontrolled shivering
- Slow or unclear speech
- Stumbles when he walks
- Cannot think clearly
- Feels very tired

Treatment:

- Quickly get the person to a dry place protected from the wind.
- If his clothes are wet, take them off and cover him with dry clothing. Wrap him in dry blankets.
- Make sure his head, feet, and hands are covered.
- Heat some stones in a fire and wrap them in cloth. Put the warm stones next to his chest, back, and groin.

> *WARNING:* **Do not warm up the person too fast as this could cause heart problems and death.**

- Do all you can to keep the person warm. If it is a child, wrap him inside your clothing against your skin (see 'Kangarooing', p. 405). Or sleep with him in your arms. If possible, have someone else lie on the other side. Or put pans of hot coals, or a few small oil lamps under the cot. (But be careful he does not get burned, or too warm.)

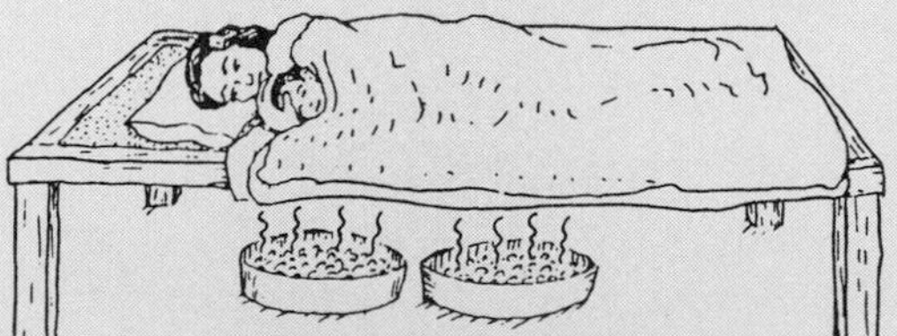

pans with hot coals

- Give him sweet things to eat and drink like sugar, candy, honey, sweet ripe fruit or fruit juice. If you do not have these things, give him starchy foods like rice, bread, plantain, or potatoes.

If the person stops shivering but still has any of the above signs, or if he is unconscious, his condition is very serious. Keep trying to warm him, but if he does not wake up, **get medical help FAST.**

Dangerously Low Body Temperature in Babies and Sick Persons

Sometimes, especially in cool weather, a baby, sick child, or person who is very old, ill, malnourished, or weak may lose so much body heat that their temperature drops below normal. The signs mentioned on the previous page may develop, and the person may die. Try to raise the body temperature by keeping the person warm as described on page 408.

Frozen Skin (Frostbite)

In freezing weather, if a person is not dressed warmly enough, her hands, feet, ears, and sometimes face may begin to freeze. **Frostbite is very dangerous.** If completely frozen, the skin will die and later turn black (p. 213). The part may have to be cut off (amputated).

Signs of frostbite:

- At first, numbness and often sharp pain in one part of the body.
- Then all feeling goes away as the part gets more frozen.
- The part gets pale in color and feels hard when touched.

Treatment of mild frostbite: If the skin still feels soft when touched, the person probably has 'mild frostbite'. Wrap the part with dry cloth and warm it against another part of the person's own body or someone else's. Try to keep moving and get out of the cold as fast as possible.

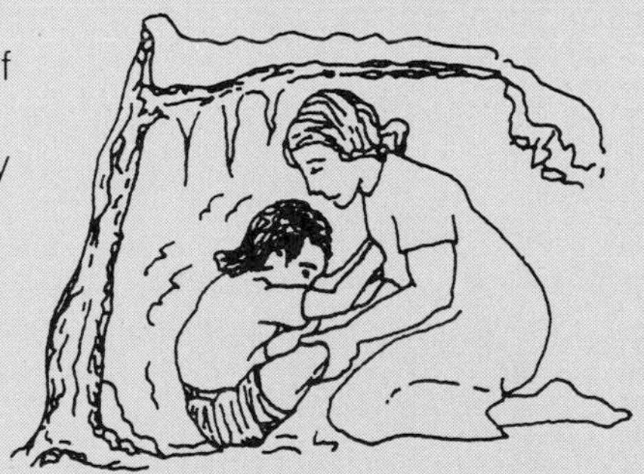

Try to cover ears and face.

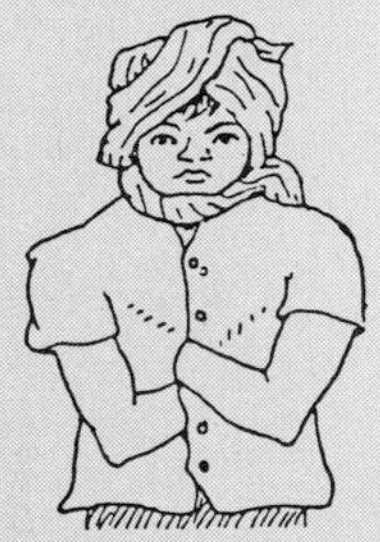

Warm hands and feet against body.

Treatment of severe frostbite: *CAUTION:* Do not start treatment for severe frostbite until you are in a place where the person's whole body can be kept warm during and after treatment. It is better to let a hand or foot stay frozen for several hours than to let it get warm and then freeze again. When you get to a warm, protected place:

- Fill a large container with warm water **(not hot)** that feels comfortable when you hold your hand in it.
- Soak the person's frozen part in the water until it gets warm.
- If the water cools, add more warm water. But take out the person's hand or foot while you do this. Remember, she cannot feel how hot the water is and you can easily burn her.
- As it gets warm, the frozen part will become very painful. Give aspirin or codeine (p. 379 and 384).
- When it is no longer frozen, the person must stay warm and rest.
- Be very gentle with the part that was frozen. Treat as you would a severe wound or burn (p. 96). Seek medical help. Sometimes dead parts of the body must be removed through surgery.

HOW TO MEASURE BLOOD PRESSURE

Blood pressure measurement can be an important skill for health workers and midwives. It is an especially useful tool in examining:

- Pregnant women (see p. 249, 251, and 253).
- Mothers before and during childbirth (see p. 265).
- A person who may be losing a lot of blood from any part of the body, inside or out (see p. 77).
- A person who might be in shock (see p. 77), including allergic shock (see p. 70).
- People over 40.
- Fat people (see p. 126).
- Anyone with signs of heart trouble (p. 325), stroke (p. 327), difficulty breathing, frequent headaches, swelling, diabetes (p. 127), chronic urinary problems (p. 234), or swollen or painful veins (p. 175).
- Persons known to have high blood pressure (see p. 125).
- Women taking (or planning to take) birth control pills (see p. 288).

There are 2 kinds of instruments for measuring blood pressure:

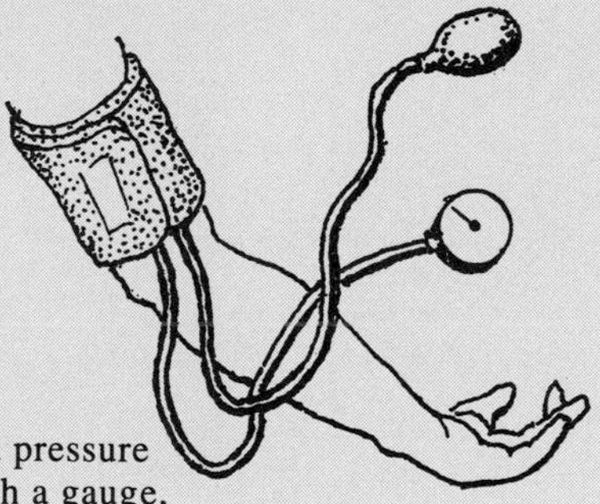

A blood pressure cuff with a gauge,

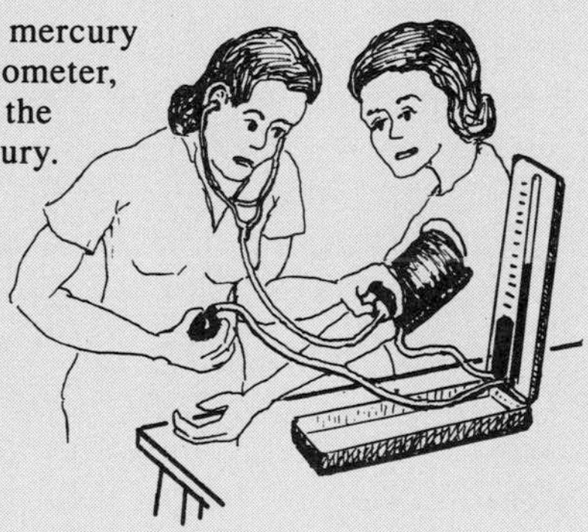

and the older mercury sphygmomanometer, which shows the level of mercury.

To measure blood pressure:

- **Make sure the person is relaxed.** Recent exercise, anger, or nervousness can make pressure rise and give a falsely high reading. Explain what you are going to do, so the person is not surprised or frightened.
- **Fasten the pressure cuff** around the person's bare upper arm.
- **Close the valve** on the rubber bulb by turning the screw clockwise.
- **Pump the pressure up** to more than 200 millimeters of mercury.
- **Place the stethoscope** over the inside of the elbow.
- **Listen carefully for the pulse** as you slowly let air out of the cuff. As the needle of the gauge (or the level of mercury) slowly drops, **take two readings:**

1. **Take the first reading the moment you begin to hear the soft thumping of the pulse.** This happens when the pressure in the cuff drops to the highest pressure in the artery (systolic or 'top' pressure). This top pressure is reached each time the heart contracts and forces the blood through the arteries. In a normal person, this top pressure reading is usually around 110 to 120 mm.

2. Continue to slowly release the pressure while listening carefully. **Take the second reading when the sound of the pulse begins to fade or disappear.** This happens when the pressure in the cuff drops to the lowest pressure in the artery (diastolic or 'bottom' pressure). This bottom pressure occurs when the heart relaxes between pulses. It is normally around 60 to 80 mm.

When you record a person's blood pressure, always write both the top and bottom pressure readings. We say that an adult's normal blood pressure (BP) is "120 over 80," and write it like this:

BP $\frac{120}{80}$ or BP 120/80

120 is the top (systolic) reading
80 is the bottom (diastolic) reading.

For health workers, it may be better to speak of the "top" and "bottom" numbers (TN and BN), rather than use big, strange words like systolic and diastolic.

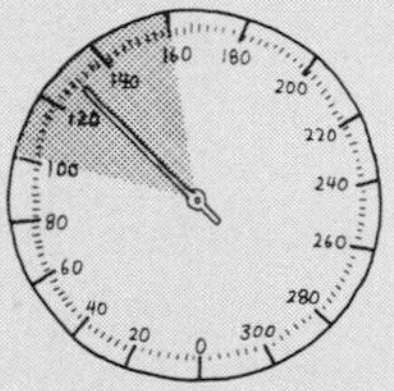

It is usually the bottom number that tells us more about a person's health. For example, if a person's blood pressure is 140/85, there is not much need for concern. But if it is 135/110, he has seriously **high blood pressure** and should lose weight (if fat) or get treatment. A bottom number of over 100 usually means the blood pressure is high enough to require attention (diet and perhaps medicine).

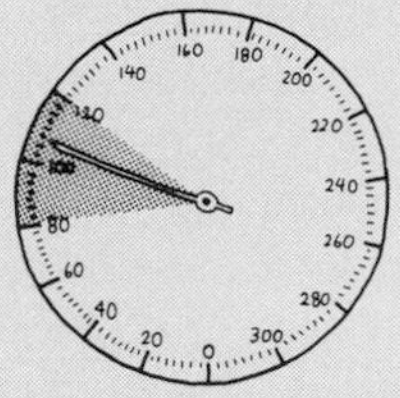

Normal blood pressure for an adult is usually around 120/80, but anything from 100/60 to 140/90 can be considered normal.

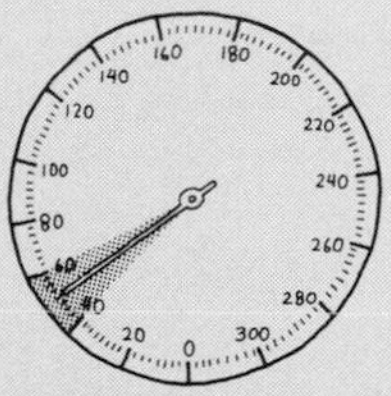

If a person regularly has **low blood pressure,** there is no need to worry. In fact, blood pressure on the low side of normal, 90/60 to 110/70, means a person is likely to live long and is less likely to suffer from heart trouble or stroke.

A sudden drop in blood pressure is a danger sign, especially if it falls below 60/40. Health workers should watch for any sudden drop in the blood pressure of persons who are losing blood or at risk of shock (see p. 77).

For more information about blood pressure measurement, see *Helping Health Workers Learn,* Chapter 19.

POISONING FROM PESTICIDES

Pesticides are chemical poisons used to kill certain plants (herbicides), fungus (fungicides), insects (insecticides) or other animals (for example, rat poison). In recent years, the increasing misuse of pesticides has become a big problem in many developing countries. These dangerous chemicals can cause severe health problems. They can also damage the 'balance of nature', which in time can lead to smaller harvests.

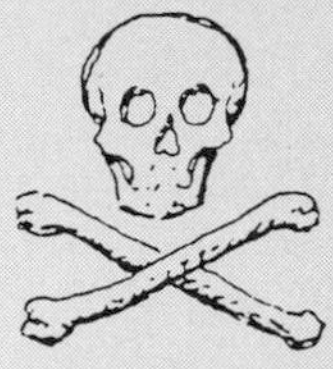

Many pesticides are extremely dangerous. Villagers often use them without knowing their risks, or how to protect themselves while using them. As a result, many persons become **very ill, blind, sterile, paralyzed,** or their children may have **birth defects.** Also, working with these chemicals, or eating foods sprayed with them, sometimes causes **cancer.**

Chemicals used to kill insects and weeds at first allow farmers who can afford them to produce more crops. But today, pesticide-treated crops often produce smaller harvests than crops produced without pesticides. This happens because pesticides also kill the 'good' birds and insects that provide a natural control of pests and are beneficial to the soil. Also, as the insects and weeds become resistant, greater quantities and more poisonous kinds of pesticides are needed. So, once farmers begin to use these chemical poisons, they become dependent on them.

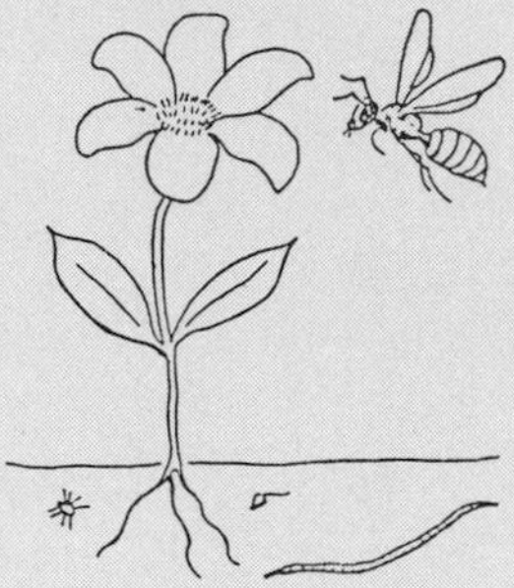

Pesticides also kill the beneficial animals—such as bees and earthworms.

As farmers' dependency on chemical pesticides and fertilizers goes up, so does the cost. When the smaller, poorer farmers can no longer afford them, they are forced off the land. As the land becomes owned by a few 'giant' farmers, and more and more people become landless, the number of malnourished and hungry people increases.

The risk of pesticide poisoning is high for these landless, poorly paid farm workers and their families. Many live in open shacks at the edge of fields that are sprayed with pesticides. The poison can easily get into their homes or water supply. This is especially dangerous for small children, who can be seriously harmed by even small amounts of these poisons. Farmers who use backpack sprayers, which often leak, are also at high risk.

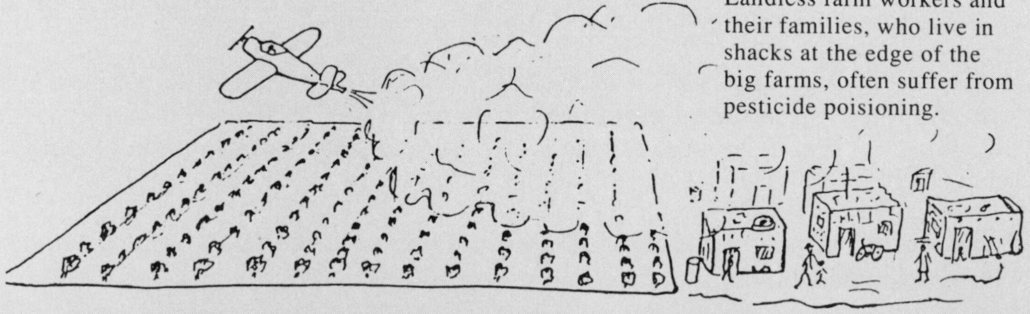

Landless farm workers and their families, who live in shacks at the edge of the big farms, often suffer from pesticide poisoning.

Laws are needed to prohibit the most dangerous pesticides and to provide clear warnings. Unfortunately, after governments in industrialized countries limited the use of many pesticides, chemical manufacturers began to sell their dangerous products to developing countries, where laws are less strict.

Some of the most dangerous pesticides are aldrin, dieldrin, endrin, chlordane, heptachlor, DDT, DBCP, HCH, BHC, ethylene dibromide (EDB), paraquat, parathion, agent orange (2-4D with 2-4-5T), camphechlor (toxaphene), poentachlorophenyl (PCP), and chlordimeform. It is very important to read carefully the labels of pesticide containers. Be sure to read the small print, because the pesticide may not be part of the brand name.

WARNING: If you use any pesticide, take the following precautions:

- Mix chemicals and load spray equipment carefully.
- Stand so that wind blows spray away from you.
- Wear protective clothing, covering the whole body.
- Wash hands before eating.
- Wash the whole body and change clothes immediately after spraying.
- Wash clothes after spraying.
- Do not let wash water get into drinking supply.
- Be sure containers with pesticides are clearly marked, and kept out of children's reach. Do not use pesticide containers for food or water.

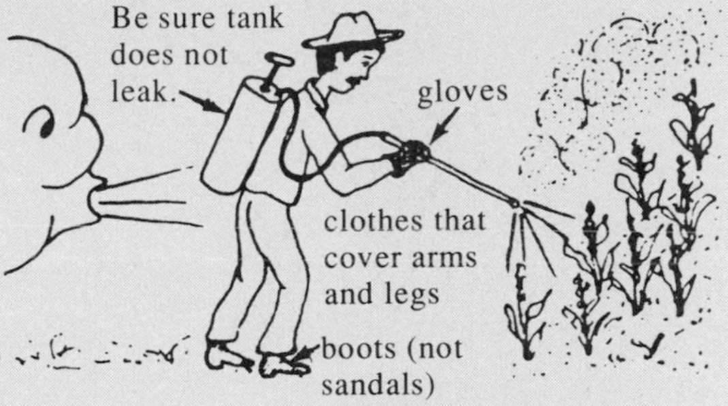
Be sure tank does not leak.
gloves
clothes that cover arms and legs
boots (not sandals)

> *CAUTION:* **Make sure that children, and women who are pregnant or breast feeding, stay away from all pesticides.**

Treatment for pesticide poisoning:

- If the person is not breathing, quickly do mouth-to-mouth breathing (see p. 80).
- Follow instructions on p. 103 to make the person vomit, and to give powdered charcoal (or egg whites) to soak up the poison inside the gut. But do not make the person vomit if you do not know what kind of pesticide he was using, or if he swallowed a pesticide with gasoline, kerosene, xylene, or other 'petroleum-based' liquids.
- Remove any pesticide-soaked clothing, and wash skin exposed to pesticide.

The above steps can help to treat the immediate problem of pesticide poisoning. But solving the underlying problem will require:

1. Education for avoiding the most dangerous pesticides, and laws to restrict their use.
2. Farm workers organizing to insist their rights are protected, and safety hazards are corrected.
3. Fairer land distribution.

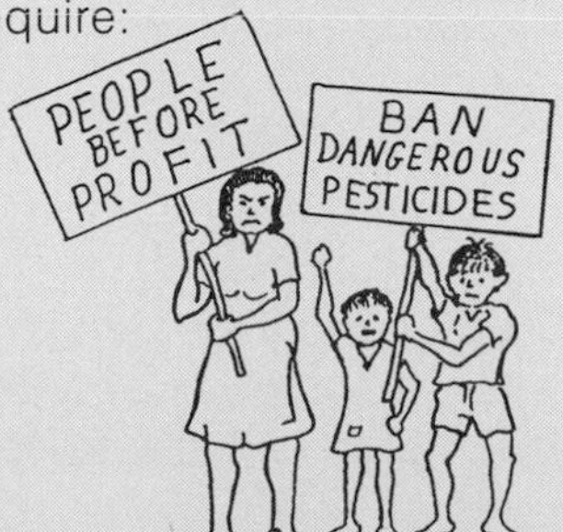
PEOPLE BEFORE PROFIT
BAN DANGEROUS PESTICIDES

COMPLICATIONS FROM ABORTION

When a woman takes action to end a pregnancy before a baby is fully enough formed to survive, this is called an ***abortion.*** (In this book we use the word 'abortion' only when the action is planned. The unplanned, natural loss of an unborn child we call a 'miscarriage'.)

Deciding whether or not to have an abortion can be difficult. In making a decision, most women will benefit from warm, respectful advice and friendly support. When abortions are done under sterile conditions in a hospital or clinic by a trained medical worker, they are usually safe for the woman. Abortions are safest when done in early pregnancy.

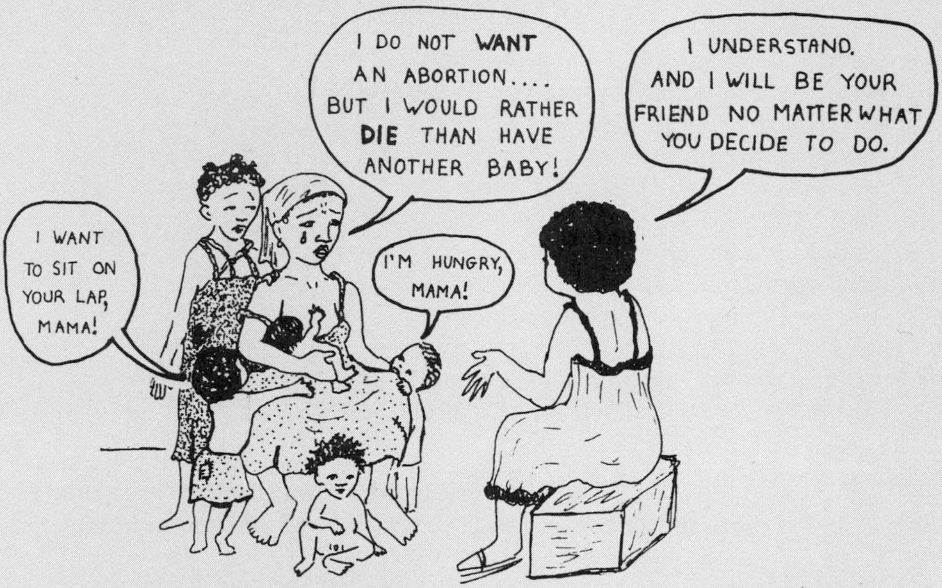

But when abortions are done at home, by untrained persons, or in unclean conditions, they can be extremely dangerous. In places where abortions are illegal or difficult to get, these 'home' abortions are often a major cause of death for women between the ages of 12 and 50.

Methods for ending a pregnancy such as putting sticks or other hard objects into the vagina or womb, squeezing the womb, or using modern drugs or plant medicines can cause **severe bleeding, infection,** and **death.**

Danger signs following an abortion:

- fever
- pain in the belly
- heavy bleeding from the vagina

If you see these signs in a woman who may have been pregnant, they could be the result of an abortion. But they could also be signs of miscarriage (p. 281), out-of-place pregnancy (p. 280), or pelvic inflammatory disease (p. 243).

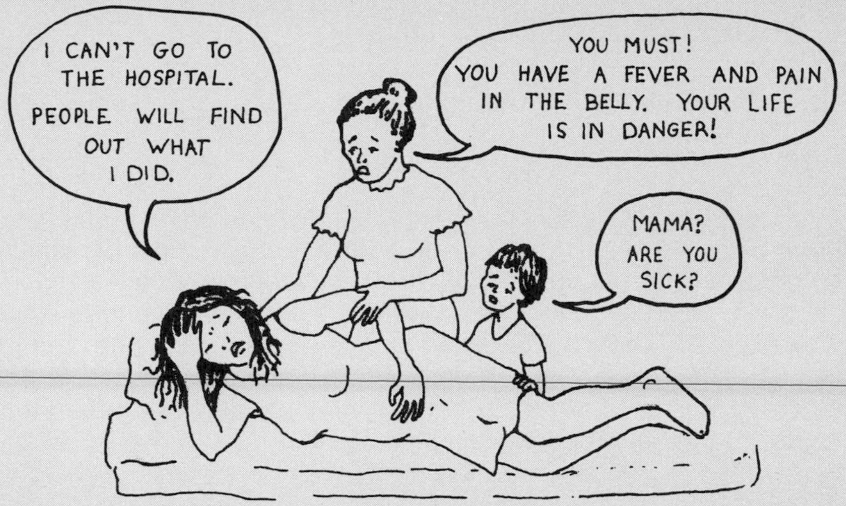

Some women with problems following an abortion go for medical help, but are afraid or ashamed to tell what really happened. Others may be too afraid or embarrassed even to seek medical help, especially if the abortion was secret or illegal. They may wait until they are very sick. This delay could be fatal. **Heavy bleeding (more than with a normal period) or infection following an abortion is dangerous. Get medical help right away!** Meanwhile, do the following:

- Try to control bleeding. Follow instructions on p. 281 for bleeding after miscarriage. Give ergonovine (see p. 391).
- Treat for shock (see p. 77).
- If there are signs of infection, give antibiotics as for Childbirth Fever (see p. 276).

To prevent illness and death from abortion:

- Give antibiotics (ampicillin, p. 353, or tetracycline, p. 356) after any abortion, whether done at home or in a health center. This reduces the risk of infections and dangerous complications.
- **Prevent unwanted pregnancy.** Birth control methods should be available to both women and men (see Chapter 20).
- Work to make your community a kinder, better place, especially for women and children. When society guarantees that everyone's needs are met, fewer women will need to seek abortions.
- Abortions done under clean and safe conditions by trained health workers should be available to women free or at low cost. That way women will not need to have dangerous, illegal abortions.
- A woman who has **any** signs of problems after an abortion—whether done at home or in the hospital—should get medical care **immediately.** To encourage this, doctors and health workers should **never make a woman who has had an abortion feel ashamed.**

DRUG ABUSE AND ADDICTION

The use of **harmful, habit-forming drugs** is a growing problem in the world today.

Although **alcohol** and **tobacco** are legal in most countries, both are habit-forming or 'addictive' drugs. They contribute to the poor health and death of many millions of people each year. *Alcohol abuse* causes enormous health, family, and social problems throughout the world. *Cigarette smoking* has for many years been a major cause of death in rich countries, and is now becoming an even bigger cause of death in poor countries. As more people in the rich countries stop smoking, the tobacco companies have turned to the 'Third World' as their new and easiest market.

Health problems related to use of alcohol and tobacco are discussed on pages 148 to 149.

In addition to alcohol and tobacco, many people in different parts of the world are using *'illegal' drugs.* These vary from place to place, and include **marijuana** (weed, pot, grass, sin semilla, mota, hashish, ganja), **opium** (heroin, morphine, smack), and **cocaine** (crack, snow, rock).

An increasing problem among poor children in cities is the **sniffing of chemicals,** especially **glue**, but sometimes paint thinner, shoe polish, gasoline, and cleaning fluid. Also, some people misuse medicines—especially certain strong painkillers, stimulants, and 'appetite control' drugs.

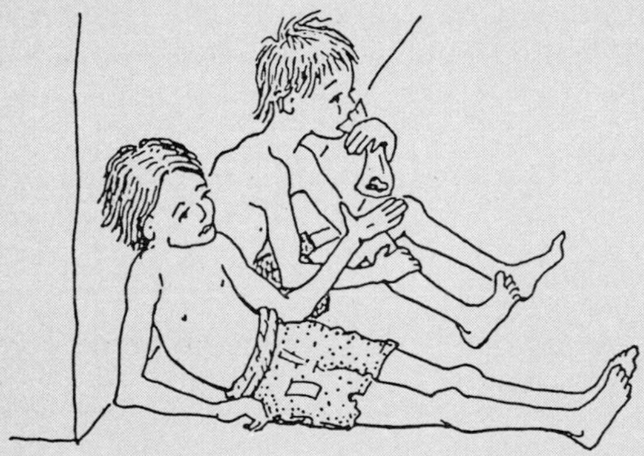

Drugs can be swallowed, injected, smoked, chewed, or sniffed. Different drugs create different effects on the body and mind. Cocaine or kolanuts may make a person feel energetic and happy, but some time later he will feel tired, irritable, and depressed. Some drugs, like alcohol, opium, morphine, and heroin, may at first make a person feel calm and relaxed, but later they may cause him to lose his inhibitions, self-control, or even consciousness. Other drugs, such as marijuana, PCP, LSD, and peyote make a person imagine things that do not exist, or create dream-like fantasies.

> *WARNING:* **Use of cigarettes, alcohol, or other drugs by pregnant women can harm their unborn child. Also, injecting drugs using the same needle for more than one person spreads dangerous diseases.** **See hepatitis (p. 172) and AIDS (p. 399).**

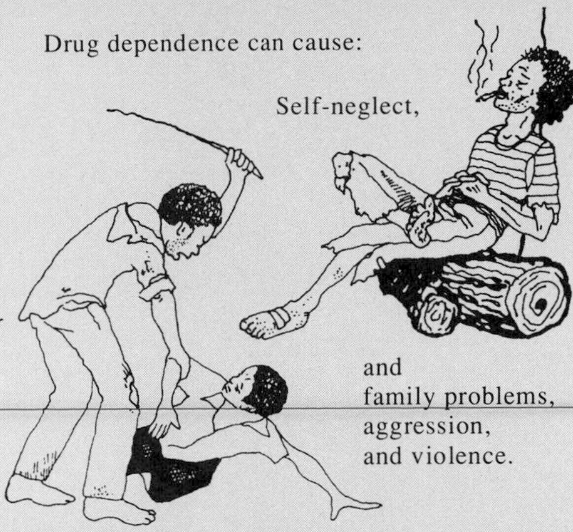
Drug dependence can cause:
Self-neglect,
and
family problems,
aggression,
and violence.

People usually start taking drugs to escape the hardships, forget the hunger, or calm the pain in their daily lives. But once they start, they often become 'hooked' or addicted. If they try to stop, they become miserable, sick, or violent. In order to get more drugs, they will often commit crimes, go hungry, or neglect their families. Thus drug use becomes a problem for whole families and communities.

Some drugs such as cocaine and heroin are very addictive; a person may try the drug only once and feel that he needs to keep taking it. Other drugs become addictive after longer periods of time. Addiction is a dangerous trap that can lead to health problems or even death. But **with determination, effort, and support, addictions can be overcome.**

When a person first gives up a drug he is addicted to, he will usually feel miserable and act strangely. This is called 'withdrawal'. The person may be extremely nervous, depressed, or angry. He may feel that he cannot live without the drug.

With some drugs, such as heroin or cocaine, withdrawal may be so severe that the person can become violent and injure himself or others. He or she may need the help of a special clinic. For other kinds of drugs, such as alcohol, marijuana, tobacco, and chemical sniffing, medical care is usually not necessary, but the care and support of family and friends is very important.

Here are a few suggestions to help solve the problem of drug use and addiction:

- Be as helpful and supportive as possible to someone trying to overcome drug use. Remember that their difficult moods are because of their addiction, not because of you.
- Members of the community who have been addicted to drugs but have overcome the habit can form a 'support group' to help others trying to give up alcohol or drugs. Alcoholics Anonymous is one such organization (see p. 429). This group of recovering alcoholics has successfully helped people all over the world to deal with problems of addiction.
- Families, schools, and health workers can tell children about the dangers of cigarettes, alcohol, and drugs. Help children learn that there are other, healthier ways to 'feel good', to act 'grown up', or to rebel.
- Work to correct some of the problems in your community that may lead people to use drugs: hunger, exploitative working conditions, and lack of opportunities to lead a better life. Help disadvantaged persons organize and stand up for their rights.

Actions that are *supportive* and *kind* work better than those that are punishing and cruel.

VOCABULARY

This vocabulary is listed in the order of the alphabet:
A B C D E F G H I J K L M N O P Q R S T U V W X Y Z

Words marked with a star (*) are usually not used in this book but are often used by doctors or found on package information of medicines.

Most names of sicknesses are not included in this vocabulary. See the Index (yellow pages) and read about the sickness in the book.

A

Abdomen The part of the body that contains the stomach, liver, and guts. The belly.

Abnormal Different from what is usual, natural, or average. Not normal.

Abscess A sac of pus caused by bacterial or other infection. For example, a boil.

Acne (pimples) A skin problem causing bumps on the face, chest, or back that form small white 'heads' of pus or sometimes 'blackheads' of dirt. Most common in young people (adolescents).

Acute Sudden and short-lived. An acute illness is one that starts suddenly and lasts a short time. The opposite of 'chronic'.

Acute abdomen An emergency condition of the abdomen that often requires a surgical operation. Severe pain in the belly with vomiting and no diarrhea may mean an acute abdomen.

Adolescent The years in which a child becomes an adult. The teens: 13 to 19 years old.

Afterbirth See **Placenta.**

Alcoholism A continual need a person cannot control to overuse alcoholic drinks such as beer, rum, wine, etc.

Allergy, allergic reaction A problem such as an itching rash, hives, sneezing, and sometimes difficult breathing or shock that affects certain people when specific things are breathed in, eaten, injected, or touched.

Amebas (also amoebas) Tiny animals that live in water or in the gut and can only be seen with a microscope. They can cause diarrhea, dysentery, and liver abscess.

Amputation Loss of a body part.

Analgesic Medicine to calm pain.

Anemia A disease in which the blood gets thin for lack of red blood cells. Signs include tiredness, pale skin, and lack of energy. See also **Pernicious anemia**.

Antacid Medicine used to control too much stomach acid and to calm stomach upset.

Antibiotic Medicine that fights infections caused by bacteria.

***Antiemetic** Vomit-control medicine. A medicine that helps keep people from vomiting or feeling nauseated.

Antihistamine Medicine used to treat allergies such as hay fever and itching. Also helps control vomiting and causes sleepiness.

Antiseptic A soap or cleaning liquid that prevents growth of bacteria.

Antispasmodic Medicine used to relieve cramps or spasms of the gut.

Antitoxin Medicine that acts against or neutralizes a poison or toxin. Often made from the blood serum of horses.

Antivenom (anti-venin) An antitoxin used to treat poisoning from a venom, such as snake poison.

Anus The opening at the end of the gut between the legs; asshole.

Aorta The main artery or vessel that carries blood out of the heart to the body.

Apoplexy An old word for stroke. See **Stroke.**

Appendix A finger-like sac attached to the large intestine (gut).

Appropriate Something that is easiest, safest, and most likely to work in a particular situation or condition.

Artery A vessel carrying blood from the heart through the body. Arteries have a pulse. Veins, which return blood to the heart, have no pulse.

Ascaris (roundworm) Large worms that live in people's intestines and cause discomfort, indigestion, weakness, and sometimes gut obstruction (blocking of the gut).

B

Bacteria Tiny germs that can only be seen with a microscope and that cause many different infectious diseases.

Bag of waters The sac inside the womb that holds the baby; amniotic sac. When it breaks, releasing its fluid, this usually means that labor has begun.

Bed sores Chronic open sores that appear in people who are so ill they do not roll over or change position in bed.

Bewitchment The act of casting a spell or influencing by witchcraft; hexing. Some people believe that they get sick because a witch has bewitched them or given them the 'evil eye'.

Bile A bitter, green liquid made by the liver and stored in the gallbladder. It helps digest fat.

Birth defects See **Defects.**

Blackhead A small plug or 'head' of dirt blocking a pore in the skin of the face, chest, or back. A kind of pimple.

Bladder stones See **Kidney stones.**

Blood pressure The force or pressure of the blood upon the walls of the blood vessels (arteries and veins); it varies with the age and health of the person.

Boil A swollen, inflamed lump with a pocket of pus under the skin. A kind of abscess.

Booster A repeat vaccination to renew the effect of an earlier series of vaccinations.

Bowel movement To have a bowel movement is to defecate; to shit; the way of passing solid waste out of the body.

Brand name Trade name. The name a company gives to its product. A brand-name medicine is sold under a special name and is often more expensive than the same generic medicine.

Breast abscess See **Mastitis.**

Breech delivery A birth in which the baby comes out buttocks or legs first.

Broad-spectrum antibiotic A medicine that works against many kinds of micro-organisms. Compare with a narrow-spectrum antibiotic, which works against only a few.

Bronchi The tubes leading to the lungs, through which air passes when a person breathes.

Bronchitis An infection of the bronchi.

Bubo A very swollen lymph node. **Bubos** is a common name for lymphogranuloma venereum.

Buttocks The part of the body a person sits on; ass, arse, rump, behind, backside, butt.

C

Cancer A tumor or lump that grows and may keep growing until it finally causes death.

Carbohydrates Starches and sugars. Foods that provide energy.

Cassava (manioc, yucca) A starchy root grown in the tropics.

Cast A stiff bandage of gauze and plaster that holds a broken bone in place until it heals.

Cataract An eye problem in which the lens of the eye becomes cloudy, making it more and more difficult for the person to see. The pupil looks gray or white when you shine a light into it.

Catheter A rubber tube used to drain urine from the bladder.

Cavity A hole or spot of decay in a tooth where bacteria have got in and destroyed part of the tooth.

Centigrade (C.) A measure or scale of heat and cold. A healthy person's temperature (normal temperature) is 37° C. Water freezes at 0° C. and boils at 100° C.

Cerebro-vascular accident, CVA See **Stroke.**

Cervix The opening or neck of the womb at the back of the vagina.

Chancre A painless sore or ulcer on the genitals, finger, or lip that is one of the first signs of syphilis.

Chigger A tiny, crawling spider or tick-like animal that buries its head under the skin and sucks blood.

Child Health Chart A monthly record of a child's weight that shows whether the child is gaining weight normally.

Childbirth fever (This is also called childbed fever, postpartum infection, or puerperal infection.) The fever and infection that mothers sometimes develop after childbirth.

Chronic Long-term or frequently recurring (compare with acute). A chronic disease is one that lasts a long time.

Circulation The flow of blood through the arteries and veins by the pumping of the heart.

Cleft Divided, separated. A child born with a cleft palate has a separation or abnormal opening in the roof of his mouth.

Climacteric Menopause.

Colic Sharp abdominal pains caused by spasms or cramps in the gut.

Colostrum The first milk a mother's breasts produce. It looks watery but is rich in protein and helps protect the baby against infection.

Coma A state of unconsciousness from which a person cannot be wakened. It is caused by disease, injury, or poison, and often ends in death.

Community A group of people living in the same village or area who have similar living conditions, interests, and problems.

***Complications** Secondary health problems that sometimes develop in the course of a disease. For example, meningitis may result as a dangerous complication of measles.

Compost A mixture of plant and animal waste that is allowed to rot for use as a fertilizer. Hay, dead leaves, vegetable waste, animal droppings, and manure all make good compost.

Compress A folded cloth or pad put on a part of the body. It may be soaked in hot or cold water.

Conjunctiva A thin, protective layer that covers the white of the eye and inner side of the eyelids.

Consciousness See **Loss of consciousness.**

Constipation Dry, hard, difficult stools (bowel movements) that do not come often.

Consumption An old name for tuberculosis.

Contact Touch. Contagious diseases can be spread by a sick person coming in contact with (touching or being close to) another person.

Contagious disease A sickness that can be spread easily from one person to another.

Contaminate To dirty, stain, or infect by contact. A syringe that has not been boiled is often contaminated and can cause infections, even though it looks clean.

Contraceptive Any method of preventing pregnancy.

Contractions Tightening or shortening of muscles. The strong contractions of the womb when a woman is in labor help to push the baby out of the womb.

Contractures Shortened or tight muscles in a joint that limit movement.

***Contraindication** A situation or condition when a particular medicine should not be taken. (Many medicines are contraindicated in pregnancy.)

Convulsions An uncontrolled fit. A sudden jerking of part or all of the person's body, as in meningitis or epilepsy.

Cornea The clear outer layer or 'window' of the eye, covering the iris and pupil.

Corns Hard, thick, painful parts of the skin formed where sandals or shoes push against the skin or one toe presses against another.

Cramp A painful tightening or contraction of a muscle.

Cretinism A condition in which a child is born mentally slow and often deaf. It is usually due to lack of iodine in the mother's diet.

Cupping A home remedy that consists of drawing blood to the surface of the body by use of a glass or cup with a flame under it.

Cyst An abnormal, sac-like, liquid-filled growth developing in the body.

D

Dandruff Oily white or grayish flakes or scales that appear in the hair. Seborrhea of the scalp.

Decongestant A medicine that helps relieve swelling or stuffiness of the nose or sinuses.

Defects Birth defects are physical or mental problems a child is born with, such as a hare lip, club foot, or an extra finger or toe.

Deficiency Not having enough of something; a lack.

Deformed Abnormally formed, not having the right shape.

Dehydration A condition in which the body loses more liquid than it takes in. This lack of water is especially dangerous in babies.

Delirium A state of mental confusion with strange movements and speech; it may come with high fever or severe illness.

***Dermal** Of the skin.

Dermatitis An infection or irritation of the skin.

Diaper rash Reddish, irritated patches between a baby's legs caused by urine in his diapers (nappy) or bedding.

Diarrhea Frequent runny or liquid stools.

Diet The kinds and amounts of foods that a person should eat or avoid eating.

Discharge A release or flowing out of fluid, mucus, or pus.

Dislocations Bones that have slipped out of place at a joint.

Douche A way to wash out the vagina by squirting a stream of water up into it.

Drowning When a person stops breathing (suffocates) from being under water.

Dysentery Diarrhea with mucus and blood. It is usually caused by an infection.

E

***Eclampsia** Sudden fits, especially during pregnancy or childbirth. The result of toxemia of pregnancy.

Embryo The beginnings of an unborn baby when it is still very small.

Emergency A sudden sickness or injury that calls for immediate attention.

***Emetic** A medicine or drink that makes people vomit. Used when poisons have been swallowed.

Enema A solution of water put up the anus to cause a bowel movement.

Epidemic An outbreak of disease affecting many persons in a community or region at the same time.

Evaluation A study to find out the worth or value of something, or how much has been accomplished. Often done by comparing different factors or conditions before and after a project or activity is underway.

Evil eye A glance or look from someone believed to have the power to bewitch or do harm to people.

Exhaustion Extreme fatigue and tiredness.

***Expectorant** A medicine that helps a person cough up mucus from the respiratory tract (lungs, bronchi, etc.); a cough-helper.

Expiration date The month and year marked on a medicine that tells when it will no longer be good. Throw away most medicines after this date.

F

Fahrenheit (F.) A measure or scale of heat and cold. A healthy person's temperature (normal temperature) is 98.6° F. Water freezes at 32° F. and boils at 212° F.

Family planning Using birth control methods to plan when to have and not have children.

Farsighted Being able to see things at a distance better than things close at hand.

Feces Stools; shit; the waste from the body that is moved out through the bowels in a 'bowel movement'.

Feces-to-mouth Spread or transmitted from the stools of one person to his or another person's mouth, usually by food or drink, or on fingers.

Fetoscope An instrument or tool for listening to sounds made by the unborn baby (fetus) inside the womb.

Fetus (foetus) The developing baby inside the womb.

Fever A body temperature higher than normal.

First aid Emergency care or treatment for someone who is sick or injured.

Fit A sudden, violent attack of a disease, causing convulsions or spasms (jerking of the body that the person cannot control) and sometimes unconsciousness.

Flu A bad cold, often with fever, pain in the joints, and sometimes diarrhea.

Flukes Worms that infect the liver or other parts of the body and cause different diseases. Blood flukes get into the blood and cause schistosomiasis.

Foetus See **Fetus.**

Folic acid A nutritious substance found in leafy green vegetables.

Follicles Small lumps.

Fontanel The 'soft spot' on the top of a young baby's head.

Fracture A broken bone.

Fright A great or sudden fear.

G

Gallbladder A small, muscular sac attached to the liver. The gallbladder collects bile, a liquid that helps digest fatty foods.

Gauze Soft, loosely woven kind of cloth used for bandages.

Generic name The scientific name of a medicine, as distinct from the brand names given it by different companies that make it.

Genitals The organs of the reproductive system, especially the sex organs.

Germs Very small organisms that can grow in the body and cause some infectious diseases; micro-organisms.

Giardia A microscopic parasite that can infect the intestines, causing frothy yellow diarrhea.

Glucose A simple form of sugar that the body can use quickly and easily. It is found in fruits and honey, and can be bought as a white powder for use in Rehydration Drinks.

Goiter A swelling on the lower front of the neck (enlargement of the thyroid gland) caused by lack of iodine in the diet.

Grain (gr.) A unit of weight based on the weight of a grain of wheat. 1 grain weighs 65 mg.

Gram (gm.) A metric unit of weight. There are about 28 grams in an ounce. There are 1000 gm. in 1 kilogram.

Groin The front part of the body where the legs join. The genital area.

Gut Intestines.

Gut thread or gut suture material A special thread for sewing or stitching certain wounds, and especially tears from childbirth. The gut thread is slowly absorbed (disappears) so that the stitches do not need to be taken out.

H

Hare lip A split in the upper lip, going from the mouth up to the nose (like a hare, or rabbit). Some babies are born with a hare lip.

Health worker A person who takes part in making his community a healthier place to live.

Heartburn A burning feeling in the lower chest or upper part of the stomach.

Hemorrhage Severe or dangerous bleeding.

Hemorrhoids (piles) Small, painful bumps or lumps at the edge of the anus or inside it. These are actually swollen or varicose veins.

Herb A plant, especially one valued for its medicinal or healing qualities.

Hereditary Passed on from parent to child.

Hernia (rupture) An opening or tear in the muscles covering the belly that allows a loop of the gut to push through and form a ball or lump under the skin.

Hex A magic spell or jinx said to be caused by a witch.

History (medical history) What you can learn through asking questions about a person's sickness—how it began, when it gets better or worse, what seems to help, whether others in the family or village have it, etc.

Hives Hard, thick, raised spots on the skin that itch severely. They may come and go all at once or move from one place to another. A form of allergic reaction.

Hormones Chemicals made in parts of the body to do a special job. For example, estrogen and progesterone are hormones that regulate a woman's period and chance of pregnancy.

Hygiene Actions or practices of personal cleanliness that lead to good health.

***Hypertension** High blood pressure.

Hyperventilation Very rapid, deep breathing in a person who is frightened.

***Hypochondria** Extreme worry or concern over an imagined sickness.

Hysteria (1) In common language, a condition of great nervousness, fear, and emotional distress. (2) In medical terms, signs of sickness caused by fear or the power of belief.

I

Immunizations (vaccinations) Medicines that give protection against specific diseases, for example: diphtheria, whooping cough, tetanus, polio, tuberculosis, and measles.

Infection A sickness caused by bacteria or other germs. Infections may affect part of the body only (such as an infected finger) or all of it (such as measles).

Infectious disease A disease that is easily spread or communicated (passed from one person to another); contagious.

Inflammation An area that is red, hot, and painful, often because of infection.

Insecticide A poison that kills insects. DDT and lindane are insecticides.

***Insomnia** A condition in which a person is not able to sleep, even though he wants and needs to.

Insulin A substance (enzyme) produced by the pancreas, which controls the amount of sugar in the blood. Injections of insulin are sometimes needed by persons with diabetes.

Intestinal parasites Worms and tiny animals that get in people's intestines and cause diseases.

Intestines The guts or tube-like part of the food canal that carries food and finally waste from the stomach to the anus.

Intramuscular (IM) injection An injection put into a muscle, usually of the arm or the buttock—different from an intravenous (IV) injection, put directly into a vein.

Intussusception The slipping of one portion of the gut into one nearby, usually causing a dangerous obstruction or blocking of the gut.

Iris The colored or dark part of the eye around the pupil.

J

Jaundice A yellow color of the eyes and skin. It is a sign of disease in the liver, gallbladder, pancreas, or blood.

K

***Keratomalacia** A dullness and softening of the eye, ending in blindness. It is caused by a lack of vitamin A.

Kidneys Large, bean-shaped organs in the lower back that filter waste from the blood, forming urine.

Kidney stones Small stones that form in the kidneys and pass down to the urinary tube. They can cause a sharp pain in the lower back, side, urinary tube, or lower belly. In the bladder they may block the urinary tube and make urination painful or impossible.

Kilogram (kg.) One thousand grams. A 'kilo' is equal to a little over 2 pounds.

Kwashiorkor (wet malnutrition) Severe malnutrition caused by not eating enough protein. A child with kwashiorkor has swollen feet, hands, and face, and peeling sores.

L

Labor The sudden tightening or contractions of the womb that mean the baby will soon be born.

Larva (larvae) The young worm-like form that comes from the egg of many insects or parasites. It changes form when it becomes an adult.

Latrine An outhouse; privy; a hole or pit in the ground to use as a toilet.

Laxative A medicine used for constipation that makes stools softer and more frequent.

Ligaments Tough cords in a person's joints that help hold them in place.

***Lingual** Of or relating to the tongue.

Liter (l.) A metric measure equal to about one quart. A liter of water weighs one kilogram.

Liver A large organ under the lower right ribs that helps clean the blood and get rid of poisons.

Loss of consciousness The condition of a sick or injured person who seems to be asleep and cannot be wakened. Unconsciousness.

***Lubricant** An oil or cream used to make surfaces slippery.

Lymph nodes Small lumps under the skin in different parts of the body that are traps for germs. They become painful and swollen when they get infected. In tuberculosis and cancer they are often swollen but not painful.

Lyophilized Powdered; a way of preparing injectable medicine so that it does not have to be kept cold.

M

Malnutrition Health problems caused by not eating enough of the foods that the body needs.

Marasmus (dry malnutrition) A condition caused by not eating enough. Starvation. The person is very thin and underweight, often with a pot belly.

Mask of pregnancy Dark, olive-colored areas on face, breasts, or middle of the belly that are normal in a pregnant woman.

Mastitis (breast abscess) An infection of the breast, usually in the first weeks or months of nursing a baby. It causes part of the breast to become hot, red, and swollen.

Membrane A thin, soft sheet or layer that lines or protects some part of an animal or plant.

Menopause (climacteric) The time when a woman naturally stops having monthly bleeding, usually between the ages of 40 and 50.

Menstrual period, menstruation Monthly bleeding in women.

Mental Of or relating to the mind (thinking, brain).

Micro-organism A tiny plant or animal so small it can only be seen with the aid of microscope.

Microscope An instrument with lenses that make very tiny objects look larger.

Microscopic Something so small that it can only be seen with a microscope.

Migraine A severe, throbbing headache, sometimes on one side of the head only. It often causes vomiting.

Milligram (mg.) One thousandth of a gram.

Milliliter (ml.) One thousandth of a liter.

Minerals Simple metals or other things the body needs, such as iron, calcium, and iodine.

Miscarriage (spontaneous abortion) The death of the developing baby or fetus in the womb, sometimes followed by heavy bleeding with blood clots.

Mongolism (Down's syndrome) A disease in which a child is born mentally slow with slanted eyes, a round dull face, and wide hands with short fingers.

Morning sickness Nausea and vomiting that occur especially in the morning in the early months of pregnancy.

Mouth-to-mouth breathing Artificial respiration. A method of helping a person who has stopped breathing to start breathing again.

Mucus A thick, slippery liquid that moistens and protects the linings of the nose, throat, stomach, guts, and vagina.

N

Narrow-spectrum antibiotic A medicine that works against a limited number of different kinds of bacteria.

***Nasal** Of or relating to the nose.

Nausea Stomach distress or upset; feeling like you need to vomit.

Navel Belly button; umbilicus; the place in the middle of the belly where the umbilical cord was attached.

Nerves Thin threads or strings that run from the brain to every part of the body and carry messages for feeling and movement.

Non-infectious disease A disease that does not spread from person to person.

Normal Usual, natural, or average. Something that is normal has nothing wrong with it.

Nutritious Nourishing. Nutritious foods are those that have the things the body needs to grow, be healthy, and fight off disease.

O

Obstruction A condition of being blocked or clogged. An obstructed gut is a medical emergency.

Ointment A salve or lotion to use on the skin.

***Ophthalmic** Of the eye.

***Oral** By mouth. An oral medicine is one taken by mouth.

Organ A part of the body that is more or less complete in itself and does a specific job. For example, the lungs are organs for breathing.

Organisms Living things (animals or plants).

***Otic** Having to do with the ears.

Ounce A measure of weight equal to about 28 grams. There are 16 ounces in one pound.

Ovaries Small sacs in a woman's belly next to her womb. They produce the eggs that join with a man's sperm to make a baby.

Oxytocics Dangerous medicines that cause the womb and blood vessels in it to contract. They should only be used to control a mother's heavy bleeding after her child is born.

P

Palate The roof or top part of the mouth.

Pancreas An organ below the stomach, on the left side, that produces insulin.

Pannus Tiny blood vessels that appear in the top edge of the cornea in certain eye diseases, like trachoma.

Paralysis Loss of the ability to move part or all of the body.

Parasites Worms and tiny animals that live in or on another animal or person and cause harm. Fleas, intestinal worms, and amebas are parasites.

***Parenteral** Not by mouth but by injection.

Pasteurization The process of heating milk or other liquids to a certain temperature (60° C) for about 30 minutes in order to kill harmful bacteria.

Pelvis Hip bones.

Peritoneum The thin lining between the guts and body wall. The bag that holds the guts.

Peritonitis A very dangerous inflammation of the peritoneum. The belly gets hard like a board, and the person is in great pain, especially when he tries to lie with his legs straight.

Pernicious anemia A rare kind of anemia caused by a lack of vitamin B_{12}. Pernicious means harmful.

Petroleum jelly (petrolatum, *Vaseline*) A grease-like jelly used in preparing skin ointments.

Pharmacy A store that sells medicines and health care supplies.

Phlegm Mucus with pus that forms in abnormal amounts in the lungs and must be coughed out.

Piles See **Hemorrhoids.**

Pimples See **Acne**.

Placenta (afterbirth) The dark and spongy lining inside the womb where the fetus joins the mother's body. The placenta normally comes out 15 minutes to half an hour after the baby is born.

Placenta previa A condition in which the placenta is too low in the womb and blocks the mouth of the womb. The risk of dangerous bleeding is high. Women who have bleeding late in pregnancy—a possible sign of placenta previa—should go to a hospital at once.

Plantain A kind of banana with a lot of starch and fiber. It is often cooked and eaten when green.

Pollen The fine dust made in the flower of a seed plant. People who are **allergic** to pollen often have hay fever at times of the year when plants put a lot of this dust into the air.

Postpartum After childbirth.

Postpartum hemorrhaging Heavy bleeding of the mother following childbirth.

Power of suggestion or power of belief The influence of belief or strong ideas. For example, sick people can feel better because they have faith in a remedy, even if the remedy does not have any medical effect.

Precaution Care taken in advance to prevent harm or prepare for emergencies before they happen.

Pregnancy The period (normally 9 months) when a woman carries a child inside her.

Premature baby A baby born before the full 9 months of pregnancy and weighing less than 2 kilos.

Presentation of an arm An abnormal position of delivery in which the baby's hand comes out first during the birth. This is an emergency needing a doctor.

Prevention Action taken to stop sickness before it starts.

Prolapse The slipping or falling down of a part of the body from its normal position; for example, a prolapsed rectum or womb.

Prophylactic The word prophylactic means preventive, but condoms are sometimes called prophylactics.

Prostate gland A firm, muscular gland at the base of the man's urinary tube, or urethra. Often in older men the prostate becomes enlarged, causing difficulty in urinating.

Protective foods Foods that are rich in vitamins and minerals. They help build healthy bodies and make people more able to resist or fight diseases.

Proteins Body-building foods necessary for proper growth and strength.

Pterygium A fleshy growth that slowly extends from the edge of the eye onto the cornea.

Pulse The number of times a person's heart beats in one minute.

Pupil The round opening or black center in the iris of the eye. It gets smaller in bright light and larger in the dark.

Purge A very strong laxative that causes diarrhea.

R

Rate The number of times something happens in a given amount of time.

Rebound pain A very sharp pain in the abdomen that occurs after the belly is pressed firmly and slowly, when the hand is removed suddenly. This pain is a sign of an acute abdomen.

Rectum The end of the large intestine close to the anus.

Reflex An automatic reaction or movement that happens without a person's trying to do it.

Rehydration Drink A drink to correct dehydration, which you can make with boiled water, salt, and sugar or powdered cereal.

Resistance The ability of something to defend itself against something that would normally harm or kill it. Many bacteria become resistant to the effects of certain antibiotics.

Resource What is needed or available for doing or making something. People, land, animals, money, skills, and plants are resources that can be used for improving health.

Respiration Breathing. The **respiratory system** includes the bronchi, lungs, and other organs used in breathing.

Respiration rate The number of times a person breathes in one minute.

Retardation Abnormal slowness of thought, action, or mental and emotional growth.

Rhinitis An inflammation of the lining of the nose, often caused by allergies. Hay fever.

Risk The possibility of injury, loss, or harm. Danger.

Rotation of crops To grow different crops one after the other in the same field, so that the soil becomes richer rather than weaker from year to year.

Rupture See **Hernia.**

S

Sanitation Public cleanliness involving community efforts in disease prevention, promoting hygiene, and keeping public places free of waste.

Scrotum The bag between a man's legs that holds his testicles or balls.

Sedative Medicine that causes drowsiness or sleep.

Septicemia An infection of the blood—sometimes called 'blood poisoning'.

Sexually transmitted disease (STD) A disease spread by sexual contact.

Shock A dangerous condition with severe weakness or unconsciousness, cold sweat, and fast, weak pulse. It is caused by dehydration, hemorrhage, injury, burns, or a severe illness.

Side effects Problems caused by using a medicine.

Signs The things or conditions one looks for when examining a sick person, to find out what sickness he has. In this book symptoms, or the problems a person feels, are included with signs.

Sinus trouble (sinusitis) Sinuses are hollows in the bone that open into the nose. Sinusitis is inflammation causing pain above and below the eyes.

Soft drinks Fizzy, carbonated drinks like Coca-Cola.

Soft spot See **Fontanel.**

Spasm A sudden muscle contraction that a person cannot control. Spasms of the gut produce cramps, or colic. Spasms of the bronchi occur in asthma. Spasms of the jaw and other muscles occur in tetanus.

Spastic Having chronic abnormal muscle contraction due to brain damage. The legs of spastic children often cross like scissors.

Spleen An organ normally the size of a fist under the lower edge of the ribs on the left side. Its job is to help make and filter the blood.

Spontaneous abortion See **Miscarriage.**

Sprain (strain) Bruising, stretching, or tearing of ligaments or tendons in a twisted joint. A sprain is worse than a strain.

Sputum Mucus and pus (phlegm) coughed up from the lungs and bronchi of a sick person.

Starches Energy foods like maize, rice, wheat, cassava, potatoes, and squash.

Sterile (1) Completely clean and free from living micro-organisms. Things are usually sterilized by boiling or heating. (2) Sterile also means permanently unable to have children.

Sterilization (1) To sterilize instruments, bottles, and other things by boiling or heating in an oven. (2) Also a permanent way of making a man or a woman unable to reproduce (have children).

Stethoscope An instrument used to listen to sounds in the body, such as the heartbeat.

Stomach The sac-like organ in the belly where food is digested. In common language 'stomach' is often used to mean the whole belly or abdomen.

Stools Shit. Bowel movement. See **Feces.**

Stroke (apoplexy, cerebro-vascular accident) A sudden loss of consciousness, feeling, or ability to move, caused by bleeding or a clot inside the brain. Also see heat stroke (p. 81).

Sty A red, swollen lump on the eyelid, usually near the edge, caused by infection.

Sucrose The common sugar that comes from sugarcane or sugar beets. It is more complex and more difficult for the body to use than glucose.

Sugars Sweet foods like honey, sugar, or fruit that give energy.

Suppository A bullet-shaped tablet of medicine to put up the anus or vagina.

***Suppressant** A medicine that helps to check, hold back, or stop something, such as a medicine to stop coughing (cough suppressant).

Suspension A powder mixed in a liquid.

Suture A stitch made with needle and thread to sew up an opening or wound.

Symptoms The feelings or conditions a person reports about his sickness. In this book symptoms are included with signs.

T

Tablespoon A measuring spoon that holds 3 teaspoons or 15 ml.

Taboo Something that is avoided, banned, or not allowed because of a cultural belief.

Teaspoon A measuring spoon that holds 5 ml. Three teaspoons equal 1 tablespoon.

Temperature The degree of heat of a person's body.

Tendons Tough cords that join muscles to bones (distinct from ligaments, which join bones with bones at joints).

***Thalassemia** A form of hereditary anemia seen only in certain countries. A child may become very anemic by age 2, with a large liver and spleen.

Thermometer An instrument used to measure how hot a person's body temperature is.

Tick A crawling insect-like animal that buries its head under the skin and sucks blood.

***Topical** For the skin. A topical medicine is to be put on the skin.

Toxemia A sickness resulting from certain poisons in the body; for example, toxemia of pregnancy and urine toxemia (or uremia).

Toxic Poisonous.

Tract A system of body organs and parts that work together to do a special job; for example, the urinary tract cleans the blood and gets rid of urine.

Traditions Practices, beliefs, or customs handed down from one generation to another by example or word of mouth.

Transmit To pass on, transfer, or allow to spread from one person to another.

Tropical Having to do with the tropics or hot regions of the world.

Tumor An abnormal mass of tissue without inflammation. Some tumors are due to cancer.

U

Ulcer A break in the skin or mucus membrane; a chronic open sore of the skin, the surface of the eye, the stomach, or gut.

Umbilical cord The cord that connects a baby from its navel to the placenta on the inside of its mother's womb.

Umbilical hernia A large, outward bulge of the navel—caused by a loop of intestine that has pushed through the sac holding the guts.

Umbilicus See **Navel.**

Unconsciousness See **Loss of consciousness.**

Under-Fives Program A plan that helps mothers learn about their children's health needs, make regular visits to a clinic for check-ups, and keep a record (Child Health Chart) of the growth of their children under five years old.

Urethra Urinary tube or canal. The tube that runs from the bladder to the hole a person urinates from.

Urinary tract The system of organs concerned with the formation and getting rid of urine—such as kidneys, bladder, and urinary tube (urethra).

Urine Liquid waste from the body; piss; pee.

Uterus Womb.

V

Vaccinations See **Immunization.**

Vagina The tube or canal that goes from the opening of the woman's sex organs to the entrance of her womb.

Vaginal Of or relating to the vagina.

Varicose veins Abnormally swollen veins, often lumpy and winding, usually on the legs of older people, pregnant women, and women who have had a lot of children.

Vaseline See **Petroleum jelly.**

Venereal disease A disease spread by sexual contact. Now called 'sexually transmitted disease' or 'STD'.

Vessels Tubes. Blood vessels are the veins and arteries that carry the blood through the body.

Virus Germs smaller than bacteria, which cause some infectious (easily spread) diseases.

Vitamins Protective foods that our bodies need to work properly.

Vomiting Throwing up the contents out of the stomach through the mouth.

W

Welts Lumps or ridges raised on the body, usually caused by a blow or an allergy (hives).

Womb The sac inside a woman's belly where a baby is made. The uterus.

X

Xerophthalmia Abnormal dryness of the eye due to lack of vitamin A.

ADDRESSES FOR TEACHING MATERIALS

Hesperian Foundation P.O. Box 11577 Berkeley, California 94712-2577 USA	Health books in basic language, in English and Spanish: ***Where There Is No Doctor, Helping Health Workers Learn, Where There Is No Dentist,*** and ***Disabled Village Children;*** slides and film strips on teaching materials and village theater; papers on community-based health work, politics of health, etc.
Teaching Aids at Low Cost (TALC) P.O. Box 49 St. Albans Herts. AL1 4AX United Kingdom	Slide sets, weight charts, aids to weight charts (flannel-graphs, etc.). Free booklist. English, French, Spanish, and Portuguese.
African Medical and Research Foundation (AMREF) Wilson Airport, P.O. Box 30125 Nairobi, Kenya	*The Defender,* a newsletter with ideas for health education methods, and an excellent series of rural health books in English.
Afrolit Society P.O. Box 72511 Nairobi, Kenya	*Illustrations for Development,* a work manual for artists to help them produce more effective illustrations on health.
Healthlink (formerly AHRTAG) Farringdon Point, 29-35 Farringdon Road London, ECIM 3JB England	*Diarrhoea Dialogue,* a newsletter about prevention and treatment of diarrhea available in English, French, Spanish, Portuguese, Arabic, Bengali, and Urdu. *ARI News,* a newsletter about acute respiratory infections available in English, French, Spanish, and Chinese. *AIDS Action,* a newsletter about measures to combat the spread of AIDS. Teaching aids about rehabilitation.
Alcoholics Anonymous World Services Incorporated P.O. Box 459 Grand Central Station New York, NY 10163 USA	Information about alcoholism and materials on how to start community support groups for persons addicted to alcohol or drugs.
Caribbean Food and Nutrition Institute P.O. Box 140 Mona P.O. Jamaica, West Indies	*Cajanus,* a nutrition bulletin; other materials in English for the Caribbean. Catalog available with nutrition education, diet management, and food tables materials.

Christian Medical College and Hospital
Vellore 632004
Tamil Nadu, India

Posters, flash cards, flannelgraphs in English and local Indian languages.

Christian Medical Commission
Box 66, 150 Route de Ferney
1211 Geneva 20, Switzerland

Contact, a newsletter about appropriate health care, in French, Spanish, and Portuguese.

Clearinghouse on Infant Feeding and Maternal Nutrition
APHA
1015 15th Street NW
Washington, D.C. 20005 USA

Mothers and Children, an international bulletin about nutrition and primary health care issues. Published 3 times a year in English, Spanish, and French.

Council for Primary Health Care
1787 A. Mabini
Malate, Manila
Philippines

General health educational materials.

Courtejoie, Dr. J.
Centre pour le Promotion de la Sante
B.P. 1800
Kangu Mayumbe (B.Z.)
Republique du Zaire

Excellent simple health books and material for villages in French, some English and Portuguese.

DEMOTECH—Designs for Self-Reliance
P.O. Box 303
6950 AH Dieren
The Netherlands

Educational material for sanitation and water systems, innovative education methods.

Development Resource Centre
c/o Concern
P.O. Box 650
Dhaka, Bangladesh

Flip charts in English and Bangla. Flannel-graph with 60 characters for health care demonstrations.

F.A.O. of the U.N.
Nutrition and Home Economic Division
Via delle Terme de Caracalla
00100, Rome, Italy

Wide variety of material, some useful at village level. English, French, and Spanish.

Health Action International Network (HAIN)
P.O. Box 1665, Central Post Office
Quezon City, Philippines

General health care information.

Health Education Department
Addis Ababa, Ethiopia

Teaching kits. Material in English and some local languages.

Helen Keller International 15 West 16th Street New York, New York 10011 USA	Material on blindness from lack of vitamin A. Information on blindness prevention and visual chart.
International Development Research Centre (IRDC) P.O. Box 8500 Ottawa, Ontario, Canada K1G 3H9	Publications, magazines, brochures, catalogs, and films on agriculture, health, and development. Materials in English, French, Spanish, and Arabic, some at no cost.
Matérial Réalisé à l'Atelier de Matérial Didactique Busiga, P.B. 18 Ngozi, Burundi	Good flip charts; a teaching plan using flip charts in French local languages.
Nutrition Center of the Philippines MCC P.O. Box 653 Makati, Metro Manila Philippines	Various written and video tape materials in English and local languages.
Nutrition Section Public Health Department, Box 3991 Boroko, Papua New Guinea	Posters, newsletters, cassettes, and booklets.
O.C.E.A.C. Service de la formation et de la documentation B.P. 288 Yaounde, Cameroun	Material in French. Some information in French and English for training experienced health workers.
Pan American Health Organization (PAHO) 525 23rd Street, NW Washington, DC 20037 USA	Various materials in English and Spanish.
Save the Children Federation 54 Wilton Road Westport, Connecticut 06880 USA	Teaching materials in English and other languages.
TAPS Appropriate Technology for Health Caixa Postal 20.396 Sao Paulo, S.P. CEP 04034 Brazil	Books, pamphlets, games, and slides on self-help and community health care. In Portuguese.

UNICEF Communication Section P.O. Box 1187 Kathmandu, Nepal	***Instant Illustration,*** a resource book of illustrations for health and development. ***New Vision,*** a comic strip magazine containing adventures of several "development" characters. Sample available.
Voluntary Health Association of India (VHAI) 40, Institutional Area, South of IIT New Delhi 110016 India	Flannel-graphs, books, flip charts; ***Where There Is No Doctor*** adapted for India, in English and local languages. List available. ***Health for the Millions*** available by subscription—articles on low-cost health care.
Women's International Network 187 Grant Street Lexington, Massachusetts 02173 USA	Flipcharts, books, and slides on women's health care.
World Health Organization 1211 Geneva 27, Switzerland	***Appropriate Technology for Health*** newsletter and other materials in English, French, and Spanish. ***International Medical Guide on Board Ship,*** a guide for teaching officers and personnel on subjects concerning health care and treatment of accidents. Flannel-graphs, books, flip charts, etc. Material in English and local languages.
World Neighbors 5116 North Portland Oklahoma City, Oklahoma 73112 USA	***Soundings,*** a newsletter on rural development communications; filmstrips and teaching aids in English and Spanish. Simple battery-operated projector equipment available. Free catalog. Flannel-graphs, books, flip charts, etc. Material in English and local languages.

INDEX

Things in this book are listed in the order of the alphabet:

A B C D E F G H I J K L M N O P Q R S T U V W X Y Z

Page numbers in **bold** tell you where to find the main reference in this book. Medicines included in the Green Pages are in the Index of Medicines, p. 341.

A

Abdomen (See Belly)
Abortion, 243, 284, **414–415**
(Also see Miscarriage)
Abscess, 419
breast, 278
caused by injecting, 67, 69, 74
liver, 144–145
of the teeth, 230–231
under the skin, 202
Acid Indigestion, 128–129
Acne (pimples), 211, 395, 419
Acquired Immune Deficiency Syndrome (See AIDS)
Acupuncture, 74, 401
Acute abdomen, 15, **93–94,** 419
(Also see Gut, Swollen belly)
Addiction, 416–417
Afterbirth (placenta), 262–264, 269, 426
AIDS, 153, 171, 236, 245, 286, 290, 396, **399–401,** 416
and pregnancy, 249
and shingles, 204
and thrush, 232
and tuberculosis, 179
Alcoholic drinks
and heat stroke, 81
problems caused by, 119, 148–149, 325, 326, 400, 416
Alcoholics Anonymous, 149, 417, 429
Alcoholism, 148–149, 416–417, 419
Allergic reaction, 23, 54, **166**
in the skin, 203
medicines for, 337, 386–387
to medicines, 54, 56, 68, 70–71, 351
Allergic rhinitis (hay fever), 165, 427
Allergic shock, 70, 105, 351, 386–387, 410
Aloe vera, 13, 129
Amebas, 144–145, 336, 368–369, 419
Amputation, 409, 419
Anabolic steroids, 51
Analgesics (painkillers), 379–380
Anemia, 124, 419
causes of, 113, 124
during pregnancy, 248–249
in children, 307, 321
treatment, 335, 392–394
Anesthetics, 380–381
Angel's Trumpet, 12
Angina pectoris, 325
Antacids, 52, 64, **129,** 248, 324, 381–382
Antibiotics, 52, **55–58,** 156, 351–365
Anti-diarrhea medicines, 156
Antihistamine, 70, 165, 204, **386–387,** 419
Antispasmodic, 235, 329, **381**
Antitoxins, 388–389, 419
and allergic shock, 70, 105
for tetanus, 389
(Also see Antivenom)
Antivenom, 70, 388–389
for scorpion sting, 388
for snakebite, 105, 388
Anus, 233, 419
hemorrhoids in it, 175
sores in it, 238, 400, 402, 403
Apoplexy, 37, 78, 288, **327**
Appendicitis, 36, **94–95**
Appendix, 94
Arms
muscles and nerves in, 37
numbness or pain in, 23, 325
Arteriosclerosis, 326
Arthritis (joint pain), 173, 324
medicines for, 51, 379–380
Ascaris (roundworm), 140–141, 420
and asthma, 167
Asthma, 167, 337, 385–386
Athlete's foot, 205

B

Babies
examining, 34
feeding, 120–121
with diarrhea, 159
with skin problems, 215
(Also see Children, Newborns)
Back pain, 173–174, 248
Bacteria, 19, 55, 420
Bacterial dysentery, 145
Bacterial infection of the blood, 273–275
Bag of waters, 256, 258, **259–260,** 420
Bandages, 85, 87, **101–102,** 336

Bathing
and hygiene, 133
newborns and babies, 7, 215, 263
postpartum mothers, 8, 276
sick persons, 7, 39
B.C.G. vaccination, 147, 180, 185
Beaded lizard bite, 106
Bedbugs, 200
Bed sores, 13, **214,** 420
Beliefs
harmful, 4, 5, 10–11
healing power of, 2
Bell's Palsy, 327
Belly
acute abdomen, 93–94
examination of, 35–36
lumps in, 280
pain in lower belly, 243
(Also see Gut, Swollen Belly)
Bewitchment, 2, **6,** 420
Bilharzia, 146
Biliousness, 329
Birth (See Childbirth)
Birth control (See Family planning)
Birth control pills, 285, **286–289,** 394–395, 410
Birth defects, 6, 247, 272, 289, **318–321,** 412
Birth kits, 254–255
Birth opening (See Vagina)
Bites
of wild animals (rabies), 181
poisonous, 104–106
that may cause infection, 89
treatment, 86
Bitot's spots, 226
Black flies, 227–228
Blackheads, 211, 420
Black magic, 5, 24
Black widow spider bite, 106
Bladder, 233
infection, 243
stones, 234, 235
Bleach, 74, 401
Bleeding
and anemia, 124
during menopause, 246
during pregnancy, 249, 281
gums, 107, 231
how to control, 13, 82–83
in an unconscious person, 78
in the whites of the eyes, 225
of the newborn, 272, 337, 394
severe, 82, 243, 246, 264, 281, 404, 410, 414
stopping after birth, 263–266, 337, 391
(Also see Blood)
Blindness, 221–222, 412
from injuries to the eye, 218
night blindness, 113, 226–227
protection for babies, 221, 237, 379
river blindness, 227–228, 378
Blisters
from medicines, 358, 361
from touching certain plants, etc., 204
with burns, 96
with chickenpox, 311
with eczema, 216
Blood
and AIDS, 399, 401
clots, 288
coughing up blood, 168
flukes, 146
in stools, 128, 144–146, 157–158, 306, 401
in the urine, 146, 234
in vomit (cirrhosis), 328
in vomit (ulcer), 128
(Also see Bleeding)
Blood pressure, 420
high, 125, 249, 288, 325–326, 395, 411
how to measure, 410–411
low, 77, 411
(Also see Shock)
Blood transfusion, 401
Blueness of skin, lips, and nails, 30
Body-building foods, 110
Boil (abscess), 202, 420
Bones
calcium for, 246
deformities of, 125, 319
hit by a bullet, 90
that have come out of place at a joint, 101
(Also see Broken bones)
Bottle feeding, 120, 154, 296
Bowel movement, 242, 420
(Also see Feces, Stools)
Braces, 315
Brain damage, 319–320
and fits, 319
from high fever, 76
from tapeworm cysts, 143
Bran, 16, 126, 383
Brand-name medicines, 55, 333, **339,** 420
Breakbone fever (See Dengue)
Breast abscess (mastitis), 278, 424
Breast cancer, 279
Breast feeding, w12, **120–122**
and birth control, 289, 294, 395
and good nutrition, 114, 116, 304
and preventing diarrhea, 154, 156
of newborns, 271, 277, 405
traditional beliefs about, 2, 7
(Also see Breasts)
Breasts
care of, 277, 279
swelling of, 278–279
Breathing (respiration), 426
difficulties, 23, 57, 168, 181, 274, 325, 410
hot water vapors 47, 168
of a sick person, 32
rate, 32
stopped, 80
(Also see Lung diseases, Mouth-to-mouth breathing)
Breech delivery, 257, **268**

Broad-spectrum antibiotics, 56, 58, 353, 356–359
Broken bones, 14, **98–99**
Bronchitis, 170
Brucellosis (Malta fever), 27, **188**
Bubos, 238, 403, 420
Bullet wound
  in arms or legs, 90
  in the belly, 15, 92–93
  in the head, 91
Burns, 13, **96–97**
  and leprosy, 192
  of the eye, 219

C

Calcium
  and rickets, 125
  danger of injecting, 53, 67
  for spider bite, 106
  for weak bones, 246
  in eggshells, 116
Callus, 210
Cancer, 25, 412, 420
  and oral contraceptives, 288–289
  and smoking, 119, 149, 168
  of the breast, 279
  of the skin, 211, 399
  of the womb, 280
Candida (See Moniliasis)
Canker sores, 232
Carbohydrates (energy foods), 110, 121, 420
Carbonated drinks, 115, **150**
Cardon cactus, 13, 232
Cascara, 16
Cassava, 117, 130, 420
  for constipation, 16, 126, 383
Cast, 14, 98, 319, 420
Castor oil, 16
Cataract, 225, 323, 420
Catheter, 239–240, 336, 420
Causes of illness, w6-w7, w10, w27, **17–19**
Cavities in teeth, 229–230, 420
Cellulitis, 212
Cereal, 152, 382
Cerebral malaria, 30, 178, 186, 367
Cerebral palsy, 320
Cerebro-vascular accident (CVA), 37, 78, 288, **327**
Cervix, 288, 420
Chancre, 237
Chancroid, 236, 238, 403
Chemical burns of the eye, 219
Chest wounds, 91
Chickenpox, 204, **311**
Chiggers, 201, 420
CHILD-to-child program, 322
Child Health Chart, w20, w24, **297–304,** 420
Childbirth
  bleeding after, 264–265
  correct use of oxytocics, 265–266
  cutting the cord, 262–263
  difficult births, 267–269, 319
  infection, 260, 276
  position of the baby, 257, 261, 267
  position of the mother, 260
  premature, 262
  preparing for, 254–256
  signs of labor, 258
  tearing of the birth opening, 269
Childbirth fever, 27, **276,** 283, 420
Children
  and diarrhea, 151–153, 159
  foods for, 112, 113, 120–122, 295
  giving injections to, 73
  growth of, 107, 297–304
  having the number you want, 283–294
  infectious diseases of, 311–315
  malnourished, 112–114, 154, 303, 305–306
  mentally slow, deaf, or deformed, 318
  problems they are born with, 316–321
  severely ill, 214
  vaccinations for, 147, 296
  (See also Babies, Newborns)
Chlamydia, 221, 234, **236–237,** 255, 360
Choking, 79, 314
Cholera, 158
Cigarettes (See Smoking)
Circulation, poor (See Varicose veins)
Circumcision, 74, 401, **404**
Cirrhosis of the liver, 108, 148, **328**
Cleanliness, 131–139
  basic guidelines of, 133–139
  in childbirth, 260, 263
  of children, 136, 296
  of equipment, 74, 401
  of mouth and teeth, 229–231
  personal cleanliness, 39, 41, 133–135
  public cleanliness, 137–139
  to prevent infection, 74, 84, 401, 414
  when injecting, 68, 74, 401
Cleft palate, 318–319, 421
Climacteric (menopause), 246
Clitoris, 233
Clubbed feet, 319
Cocaine, 416–417
Coitus interruptus, 285, **290**
Cold and hot sicknesses, 119
Cold compresses, 193–194
Colds and the 'flu', 45, 57, **163,** 308
  diet with, 123
Cold sores or fever blisters, 48, 171, 232, 402
Cold weather, 408–409
Colic (gut cramps), 35, 145, 157, 421
Colostrum, 277, 421
Coma, 78, 421
Combination medicines, 52, 385
Combined methods of birth control, 285, **292**
Comfort of a sick person, 39
Complications from abortion, 243, **414–415**
Compresses, 193–195, 421
Condom, 239, 285, 286, **290,** 396, 401–403
La Congestion, 23
Conjunctivitis, 219–221, 308

Constipation, 16, **126**
as a sign of acute abdomen, 94
during pregnancy, 248
treatment and prevention, 126, 383
Consumption (See Tuberculosis)
Contact dermatitis, 204, 421
Contraception, 284–294, 394–396
Contraceptive foam, 285, **290,** 396
Contractures, 314, 421
Convulsions, (See Fits, Spasms)
Cooperatives, w24
Cornea, 217, 218, 224, 225, 226, 228
Corn silk, 12
Corns, 210, 421
Cortico-steroids, 51, 129, 364
Cortisone, 51
Cough, 168–169
chronic, 168, 324, 400
common causes, 168
cough with blood, 140, 171, 174, 179
medicines for, 52, 384
smoker's, 149
Cradle cap, 215
Cramps, 421
gut, 12, 35, 106, 145, 147, 243, 381
heat, 81
Cretinism, 318, 421
Crop rotation, w13, 115, 117, 427
Cross-eyes, 223, 318
Crutches, how to make, 315
Cupping, 22, 421
Cuts, 84–86
CVA (Cerebro-vascular accident), 37, 78, 288, **327**
Cyst, 143, 243, 280, 421

D

Dacryocystitis, 223
Dandruff, 215, 421
Dandy fever (See Dengue)
Dangerous illnesses, w28, 42, **179–192**
Dangerous use of medicine, 50
Date of expiration, 332
Deafness
home cure for, 11
in children, 318
with ringing and dizziness, 327
Death, accepting, 330
Decongestants, 164, 165, 421
Defects, birth, 7, 289, **316–321,** 421
Deformities, 421
from birth, 289, 316–321
with leprosy, 191–192
Dehydration, 151–152, 421
and diarrhea, 46, 155
causing sunken fontanel, 9, 274
danger of laxatives with, 15, 383
medicine not to take, 52–53, 156
prevention and treatment, 152, 156, 382–383
Delhi boil (See Leishmaniasis)
Delirium, 24, 421
and malaria, 186
and typhoid, 189
Dengue, 187
Dermatitis, contact, 204, 421
Diabetes, 127, 251, 410
Diaper rash, 215, 422
Diaphragm, 285, **290,** 396
Diarrhea, 151–160
and dysentery, 144–145, 153, 306
babies with, 159, 271
causes of, w7, 17, 107, 132–133, 135, 153, 399, 400
causing sunken fontanel, 9
home cures for, 11
prevention of, w7, 46–47, 154
severe, 151, 160
treatment of, 58, 152, 155–158, 384
with blood, 144–145, 157–158, 306, 401
with vomiting, 151, 157
with worms, 142
Diet, 421
congestion and, 23
for fever, 8
for postpartum mothers, 8, 123, 276
for sick persons, 40, 123
for small children, 120–122
for specific diseases, 40, 124–130, 154–156
harmful ideas about, 123
things to avoid, 119
what to eat to stay healthy, 110–111
while taking medicines, 123
with oral contraceptives, 286
(Also see Foods, Nutrition)
Diets for specific diseases, 40, **124–130**
acid indigestion, heartburn, and ulcers, 128–129
anemia, 124
constipation, 16, 126, 383
diabetes, 40, 127
diarrhea, 155–156, 159
fat people, 126
goiter, 130
high blood pressure, 125
Digestion, 13
Diphtheria, 147, 296, **313–314**
Direct pressure, 82
Disability
how injections cause, 74, 314
in children, 74, 314, 318–321
Diseases (see sicknesses)
Dislocations, 38, 101, 316, 422
Dizziness, 327, 249
Dolor de ijar, 22
Dosage information, 340
Double vision, 227
Douche, 241, 247, 258, 281, 292, 361, 422
Down's disease (mongolism), 318, 425
D.P.T. vaccination, 147
Drinking (alcohol), 148–149, 318, 325, 326, 328, 400, 416

Drowning, 79, 422
Drug abuse, 399, 401, **416–417**
Dry eyes, 107, 113, **226,** 392
Dry malnutrition (marasmus), 112–113
Dumdum fever (See Leishmaniasis)
Dysentery, 144–145, 422
(Also see Diarrhea)

E

Ears
how to examine a sick person's, 34
infections of, 309
nodes behind, 88
ringing of, 107, 327
Earwax, 405
Eclampsia (toxemia of pregnancy), 249, 422
Ectopic pregnancy, 36, 243, 249, **280,** 414
Eczema, 216
Emergency
problems of the gut, 93–95
supply of medicines, 332
use of injections, 66
Emergencies caused by cold, 408–409
Emergencies caused by heat, 81
Empacho, 22
Emphysema, 170
Enema, 15, 76, 92, 422
Energy foods, 110–111
Enterobius (pinworm, threadworm), 141
Epilepsy, 38, **178,** 319, 389–391
Epsom salts, 16
Erysipelas, 212
Evaluation, w20, 422
Evil eye, 5, 422
Examining
a pregnant woman, 250–253
a sick person, 29–38
breasts, 279
eyes, 33, 217
eyesight, 223
for appendicitis, 36, 95
for hernia, 94, 317
for knee reflexes, 183
Excision, 404
Exhaustion, heat, 81
Expectorants, 52, 384, 422
Experimenting, w15
Extra finger or toe, 318–319
Eyes, 217–228
cross-eyes, 223
danger signs, 33, 217
dryness of, 107, 113
examining the eyes, 33
eye problems of older people, 323
eye problems with leprosy, 192
foreign objects in eyes, 48, 218
of newborns, 221, 270, 379, 392
red and painful, 219, 225
yellow, 30, 172, 274, 328, 329
Eyesight testing, 223

F

Face
dull, 318
lumpy skin on, 191
paralysis of, 37, 327
Fainting, 78, 79, 81, 325, 327
Falciparum **malaria,** 158, 186, 365
False labor, 258
Family planning, w16, 246, **283–294,** 394–396, 415
and infertility, 244
Farming, w13, 412–413
Farsightedness, 323, 422
Fatigue, 23, 124, **323,** 400
Fat people, 126, 325–326, 329
Fats, 111, 121
Feces, 132, 242, 422
and infections, 84, 96, 131
in home remedies, 11
in newborn's mouth and nose, 268
(Also see Stools)
Feces-to-mouth, disease spread from, 131–133, 140, 188
Feet
clubbed, 319
loss of feeling in, 127, 162, 173, 191–192
swelling of, 113, 124, 144, 176, 248–249, 323
Fertile days, 244, **291**
Fetoscope, 252, 255, 422
Fever
childbirth, 27, 276, 283
diet with, 8
high, 6, 15, 75–76, 335
how to bring down, 75, 76, 335
in children, 306
in the newborn, 270, 273
patterns in different diseases, 26–27, 30, 31
Fever blisters or cold sores, 48, 171, **232**
La Fiebre, 26
Filmstrips, w22
Fire wood, 135
First aid, 75–106, 422
Fits, 23, **178,** 422
caused by high fever, 76
from birth defects, 273, 319
in cerebral malaria, 186, 367
in children, 307, 319
in meningitis, 185
medicines for, 336, 389–391
(Also see Spasms)
Flannel-graphs, w22
Fleas, 190
Flies
and disease, w23, 135, 227–228, 406
before the eyes, 227, 323
Flu, 45, 57, **163,** 308, 422
Flukes, blood, 146, 377, 422
Fluoride, for teeth, 229
Foam, contraceptive, 285, **290,** 396
Folic acid, 118, 321, **393,** 422

Folk beliefs, 3, **6–8,** 123
(Also see Home remedies)
Folk disease, 21–26
Follicles inside the eyelids, 220
Fontanel (soft spot)
sunken, 6, 9, 151, 274
swollen, 274
(Also see Dehydration)
Food poisoning, 23, 103, **135,** 153, 161
Foods
at low cost, 116–118
for a person with diarrhea, 155–156
for sick persons, 41
for small children, 120–122
nutritious, 110–111, 295
plant, 116
producing, w11
spoiled, 103, 135
(Also see Diet, Nutrition)
Fractions, 59–60, 340
Fractures (See Broken bones)
Fright, 24, 422
Frostbite, 409
Frozen skin, 409
Fungus infection, 19, 58
ringworm, tinea, 205–206, 372–373
thrush, 232, 242

G

Gallbladder, 422
home cure for, 12
pain in, 36
problems, 329
Gangrene, 213
Garlic, 12, 241, 242
Gastritis, 128–129
Gelusil, 173
Generic medicines, 333, **339,** 423
Genital herpes, 402–403
Genital warts, 374, 402
Genitals, 205, 232, **233–244,** 423
sores on, 237, 402–403
German measles (Rubella), 247, **312,** 320
Germs, 19, 423
Giardia, 145, 336, 368–370, 423
and diarrhea, 153, 158
Gila monster bite, 106
Glaucoma, 33, **222,** 323
Gloves, rubber or plastic, 255, 262, 264, 401
Glue sniffing, 416
Goiter, 10, **130,** 423
Gonorrhea, 221, **236–237,** 255, 360
(Also see Sexually transmitted diseases)
Grams, measuring in, 59–60, 423
Groin, lymph nodes in, 88, 238, 423
(Also see Hernia)
Group discussions, w24–w27
Growth, children's, 107, **297–304**
Guaco, 3
Guinea worm, 406–407
Gums, 229–232
bleeding of, 107, 231
pale, 124
swelling caused by medicine, 231
Gut
cramps, 12, 106, 145, 157, 243, 381
emergency problems of, 35, 93–94
infection, 47, 131, 144–145, 153, 189
obstructed, 22, 94
out of anus (prolapse), 142
outside a wound, 92
wounds in, 92
(Also see Abdomen, Swollen belly)

H

Hair
changes with malnutrition, 107
examination for lice, 200
loss of, 107
Hansen's disease (See Leprosy)
Hare lip, 318, 423
Hay fever, 165, 427
Head
fungus infections of, 205
injury, 37, 78, 91
swollen lymph nodes on, 88
Headaches, 162, 249, 410
Health, w7, w11
Health worker, w1–w7, w29, 43, 246, 340
Heart
attacks, 23, 325
confusion with heartburn, 128
trouble, 33, 310, 325, 410
Heartbeat, 32–33, 77
Heartburn, 423
diet for, 128–129
during pregnancy, 248
medicines for, 381–382
medicines to avoid, 54, 64
Heat
cramps, 81
exhaustion, 81
stroke, 78, 81
Hemorrhage (See Bleeding)
Hemorrhoids (See Piles)
Hepatitis, 26, **172,** 416
Herbal teas, 1, 8
Herbs, curative, 12–13, 423
Hereditary problems, 18, 318–319, 321, 423
Hernia, 177, 423
during pregnancy, 256
in groin of newborn, 317
obstructing the gut, 94
Heroin, 416–417
Herpes simplex or labialis (See Cold sores)
Herpes zoster, 204, 400
Hexing, 2

High blood pressure, 125, 249, 325–326, 411
History, taking, 20, 25, 29, 44, 250–253, 423
HIV (See AIDS)
Hives, 68, 166, **203,** 423
Home remedies, 1–3
  enemas and purges, 15
  for infertility, 244
  how to tell if they work, 10–11
  questions and answers about, 6–8
  sensible use of, w2, 24
Home visits, w24
Hookworm (Uncinaria), 133, **142,** 296, 307
Hordeolum (sty), 224
Hormones, 244, 287, 394, 423
Hot and cold sicknesses, 119
Hot compresses, 193–195, 406
Housing, w10
Human immunodeficiency virus (See AIDS)
Hydrocele, 317
Hygiene (See Cleanliness)
Hypertension (See High blood pressure)
Hyperventilation, 24, 423
Hyphema, 225
Hypochondria, 329
Hypopyon, 225
Hypothermia, 408
Hysteria, 2, 24, **423**

I

Illnesses (See Sicknesses)
Immunizations (vaccinations), 19, **147,** 296, 337
Impetigo, 25, **202**
Implants (birth control), 285, **293,** 397
Indigestion
  diet for, 128–129
  during pregnancy, 248
  medicines for, 381–382
  medicines to avoid, 54, 64
Infantile paralysis (See Polio)
Infants (See Babies, Newborns)
Infection, 423
  after giving birth, 276
  and diarrhea, 154, 157
  in newborns, 182–183, 275
  in wounds, 88–89, 96, 213
  medicines for, 55–58, 335–336
  minor, 58
  of the appendix, 94–95
  of the eyes, 217, 219, 220, 221
  of the genitals, 236–239, 241–242
  of the gut, 94–95, 135, 140–146, 243
  of the tear sac, 223
  of the urinary tract, 234–235
  resisting, 108, 120, 271
  signs of a serious, 88, 194, 272–275
Infectious diseases, 18–19, 135, 423
Inferon, 51, 67
Infertility, 244
Inflamed tonsils (tonsillitis), 309
Injections, 65–73
  dangerous reactions from injections, 54, 70–71
  emergencies needing, 66
  faith in, w19, 4, 50
  medicines not to inject, 51, 56, 67
  of vitamins, 118
  risks and precautions, 68–69
  supplies for, 336
  that can disable children, 74, 314
  to prevent pregnancy, 285, 293, 396
  when to inject, 65, 67
Injury
  moving an injured person, 99–100
  of an unconscious person, 78
  severe, 33
  to the eye, 218
Insecticides, 19, 187, 373, **412–413,** 423
Insomnia (loss of sleep), 328, 423
Intestinal worms, 13, **140–145,** 423
Intestines (See Gut)
Intrauterine device (IUD), 281, 285, **290,** 396
Intravenous solution (I.V.), 40, **53,** 67, 152
Intussusception, 94, 424
Iodized salt, 130, 318
Iritis, 33, 219, **221**
Iron
  cooking pots, 117
  foods rich in, 124
  from nails in lemon juice, 118
  pills, 51, 118, 124, 307, 335, 393, 405
Itching
  caused by fungus, 205, 242
  caused by medicines, 68, 70–71, 166
  caused by plants, 204
  medicines for, 335, 386
  of hands with syphilis, 238
  of the anus (pinworm), 141
  rashes, allergies, 68, 166, 203, 236, 238
  with chickenpox, 311
  with scabies, 199
  with worm infections, 140–142, 228
IUD (intrauterine device), 281, 285, **290,** 396

J

Jaundice, 30, **172,** 274, 318, 321, 328–329, 393, 424
Jock itch, 205
Joints, painful, 101–102, 173, 310, 324

K

Kala-azar (See Leishmaniasis)
Kangarooing, 405, 408
Kidneys, 233–234, 424
Kidney stones, 235, 424
Kilograms, measuring in, 62, 424
Kwashiorkor (wet malnutrition), 30, **113,** 424

L

Labor, 258–262, 264, 424
false labor, 258
problems with labor, 267
signs that show labor is near, 258
stages of, 259–262
(Also see Childbirth)
Land
distribution of, w7, w11, 413
use of, w11, w13–w16, 115
Latido, 23
Latrines, 137–139, 153
Laxatives, 15–16, 383
misuse of, 126
Lazy eye, 223
Leadership, w5
Learning, w4, w21–w28, **322**
Legs
crossed like scissors, 320
examination of legs, 37
pain in, 288, 321
Leishmaniasis, 406
Lepra reaction, 191, 364
Leprosy, 10, **191–192,** 206, 337, 363–365
or *lepra,* 25
Lice, 134, 190, **200,** 373
Limits, knowing, w4
Liquids, 39–40, 151
Liters, measuring in, 61, 424
Liver, 36, 424
abscesses, 144–145
disease, 172, 288, 328
infection of, 172
Liver extract, 65, **67**
Lockjaw (See Tetanus)
Loss of blood (See Blood, Bleeding)
Loss of consciousness (See Unconscious person)
Loss of feeling, 38, 127, 162, 173, 191, 192, 279
Loss of sight, 225, 412
Loss of sleep (insomnia), 328
Loss of weight (See Weight loss)
Low body temperature, 409
Low-back pain, 173, 248
Low blood pressure, 411
Lumps
in the abdomen, 35, 243, 280
in the breast, 279
on face and body, 191, 228
that keep growing, 196, 280
(Also see Lymph nodes)
Lung diseases
and smoking, 149
asthma, 167
bronchitis, 170
pneumonia, 171
tuberculosis, 179
Lymph nodes, swollen, 88, 317, 424
caused by an abscess, 202
in the groin, 238, 403
signs of infection, 194
TB of, 212
with AIDS, 400
with breast cancer, 279
with brucellosis, 188 or typhus, 190
with German measles, 312
with scabies or lice, 199, 200
Lymphogranuloma venereum, 238, 420

M

Maalox, 173
Malaria, 186–187
falciparum, 158, 365
fever pattern, 26
medicines for, 337, 365–368
with sickle cell disease, 321
Malnutrition
and diarrhea, 153–155
causes of, 115, 283, 412
checking for, 109, 112–113, 297–304
during pregnancy, 248
in children, 107, 114, 305–306
kinds of, 112–114
prevention and treatment of, 108, 109, 112–113, 155–156, 392–394
problems caused by, 107, 306
signs of, 30, 37, 108, 112, 113, 208–209, 305
Malta fever (brucellosis), 27, **188**
Marasmus (dry malnutrition), 112
Marijuana, 416
Mask of pregnancy, 207
Massaging
sprains or fractures, 99, 102
the birth opening, 269
the womb, 264–265
Mastitis (breast abscess), 278, 424
Measles (Rubeola), 30, 108, 226, **311,** 392
vaccination, 147, 312, 321
Measuring
blood pressure, 410–411
in pounds and kilos, 62
medicine, 59–61, 340
Medical attention
illnesses that always need, 179–192
when to seek, 43, 159
Medicinal plants, 12–13
Medicine kit, 331–337
Medicines
brand-name, 55, 333, 339
care in giving to the newborn, 54, 272
dangerous misuse of medicine, 50–53
during or after birth, 266
during pregnancy, 54, 247
for small children, 62
generic, 333, 339
guidelines for use, w18–w19, 49–73, 339–396
healing without medicines, 45–48
how to measure and give, 59–64, 340
how to write instructions for, 63–64

limited use of medicines, w18–w19, 49
medicines not to inject, 56
reactions to, 68, 70–71, 351
uses, dosage, and precautions, 339–398
when not to take them, 54–64
Ménière's disease, 327
Meningitis, 185, 274, 307
Menopause, 246, 424
Menstrual period, 245–246, 281, 294, 394–396
Mental problems, 18, 114, 318
Microscope, 19, 144
Midwives
danger signs in pregnancy, 249
information for, 245–282
prenatal care, 250
special risk at birth, 256
things not to do, 260
things to have ready before birth, 254–255
Migraine, 162, 424
Milk
and brucellosis, 188
and diarrhea, 156
and ulcers, 129
powdered, 392
(Also see Breast feeding)
Milk of magnesia, 16, 383
Mineral oil, 16, 383
Minerals, 111, **116–118,** 425
Mini-pill, 289, 294, **395**
Miscarriage (spontaneous abortion), 246, 249, 266, **281,** 414
Models for teaching, w22
Mongolism, 318, 425
Moniliasis (thrush), 232, 242, 400
Morning sickness, 248, 287
Mosquitos, 186–187
Mothers
health after childbirth, 276, 280
health and sicknesses of children, 295–321
information for, 245–282
prenatal care, 250–253
(Also see Family planning)
Mouches volantes, 227
Mouth, 107, **229–232**
Mouth-to-mouth breathing, 78–80, 413
with newborns, 262
Moving an injured person, 99–100
Mucus, how to drain, 169, 425
Mucus method, 285, **292**
Mumps, 312
Muscles
examining, 37–38
lack of control of, 320

N

Narrow-spectrum antibiotics, 56, 425
Natural balance, 58
Nausea (See Vomiting)
Navel (umbilicus), 425
cutting the cord, 262–263
hernia of navel, 317, 318
infection of navel, 182, 272
Neck
broken, 99
stiff, 38, 182–185, 274
Needs, felt and long-term, w8–w12
Needles, 74, 399, 401
Neonatal conjunctivitis, 221
(Also see Newborns)
Nerves, 425
muscles and, 37–38
Nevirapine, 249, 400
Newborns
and tetanus, 182–183
bacterial infection of the blood, 275
bathing, 7, 263, 270
eyes, 221, 237, 270
feeding, 120, 263, 271
hernia, 317
illnesses of, 272–275
medicines for, 54, 272, 337
problems with delivery, 268
small, early, and underweight, 405
the cord, 262–263, 270
twins, 269
(Also see Dehydration)
Night blindness, 113, **226–227,** 337
Nodes (See Lymph nodes)
Non-infectious diseases, 18
Nose, stuffy or runny, 164–165, 384
Nosebleed, 11, **83**
Numbness (See Loss of feeling)
Nutrition, w11, w13–w16, **107–130,** 295
(Also see Malnutrition)

O

Obstructed gut, 22, **94**
(Also see Gut)
Older persons, 83, 214, 235, 323–330
Onchocerciasis, 227–228, 378
Opium, 416
Oral contraceptives, 285–289, 394–395
Outhouses, 137–139
Ovarian cyst, 280
Ovaries, 36, 280, 425
Oxytocics, 50, **265–266,** 319, 391
Oxyuris (pinworm, threadworm), 141

P

Pain
asking about, 29
back, 173–174, 248
chest, 179, 325
in the belly, 12, 35–36, 94–95, 128, 146, 243
in the eye, 217, 219, 221, 222
in the joints, 101–102, 173, 310, 324

in the leg, 288
in the teeth, 165, 231
in urination, 146, 235–236, 239, 242–243
medicines for, 19, 52, 75–76, 162, 335, 379–380
(Also see Cramps, Headaches)
Pannus, 220
Pap smear, 280
Papaya, 13
Paralysis
examining for, 37
from pesticides, 412
from ticks, 201
in a spastic child, 320
in leprosy, 191
in polio, 314–315
in stroke, 37, 327
in TB of backbone, 180
of face, 37, 327
Parasites, 19, 425
intestinal, 19, 140–145, 308
on skin, 19, 199–201
Patient report, 44
Pellagra, 114, **208–209**
Pelvic inflammatory disease, 237, **243,** 244, 414
Penis, 199, 232, 233, 235–240, 402–403
Peritonitis, 94–95, 129, 189, 425
Pertussis (See Whooping cough)
Pesticides
burns in eyes, 219
causing birth defects, 247
misuse of, 412–413
Pharmacist, words to, 338
Phlebitis, 288
PID (See Pelvic inflammatory disease)
Piles (hemorrhoids), 16, **175,** 423
during pregnancy, 248
medicine for, 392
the Pill (for birth control), 285–289, 394–395
Pimples, 211, 419
(Also see Chickenpox)
Pink eye, 219–221, 308
Pinta, 207
Pinworm (threadworm, Enterobius), 12, **141**
Placenta (afterbirth), 262–264, 269, 426
Placenta previa, 249, 426
Plantar warts, 210
Plants
medicinal, 12–13
that cause itching, 204
Play acting, w23
Pneumonia, 27, 41, **171,** 399, 400, 413
Poisoning, 103, 389
food, 23, 135, 153, 161
of pregnancy, 249, 422
urine, 239–240
Poisonous
bites, 104–106
plants, 204
Poliomyelitis (infantile paralysis), 314
signs of, 37
vaccination, 147, 296, 314
Population, w10, 115, 283–284
Posters, w22
Postpartum, 426
diet, 123
hemorrhage, 266, 391
Postural drainage, 169
Power of belief or suggestion, 2–5, 24, 426
Pre-eclampsia (toxemia of pregnancy), 249
Pregnancy, 247–255
anemia during, 124, 248–249, 392, 393
bleeding during, 249, 264, 281
check-ups during, w24, 250–253, 410
danger signs in, 249–251
difficulty becoming pregnant, 244
ectopic, 36, 243, 249, **280,** 414
German measles during, 247, 312
growth and position of baby, 251–252, 257
how to prevent, 284–295
how to stay healthy during, 247
how to tell the baby's birth date, 252
medicines during, 6, 54, 247
minor problems of, 174, 248, 251
nutrition during, 118, 250
record of prenatal care, 253
signs of, 247
supplies to have ready before birth, 254–255
(Also see Family planning)
Pregnancy mask, 207
Prenatal care, 250–253
Presentation of an arm, 268, 426
Pressure sores (See Bed sores)
Preventive medicine, w17, 17, **131–150**
cleanliness, 131–136
how to avoid many sicknesses, 108, 148–150, 242, 326
sanitation, 137–139
sexually transmitted disease, 239, 401–403
vaccinations (immunizations), 147
worms and other intestinal parasites, 140–146
Prolapse of the rectum, 142, 426
Prophylactic (condom), 239, 285, **290,** 396, 401–403
Prostate gland, 233, 235–236, 426
Protective foods, 110, 426
Proteins, 110, 111, 112, 113, 116–118, 121
Psoriasis, 216
Pterygium, 224, 426
Pulling out (to prevent pregnancy), 285, **290**
Pulse, 32-33, 41, 410–411, 426, inside back cover
Pulsing or throbbing of stomach, 23
Pupils, examining, 217
Purges, 15–16
misuse of, 92, 126
Pyorrhea, 231

Q

Questions to ask a sick person, 29, 44

R

Rabies, 181
Rash on the skin, 216, 236, 400
diaper rash, 215, 421
like tiny bruises (typhus), 190
of allergic reaction, 68, 166, 203–204, 358
of chickenpox, 311
of German measles, 312
of measles, 30, 311
of syphilis, 238
of typhoid, 189
preventing, 133
with itching, 199–200, 203
Reactions (See Allergic reactions)
Rebound pain, 35, **95,** 426
Rectum
prolapse of, 142, 426
Reflexes, testing, 183, 426
Rehydration Drink, 152, 311, 382–383, 400, 426
and vomiting, 161
as an enema, 15
for acute abdomen, 95
for dehydration, 9, 46, 158, 306
for newborns, 273
for very sick persons, 40, 53
Remedies (See Home remedies)
Resistance, 426
to antibiotics, w19, 57–58, 237, 351
to infection, 108, 120, 271
Resources, w8, w12, 115, 283, 426
Respiration (See Breathing)
Retardation, mental, 114, 306, 318, **320–321,** 426
Rheumatic fever, 27, **310**
Rheumatoid arthritis, 324
Rhinitis, allergic (hay fever), 165, 426
Rhythm method, 285, **291–292**
Ribs, broken, 99
Rickets, 125
Ringing of the ears, deafness, and dizziness, 107, **327,** 359, 363, 379
Ringworm, 11, **205–206,** 372
River blindness, 227–228, 378
Road to health chart (See Child Health Chart)
Rotating crops, w13, 115, 117, 427
Roundworm (ascaris), 140–141
Rubber (condom), 239, 285, **290,** 396, 401–403
Rubella (See German measles)
Rubeola (See Measles)
Rupture (See Hernia)

S

Salt
iodized, 130, 247, 318
purges, 16
using little, 120, 125, 176, 249, 325, 326
Sanitation, w10, **137–139,** 153, 427
Scabies, 34, **199–200,** 335, 373
Scales (to weigh babies), 297
Scars
on the cornea, 224, 226, 228
on the eyelids, 220
preventing burn scars, 97
Schistosomiasis, 146, 337, 377
Scorpion sting, 11, **106,** 337, 388
Scrofula, 212
Scrotum, 233, 427
small sores on, 199
swollen, 317
Seborrhea, 215
Senna leaf, 16
Septicemia, 275, 427
Serious illnesses, w28, 42, **179–192**
Seven year itch, 199–200, 335, 373
Sexually transmitted diseases (STD), 236–239, 286, 290, **399–403,** 427, 428
Sheath (condom), 239, 285, **290,** 396, 401–403
Shigella, 145, 358
Shingles, 204, 400
Shock, 30, **77,** 325, 427
allergic, 70, 105, 166, 351
from serious burns, 97
heartbeat during, 33, 410–411
in postpartum mother, 265
Shoulder, dislocated, 101
Sickle cell disease, 30, 321, 393
Sicknesses
causes of, 17–20, 107
common, 151–178
dangerous, w28, 42, 179–192
"home," 21
"hot" and "cold," 119
infectious, **18-19,** 135
non-infectious, 18
of children, 215, 272–275, 311–314
of older people, 323–330
of women, 241
prevention of, 131–150
spread of, 131–137, 140, 188–189, 237–239, 399
telling apart, 20–21, 26–27
Side pains, 22
Signs, 20, **29,** 427
Sinus trouble (sinusitis), 165, 427
Skin
cancer of, 211, 399
chart of different diseases, 196–198
diseases, 193–216, 406, 421
dryness of, 107, 208
how to examine, 34
in children, 215, 308
medicines for, 334–335, 371–374
painless sores, 191, 237, 279
TB of, 179, 212
ulcers, 212–213
Slipped disc, 173
Slowness (See Defects, Mental problems)
Smallpox, 147
Small sores with pus, 201, 211
Smoking
during pregnancy, 318, 416
problems caused by, 119, 129, 149–150, 289, 325, 326, 400, 416

Snails, 146
Snakebite, 104–105
  antitoxin, 105, 337, 388
  home cure for, 3
Soaks, 102
Social conditions, 283, 401, 415, 417
Soft drinks, 155, 161, 229
Soft spot (See Fontanel)
Solda con solda, 14
Sores
  bed sores, 41, 214
  chronic, 20, 127, 212, 213, 236, 324, 406
  large, open, 127, 213–214
  mouth, 232
  of the feet, 324
  on penis or genitals, 199, 205, 232, 237, 238, 242, 400, 402–403
  sugar or honey treatment for, 213, 214
  that keep growing, 127, 191, 211, 213, 214
  without feeling, 191, 237, 279
  with pus, 199, 201, 406
  (Also see Skin)
Sore throat, 163, **309–310**
Spasms, 183, 427
  in spider bite, 106
  in tetanus, 182–184
  (Also see Fits)
Spastic, 38, **319–320**
Sperm, 233, 244
Spermicide, 396
Sphygmomanometer, 410
Spider bite, 106
Spleen, large, 158, **186,** 393, 427
Sponge method, 285, **294**
Spontaneous abortion (See Miscarriage)
Spots before the eyes, 227
Sprains, 102, 427
Spread of disease, 131-137, 140, 190, 237–239, 399–403
Squint, 223
Starches, 110, 203, 408, 427
Starvation (See Malnutrition)
Sterile, 427
  bandages, 87
  men and women, 236, 244, 412
Sterilization, 427
  of equipment, 74, 401
  of syringes, 69, 72, 74
  to prevent pregnancy, 284, 285, 293
Steroids, 51
Stethoscope, 410
Sting
  bee, 70
  scorpion, 106
Stitches (sutures), 86, 255, 269, 423
  anesthetics for, 380
Stomach-ache, 12, **93,** 427
  (Also see Belly, Cramps)
Stomach ulcers, 128–129, 149, 381–382
Stools
  in acute abdomen (obstruction), 94
  in diarrhea (dysentery), 144–145
  like rice water, 158
  white or pale, 172
  with blood, 128, 146, 189
  with schistosomiasis, 146, 377
  with typhoid, 189–190
  with ulcer (black, tarry stools), 128
  (Also see Constipation, Feces)
Story telling, w23
Strabismus, 223
Strains, 102
Strep throat, 310
Stretcher, 100
Stroke, 37, 78, 288, 327, 410
  (Also see Heat stroke)
Sty (hordeolum), 224, 427
Suction bulb, 84, **255,** 262, 268
Sugars, 110, **111,** 382, 427
Sulfonamides, 55, 358
Sunken fontanel (See Fontanel)
Sunlight
  and acne, 211
  and rickets, 125
  and skin problems, 195
Supplies
  for childbirth, 254–255
  for the medicine kit, 334, 336
Suppressants, 427
  cough, 52, 384
Surgery
  immediate need for, 91–95, 177, 222, 267
  possible need for, 102, 175, 177, 211, 222, 225, 235, 243, 279, 280, 293, 317, 319, 329
Susto, 24
Suture (See Stitches)
Sweets, 115, 119, 122, 229, 408
Swelling
  breast swelling and lumps, 278–279
  caused by medicine, 68, 70–71, 231
  home cure for, 12
  in old age, 323
  of broken arms or legs, 14
  of hands and face, 108, 239, 249
  of strains and sprains, 102
  of the eyes, 144, 221, 313
  of the feet, 113, 124, 144, 176, 248–249, 321
  of the scrotum or testicles, 312, 317
  with infection, 194
  (Also see Lymph nodes, Swollen belly, Varicose veins)
Swollen belly
  different causes of, 20
  in children, 107, 112, 114, 321
  in giardia infection, 145
  in gut obstruction, 94
  in malnutrition, 112, 114
  in pregnancy, 248, 249
  (Also see Gut)
Symptoms, 29
Syphilis, 10, **237–238,** 403
Syringe, 72, 74, 336, 399, 401, 405

T

Taboo, 23, 428
T.A.L.C., 297, 429
Tapeworm, 143, 376
TB (See Tuberculosis)
Teaching, w2, w4–w5, **w21–w28,** 321
materials, addresses for, 429–432
Tear sac, infection of, 217, **223**
Teaspoons, for measuring, 61
Teeth, 133, **229–232**
Temperature, 30-31, 272, 409, inside back cover
(Also see Fever)
Tepeguaje, 14
Testicles, 233
swellings of testicles, 312, 317
Tetanus (lockjaw), 182–184
from a wound, 84, 89, 407
in the newborn, 182–183, 273
medicine for, 336–337, 389–390
vaccination, 147, 184, 296
Thalassemia, 393, 428
Thermometer, 31, 334
Threadworm (pinworm, Enterobius), 141
Throat
lump on the throat, 10, 130, 423
object stuck in, 79
sore throat, 163, 309–310
Throwing up (See Vomiting)
Thrush (moniliasis), 232, 242, 400
Ticks, 190, **201,** 428
Tinea, 205–206
Tinea versicolor, 206
Tobacco, 129, 416–417
Tongue, 232
Tonsillitis (inflamed tonsils), 309
Toothache, 231
Toothbrush, homemade, 230
Toothpaste, 230
Toxemia of pregnancy (eclampsia), 249, 422
Trachoma, 220
Traditions, w3, w11, 1, 2, 21
Trichinosis, 144
Trichocephalus (whipworm, Trichuris), 142
Trichomonas, 241
Trichuris (whipworm, Trichocephalus), 142
Tropical sore (See Leishmaniasis)
Tubal ligation, 293
Tuberculosis, 108, **179–180,** 337
and AIDS, 400
and children, 136
and measles, 311
medicines for, 361–363
of the lymph nodes, 212
of the skin, 212
of the spine, 173
signs of, 30, 37
vaccination, 147
Tumors (See Cancer)
Twins, 251, 256, **269,** 289
Twisted joint (sprain), 102
Typhoid fever, 188–190
fever pattern, 26
medicines for, 357–358
pulse with, 33
resistance to medicines, 58
Typhus, 26, **190**

U

Ulcer, 428
on the cornea (eye), 224–225
skin, 20, 212, 213, 324
stomach, 13, 36, 53, 128–129, 149, 382
Umbilical cord, 428
and tetanus, 182
how to cut, 262–263
infection of, 270, 272
wrapped around the baby's neck, 268
Umbilical hernia, 317, 318, 428
Umbilicus (See Navel)
Uncinaria (hookworm), 133, **142**
Unconscious person, 78, 424
breathing of, 32
difference in pupil size, 33
in shock, 77
Under-Fives Program, w20, w24, **297,** 428
Undulant fever (brucellosis), 27, **188**
Units, measuring in, 60
Uremia, 239–240
Ureters, 233
Urethra, 233, 235, 428
Urination, difficulties with, 234–236, 239–240,
324, 403, 410
Urinary tract, 36, **233–234,** 428
Urine
blood in, 146, 234, 377
brown, 172
dark yellow, 151
less than normal, 151, 236
too much or often, 127, 234
pus in, 236
Using this book, inside front cover, w28
Uta (See Leishmaniasis)

V

Vaccinations, 19, **147,** 180, 250, 296, 321, 337,
405
Vagina, 233, 428
infections of, 241–242, 370
placenta blocking, 249
tearing during birth, 269
Vaginal discharge, 241–242, 370–371
Vapors, breathing hot water vapors, 47, **168**
Varicose veins, 175, 213, 288, 410, 428
and chronic sores, 20, 212, 213, 324
during pregnancy, 248
Vasectomy, 293, 428

Veins, inflamed, 288
(Also see Varicose veins)
Venereal diseases (VD) (See Sexually transmitted disease)
Venereal lymphogranuloma, 238, 420
Ventilated improved pit latrine, 139
Verrucae (warts), 210
Village health committee, w24
Village health worker, w1–w7, w29, 43, 340
Village medicine kit, 336–337
Village storekeeper, 338
VIP latrine, 139
Virus, 19, 399–401
Vision (See Eyes)
Vital signs, 41, inside back cover
Vitamins, 110, 111, 116–118, 392–394, 405
injections of, 65, 67, 118
the best way to get, 52, 118
vitamin A, 226, 392
vitamin B, 208
vitamin C, 248, 335,
vitamin B_6, 361, 394
vitamin B_{12}, 51, 65, 393
vitamin K, 265, 272, 337, 394
(Also see Iron)
Vitiligo, 207
Vomiting, 161
during pregnancy, 248, 249
enemas and laxatives with, 15
how to cause vomiting, 103, 389
in the newborn, 273
medicines for, 161, 335, 386–387
violent vomiting, 151
with blood (cirrhosis), 328
with blood (ulcer), 128
with diarrhea, 151, 157
with urine poisoning (uremia), 239

W

Wandering eyes, 223
Warm compresses, 193–195
Warts, 210, 212, 400, 402
Water, healing with, 45–48
and cleanliness, 46, 131, 135, 137–139, 144, 146
and spread of disease, 146, 188
for fever, 75
to ease pain of burns, 96
vapors, 47, 168, 384
Weakness, fatigue, 23, 124, 323, 400
Weight
and diet, 110–111, 127
deciding dosage by, 340
homemade scales, 250
importance of losing, 125–127, 325–326
in pounds and kilos, 62
measuring medicines, 59–61
weight gain, in children, 297–304
weight gain in pregnancy, 247, 250
Weight loss
chronic, 179, 180, 400
different causes, 20
how to lose weight, 126
in the newborn, 273
sudden (dehydration), 151
(Also see Malnutrition)
Welts (hives), 68, **203,** 238
Wet malnutrition (kwashiorkor), 113
Whipworm (Trichuris, Trichocephalus), 142
White spots and patches on the skin, 206–207, 232
Whooping cough (pertussis), 168, **313**
medicines for, 336
vaccination, 147, 296
Witchcraft, 5, 24
Withdrawal
from drug addiction, 417
to prevent pregnancy, 285, **290**
Womb, 428
cancer of, 280
contractions of, 258, 266
massaging, 264–265
position of the baby in, 251, 257
Women's health care, 241
Working together, w5, w24
World Health Organization, 49, 432
Worms, 140–146, 227–228, 406–407
causing obstructed gut, 94
in children, 308
medicines for 335, 374–376
prevention of, 47, 131–134
Wounds
abdomen, 92
bullet, 90–93
chest, 91
controlling bleeding of, 82
deep, 89–92
from a broken bone, 99
how to close them, 85–86
infected, 88–89, 213, 401
knife and bullet, 89–93
medicines for, 93, 334
small, 84
that may cause tetanus, 89, 182
to the eye, 217–218

X

Xerophthalmia, 113, **226,** 306, 337, 392, 428
Xerosis (See Xerophthalmia)
X-ray, 102

Y

Yeast infection, 58, 232, **242,** 370–371, 373
Yesca, 11
Yogurt, 57, 232, 242

DOSAGE BLANKS—for giving medicines to those who cannot read (see p. 64)

Name:
Medicine:
For:
Dosage:

Name:
Medicine:
For:
Dosage:

Name:
Medicine:
For:
Dosage:

Name:
Medicine:
For:
Dosage:

Name:
Medicine:
For:
Dosage:

Name:
Medicine:
For:
Dosage:

Name:
Medicine:
For:
Dosage:

Name:
Medicine:
For:
Dosage:

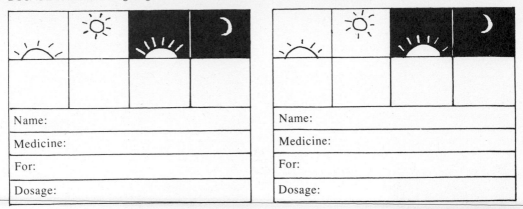

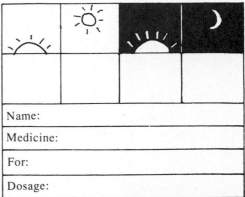

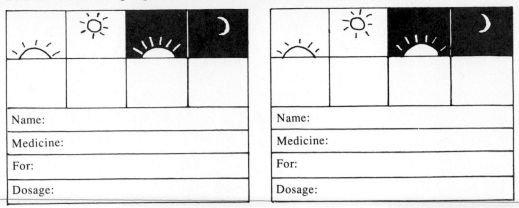

DOSAGE BLANKS—for giving medicines to those who cannot read (see p. 64)

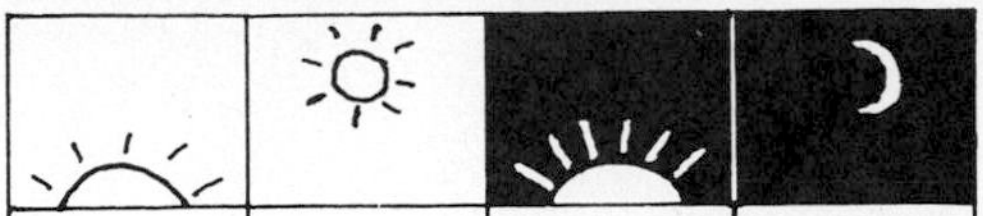

Name:

Medicine:

For:

Dosage:

Name:

Medicine:

For:

Dosage:

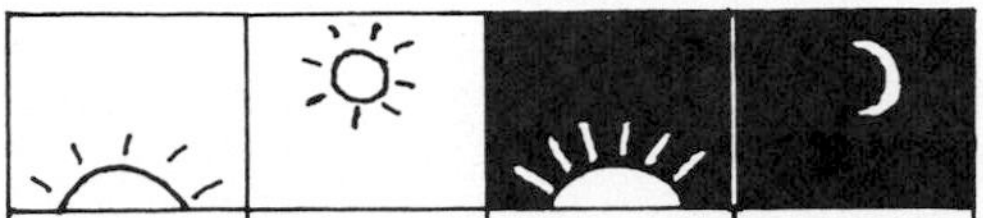

Name:

Medicine:

For:

Dosage:

Name:

Medicine:

For:

Dosage:

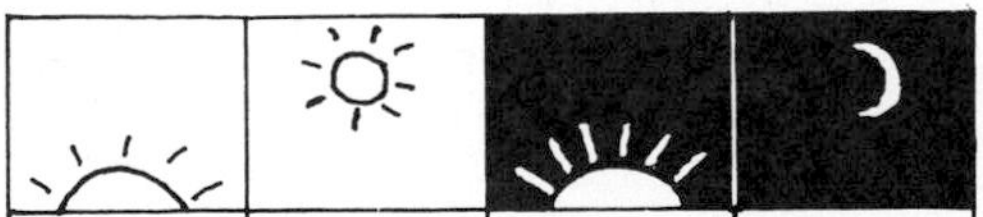

Name:

Medicine:

For:

Dosage:

Name:

Medicine:

For:

Dosage:

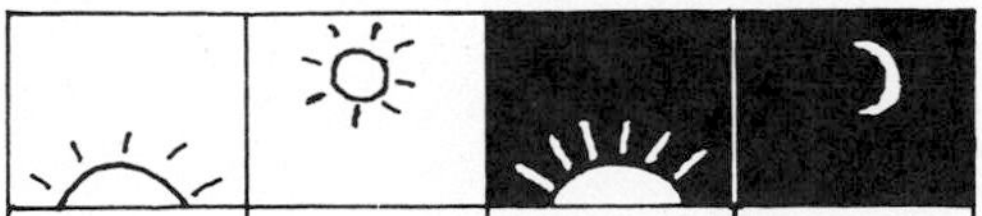

Name:

Medicine:

For:

Dosage:

Name:

Medicine:

For:

Dosage:

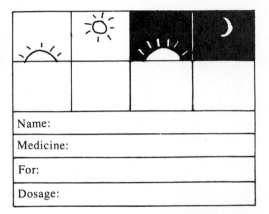

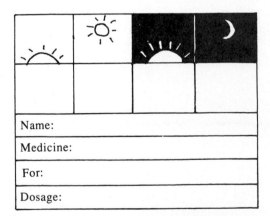

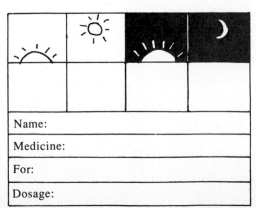

DOSAGE BLANKS—for giving medicines to those who cannot read (see p. 64)

Name:

Medicine:

For:

Dosage:

Name:

Medicine:

For:

Dosage:

Name:

Medicine:

For:

Dosage:

Name:

Medicine:

For:

Dosage:

Name:

Medicine:

For:

Dosage:

Name:

Medicine:

For:

Dosage:

Name:

Medicine:

For:

Dosage:

Name:

Medicine:

For:

Dosage:

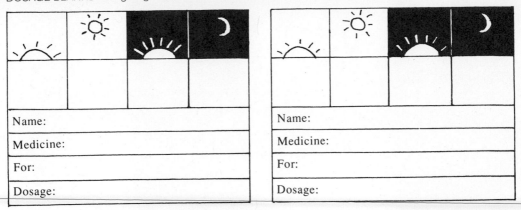

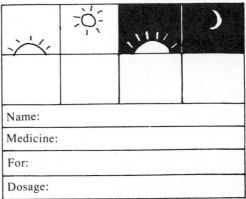

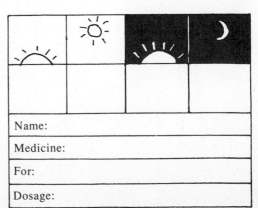

PATIENT REPORT

TO USE WHEN SENDING FOR MEDICAL HELP

Name of the sick person:______________________________Age: ______

Male ______Female______ Where is he (she)? ______________________

What is the main sickness or problem right now? __________________

____

____

____

When did it begin?____

How did it begin?____

Has the person had the same problem before? _______ When? ___________

Is there fever? _______How high? _______° When and for how long? __________

Pain?_________Where?____________________ What kind? _____________

What is wrong or different from normal in any of the following?

Skin: ________________________ **Ears:** ______________________

Eyes:_______________________ **Mouth and throat:**_______________

Genitals:____

Urine: Much or little?__________ Color?__________ Trouble urinating?_____

Describe: ____________________ Times in 24 hours:_____ Times at night: ____

Stools: Color?__________ Blood or mucus?__________ Diarrhea?_______

Number of times a day:_______ Cramps?________ Dehydration?________ Mild or severe?____________ Worms?_________ What kind? ________________

Breathing: Breaths per minute:________Deep, shallow, or normal? __________

Difficulty breathing (describe):_________________ Cough (describe): _______

________________Wheezing?_________ Mucus?__________ With blood?_____

Does the person have any of the SIGNS OF DANGEROUS ILLNESS listed on page 42?________ Which? (give details)______________________________

____

Other signs: ____

Is the person taking medicine?________ What? _______________________

Has the person ever used medicine that has caused a rash, hives (or bumps) with itching, or other allergic reactions?________ What? _______________

The state of the sick person is: Not very serious:___________ Serious: ________

Very serious:_______________

On the back of this form write any other information you think may be important.

PATIENT REPORT

TO USE WHEN SENDING FOR MEDICAL HELP

Name of the sick person:________________________________Age: _____

Male _____Female_____ Where is he (she)? ________________________

What is the main sickness or problem right now? ____________________

____

____

____

When did it begin?____

How did it begin?____

Has the person had the same problem before? ______ When? __________

Is there fever? ______How high? ______° When and for how long? _________

Pain?________Where?___________________ What kind? ______________

What is wrong or different from normal in any of the following?

Skin: _________________________ **Ears:** _____________________________

Eyes:________________________ **Mouth and throat:**____________________

Genitals:____

Urine: Much or little?___________ Color?___________ Trouble urinating?_____

Describe: ___________________ Times in 24 hours:_____ Times at night: ____

Stools: Color?_____________ Blood or mucus?____________ Diarrhea?______

Number of times a day:______ Cramps?_______ Dehydration?_______ Mild or severe?____________ Worms?________ What kind? ____________________

Breathing: Breaths per minute:_______Deep, shallow, or normal? __________

Difficulty breathing (describe):__________________ Cough (describe): ______

________________Wheezing?________ Mucus?_________ With blood?_____

Does the person have any of the SIGNS OF DANGEROUS ILLNESS listed on page 42?_______ Which? (give details)_________________________________

____

Other signs: ____

Is the person taking medicine?_______ What? _________________________

Has the person ever used medicine that has caused a rash, hives (or bumps) with itching, or other allergic reactions?_______ What? __________________

The state of the sick person is: Not very serious:__________ Serious: _______

Very serious:_______________

On the back of this form write any other information you think may be important.

PATIENT REPORT

TO USE WHEN SENDING FOR MEDICAL HELP

Name of the sick person:________________________________ Age: ______

Male ______ Female ______ Where is he (she)? ________________________

What is the main sickness or problem right now? ____________________

____

____

____

When did it begin? ____

How did it begin? ____

Has the person had the same problem before? ______ When? __________

Is there fever? ______ How high? ______° When and for how long? ________

Pain? ________ Where? ____________________ What kind? ______________

What is wrong or different from normal in any of the following?

Skin: _________________________ **Ears:** _________________________

Eyes: ________________________ **Mouth and throat:** ________________

Genitals: ____

Urine: Much or little? ___________ Color? ___________ Trouble urinating? _____

Describe: ____________________ Times in 24 hours: _____ Times at night: ____

Stools: Color? ____________ Blood or mucus? ____________ Diarrhea? ______

Number of times a day: ______ Cramps? _______ Dehydration? _______ Mild or severe? ____________ Worms? ________ What kind? ________________

Breathing: Breaths per minute: _______ Deep, shallow, or normal? ________

Difficulty breathing (describe): ___________________ Cough (describe): _______

________________ Wheezing? ________ Mucus? __________ With blood? _____

Does the person have any of the SIGNS OF DANGEROUS ILLNESS listed on page 42? _______ Which? (give details) ________________________________

____

Other signs: ____

Is the person taking medicine? _______ What? ______________________

Has the person ever used medicine that has caused a rash, hives (or bumps) with itching, or other allergic reactions? _______ What? ________________

The state of the sick person is: Not very serious: ___________ Serious: _______

Very serious: _______________

On the back of this form write any other information you think may be important.

PATIENT REPORT

TO USE WHEN SENDING FOR MEDICAL HELP

Name of the sick person:__________________________________Age: ______

Male ______Female______ Where is he (she)? ____________________________

What is the main sickness or problem right now? ________________________

____

____

____

When did it begin?____

How did it begin?____

Has the person had the same problem before? _______ When? _______________

Is there fever? ______How high? ______° When and for how long? __________

Pain?_________Where?_____________________ What kind? _________________

What is wrong or different from normal in any of the following?

Skin: ___________________________ **Ears:** ______________________________

Eyes:___________________________ **Mouth and throat:**______________________

Genitals:____

Urine: Much or little?_____________ Color?_____________ Trouble urinating?_____

Describe: ______________________ Times in 24 hours:______ Times at night: ____

Stools: Color?______________ Blood or mucus?______________ Diarrhea?_______

Number of times a day:_______ Cramps?________ Dehydration?________ Mild or severe?______________ Worms?_________ What kind? ________________________

Breathing: Breaths per minute:________Deep, shallow, or normal? ____________

Difficulty breathing (describe):_____________________ Cough (describe): _______ ____________________Wheezing?_________ Mucus?__________ With blood?_____

Does the person have any of the SIGNS OF DANGEROUS ILLNESS listed on page 42?________ Which? (give details)____________________________________

____

Other signs: ____

Is the person taking medicine?________ What? ____________________________

Has the person ever used medicine that has caused a rash, hives (or bumps) with itching, or other allergic reactions?________ What? _______________________

The state of the sick person is: Not very serious:____________ Serious: ________ Very serious:_________________

On the back of this form write any other information you think may be important.

OTHER BOOKS FROM THE HESPERIAN FOUNDATION

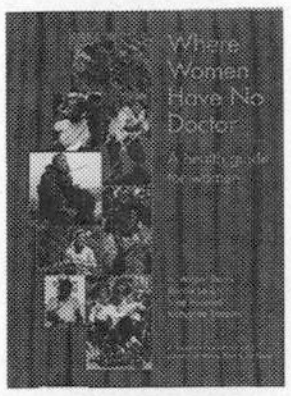

Where Women Have No Doctor, by A. August Burns, Ronnie Lovich, Jane Maxwell and Katharine Shapiro, combines self-help medical information with an understanding of the ways poverty, discrimination, and cultural beliefs limit women's health and access to care. Clearly written and with over 1000 drawings, this book is an essential resource for any woman who wants to improve her health, and for health workers who want more information about the problems that affect only women, or that affect women differently from men. 584 pages.

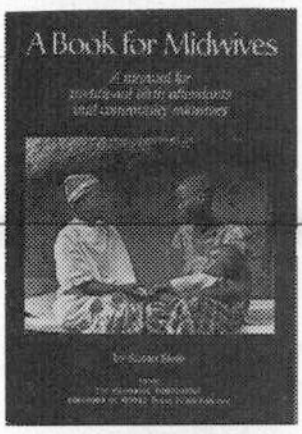

A Book for Midwives, by Susan Klein, is written for midwives, traditional birth attendants, community health workers and anyone concerned about the health of pregnant women and their babies. The book is an invaluable tool for midwives facilitating education and training sessions as well as an essential reference for practice. The author emphasizes helping pregnant women stay healthy; giving good care and dealing with complications during labor, childbirth and after birth; family planning; breastfeeding; and homemade, low-cost equipment. 528 pages.

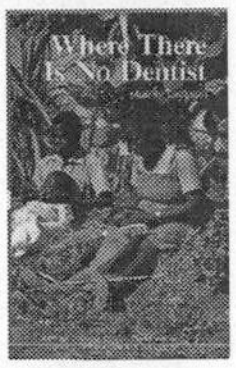

Where There Is No Dentist, by Murray Dickson, shows people how to care for their own teeth and gums, and how to prevent tooth and gum problems. Emphasis is placed on sharing this knowledge in the home, community, and school. The author also gives detailed and well-illustrated information on using dental equipment, placing fillings, taking out teeth, and suggests ways to teach dental hygiene and nutrition. 208 pages.

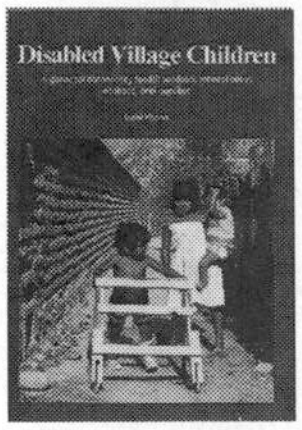

Disabled Village Children, by David Werner, contains a wealth of information about most common disabilities of children, including polio, cerebral palsy, juvenile arthritis, blindness, and deafness. The author gives suggestions for simplified rehabilitation at the village level and explains how to make a variety of appropriate low-cost aids. Emphasis is placed on how to help disabled children find a role and be accepted in the community. 672 pages.

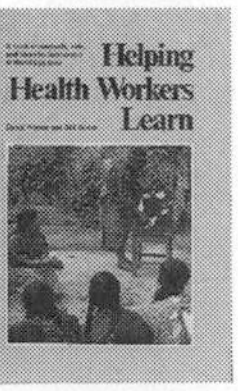

Helping Health Workers Learn, by David Werner and Bill Bower, is an indispensable resource for anyone involved in teaching about health. This heavily illustrated book shows how to make health education fun and effective. Includes activities for mothers and children; pointers for using theater, flannel-boards, and other techniques; and many ideas for producing low-cost teaching aids. Emphasizing a people-centered approach to health care, it presents strategies for effective community involvement through participatory education. 640 pages.

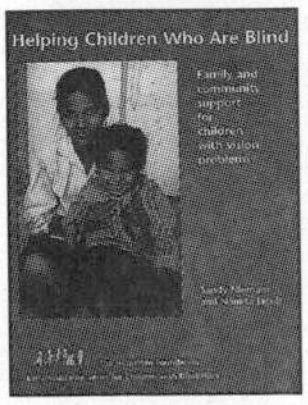

Helping Children Who Are Blind, by Sandy Niemann and Namita Jacob, aids parents and other caregivers in helping blind children from birth through age 5 develop all their capabilities. Topics include: assessing how much a child can see, preventing blindness, moving around safely, teaching common activities, and many others. 192 pages.

All titles are available from Hesperian in both English and Spanish. For information regarding other language editions, prices and ordering information, or for a brochure describing the Foundation's work, please write to us:

The Hesperian Foundation
P.O. Box 11577
Berkeley, California 94712-2577 USA
Telephone: (510) 845-4507
Fax: (510) 845-0539
e-mail: bookorders@hesperian.org
Visit our website: www.hesperian.org

INFORMATION ON VITAL SIGNS

TEMPERATURE

There are two kinds of thermometer scales. Centigrade (C.) and Fahrenheit (F.). Either can be used to measure a person's temperature.

Here is how they compare:

CENTIGRADE

This thermometer reads 40° C.
(Forty degrees Centigrade)

FAHRENHEIT

This thermometer reads 104° F.
(104 degrees Fahrenheit)

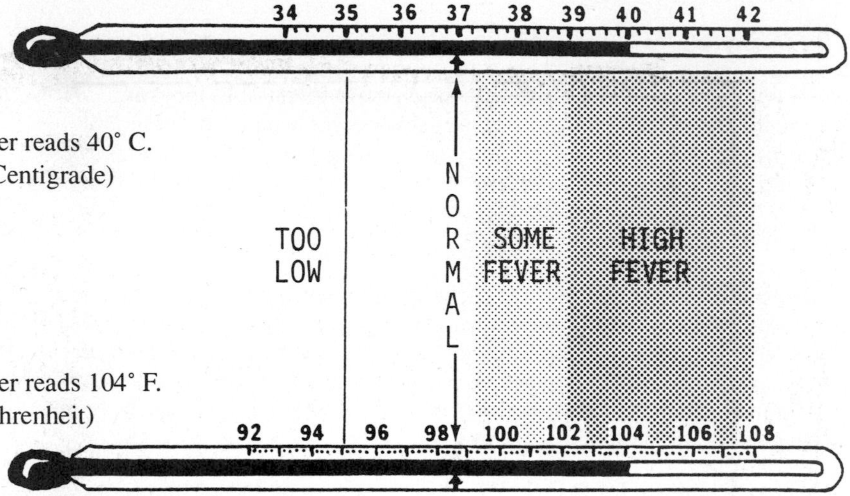

PULSE OR HEARTBEAT

For a person at rest:
- ADULTS . . . . 60-80 beats per minute is normal.
- CHILDREN 80-100
- BABIES 100-140

For each degree Centigrade (C.) of fever, the heartbeat usually increases about 20 beats per minute.

RESPIRATION

For a person at rest:
- ADULTS AND LARGE CHILDREN . . . 12-20 breaths per minute is normal.
- CHILDREN . . . . up to 30 breaths per minute is normal.
- BABIES . . . . up to 40 breaths per minute is normal.

More than 40 shallow breaths a minute usually means pneumonia (see p. 171).

BLOOD PRESSURE (This is included for health workers who have the equipment to measure blood pressure.)

For a person at rest: 120/80 is normal, but this varies a lot.

If the second reading, when the sound disappears, is over 100, this is a danger sign of high blood pressure (see p. 125).